CW01546103

HEALING THE SOUL

Volume one

The lives of Samuel Hahnemann
and William Lilley

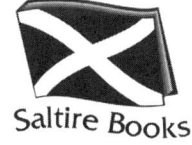 Saltire Books Limited, Glasgow, Scotland

HEALING THE SOUL

Volume one

The lives of Samuel Hahnemann
and William Lilley

DAVID LILLEY
MBChB, FFHom, LLCO

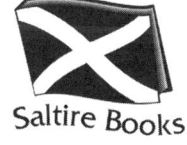 Saltire Books Limited, Glasgow, Scotland

Published by Saltire Books Ltd

18–20 Main Street, Busby, Glasgow G76 8DU, Scotland
books@saltirebooks.com   www.saltirebooks.com

Cover, Design, Layout and Text © Saltire Books Ltd 2013–4

   is a registered trademark

First published in 2014
Reprint edition 2018

Typeset by Type Study, Scarborough, UK in 9¼ on 13½ Stone Serif
Printed and bound in the UK by TJ International Limited, Padstow, Cornwall

ISBN 978-1-908127-05-1

All rights reserved. Except for the purpose of private study, research, criticism or review, as permitted under the UK Copyright, Designs and Patent Act 1988, no part of this publication may be reproduced, stored or transmitted in any form or by any means, without prior written permission from the copyright holder.

The publisher makes no representation, express or implied, with regard to the accuracy of the information contained in this book and cannot accept any legal responsibility or liability for any errors or omissions that may be made.

The right of David Lilley to be identified as the author of this work has been asserted in accordance with the UK Copyright, Designs and Patent Act 1988.

A catalogue record for this book is available from the British library.

For Saltire
Project Development: Lee Kayne
Editorial: Steven Kayne
Designer: Phil Barker
Indexer: Sue Dugen

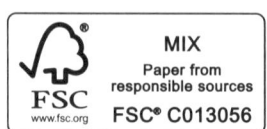

CONTENTS

About the author ix
Acknowledgements xi
Introduction 1

part one THE SCIENCE OF HOMEOPATHY
The enduring legacy of Samuel Hahnemann

1	Legacy from the past	33
2	*Similia Similibus Curentur*	59
3	The new Paracelsus	75
4	The Law of the Infinitesimal dose	93
5	Besieged and exiled	105
6	The chronic diseases	117
7	Last years in Köthen	139
8	Paris – rejuvenation and departure	161
9	Of passion and potency	193
10	Pride, prejudice and politics	227
11	Quantum medicine	257

part two THE SCIENCE OF SPIRIT
The remarkable history of William Lilley

12	The gift of healing	289
13	The Sanctuary	317
14	The move to London	347
15	Silver Birch – wisdom from beyond the grave	375
16	Healing and teaching	403
17	Controversy and initiation	431
18	A place in the sun	457

19	Miracles and magistrates	481
20	Master and pupil	507
21	Passing	535
22	The ego-self: The disease of the soul	549

Index 561

In Memory of

Lejan Tari Singh ('Dr Letari')
William Henry Lilley ('Bill')
Nancy Lilley

ABOUT THE AUTHOR

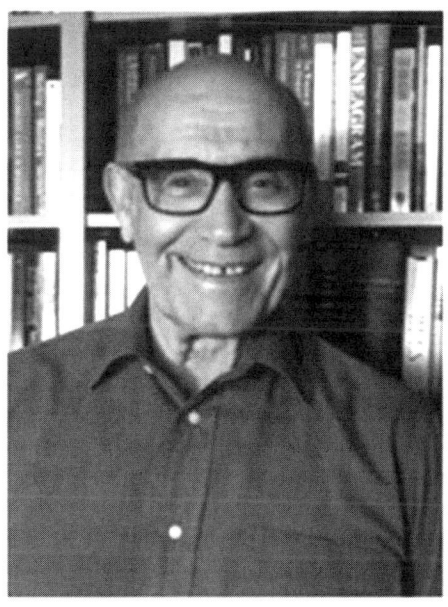

David Lilley was born into a homeopathic family in Leeds, Yorkshire, England, in 1940. His father, William Henry Lilley, was a renowned psychic healer and also a homeopathic practitioner and chiropractor. In 1949, the family emigrated to South Africa, and David's father established a successful practice in Pretoria. After recovering, through psychic and homeopathic healing, from a severe, life-threatening illness at seven years of age, David resolved to become a doctor. He studied medicine at the University of Pretoria, qualifying in 1962. After completing his hospital internship, he spent three years at the Royal London Homeopathic Hospital and the London College of Osteopathy. He obtained his homeopathic MFHom qualification in 1965, and his LLCO osteopathic qualification in 1966.

On returning to South Africa, David joined his father and he has conducted an exclusively homeopathic and osteopathic practice for the past 46 years. In 1994, he co-founded the first official homeopathic course for medical doctors in South Africa. In 1995, this course evolved into the South African Faculty of Homeopathy, of which he became the Dean.

Since 1999, David has lectured widely in the UK, and also in Ireland, Japan and Australia. In his lectures, he weaves together homeopathic art and science, analytical psychology, mythology, symbolism, chakra and colour theory, natural science and spiritual philosophy to provide a rich tapestry of perennial wisdom and knowledge.

In December 2007, David retired from his private practice in Pretoria and moved to Cape Town where he currently conducts a small, select practice and is concentrating on writing and lecturing.

ACKNOWLEDGEMENTS

This book comes late in the life of its author and owes its existence to all those who have contributed to my understanding of life and to my development as a person, as a lecturer and as a practitioner of the healing art of homeopathy; a system of therapy that has been a lifelong blessing to myself, my family and my patients.

Though this first book, covers the lives of two great healers, Samuel Hahnemann and my father William Henry Lilley, it also serves as an introduction to the texts that will follow, making this a fitting place to acknowledge those individuals who in one way or another have played an important role in my journey.

This recognition of indebtedness must embrace the thousands of patients who through their trust, friendship and loyalty enriched my life, and who through their willingness to share their lives with me taught me so much and gave me the experience that I can now share with others. I am deeply indebted to the number of outstanding nursing sisters who aided me in my work, and who, despite coming from a different paradigm of medicine, were able to accept the evidence of the healing they witnessed and embraced homeopathy with enthusiasm. Not to be forgotten are the administrative staff and all those who worked so tirelessly in the practice dispensary and laboratory. The smooth running of a busy practice depended on their efforts, and still does.

My tribute extends to all my students of the last twenty years; attending to their needs sent me foraging far and wide with an energy and motivation, which would have been difficult to sustain had they not given me the purpose. Their appreciation, their knowledge and a mountain of teaching material have been my reward. I must also extend my gratitude to the various audiences I have addressed, especially those colleagues in the UK who attended the master-classes I gave for the British Faculty of Homeopathy in Glasgow and London, and gave me so much support. Preparing for those weekend seminars gave me reason to record my concepts, and weave together the various elements that constitute a full remedy picture. Teaching married to practice has proved a potent source of learning for me.

Following these general acknowledgements, I would like to draw attention to the people who have played a special role in the course of my life. Some may have been unaware of their significance to me; many have already passed to spirit. Because the South African Faculty of Homeopathy is so much part of my life, I include in my thanks all those who have helped me in its founding and its success.

There are no words with which to express my gratitude to my parents, who from humble beginnings, through unswerving devotion to the cause of healing, and through surmounting many difficult trials and obstacles, paved the way for the work I was called upon to do. By comparison, due to their efforts, sacrifices and foresight, my life has moved forward on oiled wheels. I was blessed with two fathers, my earthly father, William Henry Lilley, who set me the example of what it means to be a man of noble spirit and a healer of the sick, and my spirit father, Lejan Tari Singh, Dr Letari, a physician seer, who from my earliest years opened my senses to the magnificence of the creation and tutored me in the mysteries of life. My mother, Nancy, was the organising power behind the throne, who made it possible for my father to devote himself to his healing work, knowing that all else was in her capable hands. Her trust in Dr Letari, my father and homeopathy was unwavering. This certitude in a woman of grounded, practical temperament instilled in me a similar trust in the action of the drops in a teaspoon of water or the little white pills that were so much part of my earliest memories; a trust that was reinforced by the benefits they bestowed.

I owe deep gratitude to those who aided and supported my father through the early years of his mission in Yorkshire and later in London: Arthur Richards, the business man who sponsored him and coached him in the ways of the world, and Maurice Barbanell, the journalist, newspaper editor and outstanding medium whose pen, support and friendship did so much towards furthering the cause and spreading the word. Barbanell cannot be mentioned without thought of the illustrious spirit-being, Silver Birch, who overshadowed Maurice throughout his life, and, imparted, through his immaculate mediumship, a wisdom of peerless purity and simplicity. It was he who warned my father of the price he might have to pay if he continued to extend himself. His teachings were as much part of my earliest years as those of Dr Letari.

In South Africa, similar gratitude must be extended to Lassie Smit, who was so instrumental in easing our transition to a new country and a new way of life, and proved a bulwark of strength to my mother at a time when her trust was tested to the very quick. Another person who played an important role was Mary Brown, my mother's spinster friend, who had worked with her as a seamstress in a textile factory in Leeds. She followed us to South Africa and devoted the rest of her life to acting as practice manager for my father; she would willingly have given up her life for him and for homeopathy. In the practice, Miss Brown, as she was always called, was affectionately known as "the battle-axe" – an uncompromising bastion protecting my father from the importunities of demanding patients. It was she who marshalled the forces that sprang to my father's aid when the law descended on him. Mary was a great support to my mother after my father's death, and died in my arms at her post in the practice reception room.

Someone who may be surprised to find his name mentioned in these acknowledgements is Fred Liebenberg, an Afrikaans orthopaedic surgeon specialising in reconstructive hand surgery. Though our lives have diverged and we have not seen one another for many years, he is never forgotten. I had very little Afrikaans when I enrolled at the Pretoria University medical school, where all instruction was through the medium of Afrikaans. *Liebenberg* and *Lilley*: the alphabetical sequence ensured that we would be allotted seats next to one another in the first practical botany class of the year. I sat silently drawing a plant specimen, insulated within a capsule of my own shyness, timidity and linguistic ineptitude. At some point, I became dissatisfied with a particular feature of my illustration only to realise that I had not thought to bring a rubber with me. Having no other option, I turned to the young man beside me and in painfully accented Afrikaans asked him if I might borrow his. He smiled, offered me the desired object, and answered me in excellent English. That was the beginning of a remarkable friendship between a Brit and a Boer; we were inseparable for the seven years of our medical training. Although he often teased me about my commitment to homeopathy, he never derided or discounted it. Ours was a friendship that was of incalculable value to me; it tided me over one of the most formative periods of my life and remains precious for the camaraderie and shared experiences it afforded us. In terms of a recurrent theme in this book – our friendship, its importance to me, and the manner in which it began, confirms that nothing in life happens by chance, and if we consider our lives in retrospect, we discover that life always provides for us.

My sister Margaret Tara, six years younger than myself, was my first muse. To this day, she is the only person to have read from the ardent, romantic writings about the Trojan War that flowed from my pen in my early twenties. Her approval and encouragement were very important to me and spurred me on. I thank her particularly for the precious memories we share of our time in London together when I was studying at the Royal

London Homeopathic Hospital (RLHH).[i] She was my inseparable companion at weekends and provided a willing and critical first audience for me when I expounded on various homeopathic topics after being enthused by my lecturers. To aid me in my preparation for the MFHom examinations, she painstakingly typed out my original sketches of the major remedies. The closeness of the bond we established then was intensified by our having been children together in a remarkable home presided over by our wise and loving spirit father, the beloved Dr Letari.

I was fortunate to attend lectures and outpatient clinics at the RLHH at a time (1964–66) when there were a number of outstanding homeopathic physicians involved in the teaching programme or working in the clinics; all willing for me to sit in with them. I cannot thank them enough for the contribution they made to my homeopathic education. As with any such group, but possibly more so among homeopaths, they represented a broad spectrum of approaches, all of which widened my own perspective. In this regard, I am particularly indebted to Margery Blackie, who was Dean at the time, Donald Foubister, John Raeside, Ralph Twentyman, Kathleen Priestman and Johanna Brieger.

In 1993, after twenty-seven years of homeopathic practice, I began my lecturing career. In this enterprise I am indebted to a number of colleagues who opened doors for me, worked with me, and supported me in various ways: Peter Frazer, who set the ball rolling, Berkeley Digby who gave me my first platform and shared it so ably with me, Ronald Boyer who enriched our South African Faculty course with his clinical expertise and French charm, and a number of our graduates and colleagues whose assistance has been so valuable to me in recent courses: Ann Haw, David Nye, Jeetesh Ranchod, Jonathan Marchand, Helen Didcot, Mary Williers, Robert Moiloa, my niece Tanya Blake, Mike Clark, Cleve McIntosh and Murray Rushmere. I thank them all for their contribution to South African homeopathy.

In considering my lecturing in South Africa, a very special person must be mentioned, Beatrix van der Westhuyzen, a modern day Miss Brown. When I met Berkeley Digby, Beatrix was on his lecture team, appointed by the pharmaceutical firm, Pharma Natura. The first time she saw me was when she attended my first presentation at the Technikon Natal in 1993. While I spoke from the platform, she was conscious of a strong Indian presence about me. So intense was this impression that contrary to what she had heard, she felt sure I was an Indian. Considering the emotions I experienced during the presentation (related in the Introduction), this

---

[i] RLHH was renamed The Royal London Hospital for Integrated Medicine in September 2010. See p235.

perception was rather significant. She had never heard of Dr Letari previously. In the course of the following years (1994–2012), Beatrix assisted me in the organisation of the lectures I delivered for the SA Faculty, of which she became a director. She collated the recordings of all the lectures I delivered to the British Faculty and supervised their editing and transfer to tape. These are now available on CD. I hope that our collaboration will continue in the years of the future should the SA Faculty be incorporated into a university.

I can speak on behalf of all my South African colleagues when I acknowledge with gratitude the role of the British Faculty and its staff in the founding and accreditation of the South African Faculty of Homeopathy and for supplying us with supportive documentation to satisfy the South African education authorities. The British Faculty Deans: Barry Rose, Jeremy Swayne and Raymond Sevar were all immensely supportive of our endeavours, and, over the years, ensured that our student assessments were conducted to the highest possible standard. I must thank the current Dean, Russell Malcolm, for arranging for Bob Leckridge to act as external examiner during the 2012 SA Faculty examinations. Special thanks must be given to Cristal Sumner, Chief Executive of the British Faculty, who was always there for us when we needed help.

The founding of the SA Faculty, was not inexpensive; we would have struggled to find the necessary finances to launch our academic programme if it had not been for the generosity of a prominent Johannesburg businessman, Louis Shill. Convinced from personal experience of the efficacy of homeopathic therapy, Louis stepped into the financial breach and ensured that the venture took off. Now in his eighties, he remains interested in the activities and fortunes of the Faculty. His timeous offer of help will always be remembered with deepest gratitude.

I wish to thank Sally Penrose, the past consultant editor of the British Homeopathic Association magazine, *Health and Homeopathy*, for approaching me to write two series of masterclass articles on leading homeopathic remedies. This provided me with an invaluable platform to develop their archetypal profiles, an exercise that afforded me great satisfaction and provided me with extra insights into the genius of the substances.

In my introduction, I have acknowledged the unstinted help and hospitality given to Paddy, my wife, and myself by Bob Leckridge and his wife Hilary in Stirling, Scotland, and Mike Jenkins and his wife Sally in London, during the time I was lecturing regularly in the UK. Bob was instrumental in instigating the project and getting it rolling. His influence on my life has been inestimable and continues to be. Mike, like Fred Liebenberg before him, was a gift to me, one I will always value.

Lecturing in the UK, brought Paddy and I into a homeopathic community that gifted us with very special friendships. These friendships soon extended to members of the British Association of Homeopathic Veterinary Surgeons (BAHVS), who kindly made me an honorary member of their association, and to members of the Society of Homeopaths. Amongst the vets, I would like to particularly thank the following colleagues for the immense support they have given me: Geoff Johnson, Mark Carpenter, John Saxon, Peter Gregory, Jane Keogh, Malene Jorgensen, Tom Farrington and never to be forgotten George Kinsella, whose memorial lecture I had the honour of giving. Geoff Johnson, like George, watches me like a hawk and delights in stretching my mind into the beyond. Lecturing to the vets has always been a special experience for me.

John Morgan, Diane Goodwin and Francis Treuherz of the Society of Homeopaths deserve special mention. John embodies the soul qualities I associate with homeopathic healing. I shall never forget the evening we spent together in Tunbridge Wells, when, at his request, I related the story of Dr Letari and my father. We cemented a friendship that will endure beyond this dimension. His encouragement in my work and his help with the expansion of our remedy base in the practice dispensary have been important, as was the provision of a Korsikovian potentiser.

Diane has promoted me, introduced me at various congresses, and in 2003, convened a short series of seminars for me in Edinburgh, which enabled me to expand on various archetypal themes. I owe Francis thanks for the copy of his book *Homoeopathy in the Irish potato famine*, which he kindly gave me a number of years ago; for hosting me when I delivered a weekend seminar to the Society entitled, *The Nine Deadly Sins*; and for escorting me round his impressive homeopathic library. His gift drew my attention to the remedy Solanum tuberosum aegrotans (rotten potato) at a time when a young girl, who had been severely abused, presented in my practice. She was compulsively cutting her wrists and most significantly experiencing repeated dreams of mutilation and bloodshed, symptoms that are characteristic of this remarkable remedy. The nosode Solanum tuberosum aegrotans (sol-t-ae.) brought her back from the brink of an emotional breakdown and over time restored her joy of life. In addition to these two colleagues, I would like to thank the many Society members I have met over the years for their kindness and appreciation.

My lecturing has taken Paddy and I to Ireland, Japan and Australia, and always we were deeply moved by the great hospitality we received.

Amongst our closest friends who have shared the adventure of my lecturing career and have urged me on to write this book are Piers Worth, a powerful intellect, who has always managed to point my nose in the right direction at the right time, indicating the authors, books and papers, that would be of value to me; Colin Brett, with whom I have shared many of my thoughts and who has always been a valuable sounding board for me; Nick Maritz and Chris McIntyre with whom I have spent so many incredible weeks in the unspoilt wilds and swamps of Botswana, who never fail to ask on seeing me "How's it going with the book?"; Tish and Neils Wessels in England, Victor Saunders in Cape Town, and Hannelie and Charl van Heerden in Johannesburg, who have for many years provided me with sanctuaries in which to introspect and prepare for lecturing; Raymond Andrews, the artist, whose many incised oil paintings on wood panels grace my home and surround me with a stimulating world of metaphor and mythology and who over 25 years ago drew my attention to the quantum nature of the homeopathic potency; Mark Bauman, who introduced me to the archetypes of the Enneagram and the teachings of Almaas; Jennifer Hepburn, whose love of homeopathy matches my own, and Geoff Woodin, a son as much as a friend to me, whose presence at my lectures always adds to my pleasure.

The support, advice and patience of my editor Steven Kayne have been of immeasurable importance to me and I look forward to our further collaboration in the works that lie ahead. I am very proud to be associated with Saltire Books.

Lastly, I wish to thank my family for bearing with me over many years of intense practice, years of preparing and delivering lectures and more recently the writing of this book. I must apologise for often having been an absent husband and father. I thank my son Dorian for successfully taking over the practice, which his grandfather established in Pretoria in 1949; my second son, Troye, for sharing many hours of philosophical discussion with me; my third son, Jason, and my daughter Brigitte for making me proud of the artisinal bakery they have created in the centre of Cape Town.

It remains only to thank my wife Paddy for the time and effort she has devoted not only to the family, but also to the smooth running of the practice, the preparatory work for every seminar and presentation I have given and the organisation of my life. Throughout our thirty-seven years together, she has been my companion, my adviser, my confidante and often my conscience. With her by my side, I look forward to the work ahead.

Note

Throughout the book the following convention is used:

Scientific names of source materials are shown in *italics* and common names in lower case. All homeopathic remedies are shown thus: Arnica montana, or as an abbreviation e.g. Calc-carb.

INTRODUCTION

Mythical beginnings

Ever since I commenced teaching homeopathy in 1993, now fully twenty years ago, I have had the urge to write about this fascinating, indispensable and mysterious subject: a gentle, natural therapeutic system that can, not only cure physical ailments, but also touch the soul. The desire was heralded many years before, when at sixteen, pursuing my love of mythology, I avidly read Homer's Iliad. The story ended with the death of Hector (hero archetype) and the reconciliation of Achilles (anti-hero archetype) and Agamemnon (tyrant archetype) and left me frustrated and wanting more. Homer's wonderful anecdotes about life on Olympus and his humorous descriptions of the very human emotions and behaviour of the gods particularly entranced me. I resolved to pick up the story from there and continue the epic to the final fall of Troy. I duly started writing with all the outrageous romanticism of an adolescent teenager. Medical studies intervened and disrupted the book's progress, but I repeatedly returned to it and during my hospital internship gave it considerable attention, ambitiously expanding my original project by starting my story many years before the war when suitors from all parts of Greece and the Aegean descended upon Sparta seeking the hand of the princess Helen, whose beauty was extolled by the gods themselves. She was born of the seduction of Leda, the Spartan queen, by Zeus, the supreme god of Olympus, who assumed the guise of a magnificent swan to achieve the consummation of his desire. Tracing the lineage of the illustrious suitors who vied with one another at the court of King Tyndareos, I was lead deeper into the great myths that I had so enjoyed as a youngster. Although not apparent to me at the time, these fabulous legends were the stuff of dreams, fantasy and the working of the deep unconscious. I was unwittingly preparing myself for the work that lay ahead, and the archetypal content of books to follow this.

A synchronistic gift

It was at this time that I experienced my first impelling evidence of the law of *synchronicity*, or meaningful coincidence. On the occasion of one of his regular appointments with my father, an elderly patient, who had been deeply committed to homeopathy since childhood, brought a very old book to the practice and placing it reverently on the desk before my father told him it was for me. Due to his advanced years and his intended move to a retirement home, this scholarly man had reluctantly concluded that he would have to sell off, or auction, his valuable library of books. With this in mind, he had been sorting through his extensive and rather eclectic collection when the book in question came to hand. Prompted by an earlier conversation with my father about the importance of archetypal themes in homeopathy, and, knowing that I was about to embark on my homeopathic studies, he instantly determined to give it to me as a gift.

This, 'greatly enlarged', third edition of the *Bibliotheca Classica or A Classical Dictionary* edited by J Lempriere, is dated 1797, the original edition having been published through Pembroke College, Oxford, in 1788. Despite its age and yellow mottled pages, it was in good condition and a veritable treasure trove of information about mythical beings and historic figures from classical Greek and Roman times, all in discursive detail and the captivating language of the time. In the front, it had a chronological table dating from the creation of the world to the fall of the Roman Empire in the West and in the East. With absolute certainty it states: "The world was created in the 710th year of the Julian period, 4004 years before Christ; and the deluge was in 2348". Indicative of its age is the use of the typed letter 'f' instead of 's' throughout the text, except in the main title and at the end of words. Hence, we read at the start of the introduction to the second edition:

> The very favourable reception which the firft edition of the *Claffical Dictionary* has met from the public, fully evinces the utility of the performance. From the confcioufnefs of this, the author has fpared no pains to render this fecund edition more deferving of the fame liberal patronage.

I soon got used to this peculiarity and to this day the book remains an invaluable reference source for me. However, far more important to me than its content, for the comprehensive compilation, *The Greek Myths* by Robert Graves, the English poet and novelist, was already at my elbow, was the tacit confirmation and approval I knew I had received from an unseen dimension at a very defining moment in my life. The significance of the cue was emphasised by the age, substance and academic tone of the work.

Archetypal correspondences

The timing was perfect; as such matters always are. My research into the Greek myths coincided with my launching into the study of the homeopathic materia medica; hence, my acquaintance with the archetypes of the materia medica and those of the Greek myths developed apace. It was impossible to overlook the remarkable similarity between the attributes and nature of *Hephaistos*, God of Fire, Volcanoes and Artisans and the remedy *Sulphur*; of *Apollo*, the sun-god, God of Light (the intellect), Prophecy, Healing, Music, etc. and the remedy Aurum (gold); of *Artemis*, Goddess of the Moon, Wild Animals, Wilderness, Childbirth and Virginity and the remedy Argentum (silver). Likewise, the correspondences between Ferrum (iron) and *Ares*, the God of War, and between Cuprum and *Aphrodite*, the Goddess of Feminine Beauty and Sexual Pleasure, were clear to see.

After my medical internship, I enrolled for the long course at the RLHH and benefited from contact with a number of physicians responsible for tuition. Among them was Ralph Twentyman, who shared my interest in Greek mythology. His observations regarding the correspondence between the archetypes of mythology and the archetypes of homeopathy, particularly the metals, clarified and endorsed my own observations. His editorship of *The British Homeopathic Journal* brought the work of Edward Whitmont, a Jungian analyst and homeopath, to my attention, and this in turn awakened an interest in the theories of Carl Gustav Jung. Whichever way I turned, I found harmony and compatibility between homeopathy, mythology and analytical psychology. Jung's concepts of the collective unconscious, the ego, the persona, the anima, the animus and the shadow, provided rich insight into the archetypal and emotional dynamics of patients and remedies. Understanding the sphere of remedy action in this way, imbeds the remedy picture in the memory and facilitates the matching of remedy and patient. As with knowledge of myth, apprehending the structures of the psyche makes analogies apparent, which confirm and expand the comprehension of remedy action.

A study of the Solanaceae, the nightshade family of plants, reveals the family's relationship to turbulence and conflict arising at the boundary between the conscious and unconscious minds; the interface where the unconscious, replete with repressed energy from the shadow, strives to find expression in the light of consciousness, and the conscious mind, rife with fears, seeks to flee existence by escaping into the shadow world of the unconscious. In this struggle between light and dark, morality and sanity may be sacrificed.

The *animus*, is the masculine principle which exists within all women, just as its feminine counterpart, the *anima*, exists within all men. The exaggerated animus state of the female Sepia archetype (the cuttlefish) illustrates dramatically the far-reaching emotional, functional and even structural effects of unconscious anima suppression. Sepia women revolting against the passive, submissive, dependent characteristics of the stereotyped female may overthrow the inherent, primordial, cultural and gender-related patterns of behaviour characteristic of women by unconscious repression of their femininity and projection of their masculinity. The effect impacts upon the endocrine system especially the ovaries and adrenal glands, and, over time, a mild, moderate or more striking degree of masculinisation may result, evidenced in outlook, manner and disposition and changes to features and form.

The ego/self interface

Observations, such as these, opened vistas not even hinted at in my medical training. I was released from the superficial, mechanistic protocols of conventional medicine and introduced to a magical world of healing that transcends orthodox treatment. The homeopathic paradigm embraces a holistic methodology focussed on the inner nature of the patient, and provides a harmless, yet highly effective, means of addressing the internal disharmony upon which all disease is founded. The inner world of human experience reveals a landscape of disease causation lying far beyond the biochemical reach of pharmaceutical drugs. The subjective plane of existence, on which we experience our joys and our heartaches, our loves and our hates, our aspirations and our disappointments; where we develop our trust, our values, our moral principles and our empathy, or, nurture our fears, our anger, our jealousy and our pride; where the dire struggle between our soul and our ego-self is contested; this plane, on which dis-ease gives birth to disease, is imponderable and susceptible only to imponderable influences. Fear, grief and despair, hatred, evil and perversion cannot be weighed and measured on the scales of medical science, neither can the diseases they foster; only their effects are measurable. The drugs of orthodox medicine, no matter how sophisticated, are crude and gross in their action, ideal for emergencies, life threatening conditions, intolerable pain and overwhelming infections; situations which present in an intensely physical manner, when only immediate action permits us to 'live to fight another day'. But the vast majority of problems bringing about the clinical encounter between patient and physician are not of this order. To bring about healing in such non-emergency cases, which constitute almost all patients seen in primary health care practice, the use of subtle, gentle and persuasive means of treatment is imperative. The remedies must be able to operate on the imponderable dimension of the soul/ego interface, at the very origin and source of disease processes, for only then can they elicit a healing response. The imponderable potencies of homeopathy have the power to bring about such a response when selected for their similarity to the unique emotional and physical picture of the patient.

Professional isolation

Though I was contemplating deeper understanding of disease dynamics, due to my unusual upbringing, described in part two of this book, these rarefied waters were familiar and comfortable. I stepped from the medical into the homeopathic paradigm with ease. It was my natural milieu. This transition, which caused my professional path to diverge steeply from that of my fellows brought to my attention the yawning gulf that, quite suddenly, separated us. When I returned to South Africa after three years studying homeopathy and osteopathy, I found myself professionally and academically isolated. Though my father had initiated the training of professional homeopaths in South Africa, there were scarcely any medical homeopaths to be found. It was many years before this changed. My isolation was paradoxically due to the conceptual freedom I had attained, untrammelled by official dictates and doctrine. My young medical peers remained tethered to idealisation of the medical model, which had so impressed us during our clinical years of study.

Medical hubris

The profound effect of those academic years cannot be underestimated. I can well remember the pride I experienced striding down the hospital corridors in my white coat with torch and stethoscope suitably conspicuous. This immature, naive self-esteem was modelled on certain larger-than-life exemplars of medical arrogance and absolutism, who lorded it over us during our student years. In the *Doctor in the House* series of films, which started just before I entered medical school and proved hugely popular during the time of my education, these inflated characters were marvellously and hilariously caricatured in the fictitious person of Sir Lancelot Spratt, a tyrannical chief-surgeon wonderfully portrayed by James Robertson

Justice. Though a figure of fancy, Sir Lancelot was scarcely an exaggeration, but, unlike many of those he parodied, he had a warm, caring side to him, which though hidden behind an overbearing, dictatorial demeanour was capable of compromise and empathy. In all fairness to him, I find imperiousness in a surgeon somehow more excusable than dogmatic authoritarianism in a physician.

Be that as it may, by the time we qualified, the contagious effects of medical hubris had swept through our ranks imbuing us all to some degree with a sense of professional superiority and exclusivity – afflictions scientific atheists and certain theologians are equally prone to. When engrained, their insidious effect is blinkered dogmatism, prejudice and a sense of unassailable rectitude, which stifle curiosity, lateral thinking, creativity and the ability to change or widen perspective: serious impediments to the advancement of a science critical to the emotional and physical wellbeing of humanity. In appraising this phenomenon, which so restricts medical thinking, I am generalising, since an entire spectrum of practitioners emerge from the medical schools of the world ranging from the most altruistic, humble and self-sacrificing to those who stand on a medical pedestal, haughty and aloof. In general, primary health care work encourages humility and compassion; but by the same token, movement away from frontline medicine into specialisation, or ascent in the medical bureaucratic hierarchy, tends to harden pride and foster monopolistic assertiveness and doctrinal inflexibility. Unfortunately, the overlords of medicine most often come from the ranks of the latter, entrenching attitudes based on a serious misconception, shared by much of the mislead public: that the official Western medical model is a healing modality and the only model possible. Medical hegemony results, promoted and exploited by the powerful pharmaceutical industry. Medical fundamentalists go so far as to declare that there can be no such thing as alternative medicine; how can there be an alternative to a medical model that is the best and works; by definition, alternative medicine cannot work.

Medicine deceives itself by the very real wonders of surgery and the signal achievements of medical technology and drug-based medicine into believing that the medical model has all the possible answers to disease and cannot be surpassed. Is this truly so? This is a question being asked by an increasing number of concerned observers, both within and without medicine and its associated professions.

The sadness is that there should be no polarisation into separate camps – on the one side conventional medicine and on the other homeopathic medicine – because each is indispensible, each has its appropriate sphere of action and each has a vital role to play. However, the highest calling of a physician must be to heal disease, which means bringing about a process of cure, which permanently restores a patient's state of health, both emotionally and physically, by simple and gentle means according to definite principles. Healing is not within the scope of conventional medicine, which lacks the means to bring about a healing process – chemical medicines cannot reach or influence the ultimate source of disease. Healing is quintessentially the sphere of homeopathy, which through utilising the energy essence of remedial substances is able to reach into the subtle regions of the psyche where the soul (the higher-self) and the ego-self (the lower-self) contend for sovereignty; an encounter that generates the turbulence at the root of all constitutional disease.

Homeopathic recluse

So I found myself professionally alone, especially after the death of my father only six years after my return to South Africa. For the next twenty-six years (1967 to 1993), I immersed myself in my homeopathic and osteopathic practice. With the addition of my father's patients to my own, my practice swelled and soon I was seeing at least thirty patients each day, successfully treating every manner of acute and chronic disease with homeopathy, and very seldom having to resort to supplementary orthodox therapy. The results would have confounded any medical sceptic and refuted the common criticism of cynics that extended consultations, placebo effect and spontaneous remissions were the reason for homeopathy's apparent successes. This intense period of practice provided me with the opportunity to put to the test all that I had learnt from my father, Dr Letari and my tutors at the RLHH, while developing my own personal skills. Professionally, I was a homeopathic recluse, engaged in solitary practice and rarely meeting with homeopathic colleagues other than when we came together for political reasons to further the cause of homeopathy in South Africa.

Emergence

However, as the 1990's dawned, destiny decided that it was time for me to emerge from my chrysalis. All the legal struggles of my father and those who followed him had at last been rewarded by the promulgation of legislation protecting the right of homeopaths to practise in South Africa. This was a huge achievement and resulted in the first institute for the education of professional (non-medical) homeopaths being established under the aegis of the Health Sciences Department of Technikon Natal (now the Durban University of Technology – DUT). In 1991 my son, Dorian, enrolled there, determined to follow in the homeopathic footsteps of his father and grandfather. Inevitably, this drew me closer to the wider world of South African Homeopathy.

Critical to my emergence was an unexpected request in 1991 from the editor of the very orthodox *CME Journal* to write an explanatory article, *What is Homeopathy?*, for its medical readership. This was included in an innovative edition devoted to a number of disciplines within the field of complementary medicine. The article was well received and, unbeknown to me at the time, evoked considerable discussion. The exercise of producing a concise account of the homeopathic system of medicine within the compass of 2,500 words proved invaluable for me; the result would serve me well when delivering introductory lectures on the subject in the future. The following year, 1992, I was asked to serve on the team of inspectors sent to evaluate the standard of homeopathic tuition at the Technikon Natal. Inexorably, I was being pushed out of my hermitage towards a stage I would otherwise have been reluctant to mount. At the institute, I met again an old friend with whom I had attended a number of homeopathic committee meetings in the past: Peter Frazer, a pharmacist and professional homeopath of considerable experience, who had been appointed as the first principal of the homeopathic department at the Technikon. He and his wife Nola were to provide my eldest son Dorian, who was then a homeopathic student, with the help and care usually given by parents when he was injured in a cycling accident. The loving energy of this couple would later manifest in the creation of a baboon rehabilitation centre near Barrydale in the South-Western Cape. Our renewed friendship and the successful CME article led Peter to invite me to give a presentation at the upcoming South African Homeopathic Congress, which was to be held in Durban at the Technikon in September 1993.

I was being gently coerced into taking what was for me a major plunge, a plunge that was to change the direction of my life. Despite my father's exceptional ability as an orator, I had always viewed public speaking with trepidation. If it had been anyone other than Peter Frazer asking me to do the presentation, I think I would have found some excuse to avoid it. However, I also knew that there was no use trying to sidestep the inevitable, so, swallowing my anxiety, I consented and forthwith directed my energy to assiduously preparing my subject. Peter had kindly, and as it turned out wisely, given me carte blanche to speak on any topic I desired. On putting pen to paper, as one still did in those days, my harboured thoughts, never shared in the thirty years since my qualification as a doctor in 1962, poured out, producing material for a six hour presentation, although I had been allotted only ninety minutes. This was to become a character trait whenever I gave presentations: I always stepped on stage armed with more detail and information than I could ever hope to give voice to. The virtue in this idiosyncrasy has been the production of rich tracts of text, which will be included in the books, which will follow this one.

The first platform

For this initiatory occasion, I thought I would begin at the very beginning, the creation of this universe, and consider the elemental archetypes (remedies) that are central to the stellar alchemy of huge stars and then pursue this to the archetypal remedies that stand central to three vital stages of planetary evolution:

- The Archaean Eon: encompassing the hot, prebiotic, chemical era and the development of first life at deep-sea hydrothermal vents: symbolised by Sulphur.
- The Proterozoic Eon: during which the aerobic *cyanobacteria* (blue-green algae) created our oxygen rich atmosphere and its protective ozone layer: symbolised by Calc-carb (calcium carbonate) of which the ancient stromatolite structures of blue-green algae colonies consists (homeopathic Calc-carb is derived from the middle layer of the oyster shell: an organic oceanic source, in keeping with the essence of the symbol).
- The Carboniferous Period (360–250 million years ago) when vast swamp forests provided the organic material for the planet's coal beds, which later became the fuel that fired the Industrial Revolution: symbolised by Lycopodium (club moss) a modern descendent of the giant Lycopods that dominated the coal swamps.

Sulphur – Calc-carb – Lycopodium: a remedial sequence that was recognised by the early masters of homeopathy. It was their experience that when Sulphur had achieved as much as it could for a patient, the remedy next indicated would often be Calc-carb, and likewise, when Calc-carb had run its therapeutic course, the remedy to follow it would often be Lycopodium. This sequence re-enacted three critical evolutionary phases of the planet: volcanism and first anaerobic life – aerobic marine life, an oxygen-rich atmosphere and the ozone layer – burgeoning plant life and the formation of the planets deposits of natural fuel. Clinical experience reveals that no matter which remedy of the three is first indicated, the best sequence remains the same, either Sulphur – Calc-carb – Lycopodium or Calc-carb –

Lycopodium – Sulphur or Lycopodium – Sulphur – Calc-carb, and the sequence may be repeated: a cycle that lifts the constitution through an ascending spiral of healing.

Following my nose and certain signposts already clear to me, I delved deeper and, like an archaeologist at a dig, unearthed facts; facts which confirmed and never refuted the findings of the materia medica; analogies abounded; cosmology and planetary evolution presented a landscape as intriguing as mythology; every corner I explored revealed cosmic congruity. The impetus of this work took me far beyond the material I needed to present and eventually I had to call a halt, and put what remained on hold to be returned to later.

I then realised that before considering the creation of the universe, I should first establish the spiritual, non-physical nature of the patient to be healed and consider the profound significance this reality must have in evaluating their life experience, their emotional profile, their health problems and their treatment. I proposed that regardless of the ailment, be it emotional or physical, superficial or dire, it was a manifestation of disease and stress at the deepest level possible, the interface between the immortal soul (true-self) and the ego-self (variously spoken of as the false-self – ego – ego-personality). In the light of this assumption, the ego-self is the disease from which the soul suffers and its nature, with all its doubts, fears, frustrations, anger, resentment, hatred, jealousy, pride, despair and lack of basic trust, lies at the heart of all mental and physical disease. I asserted that the universe issues from an all-loving, supreme cosmic intelligence, which permeates every aspect of the creation, constantly maintaining its perfection and orchestrating events with the sole object of motivating every individual soul to realise its divinity (Spirit-self). This sacred transmutation necessitates the healing and the dissolution of the ego-self, the disease from which the soul suffers. Everything that transpires in the life of the individual, no matter its nature, is perfectly attuned to this high purpose, it never occurs through chance, coincidence or luck. Life, with all its challenges and trials, is a divine prescription for the healing of the ego-based disease of the soul. In order to be aligned with this divine prescription, the homeopathic remedy must be in dynamic form, able to touch the soul/ego plane of interaction, and its archetypal essence must match the nature of the ego-self and the events to which it is exposed: *the remedy of greatest dynamic similarity*. These were the thoughts I wished to affirm with my audience.

In the meantime, my article had brought an invitation to address a group of doctors studying towards a higher qualification in Family Medicine. The talk was to be a 30-minute slot during a weekend symposium. I was asked to provide the attending medical practitioners with an introductory understanding of homeopathy. I was daunted, but realised that I had been given an ideal opportunity to test my nerves and to spread the homeopathic word on a small, but, nonetheless, important stage. Fortified with Arg-nit 10M, the previous evening, and doses of Gelsemium 200 every two hours before the ordeal (homeopathic remedies for stage-fright), clutching my notes and overhead-projection transparencies, I entered what I knew could be a hornet's nest. Contrary to my expectation, I was kindly and respectfully received and had a very polite and attentive audience that permitted me to proceed without interruption (unlike similar groups I have since addressed). Afterwards, a number of colleagues engaged me in further discussion on various aspects of homeopathy. All in all, it proved a salutary experience, and although I had been as uptight as a newcomer to Wimbledon centre court, I had broken the ice and survived.

On the big day, fortune made sure that nerves would be the least of my concerns. Being unfamiliar with Durban and having to approach the Tecknikon from an unrehearsed direction, I lost my way, eventually arriving before the lecture hall fully 10 minutes late. I can still visualise my son Dorian's anxious face as he opened the door of the car for me and exclaimed: "Where on earth have you been, Dad?" I was bustled into the packed auditorium and onto the stage before a sea of curious eyes, introduced with extreme brevity, and, with no more ado, launched into action. My trajectory took me instantly into a dimension previously unknown to me. I spoke without pause or hesitation for the entire duration of the address; words, thoughts and images streamed into my mind and I was conscious of being in a force field that bore me effortlessly forward. The concepts I had considered in my preparation took on greater clarity and aspects I had not previously recognised rose up before me. At one point, I was almost overwhelmed by what I could only describe as joyous exaltation, an intense, overpowering ecstasy which threatened to engulf me with emotion. When my time was exhausted, I had to be stopped in mid-flight otherwise I would have continued well into the evening. As I descended from my high, I found myself surrounded by those wishing to compliment me and shake my hand. I felt as if I had been in a dream and that I was not yet fully back in my body and in touch with my faculties. This continued until my wife Paddy and I were back in our hotel bedroom and I was immersed in the afterglow, sitting in an armchair nursing a welcome cup of tea. Then the deep import of my experience struck me. I remembered Dr Letari's last words to me shortly before my father's death, when in discussing my future work, he had emphasised: "the many platforms from which you will speak." The time had come; I had to begin teaching.

A significant visitor

I have always been conscious of the influence of synchronicity in my life and at this important juncture it became particularly evident and clear in its purpose. About a year before the events I have just described, late in 1992, a rather gaunt young man came to my home in Pretoria. He had made the appointment with the purpose of introducing to me the homeopathic computer programme, *MacRepertory*, originally created by David Warkentin in 1986. This programme makes the repertorising (analysis) of homeopathic case histories far simpler and more accurate and is a boon to anyone studying, practising or teaching homeopathy. In addition to the repertorising system comes Reference Works, an invaluable archive of all the major homeopathic materia medica, a mine of information derived from past and present masters of the profession, easily accessible for research and lecturing. Berkeley Digby, the young man in question, was a London trained homeopath and osteopath who had returned to South Africa the previous year after practising in London for twelve years. I was relatively computer illiterate when I met him, and he introduced me to an exciting electronic homeopathic world charged with remarkable possibilities. However, as vital as this proved, I owe him an even greater debt of gratitude. Having a nature as intense and focussed as his hollowed features indicated, in the short period of time since arriving in Johannesburg, he had launched an informal homeopathic course for medical doctors, sponsored by Pharma Natura, a Johannesburg based supplier and manufacturer of anthroposophical and homeopathic remedies. Soon after my presentation in Durban, Berkeley invited me to join him on his Johannesburg course. It was a defining moment. I gladly accepted his invitation.

Berkeley's course

There were about twelve professionals on the course, mostly doctors, but also a dentist and two pharmacists. This was a fair number given the slow trickle of doctors inclined to investigate and study other therapeutic systems. The lectures progressed well; Berkeley and I made a good team. I benefitted greatly from being associated with him: he brought me into contact with the work of the foremost teachers and researchers in homeopathy at the time, and his own eclectic interests which embraced Traditional Chinese Medicine, Acupuncture, Iris Diagnosis, Kinesiology and Eastern philosophy provided stimulation for what was seeking expression in myself. He was generous in sharing his considerable knowledge.

The course went forward into 1994, but it soon became apparent that the standard of homeopathic teaching that we were giving had transformed the original informal course into a serious and structured programme of instruction, which begged a formal outcome for the doctors attending. We decided to discontinue the course and start afresh with a well-advertised programme that would lead to a homeopathic qualification. The response was encouraging and with sufficient applications coming from the Cape Province, Berkeley and I decided to start a second course in Cape Town.

The founding of the South African Faculty of Homeopathy

After we had been active for almost a year, I contacted Barry Rose, the Dean of the British Faculty of Homeopathy, seeking accreditation with the Faculty so that on completion of the programme our students might sit the Faculty Membership (MFHom) examination. In 1995, Barry flew out to South Africa to review our curriculum and after discussions and attending part of a seminar, he granted the course accreditation. This was a major milestone and heralded the future formation of the South African Faculty of Homeopathy, registered with the South African education authorities as an official Higher Education Institution for the homeopathic education of medical doctors. In the following year, 1996, our first cohort of students graduated. Barry Rose and David Williams from the British Faculty acted as external examiners for the final, clinical section of the assessment.

On the afternoon before their departure for the airport, Barry, David, Paddy and I were sitting on the veranda of our Pretoria home during a typical Highveld summer storm when Barry prompted me to relate details of my father's unusual life. During his previous visit, he and I had found a mutual interest in the esoteric and this had led me to tell him the story of my father's development as a healer and homeopath. He had been moved by the remarkable tale and was eager that I should repeat it for David's benefit. While the storm seemed to encapsulate us and draw us closer together, an hour fled by as anecdote after anecdote came to my mind. When I finally brought the narrative to a close, David Williams drew himself up and giving me a very intent look said, "One day you must write the story of your father's life." His words were more of an injunction than a suggestion and they remained in my mind from that day to this.

A French connection

No sooner had our students graduated than Berkeley and I prepared to launch further parallel courses in Johannesburg and Cape Town. Pharma Natura was still pleased to sponsor our objectives. At this point politics intervened, but with synchronistic precision. In 1992, I had been asked to interview a French homeopath, Ronald Boyer, a medical graduate of the University of Montpellier, who had applied for the post of senior lecturer in clinical homeopathy at the Technikon Natal. He was admirably suited for the position, and had our roles been reversed, he could well have interviewed me. Following my recommendation, he was accepted and taught at the Technikon from 1992 to 1998, During the first years of his Technikon tenure, Ronald commenced teaching clinical homeopathy to medical doctors, his courses leading to the French-based CEDH qualification (Centre for Education and Development of Clinical Homeopathy).

Combining the MFHom and CEDH

With the graduation of our MFHom students, two different kinds of qualified medical homeopaths came into being, thus creating two camps. The steering committee of the South African Complementary Medical Association (SACMA), which in the 1990's represented all medical doctors practising complementary medical disciplines, approached me with concern about this, stressing the need for a common South African standard of homeopathic education for medical doctors to avoid division and dichotomy. SACMA suggested that Ronald and I should join forces, bringing the CEDH and MFHom curriculums together in a combined teaching programme. This made good sense; our students would benefit from the combination of the classical, constitutional approach of the MFHom and the clinical approach of the CEDH, and on completion of their studies, candidates would achieve both qualifications. I flew down to Durban and met Ronald to discuss the way forward. The result of our deliberations was the forging of a firm friendship and the resolve to join forces. Berkeley, confident that the course he had initiated was in safe hands and would go forward successfully, decided to leave us to carry the baton into the future while he concentrated his energy on his busy practice.

Heavy workload

The combined course proved to be well balanced. Ronald and I shared the responsibility of teaching and with courses in Johannesburg and Cape Town, our private practices and Ronald's Technikon responsibilities, we were kept busy. Looking back, I am astounded at the energy I possessed during those intense years. I started practice at 7.00 a.m. every weekday morning and continued seeing patients throughout the day with only a 30 minute break at midday for a hastily consumed fruit salad, while attending to correspondence and medical reports. On average, the afternoon session would be completed by 4.30 p.m. enabling me to do a workout at the gym before returning home for supper. By 7.30 p.m., I would be at my study desk analysing questionnaire responses from new patients, writing prescriptions for patients making their monthly progress reports, and, when these tasks were completed, preparing my lecture notes. The latter involved considerable time and effort because from the course inception it was my desire to bring together all the various elements that add colour and deeper understanding to the pictures of the major remedies. It was all a labour of love. Unfortunately, as is so common, my wife and teenage children were the sufferers: I was a present, but so very absent, husband and father.

Lectures for the laity

Not satisfied with all these efforts, I decided to give weekly evening lectures on homeopathy to my patients. For this purpose, I added a lecture room to my practice, capable of seating an audience of forty and also providing a lecture and examination room for the CEDH/MFHom course. Because my practice was drawn equally from the Pretoria and Johannesburg areas, I decided to alternate between the two cities, repeating the same lecture delivered in Pretoria the following week in Johannesburg. A patient kindly offered me a venue for the Johannesburg evenings. The project was ambitious and amounted to a lay course in domestic homeopathy together with an overview of the major homeopathic remedy archetypes. There were twenty lectures, which involved me in forty evenings of teaching, each evening being divided into two sessions of ninety minutes with a tea break between. The response was heartening. Both venues were filled to capacity throughout the course. As might be expected, mothers predominated with a sprinkling of grandparents, fathers, sons and daughters. The enthusiasm and commitment of my audience was rewarding beyond measure. It was an enriching experience for me and confirmed important conclusions I had made from my years in practice:

- The importance of educating the public in homeopathy; an objective of equal importance to educating the professions, since demand will create supply.
- The desire of the homeopathic patient to know more about the system in which they have placed their trust.
- The interest and commitment to the healing process that such knowledge generates.
- The surprisingly high level of instruction that can be given considering the non-medical background of most of the audience.
- That when well explained, the science of homeopathy appeals to the innate intelligence of those untrammelled by scientific or religious prejudice.
- A high degree of competence in domestic prescribing can be achieved; responsible homeopathic self-medication is a boon to any family.
- The ability of the patient to participate in their own healing is enhanced; they have better understanding of what the homeopath needs to know and are better able to monitor their own progress.
- The patient learns to understand the direction of cure and the dangers of suppression.
- The patient accepts that a healing process requires time to unfold; they develop therapeutic patience.
- The fascination most people have for the archetypal pictures of the major remedies.
- The ability of the informed person to recognise specific archetypes when these are lived-out in family, friends and acquaintances.

The following year, I advertised another course for parents and the numbers were such that we had to hire a lecture hall at the Pretoria University. These lectures were recorded and marketed as *The Principles of Homeopathy*.

Ronald and I worked well together; we complemented one another to a high degree. I delivered the lectures on homeopathic philosophy and the materia medica of the individual remedies, while Ronald taught their clinical application. This did not prevent our overlapping and this latitude to move into the each others territory proved beneficial in reinforcing perceptions and principles we shared, or providing healthy differences of opinion when we differed. Our friendship deepened over the years we worked together. When the lectures were in Pretoria or Johannesburg, Ronald would stay with us, and I have treasured memories of our long conversations enjoyed after the rest of the Lilley household had retired to bed.

A Scottish connection

In 1997, prompted by Barry Rose, I decided to experience the wider homeopathic world and attended the LIGA (*Liga Medicorum Homoeopathica Internationalis*: LMHI) Congress in Amsterdam. As interesting as the various presentations were, with hindsight, far more memorable to me was further evidence of the inexorable purpose of synchronicity to cue and prompt us towards predetermined outcomes. It had been arranged that on the first morning of the Congress, delegates wishing to do so, should meet in front of Central Station and from there catch a tram to the conference centre. Being alone and unfamiliar with Amsterdam, I opted to do so. There were a considerable number of us and when the tram arrived we had to board quickly resulting in a good shuffling of the group amongst the available seats. I found myself sitting opposite a short, bearded man, who though balding had his greying dark hair drawn back in a ponytail. Although we did not speak during the tram journey, we exchanged glances and the twinkle and humour in his eyes were apparent. His silvered beard made him look older than his years and gave him a venerable, wise countenance. During the seminar, we were briefly introduced and I learnt that he was Bob Leckridge, a physician working at the Glasgow Homeopathic Hospital. He possessed a warm, engaging nature, which immediately attracted me to him, and a captivating Scottish accent. We had little further contact that weekend.

On the last day, Paddy accompanied me to the seminar; she was very keen to hear the famed Jan Scholten and Massimo Mangialavori speak. She had been absent earlier because of acting as a facilitator at an NLP (Neuro Linguistic Programming) seminar in London. As we were about to leave the conference centre after the closure of the seminar, I happened to glance down the corridor between the now largely empty display stalls in the exhibition hall, and there at a distance I remarked a small figure viewing a depleted book stand. As little as I had reason to turn that way in the rush of our departure, I came to a halt experiencing a strong desire to introduce Paddy to this special person I scarcely knew. Acting on impulse, I suited action to emotion and piloted Paddy to where Bob stood. Time has erased our exchange, but both Paddy and I experienced the same warmth and impish sparkle that had previously charmed me. Little did I know it then, but this brief encounter would be the beginning of a lasting friendship and a spur to my lecturing career.

1998 would bring the final examinations for the CEDH/MFHom cohort of students. It was once again time to make arrangements with the British Faculty for the appointment of moderators and external examiners. Since the last examinations, Barry Rose had retired as Dean and his successor was Jeremy Swayne, a very erudite, scholarly man of scrupulous correctness and studied eloquence, who is now an ordained minister of the Church of England. His serious, at times pedantic, demeanour belies a nimble wit and comic ability of side-splitting proportions.

The clinical part of the MFHom examination necessitated the presence of at least one external examiner appointed by the British Faculty. Jeremy being unable to attend himself arranged for two colleagues with examining experience to take his place: Michael Jenkins, senior physician at the Royal London Homoeopathic Hospital, and, as I should have anticipated, a certain Robert Leckridge, now without ponytail.

An invitation

The examinations proved highly successful, our full complement of candidates passed. On the Sunday evening, after a tiring weekend of assessments, the examining team enjoyed a relaxing evening together at a Pretoria restaurant. I relate these details because it was an evening of great significance to me. In a quiet moment, Bob turned to me and asked me if I would like to come to Scotland to give a day of lectures to his colleagues and students. Bob was, and still is, very active in homeopathic education and there can be few, if any, of the younger generation of Scottish homeopaths who have not received their tuition through him. I agreed, and in February 1999 duly delivered a pilot lecture day in Glasgow largely on the theme of the evolution of the primary homeopathic archetypes through stellar nuclear synthesis and planetary evolution. I could not have had a more responsive and encouraging audience. Jeremy Swayne, the Dean, who had played an indirect but important role in the sequence of events, was present. The success of the day, prompted Bob to propose a truly venturesome project: a series of three day David Lilley seminars alternating between Glasgow and London, each seminar to comprise 18 hours of lectures providing me with an incredible opportunity to share my love of the homeopathic materia medica, enriched with cosmology, the doctrine of signatures, symbolism, mythology, analytical psychology and chakra science. We decided to commence the seminars that very summer, doing an initial launch in both Glasgow and London, and thereafter alternating between the two centres.

From the hospitality of Scotland, Paddy and I travelled to London for a brief holiday before returning to South Africa. There we enjoyed the hospitality of Michael Jenkins and his wife Sally. Mike, was to prove my greatest support during the time I lectured in London. He is one of the most caring and nurturing men I have ever met; his kindness and attentiveness know no bounds. Behind the pragmatic, logical mind of a specialist physician lies an intuitive nature that he would scarcely give himself credit for. He often provided a grounding influence for my forays into the mysterious and obscure. His enthusiasm for the lecture series was as keen as Bob's and he set about stirring up interest in the south.

By the commencement of the series, Bob had been elected President of the British Faculty, a post he held for six years (1999–2005), during which time his prudent, bridging influence was vital in restoring the sense of fraternity within the Faculty; a coming together that was to prove invaluable in the difficult times of conventional, medical hostility that lay ahead.

Lecturing in Britain

In all, I delivered nine seminars of this series over a period of four years, during which time Bob and Hilary Leckridge in Stirling and Mike and Sally Jenkins in London opened their homes to Paddy and myself. Our trips were looked forward to with happy anticipation and became an important part of our lives. It was a very rewarding period, which resulted in me investigating remedies and their relationships in greater depth and provided me with the ideal stage on which to express my insights. All the seminars were recorded and these recordings have proved valuable to a much wider audience. In addition, Paddy and I gained many homeopathic friends within the Faculty, the Society of Homeopaths (the association of professional homeopaths), and not least of all the British Association of Homeopathic Veterinary Surgeons (BAHVS). On a number of occasions over the past years, I have been invited to give presentations at Society and homeopathic Veterinary conferences. A memorable one given to the Society at Keele University in Staffordshire dealt with the homeopathic psychological profiling of serial killers and the likelihood of changing the course of events had the future killers received homeopathic constitutional treatment as children? Both my audience and myself were so engrossed in the topic that I went over my time limit with only Peter Sutcliffe, the Yorkshire Ripper, having been profiled and Ted Bundy and Jeffrey Dahmer still to come. When the organisers quite correctly intervened, there was an outcry from many in the filled to capacity auditorium who wanted me to continue.

South African Faculty courses

Back in South Africa, my teaching partnership with Ronald Boyer continued successfully in Johannesburg and Cape Town. In 1998, Ronald left the Technikon Natal and conveniently for our course set up practice in Cape Town. In 2001, our next cohort of students, ten in number, achieved the CEDH/MFHom qualification with Mike Jenkins and Anton Van Rhijn acting as external examiners for the British Faculty. Although the numbers sound very modest, in terms of medical homeopathy they are hugely significant; every practitioner committed to practicing this gentle art of healing is truly indispensable. Due to the small number of medical doctors interested in acquiring a homeopathic education it has not been possible for us to commence a new course every year; usually, only after our three-year course is completed do we have enough applicants to commence another.

The 2001 graduate group of students was the last to be taught by Ronald and myself. Ronald was lured away to become the President of the CEDH in the USA, based in Philadelphia; a position he still holds. His departure has been a great loss to homeopathic education in South Africa. In recognition of his service to medical homeopathy he was made an honorary member of the South African Faculty, which became a registered Higher Education Institution in 2001.

For the three courses that the SA Faculty has run since 2001, I have had the assistance of our own graduates and in addition, Robert Moiloa, the previous Head of the Department of Homeopathy at the University of Johannesburg. In early 2006, thirteen students from the Johannesburg and Cape Town courses sat the exam. The external examiner was the new Dean of the Faculty, Raymond Sevar, who has a homeopathic practice in Carlisle, Cumbria. All the candidates were successful and two achieved distinction. In July 2012, the most recent examination took place. The external examiners were Bob Leckridge from the British Faculty and Elizabeth Solomon from the homeopathic department of the University of Johannesburg. In this examination, the SA Faculty achieved its best results so far; all ten candidates passed and four merited distinction.

After 18 years of academic activity, the SA Faculty now stands at a crossroad. Escalating costs due to the administrative requirements demanded by the various government departments controlling higher education in South Africa, small student intake numbers and high running costs have made it no longer possible to maintain the Faculty as a private teaching institution. The way forward necessitates the Faculty course being incorporated into a University Health Sciences Department. As I write, this initiative is being pursued in the hope that the course that Berkeley Digby and I founded in 1994 can continue to educate medical doctors in the science and art of homeopathy, after a temporary pause.

British Faculty congress in Bath

I must now retrace my steps to 2000, the year after I commenced the masterclass series of lectures for the British Faculty. The Faculty holds a congress every two years at different venues in the United Kingdom. In 2000, the congress was held in Bath. I decided to give a presentation on a fascinating remedy, Lac caninum (bitch's milk), entitled *Lac-can – A Dog's Life*. Dog's milk was recognised as a potent medicine in Classical Greek times, but it is through homeopathic research and clinical experience that the precise indications for its use have been developed. After describing the essential characteristics of the archetype, I presented an argument in favour of the conclusion that the hugely disparate, major antagonists in World War 2, Winston Churchill and Adolf Hitler, despite their differences, represented opposite poles of a single archetype: the archetype of the Dog – Lac caninum – the Bulldog and the hybridised Wolf-type dog (e.g. Alsatian) respectively. As with serial killers, I asked whether it would not have been possible to change the destiny of the world if fortune had decreed that Hitler should have received correct homeopathic, constitutional treatment as a child: would the treatment of Adolf with Lac-can have prevented Hitler? Of course this was not to be, fate decreed otherwise, but the question remains valid and is pertinent in the treatment of all young people. Undesirable traits identified in the young, being early compensatory expressions of weakness at soul level, premonitory of mature characteristics to come and symptomatic of soul/ego contention, require healing attention from the time of their first appearance. Like life itself, homeopathy is a powerful means to fortify the soul in its task of mastering the ego-self and achieving Self-realisation: a transformation that lies at the heart of all healing. The paper was well received, stimulated much interest and proved helpful in promoting the masterclass lectures.

Another Scottish connection

It was at the Bath congress that I first met Steven Kayne, a pharmacist, Glaswegian Anglo-Scot, and at the time the first Pharmacy Dean of the British Faculty (1999–2003); a seasoned protagonist of homeopathic pharmacy, homeopathic education and homeopathic politics. He unforgettably came to my attention during his gala dinner speech, which revealed his mischievous sense of humour, agile brain and warm personality. He has always given me an impression of great strength of purpose, groundedness, clarity of vision and uncompromising directness and integrity; these qualities all mellowed by wonderful compassion and understanding and visibly attested by kindly eyes, jovial features and a powerful, stout physique. Our acquaintance grew to friendship over a number of years through meeting at various homeopathic conferences where he manned the Freeman's Homeopathic Pharmacy display tables, often with his wife, Sorelle. Steven established this family business in 1971, and his son Lee, the present Faculty Pharmacy Dean, is now Freeman's chief pharmacist.

Yet again, synchronicity assured our getting to know one another better. In 1997, due to the frequency of my lecturing sorties to Cape Town from my home base in Pretoria, I bought a flat in Fresnaye, near Sea Point, with a lovely sea view. In the back of my mind, I had the thought of one day retiring to this haven. Unbeknown to me, a few years later, Steven and Sorelle commenced yearly holidays in Cape Town, timed for late November and early December. In 2005, our respective holidays in this most beautiful of cities happened to coincide. Steven had heard me lecture on several occasions and had read the masterclass articles that I wrote for the *Health and Homeopathy* magazine, an excellent publication which epitomises much of what is needed to widen public interest in homeopathy. My contribution was some nineteen essays on key homeopathic remedies viewed from an archetypal perspective.

One evening, to celebrate our being in Cape Town together, Paddy and I took Steven and Sorelle to a restaurant on Bloubergstrand, which lies across the bay from Table Mountain. From this vantage point it is possible to delight in a magnificent sunset dominated by the iconic silhouette of the mountain. We were not to be disappointed. While savouring this breath-taking view and enjoying a sundowner on the balcony of the restaurant, Steven asked me if I would be willing to write a chapter for a book on various homeopathic topics that he was planning. The book would be titled: *Homeopathic Practice*. It was his intention to invite a number of authors with the necessary expertise to contribute to

> ... a wide-ranging book that was both a source of inspiration ... as well as a source of reference – a book that could be read rather than studied and that would appeal to knowledgeable amateur homeopaths as well as to healthcare professionals ...[1]

I readily agreed. Steven gave me a subject that was right up my alley: *The homeopathic materia medica*. The book, which fulfilled Steven's objectives, provides a happy balance between the exposition of theory and its application. My chapter was to be our first collaboration.

Synchronicity never misses a beat. Towards the end of 2006, I decided that the following year would be my last in my Pretoria practice, leaving me free to move to Cape Town, where I would continue practicing on a very small scale, giving me the time and opportunity to continue teaching and also to commence writing the books that would contain the experience of my over forty years in homeopathic practice and nearly twenty years of lecturing. During that final year of my practice, 2007, Steven and Lee Kayne also took a major step, founding Saltire Books, an independent publishing company based in Glasgow, with the intention of "serving the professional complementary medicine community". When we next met after these major decisions had come to pass, Steven approached me and said: "David, I am sure that there is a book inside you that wants to be written and Saltire Books will be proud to be associated with it." No confirmatory directive could have been more explicit; my father or his mentor Dr Letari, might as well have spoken. In March 2009, we formalised an agreement for a series of books, but it was almost four years before the completed manuscript for the first book was on Steven's desk. The main obstacle to my writing proved to be the final MFHom, SA Faculty course for which I produced a huge volume of backup literature to assure a high standard of delivery, a task which yielded splendid results and fortunately will never require repeating. I cannot thank Steven and Lee Kayne sufficiently for the patience, encouragement and support they gave me during this period of very slow progress.

This book – where to begin?

In approaching this first book, my intention was to commence with the ordered emergence of the core remedy archetypes through stellar nuclear-synthesis, followed by those which are written into the early evolution of the planet, a fascinating subject touched on in the paper I presented in Durban in 1993. This objective was reflected in the title I proposed: *The Evolution of the Homeopathic Archetype*. I anticipated being in the thick of the archetypes and their associated remedies in no time at all. But, as I soon discovered, a book, even when its subject matter is clear and specific, can possess a life of its own. No sooner had I started writing than the book asserted its influence and directed my course; I am grateful it did. The quotation from Hahnemann, which opens the first chapter, started the process in concert with my answer to a question posed by Steven when we first discussed the possibility of a book. "Who will be your audience?" It was a vital question.

The audience

On reflection, I knew I wanted to reach as wide a public as possible and particularly the many curious, educated people who desire to know more about the history, philosophy and principles of homeopathy without having to tackle a dry dissertation. Although I did not wish to write a textbook purely for the homeopathic profession, I did want to create a work that would also be of interest to many of my colleagues. I came to the conclusion that if I could craft a text, which despite my long familiarity with its topics would prove of value to myself, deepen and widen my knowledge, crystallise my concepts, be a source of information for my future lectures and provide me with an enjoyable read – and still be comprehensible to the average non-professional mind – I would be satisfied.

Hahnemann's life

When I gave what became known as my 'mothers' courses', I commenced with a short history of Hahnemann's life, and, though very abbreviated, I used his pioneering story as a framework for explaining the discovery and development of the fundamental laws and principles upon which homeopathic practice is based. Story telling provides a powerful yet comfortable vehicle for conveying information and instruction. The ladies were charmed by the narrative with all its woes, trials, triumphs and romance and expressed their pleasure. Once I had chosen the opening quote for my book, Hahnemann asserted his presence, and, mindful of the ladies' response, I resolved to start with a short account of the Master's life. Once started, I knew it was correct to do so, firstly, because this work was to be the first of a series of books and Hahnemann's life would furnish the ideal opening to an on-going story, and, secondly, because of my chosen audience, many new to homeopathy or with only limited familiarity with its history. I also reasoned that if I fashioned the story from its important highlights it would afford colleagues easy access to the essential facts and a means to refresh memory.

This reasoning ensured that the account would not be brief, because the highlights were many. It was not possible to discuss the evolution of Hahnemann's thinking without reference to his non-conforming, iconoclastic predecessor, Paracelsus, to whom Hahnemann studiously never gave credit, for fear of contaminating homeopathy in the eyes of his peers, who regarded Paracelsus as a heretic. Consideration of Paracelsus led me to Galen, from whom, despite his contempt for his work, Paracelsus inherited the theory of the four humours and their associated temperaments: the phlegmatic, the choleric, the sanguine and the melancholic – four fundamental archetypes. One of the basic tenets of homeopathy is that the symptoms of disease are an expression of Nature's healing power and therefore must not be suppressed. This concept takes us back to Hippocrates and even beyond him to the healers of antiquity. Thus, an entire chapter was expended before I even came to the birth of Hahnemann, but what a treasure trove of Paracelsian wisdom had been revealed.

Once Hahnemann's life story had been written and *the science of homeopathy* elaborated through this means, I thought I had come to the point where I could enter the fascinating and magical world of the archetype, but another tale still needed to be told.

My father's life

My father's remarkable life touched and influenced a great many people. Not only did he heal the sick through spiritual and homeopathic means, he also spread a message of love, truth, perfection and trust: knowledge of our immortal spiritual nature, of life everlasting and of the sacred journey of the soul in quest of its divinity. This message was imparted without the elaborate and implausible mythology of religious belief or need for ritual or dogma. Yet, it was numinous, replete with enlightened beings, guardian angels, ineffable beauty and majesty and a heavenly hierarchy. In conjunction with this mission, he tirelessly spread the word of homeopathy by teaching, lecturing and healing. He always led by example.

My own life, the way I practise homeopathy and the content of what I wish to share in forthcoming books are all informed by my upbringing in a home where the physical world and the spirit world were perceived as one, without division: a dimension of matter pervaded and governed by spirit. Life was understood to be a temporary sojourn in an unfamiliar environment fraught with extreme opposites, perfect for the exercise of free will and moral choice, ideal for acts of heroism or infamy: a domain for restitution or reparation.

Even while embarked on the heroic journey of Hahnemann, I pondered the possibility of including in the book something about my father's story. Because of its uniqueness and exceptional content, and not wishing to step outside any parameters Saltire Books might have, I broached the matter with Steven Kayne. Without fully knowing the esoteric nature of what I would impart, Steven accepted the proposal, and we considered including a chapter about my father's work, or simply adding an appendix.

On cue, 10th October 2011, came a directive: an email from someone I have never met, Helen Blake of Melbourne, Australia, who was doing research into the lives of the pioneers of mediumship and spiritualism. She had read about my father's spiritual work in *The Gift of Healing* by Arthur Keith Desmond, but had come to a dead end at the point when my father vacated the spiritualist platform in Britain to devote his life to homeopathy in South Africa. All she knew subsequent to that time was the account of the dramatic public demonstration in psychic surgery in the City Hall, Johannesburg, 1953, given in Maurice Barbanell's book: *The Saga of Spirit Healing*. She had experienced similar difficulties in gathering the information she needed with regard to other mediums, but wrote to me:

> . . . however, it is your father who has been most on my mind (and for quite some time now). An extraordinary man, yet in the reading he comes across so very humble.

In replying to her queries, my decision to write more extensively on my father's unusual life was resolved. In the light of my past experience, the prompt from the email, coming out of the blue, forty years after my father's passing and coming precisely when I stood at my crossroad, could not be ignored. Besides, David Williams words were not forgotten, and, as if this was not sufficient, when I was fully three quarters through my father's story, I received an email from the past Dean of the British Faculty, Jeremy Swayne, asking whether there was anything he could read about my father's work.

Including the full picture of my father's history enabled me to present two themes, which will be intrinsic to the books which follow: *The Science of Homeopathy* detailed through the life of Samuel Hahnemann and *The Science of Spirit* revealed through the life of William Lilley. The stage has been set for *The Science of the Archetype*, which will be covered in the second volume of this series.

Our spiritual nature

There was another reason for commencing my writing odyssey by combining Hahnemann's history with that of my father. From the outset, I wished to establish the perspective from which I approach science. I was fortunate that from a very early age I was cognisant of my spirit nature, that my body was a temporary vehicle for my soul, that life would afford me opportunities to develop spiritually through love and service, that I could not die and that after passing from this physical world I would be returning to my natural state of spirit, wiser and more experienced than when I entered the world. As my life unfolded, I was blessed with many experiences that confirmed this understanding. I never experienced my simple truths as being in any sense religious, philosophical or theoretical, but factual, beyond doubt and, therefore, belonging to an ineffable science that sustains and transcends conventional science.

Awareness of being an immortal spirit-being in quest of enlightenment; a visitor to an earth plane peopled by souls, all in varying degrees of spiritual development from the most coarse and unrefined to the most illumined, creates a reality that permits better understanding of human behaviour and the vagaries of life, gives fortitude in adversity and evokes empathy for the tribulations of the human state. Physical existence acquires meaning: it is for our growth; it must be rich in incident; it is not arbitrary: events are never coincidental, life happens as it must. Our spiritual progress and integrity are reflected in our responses and reactions to what life presents, and in our aspirations and our inclinations. Life provides an indispensable period of learning and testing for the growing soul, sometimes through unwelcome challenges, always through opportunities to express creativity, positivity and goodness. Earth is a school for the soul; a training ground that affords each incarnated soul unique experiences essential for spiritual development. *We are angels in training!*

Since a single lifetime can never be sufficient for the soul to achieve self-realisation, more than one lifetime is imperative. Like the seasons, the soul goes through cycles as it repeatedly passes from the spirit world through birth into physical life and then passes from physical life into the spirit world through the death of the physical body. Whenever the soul is ready, it once again enters the cycle of reincarnation. Each precious incarnation, however brief or extended, exposes the soul to essential polarities and paradoxes only possible on the earth level of reality. These demand moral choice, and a trust in the wisdom and loving power of the Creation that defies understanding. All is ordained and designed to facilitate the soul's ascent towards the Self: its essence and source.

The soul is always richer from mortal experience, no matter how perfidious or heinous its life may have been. Though seemingly removed from sentiment, remorse and pity, within the darkest soul divinity resides: an infinite power, ever drawing the struggling soul towards sublimation. Often only through hardship and suffering can the sleeping soul be awakened from its spiritual slumber or the recalcitrant soul shocked into awareness. Just as an expanding sliver of ice can split a mighty rock, so, a twinge of regret, a glimmer of selflessness, a touch of empathy or the tiniest spark of love can initiate the fracture of the blackest and hardest heart.

Life, no matter its content, is a divine prescription for the healing of the soul and the demise of the ego-self. Life is always perfect, always healing, always loving, always wise and true. Despite all appearances to the contrary, whatever is taking place in our lives at any given moment is perfect, is necessary and is tailored for our unique spiritual needs. No matter what is happening: *all is well*!

Since we are spirit beings from a spirit plane, which permeates and sustains the tangible, physical dimension, we are never alone, there are always unseen, loved ones in the spirit world, who are with us, supporting, counselling and inspiring us through thick and thin. Though we may not be consciously aware of their presence or their thoughts, nonetheless, their unfailing, loving and guiding influence always surrounds us.

Basic Trust

Knowledge of these simple truths bestows the greatest blessing of all: a state of *basic trust*. A trust, which in the face of dread and disaster, or, in the wake of harrowing events, will reaffirm and reassert itself. The soul girded with basic trust can emerge from the torrent, buffeted and bruised, and then like an Old English Sheepdog shake itself down and face life with an inner voice, which with time grows ever stronger, saying:

> You came naked and seemingly alone into this world and you will depart naked and seemingly alone. Nothing here belongs to you – not even your most dearly beloved. All that you have has been given; use these gifts wisely, selflessly, kindly and creatively. Desire to serve and life opens doors for you. Love, but do not become attached, be intensely involved, but remain dispassionate, create with joy, inspiration and to the best of your ability, but care nothing for results or rewards. You have nothing to fear; you are an immortal being immune to the hurts of this ephemeral, mortal state. Every event in your life is a blessing drawing you towards the realisation of your angelic state. Trust! – Trust! – Trust! You are as the very gods: indestructible, eternal and vested with power beyond your comprehension!

David Lilley
Fresnaye, Cape Town
September 2013

Key concepts

While it is not possible for me to make my experience that of my readers, nonetheless, in compiling this first volume, I felt it important to share the blessing of my upbringing and affirm certain key concepts. In practice, these concepts become the essential precepts that must form the foundation for any healing system of medicine. They are also the themes that will be expanded in the books that follow this volume.

- The existence of the soul, its immortality and its quest for Self-realisation.
- The creation is the work of a supreme, wise, loving intelligence working ceaselessly with purpose towards predetermined goals.
- Creation is an endless, on-going process governed by laws that ensure perfection in every detail of that which is created.
- Any imperfection perceived in the creation lies in the eye and understanding of the beholder and is the interpretation of the ego-self.
- The obstacle that lies in the path of the soul in its quest for perfection is the ego-self, the reprobate and delinquent, prodigal offspring of the soul, born of lack of basic trust.
- Life viewed through the distorted lenses of ego-perception and ego-interpretation is imperfect, unloving and threatening.
- Deluded by the misconceptions of the ego-self, the soul feels separated from its source, isolated, forsaken and vulnerable and without trust that it is significant, loveable, loved and blessed.
- The ego-self, its perceptions and interpretations (delusions) and its prejudices (exclusions) and preferences (attachments) give rise to the dis-ease of the soul, which leads to the diseases that afflict both mind and body.
- To heal any mental or physical disease it is essential to heal the soul of its ego-based dis-ease.
- Since the ego-self, the essence of all illness, sickness and disease is a dynamic force, intangible and imponderable, the curative influence necessary to bring about healing must be in dynamic, intangible, imponderable form, and its action must match as similarly as possible the singular, peculiarities of the ego-self.
- Homeopathic remedies being in dynamic, imponderable form when matched to the profile of the ego-self have the power to bring about healing at the deepest possible level: the soul dimension.

Reference

1. Kayne SB (ed). *Homeopathic Practice*. London: Pharmaceutical Press; 2008. Preface pxiii.

Part one

THE SCIENCE OF HOMEOPATHY
The enduring legacy of Samuel Hahnemann

1

LEGACY FROM THE PAST

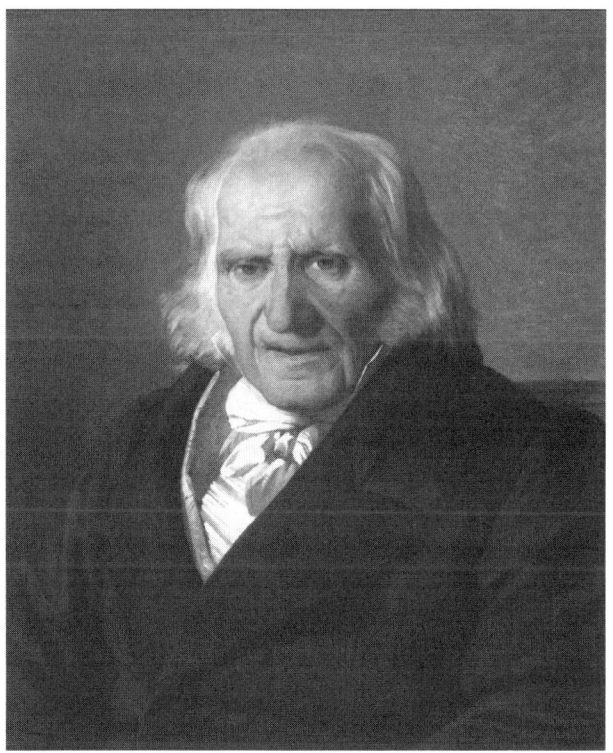

Christian Friedrich Samuel Hahnemann (1765–1843)
Courtesy of Institut für Geschichte der Medizin der Robert Bosch Stiftung, Stuttgart

Would He, the Father of all, coldly survey the torments of disease of His Dearest creatures? Would He leave open no way to the genius of mankind – otherwise so infallible – no easy, certain and dependable way of regarding disease from the right angle, of determining the use and the specific, safe and dependable results obtainable from medicines? Before I would have given credence to this blasphemy, I should have forsworn all the school systems of the world.

Samuel Hahnemann[1]

A metaphysical and scientific Law of Cure

These words, written by Dr Christian Friedrich Samuel Hahnemann fully 200 years ago, express a sentiment and a persuasion that have existed in the heart and mind of man since ancient times: that despite all appearances to the contrary, a wise and loving, omnipotent power presides over the harsh realities of life, so fraught with hardship, hazards, tragedies and disease. The conclusion of this belief is that the goodness and forethought of such a benevolent presence must have provided a means or process by which human beings can overcome, transcend and sublimate the adversities which beset them, including the ever-present spectre and experience of illness and disease. Ancient wisdom conceived that the cosmos was created for the benefit of humanity, enigmatically fashioned in every aspect and dimension to quicken the spiritual unfolding and ascent of the individual soul and that, no matter what befell, the soul would always be supported, cherished, encouraged and inspired by an ever-present, though usually undetected, loving divinity. Intimate to this concept were the immortality of the soul, the presence of eternity and the immediacy of an intelligent, enfolding universal force. Combined, these notions provided meaning and purpose to the life experience, regardless of the trials it brought, and the knowledge that this experience always unfolded according to universal law acting with sublime and positive intent. Such a law would surely embrace a 'Law of Disease' and a 'Law of Cure' and these laws would prove accessible and comprehensible to humanity.

With the advent of science and the dominance of reason and logic, these perennial truths have been largely lost to the modern mind. Newtonian physics has swept all before it and presents for man's credulity a mindless, clockwork universe, which unfolded without purpose, direction or intent. It affirms that the universe, itself the product of coincidence and chance, evolved the first simple life forms through spontaneous, chemical alchemy. Subsequently, it concludes, all the wondrous biodiversity of this planet, including the human race, came into being through random mutations of genetic material, screened by natural selection. Matter is regarded as the foundation of life. To such a science, the human being is a soulless aggregation of cells without higher destiny and all its gifts and achievements are solely the result of complex, neuronal activity. These cold and pragmatic postulates underpin the science of modern medicine and explain its mechanistic approach to both mental and physical disease and hence its reliance and dependency on surgery and powerful chemicals to extirpate, control and suppress morbid symptoms and signs. As valuable and even life-saving as these methods may prove, especially in emergency situations and overwhelming infections, they do not resolve the disease process at a causative level, nor do they stimulate and encourage the inherent capacity of the body to heal itself and bring about a permanent, curative change. Apart from resolving purely mechanical problems, the results achieved do not constitute cure – only palliation – a stopgap. Symptoms and signs driven from the surface, like unresolved emotions, become more deeply rooted and will, sooner or later, find expression and work their mischief, either in the sufferer or in their progeny. It can be confidently asserted that despite all that modern medicine can achieve, which is often remarkable and praise worthy, its premises do not provide a universal doctrine of cure and fall far short of providing the answer to Hahnemann's question, quoted above, for they do not embody a therapeutic system that is easy, certain, specific, safe or dependable.

Unfortunately, the impressive successes of orthodox medicine in palliating disease have led to professional complacency, scientific arrogance and a desire to create and maintain a medical monopoly. Despite the evidence of its shortcomings: the evolution of resistant strains of infective organisms and 'superbugs' (often a response to its indiscriminate use of anti-infective agents); its weakness in the face of viral diseases and epidemics; the ever increasing autoimmune diseases which defy chemical resolution (possibly provoked by its intense immunisation programmes); and its inability to cope with mental ill-health and chronic disease (only controlled by its use of highly expensive and toxic substances which induce dependency); the proponents of the orthodox system imperiously claim that their methods and protocols constitute the only 'scientific' and acceptable way to treat the sick. All other methods are dismissed as bogus and 'unscientific.'

While recognising and respecting the good intent, immense acumen, invaluable research and dedicated service to the welfare of the community demonstrated by conventional medicine, and intrinsic to its calling, nonetheless, it is regrettable that in the process of its development it has become one-pointed, blinkered and hide-bound, unwilling or unable to accept, or even consider, that other means of treatment exist and are deserving of open-minded investigation. Without the concepts of soul, spiritual destiny and the existence of a universal intelligence to guide its perspective, the prevailing system of medicine remains one-dimensional, at war with physical forces, which it attempts to overcome by equally powerful physical means. Like guerrilla warfare down the ages, this war of chemical medicine against disease, a shadowy, elusive adversary, unseen and not understood, other than in a naïve and superficial way, is doomed to failure and the ailing public experiences the collateral damage.

The human being, the paragon of animals, is a multi-dimensional being, existing and experiencing on many dimensions at once; dimensions which interpenetrate one another and are interdependent. To conceive that chronic disease can be circumscribed or isolated in origin or extent, even in physical terms, is absurd. To be sick in one cell of the body is to be sick in every cell of the body, because the unit of physical life is the body, not the cell, the organ, any system or the body chemistry. Nor can disease be confined to the physical plane alone; there it manifests its consequences, but not its cause. The continuity of the dimensions of existence indicates that a disease of the body is evidence of a disturbance at a more subtle and deeper level. To be sick in one dimension of existence is to be sick in every dimension of existence, because the unit of existence is the soul-ego-mind-body complex, not the emotions, the intellect or the body. The diagnostic and therapeutic procedures and the medicines of conventional medicine, despite their sophistication and ability to investigate and explain the characteristics of disease processes, to destroy pathogens and to manipulate and balance body chemistry, belong to the objective world. However, the stage upon which we enact our lives, experience our joys, suffer our griefs and fulfil ourselves creatively is primarily on a subjective plane far beyond the reach of scans, X-rays, surgery and chemical medication. It is upon this subjective stage that the causes of 'dis-ease', and consequently disease, are to be found. It is here, where we suffer, struggle and survive, that changes detrimental to health originate and cascade into the mental and physical spheres. Any curative system of medicine must be able to act at this subtle level in order to bring about permanent healing. To realise this, is, in the words of Hahnemann, ". . . to regard disease from the right angle". It constitutes a major shift in medical paradigm, which orthodox medicine has yet to achieve and until now shows no inclination to make.

This 'right angle' is not new, it was familiar to the ancients, and has been applied down the ages to the present day, through many different systems of energy-healing both in the East and in the West: a diverse spectrum of disciplines, including, amongst others, spiritual healing, acupuncture, kinesiology and herbal medicine. All of which are viewed with mistrust and disdain, if not outright contempt and hostility, by the medical orthodoxy. But, it was Samuel Hahnemann, a medical doctor from Saxony in Germany, who, in the late 1700's, formulated a clearly defined system of medical therapeutics, which at last placed in the hands of healing practitioners a means to reach into the deepest recesses of the human psyche in order to address and remedy disease at a causal level; a system which he named *homoeopathy*.

It is interesting to note that no other system of so-called alternative or unorthodox medicine, other than homeopathy, has ever managed to rouse the dominant school, known as *allopathy*, to such levels of antipathy that it would gladly seek to outlaw, abolish and destroy it. Since Hahnemann's time this enmity has not abated. By the late 1800's, homeopathy had almost been stamped out in the United States. Through the machinations of the American Medical Association, many states passed legislation making the practice of homeopathy, even by registered medical doctors, illegal. During the last century, homeopathy made a slow come-back, which increased markedly in the late 1980's and 1990's with the appearance of influential teachers who were able to impart a fresh impetus to the profession, resulting in an increasing number of defections to its cause from the ranks of the orthodoxy. As always, homeopathy's raised profile became like a red rag to the orthodox bull; its very existence seemingly a reproof and hence an insult. In the latter part of the first decade of this millennium, the occasional flurries of destructive criticism posted in medical journals and the media increased to a sustained pitch, aided and orchestrated by certain academics, who, fired by a prejudice not based on experience, attacked its precepts as unscientific and unproven with the fervour and self-righteousness of religious zealots. They 'protesteth too much,' and in so doing reveal the vulnerability of the system of medicine they so ardently champion. However, no matter what opposition and setbacks its acceptance may experience, like all truths, homeopathy will survive and spread, just as the scientific discoveries of Galileo survived the outrage and wrath of the Inquisition.

This book, and the volumes which follow, is not written as a defence of homeopathy but as a celebration and exposition of its immaculate beauty, timeless wisdom and curative power.

The First Law of Homeopathy: *the Law of Similars*

Before embarking on our odyssey into the subtle dimensions that we need to investigate in order to come to an understanding of the nature of the creation, the nature of the human being, the nature of disease and the nature of cure, it is necessary to consider for a moment the basic principle upon which homeopathic practice rests; for all that follows revolves around this vital precept.

Homeopathy is a system of medical therapeutics based upon a fundamental law of nature known as the *Law of Similars*; a law as unchanging and as constant as the laws of gravity and motion. This principle of similarity can be stated as follows: those symptoms, which a substance can cause when administered to a healthy person are the very symptoms, which that substance can cure when administered to a sick person. The law is accurately expressed by the Latin maxim, coined by Hahnemann: *similia similibus curentur*, which can be translated as 'let like be cured by like'. Stated in its simplest form, the law means: what a substance can cause it can also cure! To be given a little of the 'hair of the dog that bit you' is an idiom that captures this principle. Scorpion stings are extremely painful and can prove fatal. Amongst certain African tribes, the traditional treatment is the use of the scorpion itself as a remedy, either crushed and applied locally to the area of the sting or roasted and eaten. Though possibly crude, such examples, which abound in traditional medicine around the world, are evidence of the application of the concept of 'like cures like' that has come down to us from the remote past. The correct application of the similar principle provides the physician with the ability to bring about a cure in curable conditions and to bring relief to those cases that are beyond cure.

Homeopathy is a curative system of therapeutics, which means that it is not suppressive or palliative, nor is it replacement therapy. The term curative does not mean the mere disappearance of symptoms, but the restoration of the patient's constitution to a state of on-going vigour, health and balance, experienced both mentally and physically. To achieve this, homeopathy acts by utilising, stimulating and enhancing the body's own curative, defensive and recuperative powers.

In accordance with the Law of Similars, and in order to treat a case curatively, a remedy must be sought that has been proved to produce in healthy persons a complex of symptoms most closely resembling those of the patient requiring treatment. The remedy that fulfils this criterion by best matching or mirroring the patient's emotional and physical condition, is known as the homeopathic '*simillimum*' – the remedy most 'like.'

The word homeopathy, originally spelt homoeopathy, derives from two Greek words, *homoios*, meaning like or similar, and *pathos*, meaning disease or suffering. Brought together in one word – *homeopathy* – they indicate 'like suffering', which aptly summarises the fundamental law on which homeopathy is based.

In the light of the above, a homeopathic physician may be defined as one who adds to his or her knowledge of the basic medical sciences and diagnosis, a special knowledge of homeopathic therapeutics and in cases suited to such therapy observes the Law of Similars in selecting the required medication.

Examples of 'Like cures Like'

To get a deeper feeling and appreciation of how this principle works and how it may be applied, it will be valuable to consider some examples.

Anyone who has sliced onions in the kitchen is familiar with the coryza-like symptoms that invariably result. Allium cepa, the red onion, is an excellent remedy for many cases of typical, common winter-cold attended by copious, watery, burning nasal discharge, congested, watery eyes and paroxysms of violent sneezing. Through a similar correspondence it is also often a successful remedy for allergic rhinitis (hayfever), especially when the scent of flowers provokes the attack. However, clinical experience has made it possible to recognise a more exact onion-coryza picture, enabling a more accurate match between patient and remedy. Precision in prescribing is essential to success. Allium cepa patients are more inclined to contract a cold in cold, damp weather; the discharge from the nose burns and reddens the wings of the nose and the upper lip while the watery secretion from the eyes is bland; these symptoms are worse in a warm room and are better in the open air. Unchecked, the cold tends to involve the ears, especially the left, and descends to the larynx causing severe inflammation, hoarseness and tickling. From the larynx it progresses to the bronchi with profuse secretion of mucous and a rattling or hacking cough, which causes a very severe, tearing pain in the larynx. All symptoms are worse on the left side or start on the left and extend to the right. When symptoms evolve in this manner, Allium cepa swiftly brings relief and prevents the thick catarrh that so often follows a cold.

During the French and Italian Renaissance, arsenic was the preferred homicidal poison. The infamous Borgia family made generous use of it to silence their opponents and enemies. It was ideal, because, according to need, it could be administered to bring about an abrupt or lingering death and in those times was undetectable, so giving the impression of a natural, though unpleasant, end. Aggressive poisoning is characterised by severe gastroenteritis with nausea, retching and vomiting after the least eating or drinking and dysentery-like symptoms with agonising, griping pains and bloody, offensive diarrhoea, accompanied by utter prostration and rapid dehydration. Homeopathic Arsenicum album (Ars-alb) has proved rapidly curative in many such cases of gastroenteritis, dysentery or food poisoning when chosen simply for these unqualified symptoms. But, as with all remedies, Ars-alb has a character all of its own, with which it colours the common (generic) symptoms of a disease, drawing our attention for its use. When, in addition to the above symptoms, the patient displays the following indications: despite exhaustion, an anxious restlessness, driving them to continuously change their position and filling them with dread, despair of cure and a fear of dying, so that they fear being left alone; pains that burn like fire, yet are relieved by hot drinks, warm food and hot applications; chilled to the bones and needing to be wrapped up warmly, yet desiring the open air and coolness to the head; thirsty for cold water, yet it makes them feel worse; a need to drink frequently, but only small sips at a time; and symptoms, emotional and physical, which are worse after midnight, particularly between 2.00 a.m. and 3.00 a.m., then Ars-alb may be given with confidence. Like each of us, every remedy has a distinctive and unique fingerprint or profile.

Another homeopathic slant to the history of arsenic poisoning is that if, in those perilous times, an individual anticipated meeting such a sticky end, very small doses of arsenic, taken judiciously over a prolonged time, could so condition the body that when the homicidal dose was administered, the victim would have the necessary resistance to survive the attempt.

In modern times, disregard for the healing law of similars leaves orthodox medicine therapeutically helpless in the face of widespread viral epidemics such as the December 2012 outbreaks of winter vomiting due to *norovirus* infection. This very unpleasant, generally self-limiting, viral gastroenteritis is characterised by marked nausea, projectile vomiting, watery diarrhoea and abdominal cramps with associated prostration, weakness, muscle pains, headaches and low-grade fever. This symptom picture is identical to that caused by crude arsenic poisoning, pointing to Ars-alb as the homeopathic remedy of choice for this incapacitating condition which is highly contagious, infects thousands and has lead to schools and hospital wards being closed. All modern medicine can offer for such cases is symptomatic palliation, and, in severe cases, rehydration. Ars-alb is a well-known remedy for gastroenteritis in homeopathic households, and a remedy never missing from any homeopathic self-aid medicine kit. Its companion remedy in such outbreaks of vomiting and diarrhoea is Veratrum album (prepared from white hellebore), a plant capable of causing a very similar poisoning picture attended by severe and profuse vomiting and diarrhoea with marked prostration to the point of collapse, extreme coldness and blueness of the lips. Verat-alb is, therefore, indicated for cases that are more intense and violent than Ars-alb. Fortunately, if there is any doubt about which to choose, they are complementary and may be used in alternation. When correctly chosen both these remedies act promptly, both prophylactically and clinically, and halt contagiousness. If only orthodox medicine had the insight it could through simple means allay much suffering and disruption to society.

Other simple examples of healing by similarity are the following:

- For many people a cup of coffee taken any time after midday will cause sleeplessness that night. The type of insomnia, however, bears the individualising stamp of the substance: sleeplessness on account of unusual over-activity of the mind; a mind teeming with thoughts and ideas; with nervous excitability, so that as long as there is the least noise or light they are unable to sleep. When a patient experiences this type of insomnia, whether they have taken coffee or not, homeopathic coffee, Coffea cruda, will often be the best remedy.
- Many analgesics (pain killers) contain codeine, a derivative of opium. One of the negative side effects of such a drug is constipation due to total inertia of the lower end of the large intestine and the rectum. The constipation is very obstinate with no urge whatsoever to pass a stool. This may go on for days, even weeks. When the stool is finally passed it is in the form of dry, hard, black balls and to the patient it feels as if they are bearing down against a tightly closed rectum or anus. Knowing the law of similars, it is no surprise to hear that when faced by such a bowel problem, regardless of the cause, the homeopathic doctor will prescribe homeopathic Opium with confidence of success.
- Ipecacuanha, a member of the family Rubiaceae, to which the coffee plant and the quinine tree (*Cinchona officinalis*) belong, is a native of Brazil. Its name, derived from the colloquial Brazilian appellation for the plant, literally means 'road-side sick-making plant', indicating its reputation amongst the indigenous people. Syrup of ipecacuanha won its laurels in orthodox medicine as a simple emetic often used to induce vomiting in cases of poisoning in children and sometimes adults. In large doses it causes severe nausea and vomiting. The nausea may be overwhelming with an intense desire to vomit, but at first an inability to do so. When, after great effort, they finally succeed, the sufferer finds that the nausea persists. These are the very symptoms that require homeopathic Ipecacuanha, particularly if, despite the patient's digestive distress, the tongue remains perfectly pink and clean. Ipecacuanha has helped many adolescent girls suffering from severe menstrual pains with intense nausea and such a tongue.

Before Hahnemann

Although Hahnemann was the first to present homeopathy as a formulated system, he was not born in a void. There were influences from the past, which sowed in him the seeds that were later to germinate, shoot and blossom under the light of his insight and relentless investigations. In the forward to his major work on the principles of homeopathy, The *Organon*, he is at pains to refute any accusation that he was claiming to be the sole originator of the similar principle, or doctrine, as he termed it. He first quotes from writings attributed to Hippocrates:

> Disease is born of like things and by the attack of like things people are healed – vomiting is cured by vomiting.[2]

and then adds in parenthesis:

> (I do not bring forward the following passages from authors who had a presentiment of homoeopathy as proofs in support of this doctrine, which is firmly established by its own intrinsic merits, but in order to avoid the imputation of having suppressed these foreshadowing's with the view of claiming for myself the priority of the idea.)[3]

Among other authors he quotes are the Austrian physician Dr Anton von Stoerck (1659–1734) and the Danish army physician Dr Geog Stahl (1731–1803). Stoerck made a particularly perceptive suggestion:

> If Stramonium (thornapple) disorders the mind and produces mania in healthy persons, ought we not to try if in cases of insanity it cannot restore reason by producing a revolution of the ideas?[4]

It does not take any great stretch of the intellect to reason that if a plant (or any other substance) possesses the capacity to induce a state of mental (or physical) disturbance in a healthy person, it could by this same capacity bring order to the mind (or body) of a mentally (or physically) disturbed person. The same reasoning would also expect, as an essential corollary to this phenomenon, a very close similarity between the mental disturbance of the patient and the way in which the successful plant disturbs the mind of a healthy person, just as sound waves of similar frequency dampen and erase one another on meeting. In such a case the diseased mind presents a template of unhealthy thinking and feeling, which, to be erased, must be matched or mirrored by the plant's action upon the healthy i.e. matched by similarity. If the symptoms of the patient and those induced by the plant are diametrically opposed, then suppression not erasure results, and, as in the analogy of waves, chaotic turbulence is created, which, in the case of the patient, will be expressed on a deeper level, with ultimately greater pathology.

Stahl perceived this, and Hahnemann comments:

> ...he expressed his conviction ... in the most unequivocal terms – The rule generally acted on in medicine, says he (Stahl), to treat by means of oppositely acting medicines (contraria contrariis), is quite false and the reverse of what it ought to be. I am, on the contrary, quite convinced that diseases will yield to, and be cured by, remedies that produce a similar affection (similia similibus) . . .[4]

The Doctrine of Signatures

Long before Hippocrates (460–350 B.C.), the idea of the importance of similarity between remedy and disease was inherent in the medical folklore of many cultures throughout the world. It was based on the belief that the creator of the universe, must have provided humanity with a means of recognising the therapeutic power latent within every mineral, plant or animal: an outer sign or 'signature' denoting its curative use. Honouring this conviction, the medicine man or shaman of old, sought for correspondences between a potential remedy's characteristics of outer form, colour, odour, taste, habitat, growth, behaviour or properties and the phenomena of disease or the appearance of diseased organs: a correspondence of similarity. Greater calendine (*Chelidonium majus*), a plant with yellow flowers, or golden seal (*Hydrastis canadensis*) that produces a yellow juice would be considered good for liver disease and jaundice. In more esoteric vein, the silver splendour of the moon shining on the sea at night, evoked a correspondence between that celestial body, a symbol of the feminine principle, and the metal silver, indicating through the moon's monthly governing of the tides that silver would beneficially regulate the menstrual cycle and promote fertility. In more recent times, the shape of the body of the cuttlefish with its tentacles has been likened to the shape of the uterus with its fallopian tubes and fibriae, which would indicate its value as a remedy for uterine conditions. The healing signature of a herb may be revealed by the site most favourable to the plant's growth: Arnica montana (leopard's bane or bruisewort), the quintessential remedy for injuries with bruising, as sustained in falling, grows best on mountain slopes and in Germany is known as fallkraut (fallherb). Taken to a more subtle level, such parallels were recognised between the archetypal nature of a remedy and the archetypal nature of the patient; a parallel that we will be examining fully later on. This way of looking at the creation, although alluded to in the writings of the Greek physician Galen (see below) was first formally introduced into medical thinking and popularised by Paracelsus and subsequently became know as 'The Doctrine of Signatures.' This doctrine of similarity was critical to the discovery of many herbal remedies used successfully for the treatment of various complaints, and which subsequently became established in herbal tradition, long before the advent of pharmacology. The intrinsic beauty of this concept and the evidence it gives of a caring, controlling and guiding hand completely escapes the pragmatic mind of conventional medicine. It has been scoffed at as fanciful and without evidence. Unfortunately, this scornful attitude has seemingly been supported by many extravagant correspondences that have been made, which stretch the doctrine to the point of the ridiculous.

Another ancient correlation, which assisted the medicine men of old in choosing which substances to test for their healing potential, was the observation that the most poisonous substances generally prove to be the best remedies: the greater the poison, the greater the remedy. It was only homeopathy that later revealed the immense healing power lying latent within seemingly inert substances.

The Greek Medical Schools

To understand the medical climate into which Hahnemann was born, and in which he received his formal education, it is necessary to briefly consider the nature of medical thinking as it evolved from the Greek Classical Period and to look particularly at the lives of two very influential figures: Galen and the Swiss alchemist, Paracelsus.

The extant works of Hippocrates, the philosopher Aristotle (384–322 B.C.), and Galen allude to the curative principle of similars. However, neither Hippocrates nor Galen developed a therapeutic system based upon this precept, nor did they subject it to systematic study. Hippocrates, who may be regarded as the father of Western medicine, also stated, "The symptoms of disease are the expression of Nature's healing powers", which is a concept essential to homeopathic philosophy and natural healing. The philosopher Empedocles (492–432 B.C.), who claimed that there are only four basic forms of perceptible matter: earth, water, fire and air, probably influenced Hippocrates's approach to disease. This idea was further developed by Pythagoras (580/572–500/490 B.C.) into the theory that all illness could be attributed to four bodily fluids or humours: phlegm, black bile, yellow bile and blood, which were seen to mirror the four basic elements. Health could only be maintained if these basic humours were in perfect balance and the presence of disease indicated that one or other was in excess or diminished. The Hippocratic School of medicine adopted this theory as its fundamental axiom. The efforts of its physicians were therefore directed to either increasing or decreasing the volume of these humours in the patient's body. Medicines, diet and often bloodletting were commonly employed.

Galen (c130–c200)

Galen, an immensely egotistical, irascible man, was born in Pergamum, the capital of Mysia in Asia Minor (now Turkey). He settled in Rome in A.D. 164, and became acquainted with many eminent state officials, amongst whom was the future emperor Lucius Septimus Severus. He was the physician to four successive emperors, including the benevolent Marcus Aurelius and his profligate, tyrannical son Commodus, and was appointed physician to the Roman gladiators, in which role he honed his surgical skills and expanded his vast knowledge of anatomy. This was supplemented by the indefatigable dissection of monkeys, apes and other animals.

He entertained grandiose ideas about his achievements in medicine and esteemed himself superior to Hippocrates. He inherited the Hippocratic humours from the Greek tradition and from them elaborated his theory of the four fundamental types of human temperament and constitution: the phlegmatic (phlegm), the melancholic (black-bile), the choleric (yellow-bile) and the sanguine (blood). The phlegmatic (earth-element) is introverted, repressed, even-tempered, externally unemotional, dour, placid and apathetic, lacking drive and enterprise; the melancholic (water-element) is

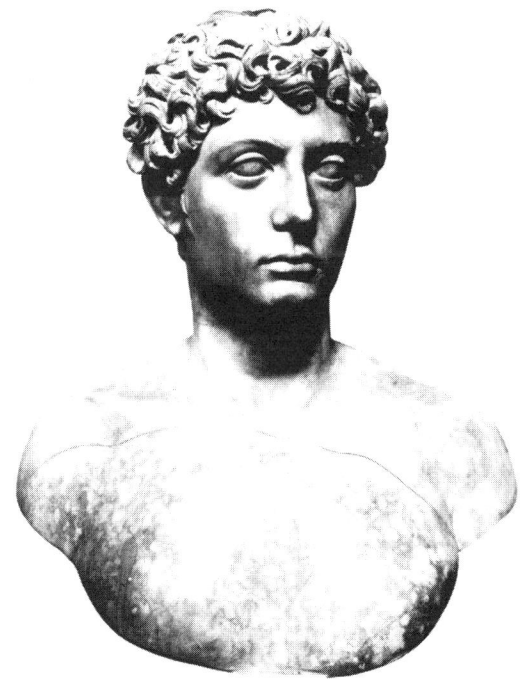

Figure 1.1 Galen (130–200 A.D.)
Credit: Science Photo Library

given to irrational fears, gloominess, brooding, sadness, pessimism, depression of the spirits and despair; the choleric personality (fire-element) is irritable, intolerant, impatient, given to volatile outbursts of anger and rage and is capable of physical violence; and the sanguine (air-element) is courageous, passionate, animated, optimistic, creative and extrovert. Galen believed that these character traits were inherent, each springing from an excess of its corresponding humour. His conclusions, and use of invasive methods to relieve this internal pressure, accounts for the popularity of bloodletting in Europe, one thousand five hundred years later.

Galen held the various medical sects of his time in deepest contempt and unsparingly employed his pen in scathing, derogatory attacks against the methodists, dogmatists, pneumatists and the empirics then flourishing in Rome. His manner was truculent, offensive and high-handed, calculated to provoke the hostility of his professional brethren. His influence in high places contributed to his unpopularity, but at the same time afforded him asylum. Medicine, down the ages, seems to recurrently produce this archetype: the unorthodox, outspoken, disputative pioneer who seeks to forcibly overthrow all that has gone before, while heaping derision upon his peers. Indeed, Galen was the forerunner of two similarly abrasive, iconoclastic figures, Paracelsus and Samuel Hahnemann. Despite the enmity of the medical fraternity, it was Galen's teachings that survived the barren Dark Ages following the fall of Rome, and, together with those of Hippocrates, became the orthodox creed of the Middle Ages, strictly laid down by the universities. He was so revered by his medieval posterity that it was deemed medical heresy to offer any degree of dissent. Even the renowned anatomist, Andreas Vesalius, could only express disagreement with Galen in a very diffident and apologetic manner.

Paracelsus

A figure that looms large in the history of medicine is a physician and alchemist with the wonderfully pompous name: Philippus Theophrastus Aureolus Bombastus von Hohenheim (1493–1541), who was born in Einsiedeln, Switzerland. Fortunately, he later assumed the humanist name Paracelsus, probably wishing to suggest his superiority or similarity to the original Celsus. He stands astride the transition between the medieval and the modern; a man, who intensely embodied the heritage of the past, the innovation of the present and the enlightenment of the future. A controversial, paradoxical, often outlandish luminary, who presided over the turbulent, birth struggles of the modern era, his own contradictory and chaotic life reflecting all the pains and passions of this emergence. His

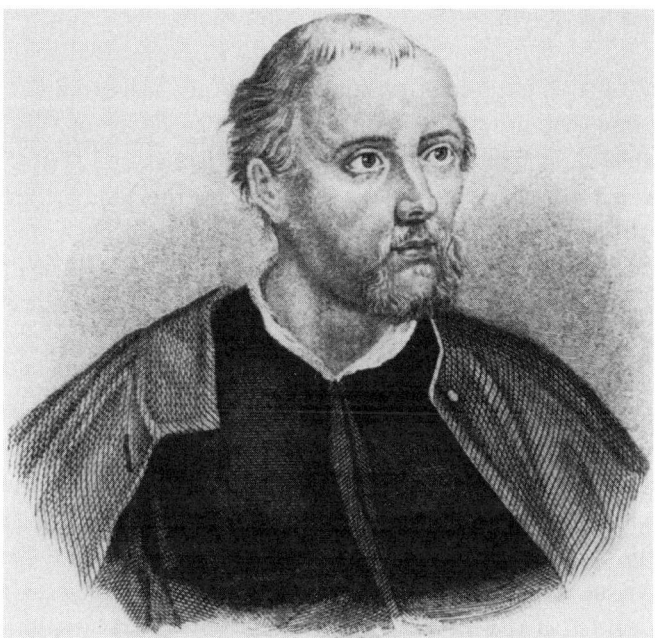

Figure 1.2 Paracelsus (1493–1541)
Credit: Science Photo Library

philosophy embraced both scientific rationalism and arcane mysticism, viewing them as not in contention but complementary. Despite his own life often being undisciplined, dissolute and vagabond, he proclaimed the absolute authority of method and experience and recognised the divine authority of a supreme being.

His father, Wilhelm von Hohenheim, was employed as a teacher in a mining school and the young Theophrastus soon acquired a passion for metallurgy, which later stood him in good stead as an alchemist. It is probable that this background also encouraged the investigations he was later to make into the pulmonary and toxic diseases suffered by miners. Endowed with a precocious and prodigal intellect and already well acquainted with alchemical knowledge, at fourteen years of age, he left home and embarked on the nomadic existence that characterised his future life. Apart from a rapid introduction to the ways of his world, his travels afforded him a wide-ranging education. Whether or not this included the successful completion of a formal, medical education remains uncertain. Those who eulogise him stoutly assert that he was fully qualified, those who vilify him are equally certain that he was an imposter. However, when he left the Italian city of Ferrara in 1515, after studying there for three years, he was certainly convinced in his own mind that he was now a doctor of medicine and he definitely held numerous medical posts throughout his life, including the hazardous position of military surgeon in Italy. This perennial traveller, now the familiar Renaissance figure of the itinerant magician-healer, or quack, sought after, investigated and tested through experience, all the traditional folk remedies in the many countries he visited. In this way, he gained a formidable and eclectic knowledge of natural remedies, most of which lay outside the territory of the orthodoxy. The basic metals always retained special therapeutic and magical significance for him.

The Luther of medicine
For Paracelsus, religion and science were inseparable. His setting was the Reformation and his kindred spirit, who was to the authority of the Church what Paracelsus was to the medical institutes, was Martin Luther. Their lives show many parallels: both came from a mining background; both were possessed of an ardent, irascible, aggressive, quarrelsome, coarse temperament; both tilted at the monumental ivory towers of the established hierarchy and did so through uncompromising, fiery invective; both were the self-appointed apostles and champions of a higher order, come to reform and redeem that which they perceived to be corrupt and false; both suffered from unmitigated hubris and spoke with divine authority, which brooked no criticism; both were intransigent in the face of powerful and dangerous opposition, which, in the case of Luther, would have gladly burnt him at the stake. But whereas Luther's religious doctrines were absolutist and bigoted, intolerant of query, preaching either salvation or damnation, and presenting man as an inherent sinner, fallen from grace, Paracelsus was always at heart an alchemist and a humanist, with a driving curiosity to unravel and understand the secrets of Nature, and an optimistic, positive view of the essence of man. As much as Luther was opposed to rationalism, Paracelsus was opposed to ritualism. If the two had ever met, given their similarity of temperament and the yawning gulf separating their vision of the spiritual nature of man, it is certain they would not have parted friends. Nonetheless, many regarded Paracelsus as the 'Luther of medicine'. Within a Christian framework, Paracelsus was a freethinker and followed no creed other than his own. Like the Neo-Platonists, he saw God in all things, the creation being a divine epiphany. From this perception, he evolved a form of pantheism, more pagan than Christian, in which the universal force of Nature individualises and manifests discretely in celestial objects, plants, minerals and medicines. He 'brought a kind of alchemical materialism to Christian philosophy.'[5]

The importance of the invisible

Paracelsus was particularly interested in diseases that afflict the mind, and in the early 1520s he wrote a book entitled: *The Diseases that Deprive Man of His Reason*. His approach to these diseases was revolutionary, for whereas his contemporaries considered insanity to be due to possession by evil spirits and the Galenists attributed it to humoural imbalance (excess of black bile, through which, it was rumoured, the devil might gain possession of the soul), Paracelsus asserted that they "develop out of man's disposition" and that "nature is the sole origin of diseases."[5] Likewise, he argued that epilepsy and mania were caused by disturbances of the '*vapours in the spiritus vitae*'.[5] Here, he anticipates Hahnemann's postulate that it is the disturbed spirit-like, vital force alone that brings about disease; only his terminology differs. When he maintains that spiritual diseases need a spiritual cure, he is advising that what is intangible and unseen in disease should be treated by that which is intangible and unseen in medicine. Over two hundred and fifty years later, Hahnemann would pronounce that disease being dynamic requires treatment in dynamic form.

Paracelsus writes with profound insight:

> The physician should speak of that which is invisible. What is visible should belong to his knowledge, and he should recognise the illnesses, just as everybody else, who is not a physician, can recognise them by their symptoms. But ... he becomes a physician only when he knows that which is unnamed, invisible, and immaterial, yet efficacious.[6]

His compassion and respect for the mentally handicapped and concern for their dignity is apparent:

> ... even if the animal body is a fool, yet the soul, his spirit, etc. is no fool ... that which is eternal within him is without folly and simplicity. ... Therefore also no one ought to be regarded as simpleton or fool, or be called so.[7]

A visionary

Like his character and habits, Paracelsus is always full of contradictions; at times a sage, possessing a wisdom and depth of insight that still eludes many philosophical and medical minds today; at times, seemingly, a superstitious fool steeped in medieval nonsense and entertaining notions that even by the standards of his day were bizarre. But care must be exercised when subjecting his observations to modern, critical scrutiny because much of what he wrote is in the form of allegory or analogy, open to more than one interpretation and often vested with hidden meaning, even prophetic. In his *Astronomia magna* (1537–8), for instance, he conjectures that one day 'pipes and crystal*s*' will carry the human voice over a distance of a hundred miles.⁸ At the time he wrote these words, they would have been considered mere fanciful musings, but today in the light of glass fibre optics they are not only visionary, but startlingly accurate. How better or more simply can this modern technology be described? Even his terminology is correct. The flexible, transparent fibre used in fibre-optic communication is familiarly called a 'light-pipe' and is made of glass (silica), which is crystal.

If we are prepared to pierce his abstruseness and selectively discard his absurdities, we discover subtle truths concealed in the flamboyance of his thoughts.

The four humours
As would happen to Hahnemann, through his vitriolic attacks upon the establishment, Paracelsus became a target for the acrimony of the medical profession and the apothecaries, a hated figure to be pulled down from his vainglorious pulpit, discredited and silenced, if not destroyed. But, even more so than Hahnemann, he was a rolling stone, always a jump or two ahead of their spite. He was utterly fearless in his diatribes, ever spotlighting the flaws in medical morality and methodology. He denounced the hallowed precepts of the Galenic school as archaic and injurious. Nonetheless, he accepted the concept of the four humours, but gave it his own slant by connecting it with the four primary flavours rather than with the four basic elements as Galen had. He also aligned the humours with Aristotle's four principles of cold, hot, moist and dry: the phlegmatic archetype was sweet, cold and moist; the melancholic was sour, cold and dry; the choleric was bitter, hot and dry; and the sanguine was salty, hot and moist. In this way he was in some measure able to disassociate himself from the teachings of Galen whom he thoroughly despised.⁹

Decrier of orthodoxy
During his brief and unauthorised period of lecturing to the medical faculty at the University of Basle in 1527, which attracted an unprecedented number of students, undoubtedly drawn by his notoriety, he allegedly added a crowning insult to the orthodoxy by publicly burning the collected writings of the revered Avicenna[i] much to the vociferous glee of his students, incited by his fiery and subversive invective. A more tempered approach would have served him better.

He railed against the acquisitive and competitive behaviour of his colleagues:

---
[i] Avicenna or Abu Ali Sina was a Persian physician and philosopher, the foremost medical thinker of his time (980–1037 A.D.) and highly respected in the time of Paracelsus.

> So great is the ill will among physicians that each denies honour and praise to the other; they would rather harm a patient and even kill him than grant a colleague his meed[i] of praise. From this, everyone can judge why a man has become a physician: not out of love for the patient, which should be the physician's first virtue, but for the sake of money. Where money is the goal, envy and hatred, pride and conceit are sure to appear – and may God protect and preserve us all from such temptations.[10]

Might one, with Paracelsian audacity, risk suggesting today that much of the current medical and pharmaceutical hostility to homeopathy stems from similar motivation?

Paracelsus shows that he is aware of a disease continuum passing from one generation to the next and that the new-born is already blighted with the full potential of all human disease. Despite this, the majority of children are born without manifest signs of disease, proving that there are healing mechanisms at work.

> Even when still in the womb, unborn, man is burdened with the potentialities of every disease, and is subject to them. And because all diseases are inherent in his nature, he could not be born alive and healthy if an inner physician were not hidden in him.[11]

He was convinced that for every illness there is a corresponding natural cure:

> For there is no sickness against which some remedy has not been created and established, to drive it out and cure it. There is always some remedy, a herb against one disease, a root against another, a water against one, a stone against another, a mineral against one, a poison against another.[12]

Days in the desert
However, he was also to discover how difficult it can be to find the correct remedy for each and every case, and that disease can develop to a point of irreversibility, rendering a case and its cure impossible. It is a very true adage in medicine and other professions, where personal expertise, credibility and reputation are interdependent, that the practitioner tends to remember his failures better than his successes. Indeed, to the over-sensitive, or over-proud, a single setback can prove unmanning. To a man who had stirred up so much antipathy in his brethren through his boastfulness and insults, this would be doubly so. This happened to Paracelsus and caused him to enter his 'days in the desert.'[13]

He was a man of passion, intensity, enthusiasm and conviction (sanguine and choleric); herein lay his strength and his vulnerability. How many of us in homeopathic practice, utterly convinced of the truth of our persuasion, have nonetheless at some time experienced a temporary lapse

---
[i] meed: a fitting recompense, a merited gift.

in faith, a niggling whisper of doubt, either in our method or our ability to apply it – a low moment, possibly precipitated by a number of difficult cases or someone dear that we have failed to help or possibly lost? In 1531, Paracelsus lost an important patient (even his name is chronicled: Christian Studer), and, whether this was the cause or not, he sank into depression and despair. Abandoning his work and his practice, he resumed his endless meanderings.

Paracelsus became a wretchedly depressed wanderer, travelling in rags through the hills and forests of Switzerland – a mad prophet who had seen too much of the world.[13] He cried out in anguish, "Where I had seen flowers in alchemy, there is but grass."

His voice was stilled. Gone were the diatribes, denunciations and disputes of the medical reformer and in his place emerged a pious penitent who saw virtue in poverty and abstinence. He writes in words later echoed by Hahnemann that he gave up medicine to ply other trades.[13]

His writings are now filled with religious admonishment expressed in a mild and gentle manner, without the hot fervour of the firebrand he had been. It was as if he had been transformed by some nervous breakdown from a state of creative ecstasy to one of religious melancholia. Given his emotional excesses, his unpredictable, swinging moods and his wild, irresponsible behaviour, this plunge into despair and religious contemplation might well indicate an underlying tendency to bi-polar disorder, responsible for the extreme contrasts in him, including his genius, his eccentricity and his fallibility. With Paracelsus' lofty views of the true scope of medicine it is impossible to reconcile his ignorance, his superstition and his erroneous observations.[14] Homeopathic analysis of his inconsistencies, his itinerant wanderings and his passionate, reformative spirit indicate that he was archetypally in the grip of a flagrant, tubercular miasmatic state. (This will be fully explained in the third volume of this series.)

Be that as it may, by 1535 his star was once again ascendant; he appears restored to his old disgruntled, irascible self, much to the discomfort of those around him, tackling both medicine and writing with renewed vigour. With his regained faith in medicine, he resumed his scathing attacks against his many opponents, inviting even more enmity.

Seek and treat the cause

He urged his colleagues to seek and address the cause of disease rather than the effects, to root out the origin of disease rather than just treat the symptoms. His sights were set on cure rather than palliation.

> The nature and force of a disease must be discovered by their cause and not by their symptoms ... for we must not merely extinguish the smoke of the fire but

the fire itself. If we want the earth to produce better grass, we must plough it, and not merely tear out the bad grass. Similarly the physician ... should direct his thought to the origin of the disease and not only to that which his eyes see. For in this he would see but the symptoms and not the origin; similarly smoke is only the symptom of the fire and not the fire itself.[15]

His medical insight penetrated to the very depths of human nature and he perceived a truth, which to this day remains unknown to most practitioners of medicine, no matter the discipline they represent and practise: ***the essential cause of disease stems from the soul***; in any healing encounter between physician and patient, therefore, ***it is the soul of the patient that requires healing.*** The healing of the body remains secondary. The highlighting and bracketed inserts in the following quote are mine.

> There are two realms in which diseases can penetrate and spread. The first is that of matter, that is to say, the body; it is here that all diseases lurk and dwell ... the other realm is not material, it is the spirit of the body (the soul and the vital force), which lives in it intangible and invisible, and **which can suffer from exactly the same diseases as the body.** But because the body has no share in this life (it cannot 'will'), **it is the spiritual active principle, from which the disease springs**.[16]

He emphasised that spiritual unfolding – i.e. soul healing – and physical healing must take place in parallel. *Spiritual counselling should always accompany the prescribing of medicines.* True, on-going healing of the body flows from healing of the soul, and healing of the soul requires alignment with the values of spirit (love and service to others).

> Medical science too (like religion) is full of mysteries and must be studied like the scriptures. These two callings – the promulgation of the word of God and the healing of the sick – must not be separated from each other. Since the body is the dwelling place of the soul, the two are connected and the one must open access to the other.[17]

Although it would be Samuel Hahnemann who would found a system of medicine capable of addressing disease at the causative or soul level through the use of highly 'dynamised', submolecular remedies; long before Hahnemann, Paracelsus perceived that to act curatively remedies had to be in an unquantifiable, imponderable form:

> Remedies should not be administered according to their weight, but according to other measurements. Who can weigh the brilliance of the sun, who can weigh air or the spiritum arcanum (soul)? No one.... The remedy should act in the body like fire.... How would it be possible to weigh the amount of fire needed to consume a pile of wood ...? No, fire cannot be weighed! However, you know that one little spark is heavy enough to set a forest on fire, a little spark that has no weight at all.[18]

This metaphorical injunction explains in easily understood terms, and with greater clarity than any scientific discourse, the inappropriateness of crude, molecular medicine to effect a cure. Since disease 'springs from the spiritual active principal' it is deviation from spiritual knowledge and values that lies at the heart of disease causation. How can chemical medicine curatively influence detrimental emotions like fear, depression, despair, anger, resentment, hate, pride, envy and jealousy? These are discordant energies that have 'no weight'; their remedy must be as 'weightless' as the trust, love and empathy that are their natural antidotes.

He stressed the need for individualisation in the assessment and treatment of all cases; that despite a common diagnosis each case is unique and needs to be treated as such.

He would have scoffed at randomised, control trials (RCT) performed on groups of patients with the same diagnosis and given the same remedy, because each patient is unique and dissimilar despite the common disease category into which they are placed and each requires a remedy chosen for this uniqueness and dissimilarity.

> If the physician is to understand the correct meaning of health, he must know that there are more than a hundred, indeed more than a thousand, kinds of stomach; consequently if you gather a thousand persons, each of them will have a different kind of digestion, each unlike the others. There are a hundred forms of health in the liver; each man has a different one.[19]

Only Nature can produce remedies that heal

He exhorts us to seek in nature for the remedies that can cure disease and not to imagine that we can compound these in the laboratory.

> Nature possesses the knowledge and makes the meaning of all things visible; it is nature that teaches the physician. Since nature alone possesses the knowledge, it must be nature that compounds the recipe. The art of healing comes from nature and not from the physician. Therefore the physician must start from nature with an open mind.[20]

Paracelsus insists that nature is the pharmacist, perfectly creating and structuring each of her remedies for it's healing purpose, nothing needing to be added or subtracted. In this, he anticipates the modern pharmaceutical focus and drive to find, isolate and concentrate the 'golden bullet' (active principle) contained in natural remedies rather than using the remedy in its entirety. For example, the cardioactive glycoside (digitoxin or digoxin) isolated from the foxglove (*Digitalis purpurea*), which although able to strengthen the contractions of the myocardium, increase cardiac output and suppress irregular heartbeats, thus bringing symptomatic relief, does not prolong the survival of heart failure patients and proves toxic especially to the gastro-intestinal tract, the liver and ultimately the heart itself.

> The art of prescribing medicines lies in nature, which compounds them herself. If she has put into gold what belongs to gold, she has done likewise with violets ... therefore understand me correctly: the virtue that is inherent in each thing is homogenous and simple, it is not split into two, three, four, or five, but it is an undivided whole.[21]

He also anticipates the homeopathic process of potentisation, by which the healing power of a remedy is released and made available for use in a dynamic, non-toxic form (to be discussed later). He uses the analogy of iron when considering the preparation of remedies. He tells us that God created iron, but not in the final form in which it can prove useful to humanity. "It must be cleansed of its dross before it can be forged."[23] Speaking allegorically, he says that the iron has to be subjected to the alchemy of fire, which is the task of the god Vulcan (Greek: *Hephaistos*).

> The same is true of the medicine. It too was created by God, but not in its finished state, but still concealed in dross. What the eyes perceive in herbs or stones or trees is not yet a remedy; the eyes see only the dross. But inside, under the dross, there the remedy lies hidden. First it must be cleansed from the dross, then it is there. This is alchemy, and this is the office of Vulcan; he is the apothecary and chemist of the medicine.[22]

Although his language is couched in the words of the alchemist, in the light of the science of homeopathy and its development under the tutelage of Hahnemann, his words are prophetic. As we shall see later, nature's remedies are not in their final form and must indeed, like iron, be subjected to the 'alchemy of fire' before they can be used curatively. This process was to be discovered by the human Vulcan: Samuel Hahnemann.

Throughout his writings, Paracelsus emphasises the need for harmony and similarity between the chosen remedy, the patient and the disease, rejecting the principle of prescribing remedies that act by contending with, and in opposition to, the disease process and its symptoms. He stated that "sames must be treated by sames" and believed that every diseased organ had its corresponding remedy in nature.[23] He was the first medical philosopher to recognise the healing power of illness and to perceive that this healing energy, even when at its most destructive, is directed towards the quickening of the spiritual aspect of the patient. Disease is often the price we must pay for the resolving of spiritual problems. Resolving these problems brings healing to the soul, and, if possible, also the body.

> There where diseases arise, there can one find the roots of health. For **health must grow from the same root as disease**, and whither health goes, thither also disease must go.[24]
>
> When a medicine is found in accordance with the star (the patient's destiny), **when hot is applied against hot, and cold against cold** (the simillimum), all this accords with the arcanum (the hidden secret of cure).[25]
>
> (The bracketed insertions are mine.)
>
> A man without a woman is not whole, only with a woman is he whole. Because woman was created from earth and he too is of earth, **both are of earth and form together a whole**.... In this sense the disease, desires its wife, that is the medicine. The medicine must be adjusted to the disease, **both must be united to form a harmonious whole**, just as in the case of man and woman. If the physician finds such a remedy, he is complete.[26]
>
> (The bold emphases in these aphorisms are mine.)

Synchronicity and healing

Long before the teachings of Carl Gustav Jung, Paracelsus introduces us to the concept of synchronicity: that all events are determined by universal law and are not random and haphazard; that what we experience as luck, chance or coincidence is not in fact fortuitous, but governed by subtle and persuasive, co-ordinating forces, which unfold destiny. The healing process, which in constitutional disease is never simply a physical change, is manifestly subject to synchronistic influence. Healing is the synchronising of that which is healing in the physician to that which is to be healed in the patient, and visa versa. There comes a time for birth, a time for sickness, a time for healing and a time for death, and all are predetermined and never accidental. In the act of healing, the readiness (knowledge and skill) of the physician and the readiness (spiritual receptivity and preparedness) of the patient are harmonised. Paracelsus considered healing, at its deepest level, to be the healing of the soul.

> If Providence has determined otherwise than you physicians intend, you will not be able to cure the patient by any remedy. But if the hour of Providence has struck, you will succeed in curing him.... Only when the hour of recovery strikes for the patient, does God send him to the physician, not before. All those who go to him before go to him in vain.... God has created remedies against diseases, and He has also created the physician; but He holds them back until the hour predestined for the patient. Only when the time has been fulfilled, and not before, does the course of nature and art set in.[27]

In the practice of curative medicine, these words resonate for the physician. Some patients, strive as we will, prove refractory to the best chosen therapy, even when their condition seems not insurmountable, whilst other patients, even though beset with dire disease, respond favourably when least expected. Knowledge of such laws maintains humility and sustains optimism.

So vocal, extrovert and controversial a figure as Paracelsus, was bound to attract the enmity of those he denounced and insulted, but also the allegiance of many who were persuaded by his convictions. He confirmed the truth of his teachings by the remarkable successes he achieved through his methods of treatment. But reports of these, embellished by many apocryphal tales of his curing the incurable, giving sight to the blind and even raising the dead, merely served to further antagonise and infuriate the orthodoxy. Such was their open hatred of him, that when, in 1541, at the age of 48, he died suddenly after a short illness, it was rumoured that his death had been precipitated by an abortive attempt on his life by assassins in the pay of his medical adversaries.

Although his teachings proved beyond the grasp of the majority of his contemporaries and provoked the derision and anger of his peers, study of his written work reveals a prodigious intellect, gifted with subtle insight into the mysteries of life, expressing a deep love and compassion for ailing humanity and an abiding reverence for God.

In the following words he emphasises and summarises the focus of his life work.

> Many have said of alchemy, that it is for the making of gold and silver. For me such is not the aim, but to consider only what virtue and power may lie in medicines.[28]

Due to his restless, emotional, disorderly and often contradictory, chaotic and irrational mind, he failed to leave for posterity a structured, organised system of therapy based on a consistent and logical philosophy, but he bestowed precious gems of insight and wisdom and brutally exposed the errors of contemporary medical thinking. Although unacknowledged, he was undoubtedly the inspirational springboard for another medical rebel and iconoclastic trailblazer, Samuel Hahnemann, who, to this day, remains a thorn in the flesh of traditional medicine.

References

1 Haehl R. *Samuel Hahnemann, His Life and Work*. Vol 1. London: Homoeopathic Publishing Company; 1922. p65.
2 O'Reilly WB. *Organon of the Medical Art by Dr Samuel Hahnemann*. Washington DC: Birdcage Books; 1997. p57.
3 Hahnemann S. *Organon of Medicine*. 6th edn. Philadelphia PA: Boericke & Tafel; 1922. p90.
4 *Ibid.*, p91.

5 Ball P. *The Devil's Doctor – Paracelsus and the World of the Renaissance Magic and Science*. London: William Heinmann; 2006. p324.
6 Jacobi J. *Paracelsus – Selected Writings*. London: Routledge & Kegan Paul Ltd; 1951. p138.
7 Ball P. *The Devil's Doctor – Paracelsus and the World of the Renaissance Magic and Science*. London: William Heinmann; 2006. p329.
8 *Ibid.*, p343.
9 *Ibid.*, p252–253.
10 Jacobi J. *Paracelsus – Selected Writings*. London: Routledge & Kegan Paul Ltd; 1951. p143.
11 *Ibid.*, p150.
12 *Ibid.*, p151.
13 Ball P. *The Devil's Doctor – Paracelsus and the World of the Renaissance Magic and Science*. London: William Heinmann; 2006. pp308–309.
14 Encyclopaedia Britannica. *Paracelsus*. Aylesbury and Slough: Hazell Watson and Viney Ltd; 1961.
15 Jacobi J. *Paracelsus – Selected Writings*. London: Routledge & Kegan Paul Ltd; 1951. p151.
16 *Ibid.*, p149.
17 *Ibid.*, p142.
18 *Ibid.*, p163.
19 *Ibid.*, p161.
20 *Ibid.*, p124.
21 *Ibid.*, p164.
22 *Ibid.*, p167.
23 Cook TM. *Homeopathic Medicine Today*. New Canaan CT: Keats Publishing Inc; 1989. p1.
24 Jacobi J. *Paracelsus – Selected Writings*. London: Routledge & Kegan Paul Ltd; 1951. p152.
25 *Ibid.*, p170.
26 *Ibid.*, p148.
27 *Ibid.*, pp155–156.
28 Holmyard EJ. *Alchemy*. London: Penguin Books; 1957.

2

SIMILIA SIMILIBUS CURENTUR

Samuel Hahnemann

Childhood

On the 10th of April 1755, Christian Friedrich Samuel Hahnemann, the second son of his parents, was born in the small town of Meissen in Saxony. This vulnerable infant, whose very survival was at first in doubt, was destined to be the prism through which ancient, medical wisdom would be focused to formulate a curative system of medicine. His grandfather, father and an uncle (see Figure 2.1) were all painters in the famed porcelain factory in Meissen, which is situated close to Dresden. He was not a physically robust child, being thin and rather delicate, with fair hair and intelligent, penetrating eyes. Of a studious disposition, he was raised in a home in which the Lutheran Protestant values of temperance, industry, thrift and piety were encouraged and observed. The strict, austere discipline of his upbringing, ministered by a stern but kindly father, accorded well with his own disciplined, committed nature and its religious overtones did not stultify his development as a far-ranging freethinker. The beauty of the neighbouring hills and the countryside surrounding the River Elbe enchanted him from an early age, and remained a source of joy throughout his life. It instilled within him a deep and lasting veneration for the works of nature.

The family were of limited means and much of his early education was conducted at home. When he was six years old, his older brother died, leaving Samuel, now the eldest son, with the responsibility, when circumstances demanded, of contributing to the family finances through work that took him away from his studies. This intermittent pattern of learning continued even after he attended elementary school. Despite his frequent and sometimes extended absenteeism, he made rapid progress and his exceptional, intellectual powers were soon recognised by his teachers. Faced with such academic ability and promise, they decided not to charge for his tuition.

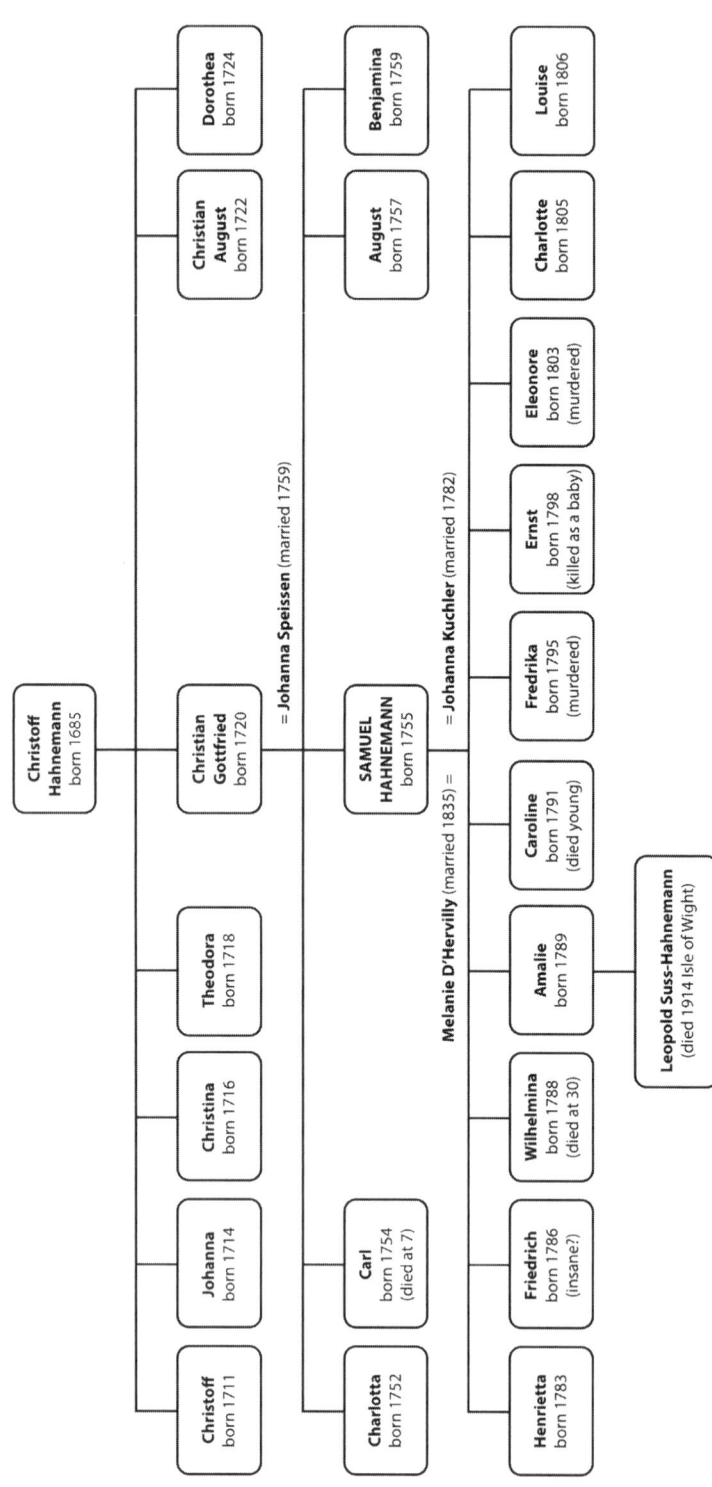

Figure 2.1 Family tree of Samuel Hahnemann

Education

From the outset he showed a remarkable aptitude for languages, eventually mastering eight: German, English, French, Spanish, Italian, Latin, Greek and Arabic. This astonishing gift of tongues gives us an insight into the fundamental workings of this brilliant mind: a mind that demanded order, structure, system, laws, principles and predictability, qualities characteristic of all languages – a platform for the pedantic, fussily meticulous and methodical nature that would emerge. It would also give him a portal into ancient and contemporary texts through which he could, at first hand, investigate and evaluate the beliefs, traditions and medical systems of other cultures.

Due to lack of finances, Hahnemann's father despaired of being able to provide his gifted son with a higher education and therefore found him work in a grocery store with a view to him becoming a merchant. The intellectual and studious youth found this work unendurable and soon returned home throwing himself upon the mercy and understanding of his mother. With her intercession and the pressing advice of Hahnemann's prime tutor, Johann Müller, Samuel's father finally gave permission for him to continue his studies. In 1771, therefore, Samuel became a pupil at The Prince's School in Meissen, where Müller had recently been appointed Rector. He was admitted without charge and supported himself by assisting Müller with his academic responsibilities and by coaching and teaching fellow students, especially in foreign languages. Such was his brilliance and his diligence, that he was granted special liberties and independence in his studies. His close relationship with Müller grew into a lasting friendship. However, his constitution remained delicate and vulnerable and as a result of 'overstudying' and too little physical exercise, he was often ill.[1]

In 1775, during his final term, he wrote a dissertation in Latin entitled *The Wonderful Construction of the Human Hand*, which he delivered to the assembled dignitaries, teachers, past pupils and parents at the School Speech Day. His choice of subject was sure indication of the direction his future education would take.

University

At twenty years of age, in the Spring of 1775, he enrolled as a student of medicine at the University of Leipzig. All he had in his pocket were twenty *thaler*,[i] the last money he ever received from his father. It seems that from

---

[i] The *thaler* was a silver coin used throughout Continental Europe for almost 400 years and minted in Saxony until 1872. It comprised 30 *groschen*.

this time, he severed all close ties with his family and rarely visited Meissen again. He now had to be self-supporting and managed to maintain himself, however meagrely, by teaching German and French to more well-to-do fellow students. His situation was further relieved by his obtaining free passes to lectures, a privilege obtained through the influence of an eminent physician, Bergrath Pörner; evidence of the high esteem in which Hahnemann was held by those who knew him. Once again he was committed to unremitting work, with very little time for the usual student frivolities and follies. However, he did not repeat the unbalanced approach of his younger years – he now attended to his physical wellbeing. He said:

> I did not forget, as of old, to procure for my body, through exercise and fresh air, that vitality and strength by which alone continual brain-work can be endured with success.[2]

This was a rule he applied throughout his long life and it became an important part of the advice he would give his future patients. It was during the two years he was resident in Leipzig that he commenced translating works from English into German. The titles he chose were all connected with medicine and therefore provided him not only with money but also an extended education.

Although the Leipzig Medical Faculty was the most renowned in Germany, Hahnemann soon became disenchanted with the standard of education provided. He was particularly disappointed by the lack of practical instruction for there was no clinic or hospital to provide clinical experience. The Faculty emphasis was on theory, both recondite, and, to his mind, fanciful. He attended only those lectures he considered to be useful.[3] He eased his frustration somewhat by taking up the study of chemistry, a subject that became a passion and always remained dear to his heart. This knowledge would later be employed in the development of certain key homeopathic remedies. Finally, however, realising that he was in a medical *cul-de-sac*, he left Leipzig for Vienna and entered the Catholic hospital of The Brothers of Mercy, to work under the senior physician, Dr Quarin, who was also a physician to the Empress Maria Theresa, the ruler of the Hapsburg Empire. He profited immensely from this period under Dr Quarin's tuition, but was so consumed by his clinical activities and continued studying that he had no time to earn from teaching, and after nine months his money began to run out.

Dr Quarin managed to secure him a post as family physician and librarian to the affluent Baron Samuel von Brukenthal, the Governor of Transylvania (now part of Hungary), in Hermannstadt. It was here, in 1777, that Hahnemann became a Freemason. Destiny yet again provided critical

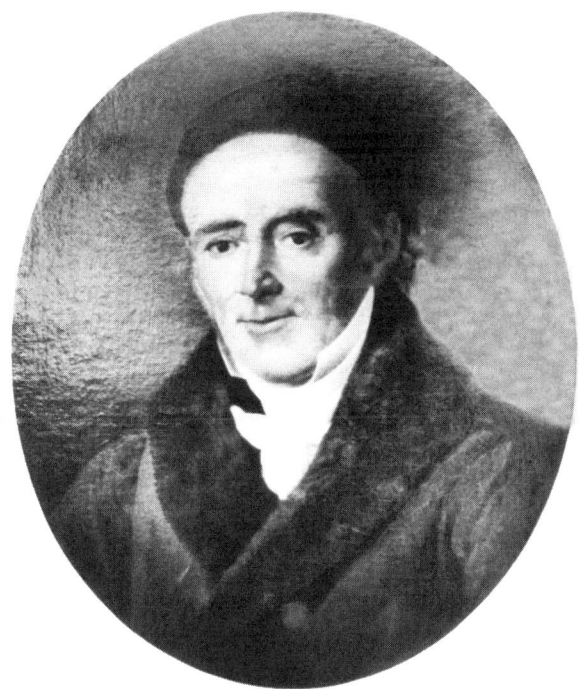

Figure 2.2 Samuel Hahnemann as a young man
Credit: Science Photo Library

elements for the work to come. Apart from the experience derived from his medical work in the town, the Baron's vast library provided him with opportunity to exercise and extend his linguistic ability and to further his knowledge of botany and chemistry. He also classified and catalogued all the library books and manuscripts as well as Brukenthal's valuable coin collection; tasks ideally suited for exercising his orderly mind. He would have tarried in these ideal conditions, but his formal education required completion and having earned enough to support himself for a while, after a year and nine months, he left Hermannstadt for the University of Erlangen, a less conservative and more free-thinking university than others in Germany, and on 10 August 1779, Samuel Hahnemann qualified as a doctor of medicine.

Marriage and early practice

He commenced practice in the small, mining town of Hettstadt and it was here that he first experienced the frustration and despair of being unable to provide the necessary care and relief that his patients needed. These were often copper-miners who slaved along the banks of the River Wipper in all weathers, and lived in impoverished and insanitary conditions, which left them prey to pulmonary disease (shades of Paracelsus). He soon came to the conclusion that many would probably have done better without him.

Opportunities for growth were limited in Hettstadt and he soon moved on to Dessau, some 50 kilometres away. Here, through his medical practice and his passion for chemistry, he soon made the acquaintance of the local pharmacist, Apothecary Häseler, and in consequence also Häseler's pretty, seventeen-year-old step-daughter, Johanna (Henriette) Küchler, with whom he fell in love and became engaged. With the prospect of marriage before him, it became essential for Hahnemann to find a secure and profitable position, hence his decision, in late 1781, to take the post of Medical Officer in the small town of Gommern, not too far distant from his betrothed. On the 17th November 1782, he and Henriette were married and, in 1783, their first child was born, a daughter named after her mother. The man Henriette married is well described by Trevor Cook in his biography of Hahnemann:

> Samuel Hahnemann was a short but erect, young man of slight build with aquiline features, a narrow, curved nose and thinning fair hair. He possessed a brilliant mind ... he was serious-minded and sensitive, pragmatic, fiercely independent ... with an affinity for nature and his homeland.[4]

Gommern – dissatisfaction with conventional medicine

Despite its promise, the rural practice at Gommern proved slow and limited, leaving Hahnemann with much leisure time. It was during this period that in addition to his continued application to chemistry, he began to translate scientific works professionally, in order to supplement his inadequate income. He also wrote his first medical essay, entitled *Directions for Curing Old Sores and Ulcers*. From this first platform, he gave vent to his dissatisfaction with current, medical practice and in scathing terms, heralding the onslaughts that were to come. He concluded that veterinary surgeons are usually more successful (in the treatment of chronic ulcers) than the most learned professors and members of the academies.

He urged for a return to nature and the use of remedies well known to 'the ordinary man.'[5] His rebellious and reforming spirit were already manifesting, as also his deep concern for public-health and the environmental conditions that contributed to ill-health, which were largely disregarded by medical authorities and practitioners: crowding, poor sanitation, the need for hygiene, fresh air, adequate sleep, exercise and correct diet. These were concepts that he would continue to pioneer throughout his life, and personal application must certainly have contributed to his own good health, sustained vigour and long life.

Dresden – translations

By 1785, the family was established in Dresden, the capital of Saxony, where they would live until September 1789. He had moved there without the promise of a post, but was soon befriended by Dr Samuel Wagner the Medical Officer of Health for Dresden, and when the latter took ill, he recommended Hahnemann as his temporary replacement. The position afforded him invaluable experience as well as exposure to the forensic aspect of medicine. When Dr Wagner died, Hahnemann applied for the permanent post, but was turned down in favour of a better-known, local physician. Hahnemann's literary work now became even more essential for the family's survival, especially with the arrival of his son, Frederich, in November 1786. This he tackled with characteristic zeal and enthusiasm, becoming the leading translator of scientific works into German. During the years 1785–1789, he published more than 2,200 printed pages, including translations, original works, and articles on medicine and chemistry: a considerable body of work. He wrote two books, one a treatise on arsenic poisoning and the other on the diagnosis and treatment of venereal disease. These were well received by the profession, despite the fact that in the former work he was uncompromising in his attack upon contemporary medicine. He expressed his conviction that practical medicine had been degraded, "... to a wretched breadwinning, a glossing over of symptoms, a degrading commerce in prescriptions ...[6]

In the latter book, *Instructions for Surgeons on Venereal Diseases* (1789). he reveals his unwillingness to accept without question the consensus opinion of the orthodoxy and his need to understand and explain the action of medicines in disease. It was believed that the success of mercury in the treatment of syphilis depended on its ability to initiate salivation, perspiration, diarrhoea and increased urination; in other words, through balancing the Galenic humours. He disputed this and pondered that the artificial disease, or 'mercurial fever,' that was induced, constituted the healing process. This work, therefore, contains Hahnemann's first suggestion that an inherent disease may be displaced by a similar, artificially induced one.

Leipzig – disillusionment and poverty

With no hope of attaining the post he had applied for, Hahnemann decided to move to Leipzig in September 1789. In order, however, to live more cheaply and at the same time to provide a better home in better air for his delicate children, Hahnemann moved after a year to the suburb of Stotteritz, four or five km. south-east of Leipzig.[7] Here, his life continued much as it had at Dresden, always struggling against poverty, and therefore immersed in translations: some 4,700 pages between 1789 and 1792 (during which time, the 'Reign of Terror' gripped France). The work he produced was peppered with corrections, additions, penetrating comments and annotations. His medical work was almost completely sidelined. He had, in any case, become thoroughly appalled by the barbaric methods of treatment practised by his colleagues. It was not only the extremely crude methods that were currently in vogue that outraged him – bloodletting, the application of blood-sucking leeches, blistering, and the prescribing of drastic laxatives and emetics to induce purging and vomiting – but also the administering of largely unknown, often extremely toxic, substances, in large doses and arbitrary mixtures, for diseases of which even less was known.

In a letter published in *Lesser Writings*, he wrote the following to Christian Hufeland:[ii]

> I could not conscientiously treat the unknown morbid conditions of my suffering brethren by these unknown medicines, which being active substances may (unless applied with the most vigorous exactness, which the physician cannot exercise because their peculiar effects have not yet been examined) so easily occasion death, or produce new affections and chronic maladies, often more difficult to remove than the original disease.[8]

This last-mentioned concern regarding the intensification of disease and its resistance to cure through chemical medication, holds true to this day due to the powerful capacity of modern drugs to suppress disease manifestations, driving the disease process more deeply into the system, rendering the patient more difficult to cure (and this regardless of knowledge of 'correct-dosage', side-effects and complications).

Hahnemann continued:

> To become thus the murderer or the tormentor of my brethren was to me an idea so frightful and overwhelming, that soon after my marriage, I renounced the practice of medicine, that I might no longer incur the risk of doing injury, and I engaged exclusively in chemistry and in literary occupations.[8]

[ii] Chistoph Wilhelm Friedrich von Hufeland (1762–1836) was an enlightened, unprejudiced and sympathetic orthodox medical contemporary and friend, who was also Editor of the respected *Medical Journal*, and prepared to publish Hahnemann's articles on his new approach to healing.

Bradford observed that Hahnemann had thus reduced himself and his family to want for conscience sake.⁹

In the same letter, he also expressed the unshakable belief that within God's plan for suffering humanity, he must have decreed some simple, gentle and certain method of healing the sick. But what was this law? If it existed, it must be based on principles quite different, or even completely opposite, to those he so abhorred in the orthodoxy: aggressive, toxic, multiple remedies, speculative and routine, with no consideration for the uniqueness of the patient. It is an old adage that tells us to 'knock and it shall be opened – ask and it shall be given!' Hahnemann was constantly knocking and asking, searching and probing with a prodigious, determined, investigative intellect, fired by curiosity and the quest for answers, honed by practice, informed by constant wide-ranging reading, weighing the wisdom of the past, scrutinising the methods of the present, refining his own concepts and hearkening to his inner promptings; activities that remained intrinsic to his nature throughout his life.

Providence – the Cinchona experiment

In 1790, the door opened for Hahnemann and the light it admitted germinated the seed of a concept, which although already long imbedded, had lain dormant, waiting for its moment. That moment came while he was translating into German a book entitled *A Treatise on Materia Medica* written by the much-respected Scottish physician, William Cullen,[iii] the second edition of which had been published in two volumes in 1789. Cullen was considered an authority on the pharmacology of medicinal substances. In his annotations to the translation, Hahnemann expressed his scepticism of the author's conclusions regarding the mode of action of cinchona, or Peruvian bark, in the cure of intermittent fever (malaria, or ague as it was then known). The eminent physician was of the opinion that the therapeutic success of the remedy rested upon its bitterness and tonic effect on the stomach. Hahnemann doubted this, regarding Cullen's conclusion as purely speculative and not based on good scientific evidence. His intense love of the laws and methods of chemistry had engendered in him a need to test theories in the laboratory of experience and not to rely on notion or conjecture. At the time, he had already achieved a reputation as 'this

---

[iii] William Cullen (1710–1790) was born in Hamilton, near Glasgow. In 1751 he was appointed Professor of the Practice of Medicine at the University of Glasgow and in 1755 moved to Edinburgh to become Professor of Chemistry and Medicine. Cullen served as President of both the Royal College of Physicians and Surgeons of Glasgow (1746–7), and the Royal College of Physicians of Edinburgh (1773–1775).

famous analytical chemist,' therefore, it is not surprising that he resolved to determine the drug's action by testing it on himself. He continued the dosage until he developed symptoms:

> I took for several days, by way of experiment, twice a day, four drachms of good cinchona. My feet and finger tips, etc. first became cold; I became languid and drowsy; then my heart began to palpitate; my pulse became hard and quick; an intolerable anxiety and trembling; prostration in all the limbs; then pulsation in the head, redness of the cheeks, thirst; briefly, all the symptoms usually associated with intermittent fever, appeared in succession, yet without the actual rigor ... but above all the numb disagreeable sensation which seems to have its seat in the periosteum over all the bones of the body – all made their appearance. This paroxysm lasted from two to three hours every time, and recurred when I repeated the dose and not otherwise. I discontinued the medicine and I was once again in good health.[10]

In a subsequent annotation he momentously writes:

> Peruvian bark (cinchona or China officinalis) which is used as a remedy for intermittent fever, acts because it can produce symptoms similar to those of intermittent fever in healthy people.[1]

These few words encapsulate a universal truth: that the power to heal and the power to perturb are directly related; that the effect a substance has on the healthy constitution demonstrates its curative power over similar disease symptoms in the sick; that cinchona can cure malaria because it can cause the symptoms of malaria when given to a healthy person. To Hahnemann's mind, steeped in the wisdom and traditions of the past, this was a revelation confirming what other medical thinkers, particularly Paracelsus, had deduced. One can only imagine the ferment that this triggered within him, estranged from his beloved profession, frustrated by his impotence in the face of disease and anchored to his interminable translations. That he immediately began to make connections is evidenced by yet another observation annotated in the same text:

> ... that in order to cure certain forms of intermittent fever, a kind of artificial fever must be produced with ipecacuanha.[10]

After his experience with cinchona (scientific name *China officinalis*), he repeated the test, firstly on members of his family and later on friends. The results confirmed his own observations of the drug effect, the response only varying in degree, revealing individual sensitivity or resistance to the substance.

Opposition to blood-letting

This crucial, life-changing experiment, in 1790, opened new vistas for him and initiated a process of investigation and deduction, always supported by practical verification, which would develop and mature during the following years and determine the focus of all his future endeavours. However, in the meantime, it did not distract him from launching into further attacks upon the pernicious practice of venesection (blood-letting) and purging that dominated medical practice. This culminated in an article written by him in a newspaper, *Der Anzeiger*, provoked by the sudden death of Emperor Leopold II of Austria, the brother of Marie Antoinette. The Emperor had developed a severe fever associated with a distended abdomen and his physician Dr Legasius had seen fit to bleed him four times before he succumbed to his illness *and his medical care*. Hahnemann wrote:

> To abstract the fluid of life four times in twenty-four hours from a man who has lost flesh from mental over-work combined with continued diarrhoea without procuring relief for him. Science pales before this![11]

His was truly a voice in the wilderness. Though his contributions to chemistry were acknowledged by academics, his repeated outpouring of critical indignation against the medical fraternity only served to build up increasing intolerance and enmity towards himself and his views.

Managing the insane

In 1792, he became the manager of an 'asylum for the insane' in Georgenthal, in the Principality of Gotha. It had only one patient, a certain notable and notorious, Herr Klockenbring, who had been the Minister of Police of Hanover and reputedly a man of eccentric and dissolute tastes. He was now reduced to a state of violent mania, possibly due to tertiary syphilis, but certainly triggered by the publication of a scurrilous article, which mercilessly exposed his blighted morality. The asylum was housed in a hunting lodge kindly provided by Duke Ernst of Saxe-Coburg-Gotha, its initial purpose probably being to provide a place of therapy for the ex-minister, who was an old friend of the Duke. This chapter in Hahnemann's life is worth recounting for, although he had but one patient, he was given the opportunity to apply methods of treatment for the insane, which had occupied his mind for some time and provides further evidence of his reforming, innovative spirit. The treatment of the insane at the time was barbaric in the extreme. Inmates were treated like animals, chained, flogged and often paraded and tormented for the amusement of spectators. Hahnemann advocated tolerance, respect, kindness, care and patience, all of which he extended to his demented charge. We have no record of the remedies he used, other than a mention of tartar emetic, but by February 1793, Herr Klockenbring was able to return to a lesser administrative post from a condition of deluded insanity.

Nomadic life

The ten years that followed were, as in the life of Paracelsus before him, a time of constant wanderings without settled abode. However, whereas Paracelsus was by nature a solitary, rolling stone, a restless, roving spirit, Hahnemann, a family man, had his nomadic existence thrust upon him, often because of financial constraints, the need to find cheaper circumstances and more remunerative posts, and the enmity of local practitioners and apothecaries, the former, jealous of his success and resentful of his criticism, and the latter, incensed because he dispensed his own remedies, despite the fact that they derided these. There may also have been a more inherent cause for his restlessness, since these wandering years coincided with a period of inner foment during which his new insights were shifting, unfolding and taking shape; possibly his outer roaming denoted his inner searching. The hardships and dangers he and his ever-increasing family must have endured travelling in Europe at that time are unimaginable. The backdrop was revolution in France and then war between the young republic and the old German states. Whatever admiration we may feel for Hahnemann's tenacity must pale by comparison with that which we entertain for his wife Henriette, almost constantly pregnant; in 1794, with five young children, four daughters and a son, and in addition, a baby boy Ernst at her breast; contending with want, war-time famine, homelessness, bone-shaking travel and all the while having to support and tend to the needs of an eccentric, irascible genius. She deserves our gratitude and our deepest sympathy, because the worst tragedy that a mother can endure loomed on the horizon.

Tragedy

In the spring of 1794, their coach, with the entire family packed inside, being driven at reckless speed on the road to Pyrmont, a favourite health resort and spar of the aristocracy, overturned on a sharp bend, causing the family severe shock and trauma. The worst injured was baby Ernst, who, although in his mother's arms, suffered head injuries and died a few days later, not yet three months old. Hahnemann writes of the event in a letter:

> The upsetting of the carriage at Mulhausen in which we nearly lost our lives (to heal our wounds we had to remain there eight days) has shattered my wife's health so much and the children have become so afraid of driving, it is impossible for me to come any further. The driver who overturned us is one of the most careless and dangerous men I have ever known. I hope no one else will suffer through him.[12]

Early writings

Although it was impossible to establish a medical practice with such an itinerant life-style, Hahnemann continued writing and during this time produced his *Pharmaceutical Lexicon*, a four-volume work on good pharmacy practice, in which he set out rules for the preparation of medicines. Many of the basic precepts he propounds are to this day part of the quality control procedures required of licensed manufacturers of homeopathic medicines. The reviews that followed its publication were universally complimentary, for example from the *Journal of Pharmacy*:[13]

> An excellent work which every apothecary ought to procure. Brevity, lucidity, decision and yet a completeness seem to distinguish this work.... This work will be of great service to the pharmacy.

Other interesting, popular works, which throw much light on Hahnemann's thinking and progressive views are *Handbook for Mothers'* and the two pamphlets published as *Friend of Health* (1792 and 1795). In the former, he proves an ardent advocate of breastfeeding for infants and of correct diet and fresh air for children and gives extensive advise on behavioural training, discipline and schooling. Extending his counsel to women, he strongly criticises the tight lacing and corsetry of the then current high fashion, with a stern warning about the consequent dangers of varicose veins, constipation and respiratory problems. In the latter, he deals with all the important issues of public and personal hygiene and shows himself to be generations ahead of his contemporaries. As always, he stresses the need for balanced diet and regular exercise. His words on exercise are worth repeating, because they so clearly and quaintly describe the benefits to be attained.

> Next to food, exercise is the most essential requirement of the animal mechanism – it is this which winds up the machinery.... Exercise and good air alone set all the humours in our body in motion to fill their appointed places, and compel every secreting organ to give off its specific secretions, give power to the muscles and to the blood its deepest red colour; they refine the fluids so that they penetrate easily into the most minute capillary vessels, strengthen the heart beats and bring about healthy digestion. They alone invite us to rest and sleep, which is a time of refreshment for the production of new spirit and energy.[14]

Who could refrain from exercising after reading this?

The frontispiece of the *Friend of Health* is an etching of a rabid dog, titled *Hydrophobia* (a feature we will have reason to return to in Volume 2). The amount of literary work Hahnemann published during these most unsettled years is remarkable – original works, essays in medical journals and translations (some 5,500 pages) – especially when we consider the difficulties, obstacles and worries that beset him and his family. All the while, during the years extending from the Cinchona experiment in 1790, his mind was constantly working on the formulation of a coherent system of medicine.

It was fully six years later, in 1796, that he published his historic *Essay on a New Principle for ascertaining the Curative Power of Drugs, and Some Examinations of the Previous Principles* in *Hufeland's Medical Journal.* In this essay, he considered the three methods by which diseases may be treated. Firstly by preventative medicine – the removal or destruction of the causes of disease, which he considered *'sublime'*. Secondly, and most commonly, by *contraria contrariis*, i.e. treatment based on opposing the symptoms of disease by remedies which act in a contrary manner e.g. laxatives for constipation, alkaline products for conditions of acidity, opium for chronic pain etc, which remains the dominant method of the orthodox school to this very day. Hahnemann wrote uncompromisingly:

> I ask my colleagues to desert this way; it is the wrong one, a false pathway ... which will lead to the abyss. The proud empiric takes it for the metalled roadway and puffs himself up with the miserable satisfaction of affording relief for some hours, without any care as to whether the evil will take deeper root under this cover. And although the greater part of our medical contemporaries still adhere to this method, I do not fear to call it injurious and destructive.[15]

The third method he described, used "only occasionally by the more conscientious physicians of deeper insight," sought to overcome the disease by 'specific' means.[16] He pointed out that this method was, however, at the mercy of chance unless based on clear principles. He stressed the need to investigate experimentally the action of remedies on the healthy, human body, because only by this means

> ... can the true nature, the real effect of the medicinal substance be discovered; from them alone can be ascertained to what maladies they are safely and successfully adaptable.[16]

He then propounded a new doctrine of healing in very clear terms:

> Every effective remedy incites in the human body a kind of illness peculiar to itself. The more peculiar, the more marked ... the more effective. One should imitate nature, which, at times, heals chronic disease by another additional one. One should apply in the disease to be healed, particularly if chronic, that remedy which is able to stimulate another artificial disease, as similar as possible; and the former will be healed – *similia similibus* – likes with likes.[16]

Considering this formal, public pronouncement of the fundamental principle of homeopathy by Hahnemann in a respected, medical journal, Dr Richard Haehl, his biographer, is probably justified when he stoutly asserts that 1796 was the year of birth of Homeopathy.[16]

Later, in the *Organon*, Hahnemann enunciated the homeopathic principle of cure more concisely:

> To obtain a quick, easy and lasting cure, choose for every attack of illness a medicine which can produce a similar malady to the one it is to cure (*similia similibus curentur*).[17]

Smallpox immunisation

It is remarkable that in the same year, 1796, Dr Edward Jenner, an English general practitioner and surgeon in Gloucestershire, first tested his theory that milkmaids were generally immune to smallpox due to being protected through their repeated exposure to pus contained in cowpox blisters on the udders of the cows they milked. Cowpox is a disease very similar to smallpox, but far less virulent. He inoculated a young boy of eight with infected material derived from blisters on the hand of a local milkmaid. This resulted in a mild fever and some uneasiness, but no marked illness. Subsequently, Jenner tested the boy's immunity to smallpox by injecting variolous material prepared from *Variola minor* lesions (the weaker of the two smallpox strains and the one routinely used at that time to produce immunity). The boy suffered no reaction or infection and a second challenge proved equally innocuous, proving that resistance had been achieved. The milder cowpox, through its similarity to the deadly smallpox (*Variola major*) had stimulated a protective, immune response. Although by comparison crude, and with the potential for serious consequences, the process of vaccination can be compared with the principle of homeopathy and a close relationship recognised, particularly as presented by Hahnemann in his published essay in which he wrote of overcoming a disease by introducing an artificial disease as similar as possible to it. Jenner, like Hahnemann, experienced a great deal of opposition to his findings from his medical colleagues, and, as a fellow sufferer, earned Hahnemann's sympathy.

References

1. Haehl R. *Samuel Hahnemann, His Life and Work*. Vol 1. London: Homoeopathic Publishing Company; 1922. p15.
2. *Ibid.*, p19.
3. Cook TM. *Samuel Hahnemann – The Founder of Homoeopathic Medicine*. Northampton: Thorson Publishers; 1981. p33.
4. *Ibid.*, p37.

5 Haehl R. *Samuel Hahnemann, His Life and Work*. Vol 1. London: Homoeopathic Publishing Company; 1922. p30.
6 *Ibid.*, p33.
7 *Ibid.*, p34.
8 Bradford TL. *The Life and Letters of Samuel Hahnemann*. London: Homoeopathic Publishing Company; 1894. p25.
9 *Ibid.*, p28.
10 Haehl R. *Samuel Hahnemann, His Life and Work*. Vol 1. London: Homoeopathic Publishing Company; 1922. p37.
11 Cook TM. *Samuel Hahnemann – The Founder of Homoeopathic Medicine*. Northampton: Thorson Publishers; 1981. p60.
12 *Ibid.*, p74.
13 *Ibid.*, p72.
14 Haehl R. *Samuel Hahnemann, His Life and Work*. Vol 1. London: Homoeopathic Publishing Company; 1922. pp 52–53.
15 Cook TM. *Samuel Hahnemann – The Founder of Homoeopathic Medicine*. Northampton: Thorson Publishers; 1981. p78.
16 Haehl R. *Samuel Hahnemann, His Life and Work*. Vol 1. London: Homoeopathic Publishing Company; 1922. p66.
17 Hahnemann S. *Organon of Medicine*. 6th edn. Philadelphia PA: Boericke & Tafel; 1922. p80.

3

THE NEW PARACELSUS

During the ensuing years, the nomadic life of the Hahnemann family continued, always with the danger of finding themselves in the path of warring armies. It was a time of long, enigmatic silences with few letters to provide us with historic continuity, but between 1797 and 1810, Hahnemann wrote a number of significant essays, which threw light on the basic elements of homeopathy. Apart from the similar principle, he stressed the need for small, much diluted, doses of remedies and called for simplicity: the use of single remedies rather than the hash of mixed drugs that his contemporaries favoured. Certain events stand out, two of which were to serve Hahnemann ill, the first earning him the reproof and wrath of his profession and the other supplying both doctors and apothecaries with ammunition to deride his scientific expertise and to refute his findings.

Scarlet fever

Whilst in Königslutter, one of his destinations, Hahnemann gained invaluable experience in the nature and behaviour of scarlet fever during a severe outbreak of the disease. Scarlet fever was at that time a serious infection often resulting in death. Hahnemann describes in *Cure and Prevention of Scarlet Fever* (1801) how he inadvertently discovered the specificity of Belladonna for the disease. Three children in a family had developed scarlet fever in its severe form, yet the eldest daughter, who was constitutionally the weakest child, vulnerable to every passing infection, "refused to sicken with the fever." Prior to the outbreak, she had been taking Belladonna internally for an inflammation of the finger joints. Deadly nightshade (*Atropa belladonna*), was a herb well known in folklore for its anti-inflammatory power. Picking up on this, Hahnemann gave homeopathic Belladonna as a preventative to the remaining children of this large family and, despite their being constantly exposed to their feverish and highly contagious siblings, not one contracted the infection. He concluded that a remedy which can speedily cure the beginning of an illness must be its best preventative.[1]

Unfortunately, seeing a means to profit from his discovery, somewhat excusable considering his large family and straitened circumstances, he unwisely advertised and offered for sale a "little book containing helpful secrets" in which he revealed his cure and prevention for scarlet fever. Given the times, this seems innocent enough, but given also the animosity and resentment which he had previously stirred up in the medical and apothecary camps by his repeated, derogatory attacks upon them, he was courting trouble. A storm of indignation descended upon him. He was attacked for demanding payment in advance, thereby intending to enrich himself even before affording any medical assistance; for keeping his remedy secret;[2] and once they knew the identity of the 'secret' remedy, that it was highly toxic and could not possibly prove effective in the minimal dose advocated by Hahnemann. This last accusation was a direct attack against the extreme dilutions he recommended for homeopathic remedies; a matter of some alarm to the apothecaries, since, if established as the norm, it would have seriously reduced their financial rewards. Hahnemann had always attracted their enmity because he did his own dispensing and furthermore advocated that it was an essential element of good, homeopathic practice that doctors should prepare and dispense their medicines themselves. One can only imagine the fury the apothecaries must have felt when they read the following tirade in Hahnemann's *Aesculapius in the Balance*:

> Away from this excessive mixing of medicines, this prescription tomfoolery! Down with the apothecaries privilege! Let the doctor have freedom to make his own medicines and administer them to his patients![3]

The treatment of scarlet fever by means of Belladonna remained a contentious matter as late as 1821, even though physicians had been reporting successes for many years, but in 1838, Hahnemann was finally vindicated when the Prussian Government made Belladonna, in small doses, the remedy of choice in the epidemics of scarlet fever which were so prevalent and devastating in those times.

Alkali Pneum

The second error was a scientific one. Unfortunately, it coincided with the scarlet fever dispute and gave his enemies further means of attacking him. During the process of a chemistry experiment, he incorrectly thought that he had isolated a new alkaline salt (*Alkali pneum*). Prematurely, and uncharacteristically, he announced his discovery, claiming that it would prove of considerable medical value and offering to make its formulation known for a price. However, when analysed, it was found by leading chemists to be common borax. Once again, his urgent need to find an added source of income betrayed him. This behaviour was in total contrast to the charity he had always shown in his medical practice: the refusal to charge the poor or to charge if he felt his treatment had proved ineffective. He had snatched at a hope of financial reward for a scientific discovery. This single lapse in chemistry, a subject that had provided an intellectual raft during the empty, medical years, must have touched this proud man to the quick. He was immediate and frank in his admission of error, but it irked him for years. Six years later, writing in a journal, he observed:

> If I had once made a chemical error – for to err is human – I was at any rate the first to retract it as soon as I had been better instructed.[4]

Torgau

From early 1805, Hahnemann's life at last became settled, the continuous odyssey came to an end. The family was established at Torgau; they had their own house with a garden, and continued there for the next seven years. This respite proved of great value to Hahnemann. He was able to establish a very successful medical practice, improve his financial position, investigate new remedies, put his newfound principles of cure to the test and elaborate the scientific details of his methods for future publication. The family had continued to increase; Charlotte, the seventh daughter, was born late that year, while Henrietta, the oldest child married and Frederich, the only son, a difficult and disappointing character, departed for Leipzig to study medicine. Five other daughters still in the house were Wilhelmina, Amalie, Karolene, Friedrike and Elionore. Hahnemann was now 50 years old and Johanna 41. The family would be complete with the birth of an eighth daughter, Louise, in 1806 (see page 60).

Judging from the letters and articles written by him during this period, it is evident that the hostile attacks of his professional opponents continued unabated. His improved finances enabled him to discontinue his work of translating and to concentrate on his own original writings. His last translation, completed in 1806, was Albrech van Haller's, *The Materia Medica of German Plants, Together with their Economic and Technical Use,* from French into German. This work had particular significance for Hahnemann, since the work dealt with some 462 plants, each described with regard to its characteristics and uses.

Preparing the way

The polemic essays he now published in the much read Hufeland's Journal were all intended to prepare the way for a major work that he was in the process of writing. It was as if, by severe criticism of the existing beliefs and methods of treatment, he wished to demolish the old structure and lay the foundation for his own. Although the harsher aspects of medical practice, which he repeatedly castigated, no longer exist, his censure was more importantly focused on the orthodoxy's mechanistic concepts regarding human life, disease and therapy; concepts which to this day remain dominant in medical thinking. Thinking that fails to recognise the unique nature of each patient's experience of disease, fails to consider the uniqueness of the individual and fails to seek knowledge of the unique power to cure implicit in natural substances; medicine that does not recognise patterns of relationship in diseases and serves expediency by suppressing and palliating rather than seeking to cure. In short, he inveighs against medicine without law and without soul!

The *Organon*

In 1810, he was ready to place before the world the fruits of his constant searching, his persistent deliberations and his painstaking observations: his philosophic and practical insight into the practice of medicine – the *Organon of Rational Healing*; later titled the *Organon of the Healing Art*, but known to subsequent generations of homeopathic students and physicians as simply: the *Organon*. In this work he sets out, in the form of aphorisms and longer paragraphs, the precepts and principles of homeopathic theory, practice and pharmacy. The book ran to five editions in Hahnemann's lifetime; the sixth was only published many years after his death, in 1921.

The first three aphorisms set the stage for what follows:

§1. The physician's high and *only* mission is to restore the sick to health, to cure, as it is termed.

§2. The highest ideal of cure is rapid, gentle and permanent restoration of the health, or removal and annihilation of the disease in its whole extent, in the shortest, most reliable, and most harmless way, on easily comprehensible principles.

§3. If the physician perceives what is to be cured in diseases ... if he clearly perceives what is curative in medicines ... and if he knows how to adapt, according to clearly defined principles, what is curative in medicines to what he has discovered to be undoubtedly morbid in the patient, so that recovery must ensue ... as also in respect to the exact mode of preparation and quantity of it required (proper dose), and the proper period for repeating the dose; if, finally, he knows the obstacles to cure in each case and is aware how to remove them, so that the restoration may be permanent: ***then he understands how to treat judiciously and rationally, and he is a true practitioner of the healing art.***[5]

Without doubt, these injunctions are principles that every student and practitioner of medicine should take to heart and make the basis of their practice. In a later paragraph he lays down the three cardinal points that must be addressed in order to achieve a cure.

> §71. . . . diseases of mankind consist merely of groups of certain symptoms and may be annihilated and transformed into health by medicinal substances, but only by such as are capable of artificially producing similar morbid symptoms (and such is the process in all genuine cure), hence the operation of curing is comprised in the three following points:
> - How is the physician to ascertain what is necessary to be known in order to cure the disease?
> - How is he to gain a knowledge of the instruments adapted for the cure of the natural disease, (i.e.) the pathogenetic powers of the medicines?
> - What is the most suitable method of employing these artificial, morbific agents (medicines) for the cure of natural disease?[6]

The body of the work answers these questions, setting out the precepts of the new healing system that he propounds, its laws and the manner of its practice. In addition, Hahnemann gives full and careful directions for the preparation of homeopathic remedies, explains the necessity for small doses and simple (non-compounded) remedies and gives instruction in the methods to be used in proving new substances. As in all his previous works, he goes to great lengths in discussing the obstacles to cure that must be removed and emphasises the importance of a healing environment, good hygiene, healthy diet and regular exercise. He insists that the prescribing of remedies must be strictly based on a study of the entire patient with particular reference to their temperament and responses to their emotional and physical circumstances. He stresses that the correct remedy must be chosen for the unique qualities of the patient, for the totality of their emotional and physical symptoms, and not simply for their disease diagnosis. Patients with the same diagnosis may require very different medication. Hahnemann also provides clear and detailed directions regarding how the physician should best proceed in questioning a patient in order to bring out the individualising characteristics of the case.

> §83. This individualising examination of a case of disease, demands of the physician nothing but freedom from prejudice and sound senses, attention in observing and fidelity in tracing the picture of the disease.[7]

Throughout the work, he reveals an uncompromisingly, critical attitude towards the therapeutic methods of conventional medicine. He stresses that its drugs, acting only by suppression, compound with existing disease and create morbid effects more deeply seated, more destructive and more resistant to cure. A study of the *Organon* gives the reader much insight into the character of its author. It reveals a wide-ranging, penetrating intellect, a pedantic, orderly mind: passionate, forceful and inflexible in presenting the principles upon which good homeopathic practice must be based; intolerant, fearless and tactless in his disparagement of the 'old-school'; and filled with deep compassion and concern for suffering humanity. Above all, the *Organon* is testimony to a clear and rational logic, pragmatic and empirical, innovative and revolutionary, able to synthesise ancient wisdom into a practical system of therapeutics and despite his theism to do so without esoteric overtones.

Given the furore caused by many of his previous publications, Hahnemann must have expected a medical outcry against the content of this most defining work, but the response was more dismissive than otherwise. Only the tiny doses he advocated attracted much criticism, because they were considered too inadequate to prove effective. We can anticipate that this proud, inveterate iconoclast must have felt piqued by such indifference. Probably hoping to elicit some reaction he wrote in *Der Reichanzeiger*:

> Is it really credible that, in these illumined times . . . a work springing purely from experience . . . was put to one side by several reviewers with empty words and expressions.[8]

Two hundred years later nothing has changed, the average, orthodox medical-mind remains impervious to enrichment from sources outside itself.

'Provings' on the healthy

The *Organon* was indeed a work springing purely from experience. During the years following the pioneer experiment with quinine (1790) and the elucidation of the homeopathic doctrine of cure (1796) and particularly while favoured by the more tranquil life at Torgau, Hahnemann had spent much time investigating the medicinal properties of various minerals and plants. The fertile valley of the Elbe and its surrounding hills and the local hedgerows provided him with many of the botanical specimens he required. Intrinsic to the application of the homeopathic law of cure is knowledge of remedy action based upon results gleaned from testing remedies on healthy male and female subjects. He emphasises the importance of the healthy state of the trialist in the *Organon*.

§107. If, in order to ascertain this (the drug's ability to alter the state of health), medicines be given to *sick* persons only ... then little or nothing precise is seen of their true effects, as those peculiar alterations of the health to be expected from the medicine are mixed up with the symptoms of the disease and can seldom be distinctly observed.[9]

To this end, he prepared tinctures of the various plant remedies in alcohol, and with characteristic thoroughness and meticulous attention to detail he tested them on himself, carefully noting all the symptoms produced.[10] Such an experiment later became known in homeopathic terminology as a *proving* (i.e. pathogenetic trial). In spite of all the medical animosity he inevitably attracted, over the years, Hahnemann drew about him a small but ardent group of admirers and supporters, both professional and lay. Many of these, together with members of his family and close friends, formed an enthusiastic and dedicated band of trialists that collaborated with him in the proving of new remedies. Under his strict supervision, this group of healthy volunteers subjected themselves to the effects of various substances drawn from the mineral, plant and animal kingdoms. The proving procedures that he laid down were exacting and rigorous, ensuring the accuracy of the observed phenomena. Even the diet and habits of the participant had to conform to Hahnemann's stringent requirements,[10] lest any negative influence should detrimentally influence the validity of the observations. Each trialist (*prover*) was required to submit a detailed account of the doses taken, symptoms experienced and any modifying influences (*modalities*) discerned, e.g. emotions, time, temperature, weather, menstrual cycle, movement, position, mental or physical exertion, etc. Hahnemann would then go through the report with them, asking questions so as to complete from their recollections that which required to be more explicit. All mental and physical symptoms and signs that could confidently be attributed to drug effect, were carefully noted and systematically assembled to form a specific drug picture.[12]

To achieve as accurate a picture of remedy (drug) response as possible, it was essential that each and every symptom experienced by the prover be appraised and teased out to reveal its every nuance, hence the necessity for regular in-depth consultations with the trial participants. Hahnemann's fussy, meticulous nature was ideally suited to such painstaking analysis. A symptom would be evaluated from every possible angle: its *manner of onset* and any *initiatory cause*; the *time* of its onset and any pattern of *periodicity*; its site (*location*) and any spread (*extension*); a description of its nature (*sensation*); all factors which aggravated, ameliorated or modified it (*modalities*); its *intensity*; and any associated symptoms (*concomitants*). This careful sifting produced what would come to be known as the *complete symptom* –

a vital element in producing a proving picture, in case taking and in matching the two.

In those early years, tinctures and low potencies were often employed for proving trials, with all the attendant risks of poisonous side effects. Certain intrepid provers knowingly exposed themselves to highly, toxic substances in their selfless determination to demonstrate a drug's healing potential. Undoubtedly, the master's driving force inspired many of these heroic provings; his desire to know, without the fallacy of supposition, the reliable symptoms of each and every substance he chose to investigate. Through refining the procedures of these early experiments, Hahnemann developed a methodology of proving remedies, which became the foundation for the exact, scientific protocols that are used today.

The compiled results of this Herculean work were published in Hahnemann's *Materia Medica Pura*, published in six volumes between 1811 and 1821[12] The subsequent English translation was contained in two volumes.

A *materia medica* is a textbook containing a systematic documentation of the knowledge of medicines, and, in homeopathy, provides a description of the nature and the therapeutic repertoire of homeopathic remedies, and also the general emotional and physical characteristics of those who are sensitive to their action.[11] The term *pura* denoted that the symptoms catalogued in the work derived solely from provings and not from cured, clinical cases or from toxicology. Later homeopathic materia medica would include invaluable material from both these latter sources. The proving symptoms (drug pictures) of 66 remedies were recorded in this major work. It is a tribute to the thoroughness and accuracy of Hahnemann's research methods that modern re-provings of certain of these original remedies, using randomised double-blind placebo-controlled methods, have simply confirmed the findings of the original pathogenetic trials conducted by Hahnemann and his helpers. To this day, the *Materia Medica Pura* remains a work of scientific importance, and the tabulated symptoms it contains have been incorporated into all major materia medica. In a footnote, Hahnemann urges the homeopathic physician to acquire a thorough knowledge of materia medica, greater than that of the simple carpenter for his tools.[12]

> What conscientious physician would consent to work away at hap-hazard on a sick person . . . no carpenter would work upon his wood with tools whose uses he was ignorant of. He knows every one of them perfectly, and hence he knows when to use the one and when the other, in order to effect with certainty what he intends to do; and it is only wood he works upon, and he is but a carpenter.[13]

To assist the conscientious physician in acquiring this essential knowledge, the proving symptoms characteristic of each remedy were set out in a carefully structured way. In his preface to the work, Hahnemann comments:

> I have arranged the symptoms of the more perfectly observed medicines in a certain order, whereby the search for the desired medicinal symptoms will now be facilitated.[14]

His chosen format commenced with vertigo, confusion, deficient mental power and loss of memory and then extended from the head downwards to the extremities, covering all the systems of the body, and finishing with disturbances of the disposition, affections of the mind. In addition he included instructions for the homeopathic preparation of the medicines, their historical use and their major clinical indications. Although modernising changes and improvements have been made to Hahnemann's original symptom layout, notably the advancement of the mental and emotional symptoms to the pre-eminent position they deserve, usually following immediately after an introductory section, the Hahnemannian order of arrangement has remained a template for all subsequent materia medica and for most repertories that developed from them.[15]

The final symptomatic picture of a remedy (medicinal substance) contained in modern materia medica consists of the following major elements:

- Symptoms derived from pathogenetic trials (provings) of the remedy.
- Symptoms cured by the specific remedy (verified by accumulated clinical experience).
- Characteristics of appearance, temperament, behaviour and constitution found to be frequently associated with sensitivity to the remedy's action, both in provings and cures.
- Symptoms gleaned from poisonings and the toxicology of the substance.

Return to Leipzig

During the winter of 1810–1811, Napoleon's hunger for conquest impinged on the settled life of the Hahnemann family in Torgau. Despite unresolved conflict in Spain, his predatory eye was focused on Moscow and to consolidate his position prior to his intended invasion of Russia, Napoleon built a defensive line along the river Elbe, from Hamburg in the north to Dresden in the south. Being at a main river crossing, Torgau was heavily fortified and French troops were encamped outside the town. The eye of the coming storm was to be centred on Hahnemann's beloved Saxony. Deeply disturbed by these events, Hahnemann wrote in a letter to Herr von Villers, a lecturer at the University of Göttingen in which he stated:

> Preparations are already made to transform Torgau into a large and terrible fortress and my people do not see any prospect of leading a quiet life here. I shall have to leave my nice, comfortable freehold residence – and move – I do not know whither.[16]

However, instead of going to Göttingen, he finally decided to return yet again to Leipzig, the intellectual capital of Germany, a decision that inevitably cast him from the proverbial frying pan into the fire, both in a military and a medical sense – for both spelt warfare. Leipzig would soon be the stage for one of the most decisive battles of the Napoleonic Wars and in Leipzig, which held no happy memories, he would be in the heartland of enemy territory, the academic centre of his medical adversaries.

Undaunted, soon after his arrival, he decided to profit from this central position by offering a six-month tutorial course in homeopathy for interested physicians at what he hoped would become an Institute for Graduated Physicians.

> In this Institute I shall elucidate in every respect the entire homoeopathic system of healing taught in the *Organon* and shall make a practical application of it with patients treated in their presence, and thus place my pupils in a condition to be able to practise this system in all cases by themselves.[18]

Dissertation on Veratrum album

As far as we know, there was not a single applicant. He therefore abandoned the idea of persuading established physicians towards homeopathic thinking and resolved to address students and young doctors, whom he was sure would not be so brainwashed by orthodox prejudice and tethered to tradition. He applied to the Dean of the Medical Faculty for the privilege of delivering lectures to undergraduates. He was informed that, as an external lecturer, to gain that privilege he would have to defend a dissertation from the Upper Chair with a respondent and pay 50 *thaler* to the Faculty. It was a challenge he relished and he set about his preparation with his usual passion and attention to detail, producing an 86-page thesis written in Latin, as was the custom of the time. The thesis was a marvel of research and erudition, concerning the white hellebore of the ancients, which he proved to be identical with the Veratrum album of the present.[17] In his choice of subject and its content, Hahnemann was careful to avoid any reference to homeopathy, any criticism of allopathy and any aspect of medicine, which might have been considered contentious. He literally swept his audience off its feet, showing to advantage his extraordinary knowledge of languages, his reading and his scholarship – particularly in the history of medicine.[18] The Dean openly congratulated him on his fine dissertation and on 29 September 1812, Hahnemann commenced lecturing twice weekly on Wednesday and Saturday at 2 p.m.

Battle of Leipzig

He had scarcely begun when world events of vast magnitude engulfed him. In that same September, the Grand Army of Napoleon retreated from its disastrous Russian campaign, grievously mauled by the ravages of the conflict, the relentless cold of winter and the pursuing enemy. Heartened by the weakened morale and strength of the French, Prussia and Austria declared war on France. With characteristic decisiveness, Bonaparte withdrew forces from Spain to reinforce his shattered army and in defiance of his foes re-entered Saxony in August 1813 and promptly defeated part of the Allied armies in a great battle at Dresden. He then moved northwest to Leipzig, and there, on 14 October 1813, confronted a vastly stronger force under the supreme command of the Austrian Prince, Karl Philipp of Schwarzenburg. On 16 October, in conditions of incessant autumn rain and impeding mud, the armies clashed in the terrible Battle of Leipzig (Battle of the Nations, as it became known). The inhabitants, including the Hahnemann family, would have taken refuge in their cellars waiting until the sounds of conflict ceased before emerging. The stress of such an experience for a 58 year-old man, the protector of his wife and daughters, surrounded by the roar and reverberation of cannons, in a battle of uncertain outcome, must have been horrific. For Charlotte and Louise, his youngest daughters, who were already of nervous disposition, the event must have proved severely traumatic.

On 18 October, the battle reached its pitch as the Allies launched a huge assault from all sides. In over nine hours of intense fighting, with heavy casualties on both sides, the French troops prevented a breakthrough, but were inexorably pushed back towards Leipzig. Later in the day, the defection of a number of Saxon regiments to the Allies highlighted Napoleon's untenable position. Realising that the battle was lost, on the night of the 18–19 October, Napoleon began to withdraw the majority of his army across the river Elster, leaving a smaller force to hinder pursuit by rear-guard action through the streets of Leipzig and then by blowing up the bridge behind them. Unfortunately, the destruction of the bridge was ill-timed; the fuses were ignited when the bridge was still crowded with fleeing French troops and the rear-guard were still holding off the Allies in the city. The huge explosion (which must have reached Hahnemann's ears) and the subsequent panic and rout resulted in the deaths of thousands of French troops and the capture of thousands more. The French were thoroughly defeated and Prince Karl rode triumphantly through the streets of the city. Napoleon withdrew from Germany, never to return, his nemesis, the Duke of Wellington, awaited him at Waterloo on 18 June 1815.

Typhus

Three days of war left chaos, devastation and disease. The number of casualties on either side was appalling, estimates ranging from 80,000 to 100,000 killed and wounded. The makeshift military hospital was filled to overflowing with the wounded, maimed and dying. The conditions and privations endured by the civilian population were severe. The incessant rain continued; food supplies were inadequate; and a new danger threatened when the drinking water became polluted. Inevitably, typhus broke out and the death toll mounted. Yet, it was this dreadful aftermath that provided Hahnemann with an opportunity to test the power of his new system of medicine against a dangerous adversary and to contrast it with the results of conventional treatment. He treated all his patients with homeopathic remedies alone and achieved remarkable results. Of the 180 cases under his care only two died and one of these was a very old man. The death rate under allopathic care was as high as 50 per cent. Considering that he had no recourse to antibiotics, his success rate would be considered impressive even by today's standards. He documented these results in a paper entitled: *Treatment of the now prevailing Typhus Fever*. There was no positive response from his allopathic colleagues.

The Master's anger

Napoleon's defeat at Waterloo, brought peace to Europe, and as the effects of the strife passed, prosperity returned and the social and cultural life of Leipzig flourished. Whereas, the *Organon* had, with few exceptions, stirred up very little animosity towards Hahnemann, his therapeutic success and his thriving practice did. The sight of the creator of the despised homeopathic doctrine receiving the accolades of the public and prospering financially irked the medical community and created increasing jealousy and ill-will. The original casual indifference and disdain shown by the establishment turned to open hostility. As today, other alternative systems of therapy, which enjoy a degree of popular interest, generally failed to ruffle academic feathers and not being seen as a direct challenge were tolerated. Homeopathy was different; it stood diametrically and uncompromisingly opposed to the existing medical system and left no room for it. It must be admitted that Hahnemann himself provoked much of the animosity he experienced. A man of great passion and intensity, filled with enthusiasm for the new system of cure he had formulated, with clear vision of the benefits it would bestow, and acutely aware of the dangers and shortcomings of current medical practice; faced by the inability or unwillingness of his colleagues to understand and embrace his concepts or even give him an ear; and repeatedly subject to their attacks, rejection and ridicule, he was filled to overflowing with hurt, frustration, intolerance, anger and bitterness, which he could not contain.

Lectures to the Medical Faculty

These emotions betrayed him and robbed him of the opportunity of influencing many of the young minds he was addressing in his lectures at the Medical Faculty. Consequent to his brilliant presentation and defence of his dissertation, these lectures commenced auspiciously. The hall was packed, not only by students but also doctors, representatives of professors and many curious people from other faculties, providing a wonderful opportunity for Hahnemann to state his case, defend its principles and win disciples. From the outset, he was unable to maintain his composure and to contain his boiling emotions thus making a laughing stock of both himself and homeopathy. The extravagant raiment he chose for the occasion and his lordly deportment, so at odds with his amiable, homely, domestic self, spoke of high affectation and eccentricity. According to Haehl:

> (He) entered the room in his extraordinary costume with an ever affected grandeur that was almost Spanish ... after reading the paragraph from his *Organon* which he was about to discuss – his professional calm and dignity soon disappeared and broke out into a 'raging hurricane' against the old methods of healing and those professional men who still clung to them.[19]

We are indebted to Dr Franz Hartmann, one of Hahnemann's most faithful students and intimate friends, for many insights into the master's life and teaching in Leipzig. Hartmann had enrolled at the Medical Faculty in 1814, at the age of eighteen, and wrote about his experiences in a series of articles published between 1844 and 1850. He attended Hahnemann's lectures to the Faculty and wrote a sad account of what transpired:

> Unfortunately the lectures were not fitted to win friends and followers for his theories or himself. For whenever possible, he poured forth a flood of abuse against the older medicine and its followers, with the result that his audience lessened every hour and finally consisted of only a few of his students. . . . Any

others were present not for the subject matter but to hear the unfortunate method of presentation, so that their sense of humour might be freely tickled.[19]

Nevertheless, this period of teaching was not without gain and proved critical to the future of homeopathy. A small core of enthusiastic students, including Franz Hartmann, looking beyond Hahnemann's tirades, recognised his deep concern for the future of medicine, the brilliance of his mind, his sincerity and the truth and value of what he taught. Having weathered 'the hurricane,' they were to prove tested and true. For the first time in his life, after years of solitary struggle, Hahnemann at last had a band of devoted, young colleagues to accompany and support him on his mission. He took them to his heart and into the fold of his family life. The close comradeship that developed was to prove essential for the survival of the group. These committed homeopathic students continued attending Hahnemann's classes and received the most important part of their medical training from him, but it remained imperative for them to continue with their formal education at the Medical Faculty in order to achieve their doctorates in medicine. They were perceived as traitors to the profession and medical heretics and the hatred and scorn, which the professors and their fellow students felt for Hahnemann, was now directed against them. Franz Hartmann gives us an engaging picture of the spirit of camaraderie that sustained them:

> We lived very happily together, caring very little for the hostile glances and remarks of our colleagues. We stuck to our studies faithfully and honestly and gathered together occasionally in our teacher Hahnemann's household some time after eight in the evening. By this we felt invigorated against new attacks, for Hahnemann was very skilful in stimulating anew our depressed spirits.[20]

Professor Dr Clarus

In counterpoise to the revolutionary iconoclast, another medical archetype often produced in the past and most prevalent in present times is the defender of the established faith, the knight of the ivory tower, the shining champion of orthodoxy, unassailably clad in the pomp and armour of scientific rectitude. Such a man was Professor Dr Johann Christian August Clarus (1774–1854), the clinical professor of the time and the loftiest figure in the Medical Faculty of Leipzig, who considered himself judge, jury and executioner in matters medical. Even when past middle age, his menacing image still lingered in Hartmann's memory:

> To him the 'carryings on' of Hahnemann and of his pupils (as he liked to call it) whom he dismissed as 'ignorant fellows,' represented a real horror, and his bitterest hatred persecuted anything that was at all reminiscent of Hahnemann

or his theories ... it fascinated him to tyrannise over students he did not like and to repudiate them in public under a cloak of scholarship and titular authority.[20]

Professor Clarus's intense enmity and influential position resulted in Hahnemann being ostracised by his academic colleagues. Certain of his more outspoken students, despite their academic ability, were subjected to discriminatory treatment by their tutors, even being failed in their examinations. Instigated by Professor Clarus, the disciplinary Court of the University ordered the confiscation of homeopathic remedies from the premises of two students, Karl Franz and Christian Hornburg. This persecution extended beyond graduation; the ever-vigilant, implacable, watchdog Clarus seizing the least opportunity to bring charges of negligence against any past student affiliated to Hahnemann. As a result, both Franz and Hornburg, who had joined Hahnemann's close band of provers, became martyrs to the homeopathic cause. Dr Franz was forced to retire from practice after one of his patients died and the most unfortunate Dr Hornburg was found guilty, after several court hearings, of 'illegal healing and prevention of proper treatment' and sentenced to two years imprisonment.[21] Three days after the verdict, he suffered a haemorrhage and died.

These persistent attacks forged an even stronger bond of brotherhood between those closest to Hahnemann. This was further cemented by the conducting of provings, which regularly brought them together with a common purpose as the now famous Group of Collaborators for the Proving of Drugs, which Hahnemann had created.[22] Many proving groups down the years and in modern times have experienced this feeling of fraternity. The benefits bestowed on a physician by being part of a proving trial are inestimable. The trialist becomes alert and observant of the nuances of emotion, thought, sensation and feeling, which are engendered by the substance taken and becomes exercised in self-analysis and in the accurate expression and detailing of the symptoms experienced during the proving. This complements clinical knowledge, and renders the physician better able to elicit and understand the symptoms of a patient. In later years, when finer dilutions (higher potencies) were employed in pathogenetic trials, provings became therapeutic to the trialist; unusual sensitivity to the action of a substance indicating a susceptibility to the curative effect of the remedy, resulting in a strengthening of the constitution of the prover.

Hartmann who continued to participate in provings after Hahnemann's death, writes of how privileged he was to have been involved with Hahnemann in this work:

Under his guidance I have proved many a remedy, together with others like Gross, Hornburg, Franz etc., and from his instructive suggestions I obtained then for the first time clear sensations which I could again express very accurately. This is not so easy a lesson as it appears at first sight, and it has never been demonstrated to me so plainly even by the later and more modern proving of drugs, as I learned it at Hahnemann's hands. It proved to be of very effectual use in my practical examination of patients. Had I learned nothing more than this from him, I should feel compelled to be eternally grateful.[22]

A name omitted by Hartmann is Johann Ernst Stapf (1788–1860), a young student who became one of Hahnemann's closest friends and supporters, and continued to correspond with the master throughout the Paris years until Samuel's death in 1843. He deserves special mention because over the years he contributed to the proving of no less than thirty-two homeopathic remedies and became an important defender of homeopathy and one of its most renowned and gifted practitioners. Between the years 1822 and 1839, he published the first scientific, homeopathic journal. Such was his reputation that Queen Victoria consulted him, at first by correspondence, and then later, in 1835, he was summoned to attend her personally. So, he became the first of a line of homeopaths appointed as physicians to the British royal household extending from that time to the present.

References

1. Haehl R. *Samuel Hahnemann, His Life and Work*. Vol 1. London: Homoeopathic Publishing Company; 1922. p60.
2. *Ibid.*, p59.
3. *Ibid.*, p74.
4. *Ibid.*, p61.
5. Hahnemann S. *Organon of Medicine*. 6th edn. Philadelphia PA: Boericke & Tafel; 1922. pp92–93.
6. *Ibid.*, pp158–159.
7. *Ibid.*, pp172–173.
8. Haehl R. *Samuel Hahnemann, His Life and Work*. Vol 1. London: Homoeopathic Publishing Company; 1922. p93.
9. Hahnemann S. *Organon of Medicine*. 6th edn. Philadelphia PA: Boericke & Tafel; 1922. p188.
10. Lilley DJ. The homeopathic materia medica. In: Kayne SB (ed). *Homeopathic Practice*. London: Pharmaceutical Press; 2008. Chapter 5, p76.
11. Swayne J. *International Dictionary of Homeopathy*. London: Churchill Livingston; 2000. p132.
12. Lilley DJ. The homeopathic materia medica. In: Kayne SB (ed). *Homeopathic Practice*. London: Pharmaceutical Press; 2008. Chapter 5, p77.
13. Hahnemann S. *Materia Medica Pura*. Liverpool: Hahnemann Publishing Society; 1880. p2.

14 *Ibid.*, p4.
15 Lilley DJ. The homeopathic materia medica. In: Kayne SB (ed). *Homeopathic Practice*. London: Pharmaceutical Press, 2008. Chapter 5, p78.
16 Haehl R. *Samuel Hahnemann, His Life and Work*. Vol 1. London: Homoeopathic Publishing Company; 1922. p95.
17 Bradford TL. *The Life and Letters of Samuel Hahnemann*. London: Homoeopathic Publishing Company; 1894. p85.
18 Haehl R. *Samuel Hahnemann, His Life and Work*. Vol 1. London: Homoeopathic Publishing Company; 1922. p97.
19 *Ibid.*, p98.
20 *Ibid.*, p100.
21 Cook TM. *Samuel Hahnemann – The Founder of Homoeopathic Medicine*. Northampton: Thorson Publishers; 1981. p124.
22 Haehl R. *Samuel Hahnemann, His Life and Work*. Vol 1. London: Homoeopathic Publishing Company; 1922. p101.

4

THE LAW OF THE INFINITESIMAL DOSE

Dilutions to potencies

Before proceeding further with the history of this remarkable man, Samuel Hahnemann, it is necessary for us to retrace our steps to 1798 and consider an important transition point in his scientific thinking: the development and use of the minimum, or infinitesimal, dose. The prescribing of extremely small doses of the similar remedy is as intrinsic to homeopathic practice as the application of the Law of Similars. It is an aspect of homeopathy, which has particularly invited the disbelief and derision of orthodox, medical opinion.

Hahnemann's move from simple dilutions to potentised remedies came about quite suddenly. The English homeopath Dr RE Dudgeon commented on this in 1853:

> We cannot fail to be struck by the sudden transition from the massive doses he prescribed in 1798 to the unheard-of-minuteness of his doses only one year later; and we can but guess the causes for this abrupt transition.[1]

From his student years, Hahnemann had been appalled not only by what he considered the harmful and barbaric methods used by the orthodoxy to drain off 'morbid humours,' which were believed to be the cause of disease, but also by the heavy doses of drugs that were employed, often in indiscriminate mixtures. His approach to the prescribing of remedies was from the start the very opposite of the prevailing method, always governed by keeping the remedy as simple as possible (a single remedy), the dosage as low as possible (dilutions) and its selection according to definite principles (precise method). As we have noted, by 1796 the method had become clear to him: like will be cured by like. Therefore, when Hahnemann commenced putting his theory into practice, he prescribed dilute, material doses of medicines selected on the similar principle. However, these small doses were still physically measurable, and, since many were derived from toxic substances capable of producing both physiological and structural changes, side effects were to be expected. And so it was. Although he enjoyed notable success, he found that due to the similarity of the medicinal effect to the symptoms already experienced by the patient, many reported an unacceptable degree of aggravation before improvement. To avoid this he experimented with increasingly dilute preparations hoping to find a level of dilution that would still cure without the risk of aggravation. As he stresses in the second aphorism of the *Organon*, the process of ideal cure must be as gentle and harmless as possible. To his disappointment he found, as we might anticipate, that when diluted sufficiently to avoid all unwanted side effects, many remedies lost their therapeutic power. It seemed an impasse!

But Samuel Hahnemann was to medical science what Albert Einstein was to physics. Faced with this obstacle, he made an 'intuitive conceptual leap!'[2] Einstein himself described this process:

> For the creation of a theory, the mere collection of recorded phenomena never suffices – there must be added a free invention of the human mind that attacks the heart of the matter.

Long before the discovery of electromagnetism, sub-atomic-particles, energy-waves and quantum physics, Hahnemann plunged into the world of the infinitesimally small, leaving behind him the world of Isaac Newton and molecular medicine. Although we know the nature of the conceptual leap that eventually resolved the problem of dilution, nowhere in his writings does he give us a clue as to the process of his thinking or how and why he came to the conclusions that he did. In order to piece this together it is necessary for us to consider the influences that informed him.

Firstly, he was a deeply religious man. Although his religious upbringing was Lutheran, his writings reveal that he was first and foremost a theist with a profound belief in an omniscient, omnipotent and omnipresent deity, a Creator, who benevolently and wisely presides over the affairs of humankind. This knowledge coupled to his utter conviction of the truth of the similar principle and the necessity of the minimal dose, left him with no doubt that there must be a solution; it was only a matter of thinking it out.

Secondly, there was his intense love of chemistry and experimentation, undoubtedly influenced and enriched by an intimate knowledge of alchemical techniques, which he would have stoutly denied, but which is clearly revealed in his later elaboration of certain strange, yet key homeopathic remedies e.g. Hepar-sulph and Causticum. The original intent of 'The Great Work' of the alchemists was the transmutation of base metals, such as copper and lead, into the noble metals, silver and gold; the formulation of an elixir of life which would prove a panacea able to cure all diseases and bestow immortality; and the discovery of a universal solvent. The transmutation of lead to gold became likened to man's spiritual growth and ascent from a primitive to an enlightened state; a process of internal alchemy, which Jung was later to equate with the individuation process of the human soul. Thus, a mystical component, compounded of astrological and religious influences vested the practical techniques of alchemy with esoteric significance. This lead to the search for the 'philosopher's stone,' a mythical substance regarded as essential to the realisation of these goals. These alchemical strivings eventually gave birth to modern chemistry, which owes so much to the methods developed by the alchemists and the remarkable discoveries that they made in the course of their experiments, e.g. the discovery of phosphorus. Alchemy sought to bring about transmutation through processes of refinement, separation, dissolution, distillation, dilution and filtration. All of which symbolised purification, sublimation and transcendence – transformations from the gross to the refined and a dematerialisation that empowered and ennobled. This was exactly what would occur in the special diluting process that Hahnemann was to evolve.

Finally, there was Paracelsus!

His memory still loomed large in the 18th century and his works must have been well known to Hahnemann. What influence did he have upon Hahnemann at this vital juncture? After all, was it not Paracelsus who said that medicine is

> ... not in its finished state, but concealed in dross – what the eyes perceive in herbs and stones or trees is not yet a remedy; the eyes see only the dross – but inside, under the dross, there lies the remedy – first it must be cleansed from the dross, then it is there. The remedy has to be subjected to the **'alchemy of fire'** – this is alchemy, and this is the office of Vulcan; he is the apothecary and chemist of medicine.[3]

Fire denotes destruction, but viewed positively, it represents destruction of the old and release or creation of the new, as in the myth of the phoenix – hence, creative and regenerative energy or power. It also symbolises purification, renewal, transformation, revelation, and physical and spiritual transcendence. In unravelling the Paracelsian metaphor of alchemical fire, to which the remedy must be subjected before it can be revealed, cleansed and made accessible for use, we must conclude that the remedy has to be subjected to creative energy or power. In the event, this is exactly what Hahnemann did: a process he termed 'potentisation'.

We can surmise that in addition to his own genius, it was a confluence of all three of these promptings that inspired Hahnemann. While the principle of 'like curing like' came to him from the past, the concepts of proving substances on healthy people and the potentisation of remedies belonged solely to Hahnemann and both are a testimony to the brilliance of his mind.

Divining that a specific curative power exists in all medicinal substances and that it must in some way be wrested from its physical form, like a metal from its ore, and knowing that simple dilution was not sufficient to access that power, he concluded that he must subject each progressive stage of dilution to a period of friction or agitation, since direct heating would disorganise and degrade the substance. In this way he sought to convert inert, latent or toxic energy into curative energy, without loss of healing power – and he succeeded!

Potentisation

Soluble substances

So, as in the imagery of Paracelsus, the homeopathic Hephaistos (Vulcan) set to work. Taking the *mother tincture* (pure alcohol extract, denoted by the letters MT or the symbol Ø) of a plant material, he diluted it by adding one part to 9 parts of pure alcohol, a dilution factor of one tenth ($\frac{1}{10}$ or 10^{-1}). This dilution was poured into a glass bottle until three-quarters full. The bottle was corked and then vigorously struck against the palm of the hand or a hard, but resilient surface, e.g. a leather bound book, for a specific number of strokes, causing the contents to strike alternatively against the cork and the bottom of the bottle with as much force as possible. In this manner, the remedy was thoroughly mixed with the alcohol or solvent, molecular collision was caused and mechanical (kinetic) energy was imparted to the mixture. But more important than these physical results was the dynamic imprinting of the medicinal image of the remedy upon the substrate of the solvent. Figure 4.1 depicts a diagrammatic representation of the potentisation process.

This vigorous agitation of the remedy he termed 'succussion'. The first succussed dilution was defined as the 1X potency –X denoting the decimal scale of dilution that had been employed, and potency, denoting the curative energy or level of the remedy. In some European countries the decimal scale is denoted by the letter 'D' placed before the number, thus: D1.

Hahnemann then proceeded to further reduce the physical strength (toxicity) of the original tincture by repeating the entire process by adding one part of the 1X succussed dilution to 9 parts of pure alcohol and subjecting the resulting one-hundredth ($\frac{1}{100}$ or 10^{-2}) dilution to another period of

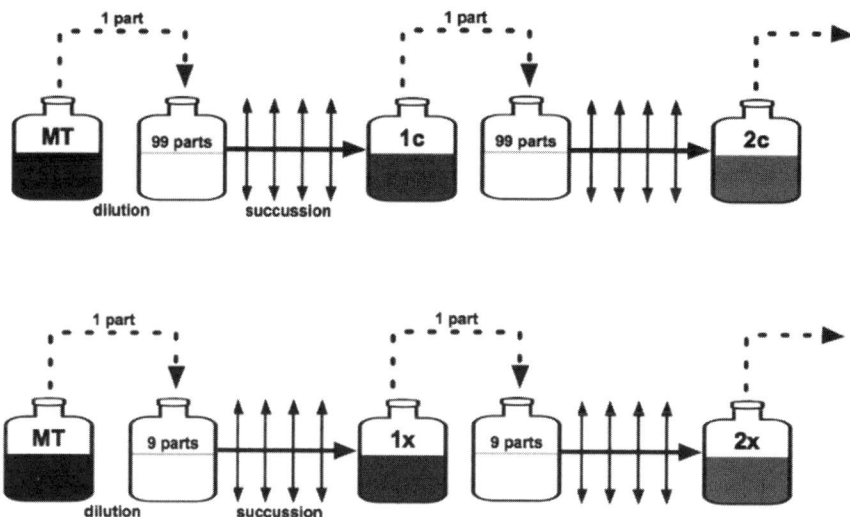

Figure 4.1 Diagrammatic representation of the potentisation process

succussion. This produced the second decimal or 2X potency. In this manner he continued the process of potentisation – a process of *serial dilution with succussion*, – whereby each potentised dilution was prepared from the dilution that immediately preceded it, each step being followed by succussion. The next potentised dilution was the one-thousandth (3X or 10^{-3}); the next was the ten-thousandth (4X or 10^{-4}); the next was the one hundred-thousandth (5X or 10^{-5}); and from this the one-millionth (6X or 10^{-6}) was prepared. Thus an exponential and infinite scale of potentised dilutions became possible.

In addition to this decimal scale, Hahnemann also developed the *centesimal scale of dilution*, which commenced by taking one part of the mother tincture (MT or Ø) and adding to it 99 parts of alcohol as the diluent, a dilution factor of one-hundredth, and following this by succussion. This produced the first centesimal potency (10^{-2}), known as the 1C potency. Further serial dilutions with succussion proceeded as for the decimal scale, but at each step of dilution 99 parts of alcohol were added to one part of the previous potency (whereas, 9 parts were used in the decimal scale). Through using the centesimal scale, the potency of the remedy can be lifted more rapidly; the 1C (10^{-2}) potency is already mathematically equivalent to the 2X potency (10^{-2}) and the 3C (10^{-6}) is mathematically equivalent to the 6X (10^{-6}) potency; therefore, exponentially, the 30C (10^{-60}) potency is equivalent to the 60X (10^{-60}) potency.

However, whereas the 6X (10^{-6}) has been through six steps of dilution and succussion, its mathematical equivalent, the 3C (10^{-6}), has only been subjected to three steps. Therefore, the 6X must be regarded as more *dynamic* in its action than the equivalent 3C – and this is born out in practice (the term 'dynamisation' is often used as a simile for potentisation). This difference in dynamic potential is significant when prescribing the lower potencies e.g. up to the 12X, but less so thereafter. For practical reasons the higher, and particularly the highest potencies, are prepared using the centesimal scale (the use of the terms low, medium or high potency, refers to the level of potentisation reached through serial dilution with succussion).

Insoluble substances

Of course, the above method of potentisation can only be used for substances, which are soluble in water or alcohol. Hahnemann developed a method for potentising insoluble substances. This differs from the technique for soluble substances only in the initial stages, since once the insoluble substance has been potentised to the 6X or 3C (10^{-6}), it can be colloidally dispersed in a diluent, water or alcohol, and further potencies can then be prepared in liquid form, via either the decimal or centesimal scales. Hahnemann chose sugar of milk (lactose) as his preferred carrier or diluent for insoluble substances because it was relatively inert and would not interact with the substance being potentised and the sugar content would act as a preservative. Using the decimal scale, he added 1 part of the mother substance e.g. pulverised quartz (for Silicea) or gold dust (for Aurum met.) to 9 parts of lactose and ground the mixture in a mortar and pestle for one hour to produce the 1X potency in powder form. This dry method of potentisation he termed 'trituration' and the resultant powder potency was called a 'triturate'. In modern laboratories, a ball mill can perform the laborious task of trituration. The mill comprises a ceramic pot containing a large number of ceramic balls of varying diameter. The ball mill is charged with the mixture of powdered substance and lactose and mechanically rolled for one hour so that the balls grind the mixture thoroughly. When large amounts of potentised material have to be prepared, such mills become indispensable. In modern practice, the laborious preparation of triturates by hand is impractical. Though many homeopaths are convinced that hand made potencies prepared by succussion or trituration remain the best, in practice, the higher potencies, which can feasibly only be produced by mechanical means, prove clinically effective.

As with liquid potencies, further potentising of insoluble substances proceeds by means of serial dilution, each potency being prepared from the one immediately preceding it (1 part to 9 parts lactose), but with each step being followed by trituration instead of succussion. After six such procedures, beginning with the raw substance and lactose, the 6X triturate (one millionth potency) is achieved and at this level of dilution any insoluble substance becomes soluble (can be colloidally dispersed) in alcohol or water. Although potencies beyond 6X can be prepared by continuing serial dilution with trituration (seldom done beyond the 12X), it is more practical to change from the 6X triturate to the liquid method of potentisation. To achieve this one part of the 6X triturate is dispersed and succussed in nine parts of alcohol and this colloidal solution forms the base for the following liquid potencies, prepared as described above. Because of this double step of dilution which is needed to progress from powder to liquid form, the first liquid potency prepared from an insoluble substance will be the 8X potency, or if the centesimal scale is used, the 4C potency.

Hahnemann's initial use of potencies

The potentising methodology described above gives the sequence of steps required to produce all the potencies of the homeopathic decimal and centesimal ranges, from the lowest to the highest, a scale, which in theory is infinite. But in 1798, Hahnemann's first sortie into the dimension of the infinitely small was very modest. It included only the 2X, 4X and the 2C potencies. A year later, in 1799, he had begun to venture further by developing and using the 5X, 6X, 3C and 8X. By 1800, he had advanced to the 10X and in 1803 a major leap took him to the 12C potency (the mathematical equivalent of the 24X).[4]

Avagadro constant

Scientifically, in achieving the 12C potency, Hahnemann had reached a critical point in the process of serial dilution. Mathematics reveals to us that in the sequence of serial dilution, a point is reached after 23 steps on the decimal scale (a dilution of 10^{-23}) when it can be mathematically proven that any further dilution cannot be expected to contain a single molecule or atom of the original medicinal substance from which it is derived. In scientific terms, this is known as the *Avogadro Constant*. Therefore, the 24X or 12C (10^{-24}) homeopathic potency, and any potency higher, contains no residual medicinal atoms whatsoever. Today, the 12C is regarded as still being at the lower (less potent) end of the potency scale. Most experienced homeopaths regularly use potencies far higher than this, e.g. 200C (10^{-400}); M (10^{-2000}); 10M ($10^{-20,000}$), all of which are devoid of medicinal substance. Since in practice *the curative power* of potencies continues to increase exponentially on a scale that extends infinitely beyond 10^{-23}, we can be certain that after the lowest potencies the remaining medicinal atoms still present in serial dilution up to 10^{-23} are irrelevant to the potentising process, which must be energy based.

Subtle, spiritual power

Serial dilution with succussion is a process of dematerialisation and the progressive release and imprinting of the carrier substance with a specific energy pattern, an ethereal medicinal template or subtle power derived from the potentised substance. We may not know the exact science of what transpires in the process of potentisation and we may never know how the energy pattern of a potentised substance can be indelibly inscribed and carried forward in lactose, distilled water or absolute alcohol, but we do know from 200 years of practical application that this is exactly what happens.

His biographer, Richard Haehl, considering the thinking behind Hahnemann's shift from mere dilution of remedies to potentisation, observes:

> ... with time there emerges ever more clearly the view that, by shaking and trituration, a uniform mixing, dilution and weakening of the medicinal substance is not all that is achieved; on the contrary, the material part of the medicine is thereby more and more eradicated and as a consequence the spiritual part of the medicine (not perceptible to human faculties) is released and extraordinarily increased. This is dynamisation.[5]

Hahnemann's later use of potencies

1805 brought the 18C into use, which Hahnemann found so effective that it remained his highest and most frequently used potency until 1816 when the 30C is first mentioned in his writings. Subsequently, this potency became his enduring favourite. Another preferred potency was the 24C. A careful audit of his prescribing towards the end of his career reveals that more than three quarters of his healing work was achieved through using the centesimal potencies 12, 18, 24, and 30.[6] Though, as we shall see, he did on occasion use potencies higher than the 30C, and in 1825 even went so far as to recommend Thuja 60C as being particularly effective in the treatment of gonorrhoea, nevertheless, 30C generally remained his optimal potency.

One can only imagine how Hahnemann must have felt when he first put these new potentised dilutions to the test. Given his intense faith, pragmatic thinking and meticulous method of preparation, it is highly probable that he fully anticipated success: he was not to be disappointed. Far from losing efficacy in the process of serial dilution, he found that, when chosen on the basis of similarity, the remedy's action was not only potentiated, but also accelerated and more profound. Even more significant was the discovery that the further he proceeded with successive serial dilution and succussion, the more curatively potent the remedy became. He therefore called the process of preparation 'potentisation' and the prepared dilutions 'potencies'.

He had discovered the vital **Second Law of Homeopathy** known as The Law of the Infinitesimal Dose – which states:

The curative power of a homeopathic potency increases in direct ratio to its degree of serial dilution with succussion (i.e. its degree of potentisation).

The Second Law of Homeopathy: *the Law of the Infinitesimal Dose*

To the uninitiated, this Second Law of Homeopathy, understood as stating that the weaker a substance becomes the more healing power it possesses, sounds absurd and illogical. It would be if it stated that the pharmacological strength of the homeopathic remedy was increased in direct ratio to its degree of dilution. The Law of the Infinitesimal Dose, however, expresses the ratio that exists between a remedy's curative power (not drug power) and its degree of potentisation *when prescribed according to the Law of Similars*. The two laws must be seen as interdependent! It is only when the remedy is selected according to its resemblance to the symptomatic picture of the patient that the healing power released through potentisation can prove effective. When close similarity exists between a remedy's picture [developed through provings] and the patient's clinical picture, the higher potencies, 30C and above, hold such patient-specific influence that they are able to thoroughly and beneficially penetrate and pervade the entire constitution of the patient, both physically and emotionally.

Benefits of potentisation

Potentisation brought all-important benefits to the science and practice of homeopathy, enabling Hahnemann to further develop the therapeutic scope of the law of similars:

- Potentisation intensifies (modulates) the curative energy and action of the similar remedy: as the potencies rise, energy packets of higher and higher frequency bearing the characteristic pattern of the remedy are released into the carrier medium, indelibly imprinting it.
- While affecting the entire organism, the lower potencies or frequencies exert their influence especially on the lower levels of the body's energy system, an influence that has a physical emphasis, more focused on organs and tissues.
- The higher potencies or frequencies are able to touch not only the physical but also the mental and emotional spheres, enabling the homeopath to treat even the deepest psychological disturbances.
- The use of a wide spectrum of potencies in pathogenetic trials (provings) produces a far more complete spectrum of remedy symptoms, ranging from the physical to the psychological.
- Substances previously too toxic for clinical use are rendered harmless and yet retain their curative power, which is progressively augmented during potentisation Examples of such remedies and their sources include Belladonna (deadly nightshade), Lachesis (Brazilian pit viper) and Mercury (the element).
- Essentially inert substances, which do not readily interact with the body, are rendered clinically active and curatively potent. Examples include Silicea (quartz) and Lycopodium (club moss).

Orthodox enmity

With the acquisition of the potentised form of the similar remedy, Hahnemann found that a new world of healing potential opened for his use. This, together with his growing experience in practising his new system of medicine and the widening clinical scope provided by his ever-expanding arsenal of remedies, brought him success and fame. His reputation spread and his practice in Leipzig thrived. The level of his success and the increasing public interest in his healing ability, coupled to his scathing attacks upon the methods of the orthodoxy and the ethics of the apothecaries, mixed envy with hatred, and provided fuel for an all-out attempt to stifle him, or, at least, expel him from Leipzig. It needed only the slenderest evidence of vulnerability for his enemies to vilify him. His peculiar destiny provided the opportunity.

References

1. Dudgeon RE. *Lectures on The Theory and Practice of Homeopathy*. New Delhi: B Jain Publishers; 1978. pp395–396.
2. Herr BJ. What is Homeopathy? Available online at: http://tinyurl.com/cnur55h
3. Jacobi J. *Paracelsus – Selected Writings*. London: Routledge & Kegan Paul Ltd; 1951. p167.
4. Morrell P. *Hahnemann & Homeopathy*. New Delhi: B Jain Publishers; 2003. p144.
5. Haehl R. *Samuel Hahnemann, His Life and Work*. Vol 1. London: Homoeopathic Publishing Company; 1922. p324.
6. Morrell P. *Hahnemann & Homeopathy*. New Delhi: B Jain Publishers; 2003. p153.

5

BESIEGED AND EXILED

The saga of Prince Karl Philipp

As we have related, on 19 October 1813, Prince Karl Philipp of Schwarzenburg (1771–1820), the renowned Austrian *Feldmarschall* and cousin of the King of Saxony, rode in triumph through the streets of Leipzig after his troops had inflicted a decisive defeat upon Napoleon. His military success and fame grew in subsequent campaigns against the French, culminating in the 'Battle of Paris' and the capture of the French capital on 13 March 1814, a victory which contributed to the final overthrow of Bonaparte. In recognition of his achievements, he received many honours and rewards, both from Austria and other grateful, foreign states, amongst which was an extensive country estate where he lived in great luxury with his adored wife, the Countess Nani of Hohenfield. Scarcely three years after conquering Paris, on 13 January 1817, when not yet 46, the Prince suffered a stroke, which paralysed his right side and left him with chronic insomnia and incapacitating lethargy. He had a reputation for very heavy drinking, but the stroke was thought to have been precipitated by the death of his beloved sister, Caroline, a short time before.

All the efforts of his doctors, the Royal Physician Field Surgeon Major Dr Jos Edler von Sax and the Imperial Regimental Surgeon Dr Mathias Marenzeller, failed to alleviate his suffering. Hahnemann's fame as a physician had already reached the court of the Austrian Emperor, Franz 1. Faced with such a difficult case and such an illustrious patient, Dr Marenzeller, who was favourably inclined towards homeopathy, proposed that Hahnemann should be consulted. As was the custom of the aristocracy, Hahnemann was requested to travel to Austria to attend the afflicted Field Marshall on his estate. Ironically, in the previous year, 1819, due to the machinations of the Imperial Medical Adviser von Stifft, an ardent opponent of the new method, the practice of homeopathy had been banned in Austria. Undoubtedly, had Hahnemann acceded to the request, some means would have been found to surmount this legal obstacle, but in the event, while consenting to treat Prince Karl, he stubbornly refused to be persuaded to leave Leipzig, and insisted that the patient should be brought to him.

So, despite his weakened condition, Prince Karl came to Hahnemann in Leipzig, with his two physicians in tow and a large retinue of servants in attendance and took up residence on a fairly large estate outside the city. This willingness on the part of the very influential prince says much for the renown and reputation that Hahnemann had attained in Central Europe. In consequence, a great deal of professional and popular interest was generated by Hahnemann's treatment of the prince.

No less a figure than Johann Wolfgang von Goethe, the great German literary figure, philosopher and polymath, commented on the anomaly of the situation:

> In this place a curious game is being played by refusing and damming up innovations of every kind. E.g. it is forbidden to cure by magnetism (Mesmer) and nobody is allowed to practise by Hahnemann's method.... But now Prince Schwarzenburg, very ill and probably incurable, has confidence in this new Theophrastus Paracelsus and begs leave of absence from the Emperor to seek a cure across the border.[3]

Goethe was very interested in homeopathy and in the fortunes of its discoverer. He had personally benefited from homeopathic treatment and referred to Hahnemann as "the wonder physician" and again as "the world famous physician".

Referring once more to the Schwarzenburg saga, he wrote in September 1820:

> I believe more than ever in this wonderful doctor's theory as I have experienced, and continue to experience, so clearly the efficacy of a very small administration. It should benefit Prince Schwarzenburg, just now staying in Leipzig for this very cure, as much as me; the doctor's fame and reward will not by any means suffer.[3]

That such a brilliant mind as Goethe's should have been deeply impressed with the homeopathic concept of healing and embraced it with such enthusiasm is significant and a reflection upon the lesser minds of today that struggle to perceive its validity.

He was correct in his evaluation of both Prince Karl's condition and his probable response to homeopathic treatment. He *was* incurable, suffering from advanced arteriosclerosis ('hardening of the arteries') and, whereas his condition had previously proved resistant, he did experience an initial, heartening improvement in his overall health, and that despite being displaced from his customary environment and distanced from the tender ministrations of his Countess. He expressed this in letters to his wife and friends in Austria informing them that his attacks had been alleviated and his condition was improving.[1] The example of Austria had alerted the prince to the fact that his physician stood on shaky, legal ground, and therefore, anxious to ensure that his treatment would continue and also to make a show of gratitude, he wrote to King Friederich of Saxony 'humbly' requesting that Hahnemann should not be refused by a decree of Government the right of treating patients in accordance with his new system. The polite, but politically cautious, response from the King assured the prince that Hahnemann would not in any way be hindered in his efforts to cure 'his dear friend', with this new method of treatment.[2] An attached letter from the King's secretary, however, explained to the prince that while there was no intention of forbidding Dr Hahnemann the right to practise homeopathy, in response to complaints from the apothecaries, the City Council was on the point of forbidding him the right to dispense his own medicines. The same document courteously congratulated the prince on his restoration to health.

Oh! that Providence should have then decreed that by some miracle Prince Karl's arteries could have been restored to their former supple elasticity. It might have smoothed the way, but this was not to be. Even when shouldering the responsibility of truth and right, the path of the hero is often arduous. Finding his strength quickening and able once again to take regular walks, Prince Karl lapsed into his former drinking habits. To this was added the interfering and dissuading influence of Dr von Sax, an inflexible allopath, who brought about inconsistency in the treatment regime and even persuaded the prince to continue with further bloodletting. Hahnemann, in the company of Dr Marenzeller, now a supporter of homeopathy, happened upon this scene and after what must have been an acrimonious altercation, removed himself and never visited the patient again. Five weeks later, and nearly six months after his arrival in Leipzig, Prince Karl died of another stroke, on 15 October 1820. Undismayed by the snide remarks and accusations of the allopaths, whose jubilance at the unfortunate outcome was only matched by their previous envy, Hahnemann proudly and defiantly walked in the cortege that followed the Prince's coffin through the streets that had so recently been the stage for his victor's triumph.

The autopsy was attended by homeopathy's most rabid antagonist – the ubiquitous Dr Clarus. It confirmed the diagnosis of a cerebral vascular accident, and revealed a gravely damaged heart and widespread arteriosclerosis – an incurable condition, with death as its consequence. A straightforward and uncomplicated conclusion, one would have thought. However, Dr Clarus abused his position and availing himself of the opportunity, used the post-mortem statement as a platform for an extremely personal attack against Hahnemann. After beginning unctuously that he, Clarus, did not envy the celebrity acquired by his colleague, he forgets his mandate and launches into a condemnatory tirade against homeopathy, claiming that it brought great injury by delaying the application of more powerful measures.[3] He omits to mention that the dead prince received 'more powerful measures' both before and after his homeopathic treatment and it would have been too much to expect him to mention the short-lived improvement the prince had experienced on commencing homeopathic therapy. These days, little has changed – benefit experienced under homeopathic treatment is explained away by the so-called placebo effect – a psychosomatic, expectancy response – and when a cure is achieved, it is explained away as being the result of spontaneous remission or mistaken diagnosis.

The apothecaries make their move

With Prince Karl's death, the considerable forces arrayed against Hahnemann swung into action. Although his medical brethren would have willingly brought him down, it was the apothecaries who possessed the means. They ridiculed the homeopathic potencies as being mere 'nothings' and totally ineffective, but, nonetheless, they wished to impose upon homeopaths the dispensing restraints that applied to allopathic drugs. This would give them almost complete control over the dispensing of homeopathic remedies, a process for which they had no understanding, training or sympathy. The homeopath would only be permitted to dispense in rural areas at considerable distance from the nearest town; in emergency situations when immediate dispensing was imperative; in areas where there were no apothecaries; or without charge to the poor. The Saxon Government finally yielded to the pressure of the apothecaries and issued this prohibition by royal edict. But the wolves were not sated. They came forward with a further complaint and representation for the imposition of even tighter restrictions, because they feared that Hahnemann would abuse the privileges retained within the edict. This was refused, but the petitioners were advised to 'report individual cases of misuse occurring from this cause.'[4]

This was a struggle that would continue to dog Hahnemann and his disciples throughout his life. To the end, he resolutely defended the right of homeopaths to dispense their own remedies. Paradoxically, it remained for a medical adversary, the Professor of Medicine, Dr Riecke, of Tübingen, to make a speech in support of this right, in 1833:

> The homeopathic doctor must above all prepare his drugs himself – not a very difficult matter considering the simplicity of their composition. Now since all homoeopathic doses have neither chemical reaction, nor colour, nor smell, nor taste, there can be no imaginable means of being convinced of the genuineness of such a dose unless it be the doctor's consciousness of care in the preparation. . . . Homoeopathy here stumbles against medicinal laws allowing only the apothecaries to prepare medicines.[5]

On every professional level, the animosity and envy of the medical fraternity was brought to bear on Hahnemann. He was ostracised at the University, he was attacked in the press by a group of thirteen doctors for claiming to be the first to advise Belladonna as a treatment and prophylaxis for scarlet fever, his students were threatened and persecuted and the apothecaries watched his every step. Life in Leipzig had become intolerable and Hahnemann decided that he could no longer stay. In a letter to Dr Billig, written from Leipzig in February 1821, he gives his reasons:

> By the public proceedings directed against me by the Saxon medical men, you will have learned (I am sure with grief) how bitterly my method of treatment and its author are persecuted in this country. This persecution has now reached its climax, and I should be doing an injury to the beneficent art, and imperilling my own life, were I to remain longer here and not seek protection in some foreign country.[6]

Köthen – a safe haven

After much uncertainty, he finally decided to move his family to the small, country town of Köthen in the minor, but autonomous, central German principality of Anhalt-Köthen. Today, such a move, a mere 50 kilometres North-West of Leipzig, would be regarded as merely a relocation from one part of Germany to another, but in Hahnemann's time it was equivalent to entering a 'foreign country.' For Hahnemann, given his intense love for his Saxon homeland, it was a severe dislocation. It came on the heels of a forced capitulation, exacerbated by having to relinquish his University post, a stage which he so enjoyed and which he had fought so hard to attain. He was forced to distance himself from his students, abandon his successful practice and yet again uproot his family. He never reconciled himself to life in Köthen, so removed from the stimulating, if threatening, intellectual energy of Leipzig. Writing fully 10 years later, in 1831, he refers to 'this miserable hole, where for the first five years not two people of repute in the town had need of me.'[7] Fortunately, the nine years he had spent in Leipzig, despite all his tribulations, had proved lucrative and the Hahnemann family would not experience privation again. Hahnemann vowed to leave his eight heirs enough for each of them to live on the interest without working.[8]

The principality was ruled by the kind-hearted and broadminded, Ferdinand, Duke of Anhalt-Köthen. He was a patient of Hahnemann's and also a brother Freemason. He gladly extended permission for Hahnemann to settle down in Köthen and furthermore granted Hahnemann's request (or demand as Haehl expresses it) that he be given leave while practising there to prepare and administer his medicines without the intervention of the apothecaries. Early in June 1821, the family convoy of eleven wooden wagons loaded with the Hahnemann family possessions arrived in Köthen (twenty-eight years before, a single wagon had sufficed when they departed from Georgenthal).[9] After all the storms, Hahnemann had at last reached the tranquil waters of a provincial retreat.

The house in which Hahnemann lived from 1821 to 1835 is situated in the Wallstrasse and has now become a Hahnemann museum. It is a double story, corner building and in Hahnemann's time had a small garden in the rear with an ivy-covered arbour, next to which he built a summer house where he could write and at the same time enjoy closer contact with nature. It was here that he would produce the third, fourth and fifth editions of the *Organon*; the second and third editions of the *Materia Medica Pura*; and his monumental work *The Chronic Diseases, Their Peculiar Nature and Their Homoeopathic Treatment* (see Chapter 6) in which he elaborated for the first time his concepts of *vitalism* and the *chronic miasms*.

Hahnemann in his sixties

Hahnemann was now 66 yrs of age, and, with the perspective of the times, deemed himself an old man. In fact, he was but three-quarters of the journey along his life's path and still vital in both mind and body. This energy, which never deserted him, was maintained and invigorated by the continuous application of his prodigious intellect and regular exercise. He had already experienced family tragedy and loss, the death of baby Ernst and, in 1818, of his second daughter, Wilhelmine, who had married a music director.

Samuel Hahnemann was a complex being, a multifaceted blend of quite extreme opposites: at once brilliant yet naive, reserved and expansive, cautious and impetuous, diffident and arrogant, homely and grandiose, conservative and eccentric, sensitive yet tactless, serious and humorous, warm and caring yet at other times so removed and seemingly indifferent. And not least of all were the stark contrasts that existed between his abrasive truculence and his tender vulnerability, his utter conviction and his curious uncertainty and his absolute faith in Providence and yet his perennial paranoia; surely, echoes of his predecessor, Paracelsus?

Ernst George, Baron von Brunnow, gives us an intimate picture of the master in his early 60's, while still in Leipzig:

> Locks of silver-white hair clustered round his high and thoughtful brow, from under which his animated eyes shone with piercing brilliancy. His whole countenance had a quiet searching, grand expression; only rarely did a gleam of fine humour play over the deep earnestness, which told of the many sorrows and conflicts endured. His carriage was upright, his step firm, his motions as lively as those of a man of thirty. When he went out his dress was of the simplest; a dark coat, with short small clothes and stockings. But in his room at home he preferred the old household, gaily-figured, dressing gown, the yellow stockings and the black velvet cap.[10]

Viewing his sculpted bust of 1829, cast in bronze by Dietrich, one is struck by the nobility, intelligence and strength of his features, dominated by a broad expanse of brow, an aquiline nose, a stubborn forward thrust of the lower lip and a resolute jaw, all framed by a profusion of locks encircling his bald pate.

Hartmann describes how Hahnemann presided over the evening *soirée*, which began at eight o'clock at his home in Leipzig, when family, friends, students and learned minds would gather round him, like children at the feet of an august and paternal figure. On these occasions, he shed his

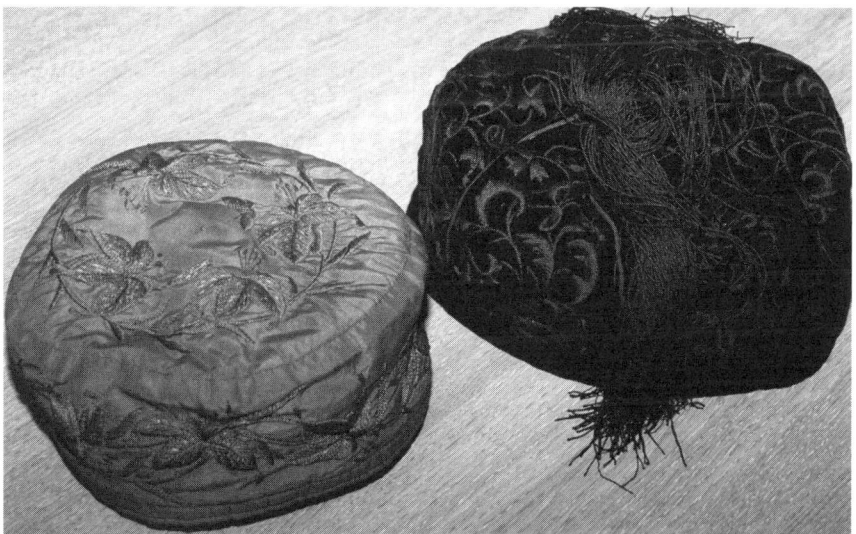

Figure 5.1 *Two silk and velvet caps belonging to Hahnemann*
Faculty of Homeopathy Collection

serious demeanour and revealed an engaging and delightful sense of humour, familiarity and openness that charmed his audience. He sat in his armchair wearing a velvet cap (examples of which are shown in Figure 5.1) and dressing gown, with a glass of light Leipzig white beer and his pipe.

Both cap and the long pipe, which was seldom out of his hand, were essential props to his comfort and relaxation. When expounding animatedly on the doings of his orthodox colleagues, he would move the little cap too and fro on his head and puff out clouds of tobacco smoke, which enveloped him like a fog.[11] If the pipe should go out, one of his ever-watchful daughters would immediately re-ignite it. He particularly liked to converse about the natural sciences and foreign cultures, with a singular preference for the Chinese, and invited and encouraged others to voice their thoughts and opinions. The guests would depart by 11p.m.

Ducal patronage and protection

In Köthen, due to the reputation that preceded him and his connection to Duke Ferdinand, he was soon able to establish a successful and profitable practice, which he set up in his new home. Initially he was assisted by two young doctors who had accompanied him from Leipzig, Dr August Haynel and Dr Theodore Mossdorf, the latter being engaged to Hahnemann's youngest daughter, Louise. Eleonore, Charlotte and Louise, acted as receptionists and were responsible for the filing of correspondence and case reports. Hahnemann never saw eye to eye with Mossdorff, and Henriette never approved of him as a husband for their "little *Louischen*". She proved right, and both were undoubtedly relieved when he and Louise finally divorced and he passed out of their lives. Haynel remained a member of the family for more than ten years, proved a number of remedies for Hahnemann, and eventually emigrated to America where he practised homeopathy in various cities, finally dying in Dresden in 1877 at 81.

The Duke continued to be an enthusiastic patient and very soon persuaded his wife, the Duchess Julie, to seek Hahnemann's help. The Duke's health improved so markedly that in 1823 he wrote:

> While expressing to you my thanks for your medical help this year, and for the last two years and assuring you of my complete satisfaction, I wish you to accept the enclosed trifle as a slight recompense for your medicine and your services. May heaven preserve you in good health for many years to the benefit of suffering humanity.[13]

The Duke was so delighted at his restored health and so admiring of Hahnemann's work that he ordered the local newspaper to publish a report on the successful outcome of his treatment and express his gratitude publicly. On May 13, 1822, the Duke had made Hahnemann *Hofrath*, an honorary title bestowed by princes on persons they particularly wished to distinguish.

The Duchess also responded well to Hahnemann's treatment and the two established an affectionate relationship:

> *My best thanks, my dear Hofrath, for your kind wishes on my birthday.*
>
> *I owe to your exertions one of the pleasantest gifts on entering on a new year, improved health.*
>
> *I hope to preserve this to your praise and credit.*
>
> *With sincere pleasure,*
>
> *Yours affectionately,*
>
> *Julie, Duchess of Anhalt.*[12]

Under the protection and patronage of the Duke and Duchess, Hahnemann spent the following years of his life in the calm and relaxing, rural atmosphere of Köthen. Though he resented the need to seek refuge there and by association felt an undying resentment against the town itself, it was to furnish him with circumstances ideal for the work still to be done. The Duke provided him with a substantial, retaining salary that was independent of his private practice. He could at last relax about his finances, practise according to his desire and know that his family would be comfortably cared for. For Frau Henriette, now a rather corpulent, elderly lady, Köthen must have seemed a haven sent from heaven.

Different horizons

With varied intensity, the attacks against homeopathy continued to wax and wane, as they have to this very day, but although still possessed of youthful vigour and an incisive, enquiring mind, age had, indeed, changed Hahnemann. He no longer had any relish for such battles and he left to the young bloods that were emerging, the task of championing the new science of healing. He remained silently in the background, passively unresponsive to hostile provocation. In the years to come, he only became embroiled when disputes arose within the homeopathic fraternity, often, unfortunately, still displaying his customary lack of diplomacy and objectivity, lending his ear to one or other party and often thereby contributing to the discord rather than resolving it. He was never skilled as a mediator or medical politician. His withdrawal from the epicentre of antagonism against homeopathy and equally from the heartland of homeopathy's germination and spread, lost to the cause a unifying, central figure and very soon disagreements developed amongst homeopaths of differing tendencies and persuasion. A pattern of internecine conflict within the homeopathic family was established from the very outset and at times still tends to plague the profession.

From his central position in the vanguard, surrounded by his immediate students and in the background supported by an increasing number of converts, he abruptly retired from the fray. At the time, the feud was at its height. He knew all too well the trials that would beset his disciples, he himself had long been the butt of professional opposition, yet there is no evidence that he in any way concerned himself with their plight or assisted them before or after his departure. Although himself immune to any consequences arising from the verdicts, he left to their own fate two of his closest friends who were facing trial for practising illegally. This indifference was foreshadowed by a previous incident when in submitting his defence in support of his right to both prescribe and dispense, he denied being a mouthpiece for his pupils and pointedly emphasised that he was not associated with them and did not represent them.

Haehl reports that in contemplating this anomaly, Georg Otto Kleinert wrote:

> That homœopathy assumed defined shape and developed strength to live and overcome obstacles is much more the result of their (the students and disciples) labours than that of Hahnemann.

He could not have been more effusive in their praise:

> In spite of every species of adversity, not infrequently proceeding from the master himself, they stood like beacon-lights of fidelity, and, when it became necessary, distinguished between the precious doctrine and its prophet, between the jewel and its setting.[13]

There can be no doubt that a marked and profound transformation had been unconsciously and irresistibly unfolding within the Master, and, synchronising with events, inevitably drew him into the next chapter of a life crucial for humanity. Such inexorable forces could not tarry for what in the scales of destiny were petty and circumscribed upheavals. His seeming indifference to the welfare of those closest to him and to the survival of homeopathy was due to his inner vision already shifting its attention to more distant and deeper horizons. Homeopathy had taken root, its continuance assured, his followers up to the task of defending and disseminating it, and, it must be admitted, more able in this than he. His attention was needed elsewhere for the uncovering and elaboration of a theory of disease causation that would shake even the credulity of his staunchest adherents.

The withdrawn energy, charged with all the passion and intensity that had previously sought to overthrow singlehandedly the entire edifice of conventional medicine and establish in its place a gentle doctrine of healing, now, fostered by the security and calm of Köthen and undisturbed by the distant tremors in Leipzig, addressed the deepest aspects of the nature of disease and the process of cure.

References

1. Cook TM. *Samuel Hahnemann – The Founder of Homoeopathic Medicine*. Northampton: Thorson Publishers; 1981. p120.
2. *Ibid.*, p121.
3. Haehl R. *Samuel Hahnemann, His Life and Work*. Vol 1. London: Homoeopathic Publishing Company; 1922. p113.
4. *Ibid.*, p114.
5. *Ibid.*, p115.
6. Bradford TL. *The Life and Letters of Samuel Hahnemann*. London: Homoeopathic Publishing Company; 1894. p122.
7. Haehl R. *Samuel Hahnemann, His Life and Work*. Vol 1. London: Homoeopathic Publishing Company; 1922. p118.
8. *Ibid.*, p119.
9. Cook TM. *Samuel Hahnemann – The Founder of Homoeopathic Medicine*. Northampton: Thorson Publishers; 1981. p133.
10. Bradford TL. *The Life and Letters of Samuel Hahnemann*. London: Homoeopathic Publishing Company; 1894. p110.
11. Cook TM. *Samuel Hahnemann – The Founder of Homoeopathic Medicine*. Northampton: Thorson Publishers; 1981. p110.
12. Bradford TL. *The Life and Letters of Samuel Hahnemann*. London: Homoeopathic Publishing Company; 1894. pp131–132.
13. *Ibid.*, p138.

6

THE CHRONIC DISEASES

A profound and controversial text

The years in Leipzig had provided him with considerable practical experience in the use of homeopathy over a wide spectrum of clinical conditions, both acute and chronic. He had fully tested and proven the principles he had laid out in the early editions of the *Organon*. He had revealed how disease should be treated. He now began to ponder how disease first arose and why. Why disease manifests in so many different forms? Was there a presiding and integrating law behind the evolution of these varied manifestations? What was the nature of the energy or force that maintained the body in its state of health, and why, and how, did it become so perturbed that its regulatory power failed – so that even a simple wound might fester and fail to heal? Why and how did the infinitesimal dose have the power to restore the balanced function of this regulating force? Was the healing power released by potentisation related to it? What role did the emotional life play in the development of disease and was it able to detrimentally impinge on the function of this vital force.

In seeking the answers to these questions, he pushed back the obscuring shroud of medical ignorance and revealed a landscape of subtle yet immense proportions, which continues to unfold to this day. After years of silent research and practical application, he finally presented the fruits of his investigations in his last great medical work, *Chronic Diseases: Their Peculiar Nature and Their Homœopathic Cure*, which was published in 1828. The theories he postulated remain at the cutting edge of homeopathic philosophy and are increasingly valued in homeopathic practice. Modern medicine still remains in ignorance of this wisdom, and, without a major shift, its materialistic paradigm is unlikely to recognise or fathom it. His thoughts were so far ahead of his time that few, even among his most ardent followers, were able to accept his conclusions. To many, it seemed that the old man had lost his way and had yielded to the fancies of his imagination. Others misinterpreted aspects of his argument and so added to the general confusion. To the allopaths, it's content was an even greater cause for mirth and mockery than the infinitesimal dose had been.

The great controversy generated by this book served to further disrupt the ranks of his followers and contributed to the creation of different paths that developed within the homeopathic discipline.

Haehl comments on this furore:

> Few books have stirred up more excitement in the medical world than Hahnemann's *Chronic Diseases*. His conception of these diseases and, in particular, his Psora Theory, aroused the criticism of friend and foe to a tremendous extent from the very moment of their publication. At this point many of his adherents and students refused to follow him any further.[1]

Some critics, dismayed by the disunity it created, and weighing this rather than the book's defining importance, declared that it might have been better for the homeopathic cause had it never been published. It is only in recent times that Hahnemann's theory of disease causation has become pivotal to homeopathic philosophy and a major influence in many homeopaths' prescribing strategy.

The *Psora theory* to which Haehl refers, was central to Hahnemann's argument and postulated a disease continuum of latent disease potential that is handed down from generation to generation.

His deliberations during the latter years in Leipzig and the early years in Köthen were concentrated on unravelling the enigma of disease causation. He was convinced that such an understanding would make it possible to treat disease in a logical and structured way, particularly when dealing with chronic disease. He knew full well the importance of incorrect diet, lack of exercise, poor living conditions, negative environmental influences, pollution and the ill effects of emotional and physical trauma – the 'morbific agents' that he had spoken of in his *Organon* – all of which had to be taken into consideration in the management of any case of disease, but he further intuited the existence of something more fundamental, something insidious and hidden, a pernicious undercurrent that sustained the visible manifestations of disrupted health and was responsible for the peculiar susceptibilities of individuals.

Relapsing chronic disease

In his early practice of homeopathy, Hahnemann observed that despite removing all hindrances to cure, and successfully treating acute conditions, such cases showed a repeated tendency to relapse, presenting either a recurrence of similar or more severe symptoms, or in many instances the emergence of a changed or different clinical picture. It was as if some underlying condition, which had remained unaddressed by even the most carefully selected and successful remedy, continued on its inexorable course. His experience with cases of chronic disease proved similar: initial improvement would be followed by relapse and previously successful remedies inexplicably lost their efficacy.[4]

In the theoretical section of *Chronic Diseases*, he expresses this in uncompromising terms:

> Their beginning was promising, the continuation less favourable, the outcome hopeless.

but he adds, with emphasis:

> **Nevertheless, this teaching** (the homeopathic method) **was founded upon the steadfast pillar of truth and will evermore be so.**[2]

His followers, confronted by the same therapeutic stalemate, consoled themselves that this was due to the still limited number of homeopathic remedies at their disposal. The Master, however, gifted with a deeper insight, and also with proof that the continuous addition of new and valuable remedies to the materia medica had not advanced a solution, was not in the least satisfied with this explanation, and bent his mind to find the answer.

> This very serious task has occupied me since the years 1816 and 1817, night and day: and behold! the Giver of all good things permitted me within this space of time to gradually solve this sublime problem through unremitting thought, indefatigable inquiry, faithful observation, and the most accurate experiments made for the welfare of humanity.[3]

Miasms

With his characteristic thoroughness, he set about searching for patterns of disease in patients and in their family histories to explain and solve the problem of this phenomenon. After a period of intensive investigation, his conclusion was that like waves on a vast ocean, both the manifestations of acute illness and the symptoms and signs of chronic disease were superficial expressions of a deeper, hidden, destructive force, and that only treatment which addressed this underlying condition would prove permanently curative.[4]

In keeping with the language of his time, Hahnemann called this morbid influence, or force, a *miasm*, an expression for something noxious and ubiquitous in the atmosphere, like an infectious or toxic vapour. The term *miasm*, is therefore, aptly described as being:

> The concept of an undermining, pervasive process of contamination or pollution of the system, a blight or stigma, acquired or inherited, which renders the individual susceptible to certain patterns of illness.[4]

Hahnemann perceived the miasmic influence to be inherent in every constitution, present from birth, progressive through life, transferred by inheritance and exacerbated and increased by acquired disease and the travails of physical existence. An unbroken continuum extending from the distant past, from our very origin as a species, through the generations to the present time and responsible for the multiple expressions of disease that afflict us. The concept of such a disease continuum was totally new to medical thinking and proved difficult for his contemporaries to understand, even for those who otherwise supported him. To this day, diseases are placed in categories without conceiving, in the words of Hahnemann, that:[5]

> They must all have their foundation in the original malady and can only be part of a far greater whole.

> The original malady sought for must be also of a **miasmatic**, chronic nature clearly appeared to me from this circumstance, that after it has once advanced and developed to a certain degree, it can never be removed by the strength of any robust constitution, it can never be overcome by the most wholesome diet and order of life, nor will it die out of itself. But it is ever more aggravated, from year to year, through transition into other and more serious symptoms, even till the end of man's life, like every other chronic, miasmatic sickness.[5]

He likens the nature of the original, underlying disease-cause, or miasm, to that of syphilis, which was known at the time to possess just such chronicity and the capacity, overtime, to unfold ever-worse manifestations of its otherwise hidden presence, irrespective of how strong the constitution or how virtuous the habits, until finally it encroached on sanity and life itself.

In *Chronic Diseases*, Hahnemann identifies the presence of three major chronic miasms: the first and most fundamental, he named the 'Psoric Miasm'. At the time, 'psora' was a common generic word used to describe a wide array of different skin diseases. It derived from the Hebrew word *tsorat* – meaning a groove or fault, a pollution or stigma – therefore, an ideal term for his vision of a primal blemish from which all other diseases arose and which first betrayed its presence by producing an itching irritation of the skin. He termed it a *non-venereal chronic disease* to distinguish it from the other two miasms he recognised: the *Sycotic Miasm* and the *Syphilitic Miasm*, which he directly connected to the venereal diseases, Gonorrhoea and Syphilis, respectively.

His exposition of the nature of *Psora* and its widespread ramifications, so diverse and multifaceted that he called it 'hydra-headed,' and his identification of gonorrhoea and syphilis as being critical elements in the development of the miasmatic continuum are profound, but also astounding, not only for his innovative thinking, the product of acute powers of observation and deduction, but also because his conclusions predated the germ theory of Louis Pasteur and Robert Koch and the genetic model of Gregor Mendel. Whereas, previously, the symptoms and signs of gonorrhoea and syphilis had been lumped together as a single venereal entity, Hahnemann perceptively recognised the indications that they were undoubtedly two separate sexually transmitted infections, each leaving in its wake its own peculiar disease legacy.

Psora

The greater part of *Chronic Diseases* is devoted to the subject of *Psora*: its origin, expression and cure. Hahnemann understood *Psora* to be the mother of all disease, ancient in its beginnings and tenacious, inveterate and subversive in its nature:

> **Psora** is that **most ancient, most universal, most destructive**, and yet **most misapprehended** chronic miasmatic disease, which for many thousands of years has disfigured and tortured mankind, and which during the last centuries has become the mother of all the thousands of incredibly various acute and chronic (non-venereal) diseases, by which the whole civilised human race . . . is being more and more afflicted.[6]

And he adds, with a vision as all encompassing as the miasm he descibes:

> **Psora** is the **oldest** miasmatic disease known to us . . . the most ancient history of the most ancient people does not reach its origin . . . not to be extinguished before the last breath of the longest life, unless it is thoroughly cured, since not even the most robust constitution is able to destroy and annihilate it by its own innate strength. Without the aid of art it is ineradicable.[6]

He understood it to be a constitutional disease, pervading the entire system, which despite its antiquity and extent, was first manifested externally as an itch or eruption upon the skin – hence its other appellation: the *Itch Miasm*. This was its most innocent and elementary form, so misleading in its simplicity as to delude the physician into thinking it easy to treat by external means. Like an iceberg, it gave little indication of the dangers beneath. Though seemingly slight and superficial, it nevertheless represented and was sustained by the internal state of *Psora*, which he therefore referred to as the 'Internal Itch.' The itching eruption, often in the form of fluid-filled vesicles, provided a safety valve for the miasmic force beneath and displayed the self-healing activity of the body's *vital force*: the autonomous, regulating and harmonising life energy that maintains the healthy balance of all the functions of the material body. The rash announced not only a healing response, but also a deep and thorough disturbance of the vital force, which necessitated this response. It constituted, the "outwardly reflected picture of the internal essence of the disease, that is, of the affection of the vital force."[7]

He compared the development of chronic miasmatic disease to that of, what he termed, the *acute miasms*, or children's illnesses (exanthemata or eruptive fevers), such as measles, chicken pox and scarlet fever. In these conditions, there is:

- Firstly the moment of infection.
- Secondly, a silent, incubation period, during which the infective organism progressively permeates the entire system.
- Thirdly, after this latent stage of saturation, the disturbed vital force produces a curative response to counter and eliminate the infection by fever and an eruption characteristic of the invading contagion ("... whereby nature externally demonstrates the completion of the internal development of the miasmatic malady throughout the whole organism").[8]

He emphasises the fact that the 'malady' or miasm, be it acute or chronic, is first imbedded centrally and then through the action of the vital force announces its presence peripherally. He identifies a similar sequence in far more severe conditions such as smallpox and rabies and asserts that chronic miasmatic disease observes the same course, first establishing itself throughout the entire economy prior to its effect being projected outwards by the defensive reaction of the vital force. However, whereas, in acute miasms the thoroughly developed eruption, or other form of externalisation, ensures that healing will be complete and without complication, in chronic miasms these external manifestations, while relieving and hindering further inroads of disease, fail to resolve the centrally based condition, which, without homeopathic treatment, persists and progresses throughout life.

Referring specifically to *Psora* he writes graphically:

> Only when the whole organism feels itself transformed by the peculiar chronic-miasmatic disease, (does) the diseased vital force endeavour to alleviate and to soothe the internal malady through the establishment of a suitable local symptom on the skin, the itch vesicle. So long as this eruption continues in its normal form, the internal Psora with its secondary ailments, cannot break forth, but must remain covered, slumbering, latent and bound.[9]

As long as the external eruption or other peripheral expression of *Psora* remains undisturbed, the causative disease, although still active and slowly increasing, is held within bounds and the general health of the sufferer remains good. Its expression is restricted to the least harmful level – the skin. As the internal condition advances, it necessitates a corresponding increase in the skin symptom, even to a point where it may become generalised, covering most of the body, but still limited to the skin. However, if the external relieving condition should be suppressed by allopathic means and the skin clears, the disease will be pushed back upon itself, remain latent for a varying time and then according to its nature and the constitution of the patient, break forth with renewed vigour, often striking at a deeper and more harmful level.

He also recognised that even in the absence of suppression through medical intervention, the inexorable advance of untreated *Psora*, must reach a point where it can no longer relieve itself satisfactorily upon the surface, and would then, by its own impetus, inevitably move inwards with more dire consequences due to disruption of body function. The disappearance of the surface symptoms (often seen in cases of eczema at puberty) would delude both the physician and the patient into thinking that a spontaneous remission or cure had taken place. The further history of the patient would prove otherwise.

In the light of this, it is understandable that Hahnemann, in *Chronic Diseases*, sternly and repeatedly warns against the dangers of suppressing the external manifestations of miasmatic disease. The deleterious effect of such suppression applies not only to the external phase of *Psora*, but also to those of gonorrhoea and syphilis.

Sycosis

Hahnemann called the chronic miasmatic disease linked to mal-treated, suppressed or neglected gonorrhoea, *Sycosis*. The word is derived from the Greek, *'sykon,'* meaning fig. *Sycosis* therefore means 'fig-wart' disease, a name that aptly describes the warty excrescences that often flourish on the external genitalia of those suffering from the miasm. Another external manifestation of the sycotic miasm is catarrhal discharge. In gonorrhoea, caused by the sexually transmitted organism *Neisseria gonorrhoea*, after an incubation period lasting from 4 to 6 days, a yellow-green, purulent, itching, urethral discharge appears, which (as in the case of the eruption in *Psora*) manifests when the vital force reacts to the perfusion of the entire system with gonorrhoeal miasmatic energy and attempts to force its invasive effect outwards, away from the vital organs.

Syphilis

Similarly in syphilis, transmitted by a pale, thread-like, spiral organism, *Treponema pallidum*, the vital force protects the body to the best of its ability by externalising the disease through an ulcerous lesion on the skin or mucous membrane, called a chancre. Hahnemann noted that if any of these external manifestations were suppressed by the crude methods popular at the time, the disease would move deeper and eventually reappear in an exaggerated and *miasmatic* form. Also, like *Psora*, left untreated homeopathically, both the sycotic and syphilitic miasms would steadily progress penetrating ever more deeply into the patient's constitution.

In considering the allopathic approach to these diseases, he pinpoints two weaknesses, which, to a greater or lesser degree, still exist to this day. Firstly, to regard the outward clinical presentation of a case as constituting the disease in its entirety, and therefore, to concentrate on the control or removal of this and to be satisfied when this objective is achieved, and secondly, failure to recognise in the 'new' conditions that later arise, the secondary consequence of such manipulative suppression, and the uncured continuity of the underlying condition, which has neither been addressed nor eliminated.

> In their narrowness of mind ... all the sufferings, which follow the one-sided destruction of the cutaneous eruption, which belongs to the natural form of the Psora, they passed off as a newly arisen disease, owing to quite a different origin.[10]

While no one today would consider the urethral discharge as representing the entirety of gonorrhoea or the chancre to be all that there is of syphilis, nonetheless, in practice so much of modern medicine reflects the same narrow perspective that Hahnemann detected, treatment being confined to dealing with the presenting features of a clinical condition, rather than treating the patient in their entirety.

Miasmatic treatment

In *Chronic Diseases*, Hahnemann not only identifies the existence of the three major miasmatic currents existing beneath the surface of every disease, he also provides a means to address these hindrances, which had previously frustrated his efforts to bring cases to a successful conclusion.

The materia medica section gives the emotional and physical, symptomatic pictures of what he deemed the most important 'ant-psoric remedies' (remedies most frequently indicated in the treatment of *Psora*) – some 48 remedies in all. This range includes some remedies, which today would be regarded as predominantly *anti-sycotic* or *anti-syphilitic* rather than anti-psoric, e.g. Aurum (gold), Nitric acid, Mezereum, Guaiacum, but at that time when the scope of each miasm was still emerging for him, he presents *Psora* as almost all-encompassing, its grossest form even culminating in the ghastly picture of leprosy. In reconciling his conclusions with modern understanding, it must be remembered that the full extent of the chronic forms of syphilis was at the time still unrecognised, as was the relationship between leprosy and tuberculosis. Knowing *Psora* to be the origin or 'mother of all disease', its presence being essential before either *Sycosis* or *Syphilis* can take root, Hahnemann attributed to its inroads far more serious and widespread, pathological states than contemporary homeopaths do, given our current knowledge of bacteriology and pathology. Today, *Psora* is understood to be the initial layer or foundation of all disease, but in its uncomplicated form is limited to psychosomatic illness and diseases that are restricted to disturbed function without the presence of organic change. *Psora* does not incline, like *Sycosis*, to proliferation of tissues (warts and other excrescences) and catarrhal discharges (thick and pus-like), or, like *Syphilis* (and leprosy), to ulceration and destruction of tissues.

Psora – Sulphur

Of the anti-psoric remedies that Hahnemann used in addressing the deeper aspects of the chronic miasm *Psora*, the most central and fundamental was Sulphur, a remedy which came down to him from antiquity as an outstanding, topical remedy for skin diseases. Because he discerned that *Psora*, in one form or another, was present or latent ('slumbering') in all his patients, he often initiated treatment with Sulphur. He found it to be a remedy, which could at once clear the decks of previous allopathic interference and suppression, address the psoric elements of the case, and bring greater clarity by evoking symptoms. These 'new symptoms' when added to the original picture, often indicated the remedy most likely to follow in the treatment of the patient. This ability of Sulphur to act centrifugally, throwing things (including symptoms and signs) outward onto the surface, is not surprising considering the element's involvement in volcanic activity; its tell-tale noxious odour always pervading the vicinity of geysers and volcanic vents.

He did not propose that Sulphur was a cure-all, but rather an initiator to prompt a curative reaction and to facilitate the response to subsequently chosen remedies. He recognised that in the majority of psoric cases, Sulphur, on its own, is not sufficient; most often several remedies in sequence prove necessary to achieve a complete cure.

Syphilis – Mercurius

His remedy of choice in treating the syphilitic miasm was a preparation of mercury, which he developed and called Mercurius solubilis. The indication for this remedy also dropped into his lap, because the orthodox school had for generations been making great play with mercury in the treatment of syphilis, and its value in such cases was beyond doubt, despite the horrific symptoms of toxicity, which the hefty allopathic doses provoked. Moreover, the toxicology of this remarkable substance so accurately mimicked the many faces of the mercurial, syphilitic disease that its homeopathic suitability for the condition was clearly apparent. However, it would only be the potentised form of mercury that could keen the body's immune system, alert it to the presence of its almost invisible invader and cause it to mount an effective defensive response, without the danger of suppression and poisoning.

With Sulphur and Mercurius in place for *Psora* and *Syphilis*, Hahnemann lacked only the signature remedy for *Sycosis*. Providence once again smiled on him, as she had in the critical cinchona experiment of so many years before, but this time the inspiration came not through an experiment, but ironically, considering the nature of the miasm, in the shape of a gentleman of the Church.

Sycosis – Thuja

A young clergyman sought Hahnemann's advice regarding an irritating, greenish, urethral discharge with inflammation and swelling of the genitals. On questioning, he stoutly denied any sexual contact that could have accounted for his affliction. Respecting his honesty, Hahnemann refrained from prescribing and asked him to report again in three days. On his return, all symptoms had passed away and he confessed to an unusual feeling of wellbeing. He then recalled that whilst sauntering through a garden he had broken off and chewed a sprig of *Arbor vitae*; the discharge had commenced shortly afterwards. This episode led to provings, which confirmed that Thuja was capable of producing phenomena identical to gonorrhoea, including its chronic consequences, and was the pre-eminent remedy for the gonorrhoea-related sycotic constitution (*Sycosis*).[11] In his introduction to the symptom picture of the remedy, contained in his *Materia Medica Pura*, Hahnemann writes:

> The pure effects of this uncommonly powerful medicinal substance will be regarded by the homoeopathic practitioner as a great addition to his medicinal treasury, and he will not fail to make a useful application of it in some of the most serious diseases of mankind, for which hitherto there has been no remedy.[12]

Thuja occidentalis, one of several world trees given the designation *Arbor vitae*, tree of life, is the northern white cedar or marsh cedar, a very attractive conifer, often used as an ornamental tree to beautify formal gardens. In *Chronic Diseases*, under the heading *Sycosis*, Hahnemann strongly advocates the use of Thuja in the treatment of the sycotic miasm:

> The Gonorrhoea dependent on the Figwart Miasm . . . (the whole Sycosis) . . . (is) cured most certainly and most thoroughly through the internal use of Thuja, which in this case is homeopathic.[13]

And, further on, he advises that after Thuja has exhausted its action, it should be followed by Nitric acid in order to complete the cure. Since Hahnemann wrote these words, experience with these two remedies has repeatedly confirmed their remarkable anti-sycotic healing power.

He warns that if the external lesions of *Sycosis* or *Syphilis* have been *badly treated* (suppressed), the universal, underlying, previously latent, *Psora* will tend to emerge and complicate therapy. In such cases, treatment of the dominant psoric state with specifically indicated anti-psoric remedies should be given before the sycotic or syphilitic elements of the case are tackled.

Under-evaluation of *sycosis* and *syphilis*

Hahnemann felt that the miasm of *Syphilis*, while infinitely less important than *Psora*, was nonetheless, more prevalent than *Sycosis*, which he discounts as being

> . . . that miasma, which has produced by far the fewest chronic diseases, and has only been dominant from time to time.[14]

This overmodest perception of *Sycosis*, which we now know symbolises and expresses all that is excessive, profligate and reprobate in human society and hence covers a wide terrain within the landscape of disease forms, resulted from his placing so much emphasis on his newly conceived concept of *Psora* and limiting his interpretation of *Sycosis* to its venereal aspect. This resulted in many manifestations of disease (e.g. leprosy), which today would be regarded as evidence of other miasmatic influences, being attributed to *Psora*. The problem of miasmatic classification was further complicated by the ability of syphilis to appear in so many different guises.

In the early 1800's, there was as yet little understanding of the dread, chronic nature of syphilis, which after imbedding itself in the constitution can lie dormant for as much as 15 to 20 years before stirring and rising up to destructively attack the tissues of its host. This ability of syphilis to recede into the depths, leaving no trace of its presence on the surface, yet biding its time, provides wonderful confirmation of Hahnemann's remarkable insight into the nature and potential of miasmatic disease. But at the time, the various forms that tertiary syphilis can assume were largely unsuspected by Hahnemann and his contemporaries. In consequence, he entertained unrealistically optimistic expectations about its treatment:

> There is no chronic miasm, no chronic disease springing from a miasm, which can be more easily cured than this (Syphilis).[15]

This error must be evaluated in the light of the limited medical knowledge of the time.

Characteristic of the pre-eminence he gave to *Psora* is the grand flourish with which he closes a long list of symptoms attributed to the miasm.

> These are the characteristic secondary symptoms of the long unacknowledged, thousand-headed monster, pregnant with disease, the Psora, the original miasmatic malady which now makes its manifest appearance.[16]

As an initial overview, his allocation of so much to *Psora* was not incorrect, since it was the presence of *Psora* that made other miasmatic contaminations possible; hence, all the various expressions of more complex disease (many of which still required unravelling) could legitimately be regarded as *secondary* to *Psora*, but further refinement and differentiation would prove necessary to develop miasmatic theory into a science. In *Chronic Diseases*, Hahnemann certainly laid that foundation.

Misunderstanding and consternation

Reading the theoretical section of *Chronic Diseases* today, it is hardly surprising that the work created such misunderstanding and consternation amongst his followers. His far-ranging mind had left them far behind. Indeed, it would seem that his intuitive vision and understanding of the concept of the chronic miasms had in some degree even outstretched his own intellectual grasp – and also his ability to clearly explain and define the theory supporting his observations.

> Psora (Itch Disease), like Syphilis, is a miasmatic chronic disease and its original development is similar. The Itch Disease is, however, also the **most contagious of all chronic miasmata**, far more infectious than the other two chronic miasmata, the venereal chancre disease and the figwart disease. But the **miasma of the itch needs only to touch the general skin**, especially with tender children.... No other chronic miasma infects more generally, more surely, more easily and more absolutely than the miasma of Itch; as already stated it is the most contagious of all.[17]

In trying to convey his perception of the origin and fundamental cause of all disease represented by the ubiquitous, *Psora*, and likening its development to the infectious venereal diseases (especially syphilis), in this paragraph he incorrectly leaves the reader, and his critics, with the impression that he ascribed the multitude of psoric ills to infection with the prevalent and highly contagious scabies or 'itch mite' (*Sarcoptes scabiei*); while in truth, the majestic sweep of his vision was far wider and deeper.

Whatever his intention, his manner of presentation certainly misguided his audience into coming to this ludicrous conclusion. Even his closest associates, Dr Stapf and Dr Hermann Gross, the co-publishers of the *Archiv für die homöopathische Heilkunst,* who were the only persons he had informed about the research he was doing prior to its publication in *Chronic Diseases*, were concerned when they read the text and alarmed that it would expose both Hahnemann and homeopathy to further ridicule and stir up even more incredulity and animosity in the medical world.

Sadly, among those who defected from Hahnemann, was Ernst Georg, Baron von Brunnow, the same who left us such an intimate and tender portrait of Hahnemann at home, surrounded by his students in Leipzig, and who had translated the *Organon* into French in gratitude for having had his sight restored by Hahnemann after orthodox medicine had failed. Hahnemann, in a reciprocal gesture of appreciation, had publically dedicated the new work to the Baron. It must have proved extremely hurtful to the Master when Brunnow wrote in his criticism of its contents:

> Hahnemann's complete isolation from doctors with different views and the hitherto almost unconditional loyalty and veneration of most of his adherents are probably the chief factors responsible for the way in which this man of genius pushed his theories to the extreme.[18]

Haehl, commenting on the furore that developed and the divisions it created, hoped that with advancing medical science and better understanding of disease causation:

> ... we may perhaps succeed in making clear to it what Hahnemann really wished to say. Perhaps the moderns will recognise the true kernel of enduring value,

which, enveloped in much that is incomprehensible, vague, untenable and obsolete, is contained in this work by a more than seventy years old explorer of rare acumen.[19]

An enduring legacy

As it proved, there was more than just a kernel of enduring value contained in Hahnemann's impassioned and inspired, but ill-expressed and ill-explained thesis, and far less that was untenable and obsolete than Haehl supposed. Indeed, although still disputed by certain schools and still often misunderstood, and though others have piggy-backed their own miasmatic concepts onto that of Hahnemann, his theory of the so-called, *Classic Chronic Miasms* – *Psora*, *Sycosis* and *Syphilis*, to which were subsequently added the miasms of *Tuberculosis* and the cancer miasm, *Carcinosis* – has not only endured and been further analysed, developed and clarified, but now forms the strategic backbone of therapy for a great number of seasoned homeopaths.

In following volumes in this series, detailed consideration will be given to the theory of the chronic diseases, as well as its practical application in medical practice, but now, sifting through the often impenetrable and labyrinthine complexity of Hahnemann's exposition in *Chronic Diseases*, it is possible to recognise and collect the nuggets of wisdom that form a template for a disease-causation theory of unprecedented insight and scope.

Some of the critical elements that he postulates, couched largely in Hahnemann's language and presented sequentially, are the following:

- The presence in all forms of life of an animating, regulating, *vital force*, which in health maintains the physical body (organism) in a state of functional harmony and balance, or homeostasis.
- This *vital force* is a self-regulatory, self-acting (automatic) instinctively perceiving energy, which governs, maintains, balances, protects, defends and restores.
- In disease, the *vital force* is disturbed and it is the disturbed *vital force* alone that produces symptoms and signs.
- These symptoms and signs result from the efforts of the *vital force* to externalise its disturbance and to confine it to the least harmful level of the organism.
- The initial disturbance of the vital force originated in antiquity and is called *Psora*.

- The appearance of *Psora* in the human race marks the start of a continuum of disease, which is all pervading, present at birth and progressive throughout life.
- Not even the most robust constitution through its own unaided efforts can overcome and extinguish this continuum.
- *Psora* is universal – no human being is free of *Psora*.
- *Psora* disturbs the *vital force* in its entirety, resulting in a pervasive disturbance of the entire organism in every cell, tissue and organ – an *'Internal Itch'* is established – it is never localised (no matter how circumscribed its outward expression may be).
- The initial expression of the disturbance of the *vital force* responsible for *Psora* ('Internal Itch') is an external itch.
- The external itch constitutes the least harmful expression of the *'Internal Itch'* and is evidence of the healing activity of the *vital force*.
- *Psora* is potentiated by bad diet; lack of hygiene, fresh air, and exercise; pollution (Hahnemann includes the immoderate use of tobacco, coffee, tea and alcohol); injury; mental and physical exhaustion; and emotional stress or trauma.
- *Psora* is essentially a state of susceptibility or vulnerability to *'attack'* (challenge, stressors).
- The presence of internal *Psora* results in lowered resistance to infestation of the skin by infective agents (parasites) e.g. scabies.
- The outer manifestation of scabies is a vesicular eruption (containing the mite *acarus*), which is highly contagious and carries psoric, miasmatic energy.
- The degree of vulnerability to scabies depends on the degree of *Psora* already present in the infected individual.
- Although the scabies organism remains localised to the skin, the attendant psoric miasmatic pollution permeates the entire body becoming a centrally-based disturbance of the *vital* force, adding to the already present – innate – psoric miasmatic state.
- After a latent period the *vital force* reacts, externalising the miasmatic energy as an itch or eruption on the skin (not scabies): the least harmful level of expression.
- While ever the skin lesion is manifest, the internal *Psora* remains dormant or is contained and only progresses slowly – the internal health remains unperturbed.
- Suppression of the external itch or eruption will potentiate the *'Internal Itch,' Psora*, which after a latent period will manifest on a deeper, more harmful level: the miasmatic disturbance of the *vital force* is increased.

- Deeper psoric inroads lead to "disturbances of the mind and spirit (soul) of all kinds" (Hahnemann's emphasis).
- The presence of *Psora* results in increased vulnerability to emotional impingement (stressors).
- The specific, general remedy for *Psora* is Sulphur.
- A sequence of anti-psoric remedies may be required to complete a cure.
- The presence of *Psora* emotionally and physically predisposes the individual to gonorrhoeal infection (increased susceptibility).
- Gonorrhoeal infection is followed by an initial latent phase during which the gonorrhoeal energy pervades the entire organism and becomes miasmatic.
- After the latent incubation period, the disturbed vital force reacts, externalising the condition as a yellowish-green purulent discharge from the genital mucous membranes – the least harmful level of expression.
- The combination of *Psora* and miasmatic pollution with gonorrhoea gives rise to the miasm *Sycosis* (figwart-disease), which "rules the whole organism".
- The outer, relieving manifestation of *Sycosis* is catarrhal discharges (increased secretions) and warty excrescences (overgrowth of tissues).
- Topical or systemic chemical (and here we must include antibiotic) removal of these relieving symptoms will drive the miasm deeper resulting in more severe and chronic secondary *Sycosis*, even when the infection of gonorrhoea is 'cured.'
- The specific, general remedy for *Sycosis* is Thuja, followed when necessary by Nitric acid.
- The presence of *Psora* (complicated by *Sycosis*) emotionally and physically predisposes the individual to syphilitic infection (increased susceptibility).
- Syphilitic infection is followed by an initial latent phase during which the syphilitic energy pervades the entire organism and becomes miasmatic.
- After the latent incubation period, the disturbed vital force reacts, externalising the condition as a superficial ulcerous lesion on the skin or mucous membrane – the syphilitic chancre – the least harmful level of expression.
- The combination of *Psora* and miasmatic pollution with syphilis (in the presence of *Sycosis*) gives rise to the miasm *Syphilis*, which in turn, "rules the whole organism."
- Topical, or systemic, chemical removal of the external manifestations of syphilis will intensify the miasm of *Syphilis* and drive it deeper into the constitution, even when the disease of syphilis is 'cured.'

- The specific, general remedy for *Syphilis* is Mercurius.
- The sequence of miasmatic evolution is always *Psora* → *Sycosis* → *Syphilis*; thus creating predictable miasmatic layers.

Miasmatic continuum

When, as above, the fundamental observations of this great mind are extracted from the ponderous text and assembled sequentially, a very clear and practical understanding of the concept of the miasmatic continuum of disease emerges; a concept which has been expanded and elaborated by subsequent generations of homeopathic minds, but never refuted.

Throughout the theoretical section of the book, Hahnemann repeatedly returns to the dangers inherent in the suppression of disease symptoms and signs and exhorts the physician to avoid employing methods of treatment that only mask the underlying cause.

> ... with what fury the internal Psora manifests itself when the external, local symptom which serves to assuage the internal malady is hastily removed ... it must be a matter of conscience for the physician who loves his fellow man to direct all his endeavours to cure, first of all the internal malady, whereby (the external expression of disease) will at the same time be removed and destroyed and all the subsequent innumerable lifelong, chronic sufferings springing from the Psora be prevented or, if they are already embittering the life of the patient, be cured.[20]

These words apply equally, if not more so, to the far more morbidly powerful sycotic and syphilitic miasms.

Finally, it may be added that the continuum nature of disease ensures that no constitution is free of the influence of the three major chronic miasms *Psora, Sycosis* and *Syphilis*. They are present in every individual from birth to death and responsible for the many and varied expressions of disease that trouble and torture humanity. In every case of disease, either one or other miasm will be dominant or there will be evidence of the compounding of these miasms, "conjoined in threefold complication," or of the creation of the mixed miasmatic pictures of *Tuberculosis* or *Carcinosis* (to be considered later).

Although Hahnemann does not unequivocally state that the chronic miasms and their diseases are inherited from one generation to another – the pioneer work of Gregor Mendel (1822–1884) on inherited traits was yet to come – yet a study of his work leaves no doubt that he perceived the disease continuum as flowing through the generations and to be the underlying cause of disease susceptibility. Likewise, although he does not directly lay the responsibility for the evolution of *Psora* upon psychological or emotional causes, but rather concentrates on the infective aspect (e.g. scabies), nonetheless, he is at pains to emphasise the extreme sensitivity of the psoric state to the impingement of injurious emotions – far greater than exposure to even the harshest physical circumstances – and of the on-going havoc these wreak upon the constitution.

> Yea, an innocent man can, with less injury to his life, pass ten years in bodily torments in the Bastille or on the galleys rather than pass some months in all bodily comfort in an unhappy marriage or with a remorseful conscience.

He identifies the significance of emotional trauma in the development of tuberculosis or cancer or emotional illness when underlying miasmatic disease is present:

> The sudden death of a son causes the tender mother, already in ill health, an incurable suppuration of the lungs or a cancer of the breast. A young affectionate maiden, already hysterical, is thrown into melancholy by a disappointment in love.

And he states further:

> By far the most frequent excitement of the slumbering Psora into chronic disease, and the most frequent aggravation of chronic ailments already existing, are caused by grief and vexation.[21]

It is but a small step to intuit that sudden, severe, or prolonged negative emotions could prepare the ground for the increased susceptibility to infections and parasitisation, which Hahnemann surmised was the original cause of *Psora* being the universal mother of chronic diseases. Once the cycle was established – a physical state first weakened by erosive or destructive emotions and in consequence vulnerable to attack by opportunistic organisms (e.g. scabies) – *Psora* would become a self-perpetuating sequence of interweaving emotional and infective causes, escalating progressively over millennia. It was Hahnemann's observations regarding the central importance of disturbed emotions in the development of miasmatic disease that laid the foundation for the modern homeopathic focus of unravelling the psychopathological aspects of a case in order to find the most similar remedy; matching remedy and patient at the deepest level possible.

When that which is incomprehensible and vague in *Chronic Diseases* is pushed aside, the insights of genius are revealed; insights which have provided subsequent generations of homeopaths with a means of understanding the multifaceted manifestations of disease and their relationship, one to another, despite the seeming disconnectedness emphasised by modern, generic classifications. This understanding enables the homeopathic physician to recognise the disease layers present in each case of chronic disease and to devise a structured strategy of therapy to address the complexity of such cases and provides a means to evaluate therapeutic response – which should reveal a miasmatic recession in the reverse order of evolution: *Syphilis* → *Sycosis* → *Psora*.

Eccentricity

However, even genius may lapse, especially when moved by an eccentric, Paracelsian-like rush of self-esteem or distracted by a proverbial bee in the bonnet. The first instance is revealed in a footnote to an exhaustive list of symptoms of latent *Psora*, in which he states with great satisfaction that it was easier for him to recognise the presence of *Psora* in others, even when *as yet slumbering*, simply by comparing them with himself,

> . . . who, as is seldom the case, have never been afflicted with the Psora, and have, therefore, from my birth even until now in my eightieth year been entirely free from the (smaller and greater) ailments enumerated here . . . although I have been, on the whole, very apt to catch acute epidemic diseases, and have been exposed to many mental exertions and thousand fold vexations of the spirit.[22]

Many have smiled knowingly at this gentle conceit, but in mitigation, his rude health, which would continue into his deep eighties, enjoyed against a background of repeated professional and personal trials, surely entitled a man approaching his eightieth birthday to conveniently forget the occasional tweaks and twinges of *Psora*, which must afflict us all from time to time.

The distracting bee, just as eccentric and just as charming as his total freedom from *Psora*, was his obsessive concern about the excessive drinking of warm coffee and Chinese tea, which he was certain palliated many of the symptoms of *Psora*, and was therefore partially responsible for *Psora* spreading,

> . . . such innumerable, such obstinate chronic sufferings among mankind; for Psora alone could not have produced this effect.[23]

So absorbed had he been with this conviction that in 1803 he produced a small book on the subject entitled *The Effects of Coffee*. In *Chronic Diseases*, he compulsively revisits this contentious subject in another footnote, but sensible to the doubt with which many colleagues had received his minor work, softens his previously adamant and extreme stance by admitting that he might have made "perhaps too prominent" the role of coffee and tea in the cause of chronic disease. Given the current vast consumption of caffeine-loaded beverages, the multitude of 'hyped-up', overstressed individuals in modern society, the widespread dependence on tranquilisers and sedatives and the ever increasing incidence of stress-related disease, Hahnemann's pet concern may not appear as misconceived now as it appeared during his lifetime.

Chronic Diseases reveals a man of noble spirit, great erudition, profound insight, deep compassion for human suffering and an inexhaustible drive and commitment to unravel the enigma of a species singularly cursed with a host of diseases capable of producing the most horrible afflictions. With the completion of this last major work, rich in clues towards meeting the challenge of disease, his protected life in quiet, rural Köthen and his advanced years, one might expect that Providence, content with the service that this warm, idiosyncratic, and industrious man had rendered his fellow man, would at this point have designed a tranquil, restful, final chapter to his life. Such was not to be, for a most remarkable future still lay before him.

References

1 Haehl R. *Samuel Hahnemann, His Life and Work*. Vol 1. London: Homoeopathic Publishing Company; 1922. p137.
2 Hahnemann S. *Chronic Diseases*. Vol 1. Calcutta: C. Ringer & Co. Original; 1835. p20.
3 *Ibid.*, p21.
4 Lilley D. The Chronic Miasms. In: Owen D. *Principles and Practice of Homeopathy*. London. Churchill Livingstone; 2007. Chapter 7, p220.
5 Hahnemann S. *Chronic Diseases*. Vol 1. Calcutta: C. Ringer & Co. Original; 1835. p22.
6 *Ibid.*, p54.
7 Hahnemann S. *Organon of Medicine*. 6th Edition. Philadelphia PA: Boericke & Tafel; 1922. §7, p96.
8 Hahnemann S. *Chronic Diseases*. Vol 1. Calcutta: C. Ringer & Co. Original; 1835. p44.
9 *Ibid.*, p49.
10 *Ibid.*, p53.
11 Farrington H. *Homeopathy and Homeopathic Prescribing*. American Institute of Homeopathy; 1944. p191.
12 Hahnemann S. *Materia Medica Pura*. Vol 2. Liverpool. Hahnemann Publishing Society; 1881. p649.
13 Hahnemann S. *Chronic Diseases*. Vol 1. Calcutta: C. Ringer & Co. Original; 1835. p92.
14 *Ibid.*, p94.

15 Haehl R. *Samuel Hahnemann, His Life and Work*. Vol 1. London: Homoeopathic Publishing Company; 1922. p142.
16 Hahnemann S. *Chronic Diseases*. Vol 1. Calcutta: C. Ringer & Co. Original; 1835. p88.
17 *Ibid.*, p48.
18 Haehl R. *Samuel Hahnemann, His Life and Work*. Vol 1. London: Homoeopathic Publishing Company; 1922. p149.
19 *Ibid.*, p138.
20 Hahnemann S. *Chronic Diseases*. Vol 1. Calcutta: C. Ringer & Co. Original; 1835. p31.
21 *Ibid.*, p115.
22 *Ibid.*, p54.
23 *Ibid.*, p28.

7

LAST YEARS IN KÖTHEN

The inveterate physician

With *Chronic Diseases* completed, and now somewhat distanced from the continued warfare against homeopathy, Hahnemann, in his seventies, directed his still considerable energy towards conducting a very extensive and steadily increasing practice. At a time of life when many have chosen to retire from the rigours of professional life in order to enjoy their latter years at leisure, this indefatigable and enthusiastic physician, without thought of recreation or rest, immersed himself in service to his patients. To his time spent in daily consultation was added an evening marathon of answering the numerous letters from patients all over the world. His day extended into the night. This all-consuming commitment to homeopathic practice seemed to suit his reclusive nature well, but made him less accessible to colleagues, friends and family. However, he still managed to correspond regularly, and at length, with a few chosen intimates, such as Stapf, Gross, Hering and Bönninghausen.

* * * * *

Clemens Maria Franz von Bönninghausen

Bönninghausen (1785–1864), a personage most important to the early development of homeopathy, had become one of Hahnemann's closest friends. He was born in the Netherlands in 1785 to a noble, military family, which traced its lineage back to Austria. Such was the compass of his intellect that during his studies in law at the Dutch University of Groningen, he also attended key lectures in natural history and medicine in order to broaden his knowledge. It was these additional studies that would pave his future course in life. On qualifying as a lawyer, he entered the Dutch Civil Service in 1807 and in recognition of his unusual abilities, both personal

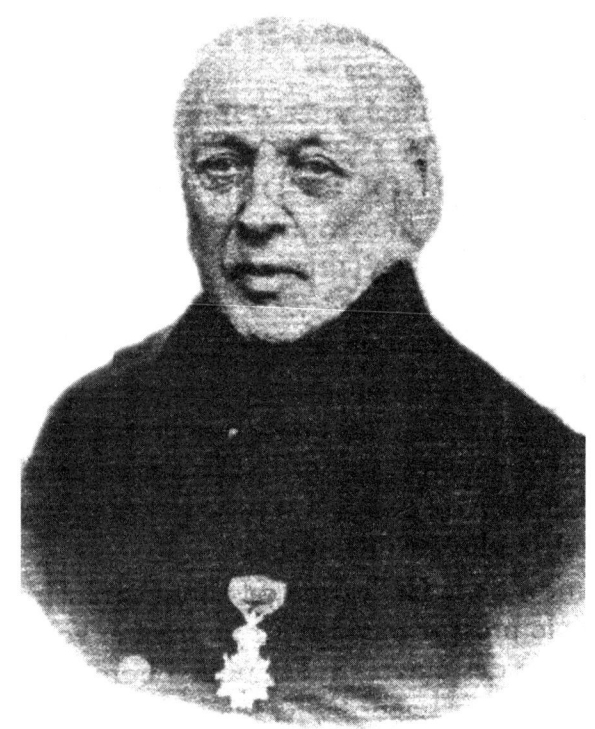

Figure 7.1 Clemens Maria Franz von Bönninghausen (1785–1864)
Credit: Science Photo Library

and intellectual; he was rapidly advanced through the bureaucratic ranks to become Secretary General to Louis Bonaparte, who was then King of the Netherlands. He became very close to the King, enjoyed working with him and developed a great respect for the monarch. When Louis Bonaparte finally abdicated his royal appointment in 1810, Bönninghausen lost interest in the otherwise tedious nature of his civil service work and decided to move on. Instead of seeking another legal position, he chose to pursue his interest in agriculture and particularly the study of botany.

Having married in the autumn of 1812, he retired in the spring of 1814 to his ancestral estate at Darup in Westphalia with the purpose of developing its resources and gaining experience in modern agricultural methods. He was extremely successful in his endeavours and eventually extended his labours to the improvement of farming and the lot of the peasantry throughout Westphalia, and also established the first formal agricultural society for the area. In consequence, due to the respect he earned in the community and his legal background, at the age of thirty-one, he was offered and accepted the position of President of the Provincial Court of Justice for the Westphalia district. Six years later he was appointed Commissioner-General of the newly created Deeds' registry for the Rhineland and Westphalia. This latter appointment necessitated constant travelling through these provinces and afforded him the opportunity of studying the abundant and varied riches of the indigenous flora of the region. A scientific botanical book was the product of these studies and his recognised expertise led to him being made Director of the Botanical Gardens at Münster. His distinction in the botanical world was honoured by two species of plants being named after him.

Tuberculosis

In the autumn of 1827, Clemens von Bönninghausen fell seriously ill with what was diagnosed independently by two of the most respected physicians in the area as 'purulent tuberculosis.' Despite all the ministrations of his medical attendants, by the spring of 1828 his condition had become desperate. Anticipating his imminent death, Bönninghausen wrote a letter of farewell to one of his close botanical associates, Dr A Weihe. Unknown to Bönninghausen, since all their contacts and correspondence had been confined to botanical matters, Weihe was not only medically qualified but also an experienced homeopathic physician. Deeply concerned by the news, Weihe immediately wrote back and requested his friend to give him a detailed description of his symptoms in the hope that he might be able, even in this dire extremity, to help him through the new form of healing he was now practising. Grateful for some possibility of help, Bönninghausen furnished him with as full a picture as he was able and then conscientiously followed Weihe's advice by taking the remedies he prescribed. Within a remarkably short time, considering the severity of the condition, Bönninghausen began to feel his health gradually returning, indeed, so much so, that by the end of the summer his cure was complete.

Homeopathic studies

Given his deep interest in botany, his university exposure to the medical and natural sciences and his life-changing return from the very brink of death, it is small wonder that this highly intelligent and strongly motivated man of forty-three should now devote his considerable energy to studying and furthering the cause of homeopathy. Having personally experienced its subtle and gentle healing power, his greatest urge was to promote its practice and bring relief to those, who like himself, found themselves beyond the help of the orthodoxy. Because he was medically unqualified, he knew that if he should personally treat patients, he would be risking attack from the medical establishment. Being a founder member of the local Medical Society, he was very familiar with the Münster physicians. He therefore attempted to kindle interest in homeopathy among them. All his efforts proved in vain. His enthusiastic exhortations were met by stubborn, conservative prejudice. Despairing of any help from this quarter, he resolved to champion the cause himself. To this end, he first set about laying for himself a sure foundation of knowledge. With assiduous zeal, he revisited, refreshed and expanded his studies in the medical and natural sciences, acquired a thorough understanding of the theory and principles of homeopathy, and studied in depth all the documented homeopathic remedy provings. His considerable knowledge of botany proved of great assistance to him. In addition to the *Organon*, both Hahnemann's *Materia Medica Pura*, the final volume of which had been published in 1821, and *Chronic Diseases*, recently published in 1828, were available to him.

Bönninghausen's *Repertory*

It was at this point that Bönninghausen's intense enthusiasm for the cause moved him to contact the Master himself. Thus began a warm and intimate friendship, which endured until Hahnemann's death, keened by their common goals and compatible minds and sustained by regular correspondence. Their individual qualities complemented one another and in Bönninghausen, Hahnemann found not only a knowledgeable friend and sympathetic confidant, but an astute and energetic mind gifted with both a lawyer's perspicacity and need for order and system, and a botanist's love of differentiation, accuracy and attention to detail. Faced by the already daunting body of homeopathic literature, Bönninghausen brought both these attributes to bear on the task of rendering the material of the materia medica more easily accessible to the practitioner. The practical mind that had so ably brought method and mode to agriculture in Westphalia at once perceived that the prime objective of this task must be to identify, highlight and index the characteristic peculiarities of each remedy and compile a reference work, which would enable the homeopath to more easily and surely differentiate and single out the remedy required to match most accurately the symptom picture of the patient to be treated. The result of his devotion to this work was the creation of the first homeopathic *repertory*: a repository of indexed symptoms derived from the materia medica, entered as specific headings, or *rubrics*, each descriptive of a specific symptom, under which all the remedies known to have produced or remedied that symptom were listed. *Sub-rubrics* appended to these main headings covered the modifying influences, or *modalities*, known to ameliorate or aggravate the specific symptom [e.g. time; heat; cold; wet; dry; touch; pressure; etc] each with a list of its related remedies. He also recognised that certain symptoms or disorders are commonly found associated with one another and these he grouped together as *concomitant* symptoms.

Considering that Bönninghausen first made acquaintance with the homeopathic method when he personally experienced its efficacy in 1828, it is remarkable testimony to his understanding, versatility and industry that as early as 1832 he produced his first repertory: *Repertory of the Antipsoric, Medicines*. Hahnemann gave his stamp of approval by writing a preface to the book in which he offered guidance regarding the frequency of dosage of a remedy. By 1835, Bönninghausen had added a further repertory to this seminal work, clumsily entitled: *Repertory of the Medicines which are not Antipsoric*. These works have stood the test of time and were later combined and augmented by the American homeopathic physician Dr C M Boger as *Bönninghausen's Characteristics and Repertory*. Maintaining his focus on practicality and ease of use, Bönninghausen was later (1846) to write an important manual for day to day application in homeopathic practice: *Therapeutic Manual for Homœopathic Physicians, for use at the sick bed and in the study of the Materia Medica Pura*. This became popularly known as *Bönninghausen's Pocket Book*. Both the repertory and the pocket book provided blueprints for many similar manuals and repertories that were to follow, all of which would contain considerable material derived from them. His repertory remained *the* reference book of its day until Kent's repertory was published in 1877. It proved of great value to Hahnemann during the last ten years of his practice, lightening the work of finding the most similar remedy.

Hahnemann had such regard for a particular book of Bönninghausen's, which he had written for the general public that in a letter to Dr Schreeter – in which he writes of the difficulties experienced when treating persons of the upper classes who will not take orders, refuse to listen to good advise and fail to adhere to the strict rules of healthy living, essential for their cure – he finishes with the following stern declaration:

> All my patients of rank affected with chronic diseases must have read the *Organon* and Bönninghausen's *Homœopathy (Homœopathy, a Manual for the Non-Medical Public*), otherwise I will not undertake their treatment.[1]

Haehl emphasises the esteem in which Hahnemann held Bönninghausen and his written works:

> Up to his death, Hahnemann remained in closer touch with Bönninghausen than any other disciple or student, and nobody was held in higher esteem by the Master than he, who by different writings has contributed so effectually to the perfection and expansion of homœopathy.[2]

Renowned homeopath

Bönninghausen spent the years between 1828 and 1843 largely on these literary labours and acquiring a phenomenal knowledge of the materia medica. His was a rare mind, possessing an almost encyclopaedic memory of remedies and their differentiating characteristics, a gift of inestimable value at the bedside. Bönninghausen tried to keep his steadily increasing practice of homeopathy as unremarkable as possible because of the danger of coming to the attention of the medical authorities. But once he was published, and word of his therapeutic successes began to spread, anonymity became impossible. His fame extended beyond Germany and he became recognised as an authority on homeopathy. Physicians from other countries approached him for advice in dealing with difficult cases and some even journeyed to Münster to consult with him.

Honorary physician

He continued with his official duties as Commissioner-General, but was increasingly obliged on his frequent travels in that capacity to interrupt his commission in order to render medical advice to colleagues and patients. Inevitably, this came to the ears of local orthodox physicians and aroused their jealousy and animosity. Considering the wrath of officialdom that had repeatedly descended in similar circumstances upon the venerable head of the medically qualified Hahnemann, it might have been expected that history would repeat itself, and worse, in the case of a medically unqualified practitioner. But Bönninghausen lived a charmed life and besides enjoyed huge social standing. He was a landed aristocrat, holding an influential government appointment, highly respected and esteemed in the entire region of Westphalia and the Rhineland, and gifted with an exceptional legal mind and a thoroughly charming and engaging manner. His was a nature always contained, cordial and considered, blessed with an affability and diplomacy, which smoothed his way forward rather than precipitating him onto the rocky and often perilous terrain that Hahnemann's disputative character so frequently invited. Faced with such pre-eminence, the mutterings and complaints of the medical fraternity never rose above a swell. In mid 1843, before any serious threat could arise, as if fortune wished to confirm the favour in which she held him, by a curious coincidence of events, Bönninghausen, who had just completed, after many years of toil, the setting up of the Deeds' Register, received notification that his medical accomplishments and success were to be honoured by a cabinet order issued by His Majesty, King William IV, dated July 11 1843 – on the very day his friend and mentor, Samuel Hahnemann, was laid to rest at Montmartre cemetery. The order, quite exceptionally, granted him the authority to practise medicine, and this without having to undergo the rigour of any qualifying examination.

The Lesser Writings

Without further ado, Bönninghausen requested that he be given leave to retire from his civil responsibilities. This was granted, and at last he was able to enter into full-time homeopathic practice in Münster. His years of study and preparation served him well and within a remarkably short time he had established a large, thriving practice and become known as a practitioner of exceptional ability, a master of the materia medica and an authority on the homeopathic method of healing. That the high opinion in which he was held was fully justified is evidenced by the quality and content of the many contributions he made to various journals. These have fortunately been preserved for us, translated from the original German by Professor LH Tafel and brought together by Dr TL Bradford, in a valuable book titled: *The Lesser Writings of von Boenninghausen*. In modern parlance, Bönninghausen's literary style is far more 'user-friendly' than that of Hahnemann. He is able to communicate understanding of complex concepts in a lucid and intelligible manner devoid of obscuring elaboration and provides good solid, practical advice on many aspects of homeopathic practice, including the use of potencies and the preparation of these. His observations and arguments are always expressed with great care, confidence and clarity. He was an ardent champion of the use of the higher potencies. He built on the foundation laid by Hahnemann and gained experience with far more highly dynamised dilutions than those generally used by the Master. With experience, the 200th centesimal potency became and always remained his particular favourite, although it was by no means the highest potency that he used.

Homeopathic protagonist

Despite the remarkable results that homeopaths were achieving, the majority of old-school physicians remained adamantly sceptical about the therapeutic power of the infinitesimal dilutions of homeopathy. As if anticipating current medicine's discounting of all positive response to homeopathic treatment and attributing any improvement in a patient's wellbeing to the so-called placebo effect, homeopathy's detractors in the mid-1800s advanced various objections against drawing favourable conclusions from any benefits experienced by homeopathic patients.

In an article written in the *Allgemeine Homœpatische Zeitung*, Bönninghausen identifies two of the objections used by antagonists of homeopathy when refuting the curative role of the homeopathic remedy even when faced by positive therapeutic results. He writes:

> These objections are: first, that cures are due to a *trusting confidence* of the patients in their physician, the *moral effect* of which is rated too highly; and *secondly* to *homœopathic dieting*, which brings back the patients to a natural mode of living, and is supposed to be able to restore health by dieting alone, *without any medicine*.
>
> We dynamists [homeopaths], if we were inclined to retaliate, would be fully justified in asking the materialists [allopaths] why they do not labour to gain with their patients as great and mighty a confidence and prescribe the same diet with all their patients, throwing aside all medicine as useless? But . . . we know as well as our opponents that there are many, especially *chronic* diseases, which can never be thoroughly and permanently eradicated by the vital force alone, as also *acute* diseases where the regular course can only be mitigated and aborted by suitable medicines, and where a fatal issue can only be safely averted by the same.

During his early years as a homeopath, when it had been wise for him to limit his practice, and while he was testing the efficacy of the various potencies, it is not surprising that being a gentleman farmer, Bönninghausen developed much of his clinical and prescribing skills from treating animals. In this he proved highly successful. Indeed, he can be considered *the* pioneer of veterinary homeopathy.

He argues from great experience when he adds to his above remarks:

> But all these excuses and objections are at once cut off in the *homœopathic cures of animals*. These cures, and only these, give us the surest and most irrefutable information what, and how much, medicines, and also high potencies, are able to do, quite *independent of all moral faith and of all dieting*, both of which are here entirely eliminated, so that not the remotest suspicion can be admitted in any of them.[3]

Knight of the Legion of Honour

In 1848, Bönninghausen founded the Society of the Homœopathic Physicians of Westphalia and the Rhine. He was well known to the leading American homeopaths, Dr Constantine Hering (of whom we shall have more to say) and Dr Adolph Lippe, both of whom regularly corresponded with him, and Dr Carroll Dunham. Bönninghausen maintained a worldwide interest in the progress of homeopathy and especially that of America, where, under the impetus of Hering, it was spreading rapidly. In 1854, The Homœopathic Medical College of Cleveland conferred upon him the honorary degree of doctor of medicine, and on 20 April, 1861, he received his highest accolade when, in recognition of his reputation and professional standing, the Emperor of France, Napoleon 111 made him Knight of the Legion of Honour.

After the death of Gross, Bönninghausen joined Stapf as associate editor of the *Archiv für die Homöopathische Heilkunst.* When Stapf in turn died, Bönninghausen remained the sole commanding voice of homeopathy in Europe. He was a towering figure and guiding influence until his death from a stroke on 26 January 1864, at the age of 79.

Bradford, the homeopathic historian, to whom we owe so much knowledge of the early homeopaths, provides us with these warm, respectful words to close our consideration of this worthy man and outstanding physician.

> His fame as a successful practitioner and as the acknowledged master of our Materia Medica, brought him many visitors from among professional men, these his genial cordiality converted into warm and steadfast friends. Advancing years dealt with him tenderly and death has at last overtaken him at his post of duty, still earnest in his labours, warm in his friendships and at peace with God and man.[4]

He was blessed with seven sons of whom the eldest two, Karl (1826–1902) and Friederich (1828–1910), followed in their father's homeopathic footsteps after first qualifying in medicine. Karl was to marry Sophie, the adopted daughter of Hahnemann's second wife, Mélanie. After the marriage, he settled in Paris where he practised homeopathy together with his widowed mother-in-law.

Together, Hahnemann and Bönninghausen represent the two enduring limbs of professional homeopathy: the medically qualified homeopathic physician and the non-medically qualified, homeopathic practitioner. Their friendship, their mutual respect and their shared, intense and unremitting commitment to furthering the art and science of homeopathy stand as an example to members of the two professions today, which, if promoted and adhered to, must unite them, benefit homeopathy and preserve it as the medicine of choice for modern society.

* * * * *

Hahnemann's Jubilee

The year 1828, in which Bönninghausen escaped from his close brush with death and in consequence embraced homeopathy, was the year in which a decision was made amongst leading followers of Hahnemann to hold a festival on 10 August 1829 to commemorate the jubilee of the Master's medical graduation from the University of Erlangen in 1779. Stapf, as editor of his *Archive*, was largely responsible for spreading the word and rousing interest. It proved a great success, drawing together at least four hundred attendees, mostly doctors, from almost every European country, in one accord: to demonstrate their gratitude and their respect for the founder of homeopathy. A happy result of this common purpose was the founding of the Society of Homœopathic Physicians, which from then on would hold annual general meetings on every 10th of August. The society was created to provide a rallying centre for those united in promoting homeopathy and resisting the antagonism of the orthodoxy. This was timely, since in recent years disagreements and discord within the homeopathic fraternity had begun to mount and were threatening to create opposing factions within the profession.

Stapf presented Hahnemann with a red, velvet case containing gold and silver medals and a special edition of the *Lesser Writings of Samuel Hahnemann* inscribed with the following words:

> May through these pages the spirits of bygone days pass before you once more. At the same time rejoice in what you have accomplished and fought for in the past, full of labours, now crowned with fame and affection.[5]

Duke Ferdinand and Duchess Julie of Anhalt-Köthen sent a gift of a gold snuffbox with the initials 'S.H.' in diamonds, together with personal letters.

Hahnemann was deeply touched by all the demonstrations of love and respect. In a letter of appreciation to his friend Stapf, who was the main architect of the Jubilee, he wrote:

> I can bear much joy and sorrow, but I was hardly able to stand the surprise of so many and such strong proofs of the kindness and affection of my pupils and friends with which I was overwhelmed on the 10 August.[6]

The death of Frau Johanna Henriette

The uplifting energy of the jubilee was still alive in the homeopathic community when, on 31 March 1830, Johanna Henriette Hahnemann was taken ill and quite unexpectedly died in her 67th year. Earlier in the month, she had developed a high fever and what appeared to be a bronchial infection complicated by an abscess on the liver. Her condition steadily declined and within the space of four weeks death supervened. Her departure brought forty-eight years of married life to a close.

Although married to a man of strong, determined character, Frau Henriette, as Hahnemann liked to call her, was no timid, wilting violet. She was a strong-willed woman, resolute and extremely industrious. She had to be! She bore Samuel eleven children and in the earlier years of their marriage, she, the well educated daughter of a prosperous apothecary, brought up in comfort and security, endured privation, need, a constantly disrupted, itinerant life and the death of her baby, Ernst. Later, when the family were at last blessed with prosperity and a stable existence, she suffered the divorces and deaths of daughters and the unpredictable behaviour of her mentally unstable son, Friedrich. She steadfastly and uncomplainingly shouldered her burdens, providing her genius husband with the companionship and support he needed on the arduous path he had chosen, and giving him the confidence that he could leave all domestic demands and problems in her diligent and able hands, while focusing his mind exclusively on his professional objectives. It was largely she who attended to the education of the children and the bringing up of her daughters to become exemplary German housewives, as she was herself.

Given this background, it should not be weighed against her that she was, either through nature or force of circumstances, more practical than romantic, domineering and officious, and ruled the Hahnemann home and finances with an iron hand, to which even her husband was subordinate. She had no aspirations, social or otherwise, outside her circumscribed, yet extremely busy, domestic life and appears to have remained much in the background during the homeopathic soirées held in her home, never cultivating any personal friendship with those closest to Hahnemann. Hence, her passing was only felt by her immediate family and especially by her seventy-five year old husband. He always spoke of her with love and esteem. Often in the evenings when he broke off from his work, he would retire to the parlour and she would play something for him on the piano.

> Even if she were (as had been reported) fond of power and imperious, she must have possessed excellent qualities which were highly valued by her husband. Her energy was, no doubt, often a support to him in his stormy life,[7]

It is certain that Hahnemann must have cherished many precious memories of her and would deeply miss her.

The day after her death, Duchess Julie expressed her concern for the old man in a letter of condolence to him:

> I have learned with the greatest distress, my dear Hofrath, of the sad blow which has fallen on you this night. The news was all the greater shock to me since I had no suspicion of the illness of the departed. I beg you to be assured of my most hearty sympathy, and to grant my earnest request that under this severe shock, you will not neglect your health, which is so necessary to the welfare of mankind.[8]

But providence did not leave him alone and unsupported in the work that lay ahead, his two youngest daughters, Charlotte and Louise (*"Lotchen"* and *"Luischen"*) stepped into the gap left by Frau Henriette and devoted themselves to maintaining the home in Köthen as their mother had done and to assisting their father in his practice.

Hahnemann's life continued at the same unremitting pace. Word of his cures spread everywhere and patients from all walks of life came from far and wide to consult him. He did not visit patients in Köthen. Those from distant parts had to find accommodation in the town and remain there until he was satisfied with their progress. This they were willing to do; for many, the grand old man was their last hope. However, it was particularly amongst the elite that his reputation grew and at the time it became a mark of discernment and correct form to be an adherent of homeopathy and to be under homeopathic treatment. Much of the successful propagation of homeopathy was owed to the zeal of informed members of the gentry. But the more ground homeopathy gained, the more hostile became its antagonists – as always: execration rather than investigation.

Cholera

Almost as if wishing to put homeopathy to the test and prove its efficacy to the sceptical medical world, in 1831, Asian cholera:

> ... the mysterious and murderous pest, left Asia, and with tremendous speed and terrible power drew nearer and nearer to the countries of Western Europe.[9]

Innumerable victims fell before this onslaught and allopathy possessed neither preventative nor curative measures with which to stem the tide. As news spread of its inexorable approach, anxiety and unrest mounted, stirring historic memories of the black plague that had swept out of the East in the mid-1300s. If his mind had been staid for a time by grief, this was set aside as Hahnemann pitted his wits against the challenge. Without the possibility of first hand observation of cholera cases and relying entirely on the descriptions of the symptoms and course of the disease provided by his students and friends to whom he urgently appealed for details, his brilliant mind soon apprehended its nature, its prevention and the most likely remedy to successfully treat each stage of the disease. In opposition to general medical opinion, even that of the highly respected Hufeland, and long before the advent of bacteriology, Hahnemann perceived that the cholera must be due to an infective agent ('living miasma' transferable by contact from one person to another). With prophetic insight he pronounced:

> The most striking infections took place and made astounding progress ... whenever in the stuffy spaces of ships, filled as they are with musty aqueous vapours, the cholera miasm found an element favourable to its own multiplication and throve to an enormously increased swarm of those infinitely small, invisible living organisms, which are so murderously hostile to human life and which most probably form the infectious matter of cholera.[10]

The results of his research were written up in four separate pamphlets, which he presented to the publishers for as wide a distribution as possible without asking for any remuneration for his work. The homeopathic remedy he advocated for use, which matched most perfectly the symptoms of the current epidemic, was Camphor, a remedy derived from the ethereal oil of the magnificent camphor tree and run up into homeopathic potency.

The previous year had seen the death of Duke Ferdinand of Anhalt-Köthen under whose protection and patronage Hahnemann had remained secure from medical censure. His local allopathic opponents hoped that with the Duke's passing, Hahnemann would be vulnerable to attack. They were proved right; Heinrich, the new duke, unlike his brother was prepared to lend them a sympathetic ear. The members of the Köthen medical council wasted no time in bringing to his attention what they claimed were derogatory statements contained in the pamphlets inferring that allopaths were ignorant regarding the propagation and prevention of cholera, and pointing particularly to Hahnemann's condemnatory remarks about accepted allopathic treatment, which they felt were uncalled for and would undermine their authority. The Duke yielded to their obsequious pleas and in consequence the sale of *Cure of Cholera* was forbidden in Köthen, and thus, as would happen repeatedly in the future, the voice of reason was stifled. Hahnemann refused to be intimidated and had his pamphlets published in Leipzig.

Hahnemann advised that the Camphor dose should be given as speedily as possible, at the very onset of the disease, as it particularly suited the acute phase, and must be repeated frequently on account of the dangerous impetus of the illness and because, although powerful, Camphor's action was transient and relatively superficial. He stressed that in this role

Camphor did not act as a mere palliative; it brought about a successful and permanent cure.

If the disease had already advanced into its later stages then the time for Camphor had passed and Hahnemann then recommended the use of Cuprum (copper) or Veratrum album (white hellebore) depending on the presentation: Cuprum being renowned for its efficacy where blueness of the lips and skin and severe cramping pains were predominant and Veratrum being indicated where cold sweat, coldness of the body and profuseness of the vomiting and diarrhoea were conspicuous. In other cases, he recommended Bryonia alba (white bryony) and Rhus toxicodendron (poison oak) to be given in alternation with one another.

Father Veith, a prominent Viennese cleric and homeopathic enthusiast of considerable skill, brought to Hahnemann's attention the remarkable value of *Phosphoric acid* for cholera in the stage of collapse: cases desperately weakened by loss of body fluids through persistent diarrhoea.

Hahnemann also recognised the value of Carbo vegetabilis (vegetable carbon) during the convalescence stage to hasten the return of strength and bring about full recovery.

Considering the infinitesimal doses, so derided by the allopaths, yet used so successfully in the homeopathic treatment of cholera, it is interesting to note that copper, merely worn as a pendant next to the skin, had long been known to act as a preventative – a custom that is still followed in India. When administered in this way, the protection afforded obviously derives from incredibly small doses!

In the *Organon,* Hahnemann had shown himself to be an ardent advocate of preventative medicine and the pamphlets, in addition to specific remedial measures, gave clear directives of how to protect against further spread of the disease.

> ... in order to make the infection and spreading of cholera impossible, the garments, the linen, etc. of all strangers arriving there had to be kept in the quarantine (whilst their bodies were cleansed by speedy baths and provided with clean clothes ...) and retained there for two hours in a stove heat of 80°.... This represents a heat at which all known infectious matters and consequently the living miasma is annihilated.[11]

Thus, the seventy-six year old doctor threw down his homeopathic gauntlet in the face of a devastating disease and, like David before monstrous Goliath, armed only with the tiny sling of his carefully selected remedy in infinitesimal dose, engaged the enemy. The results were remarkable. Whereas, almost 50% of all allopathically treated patients died, in various homeopathic groups the percentage of deaths was by comparison minimal e.g. 6 deaths out of 154 cases; 31 out of 631; 1 out of 27, etc. These results created a great stir, especially in Austria where, as will be remembered, homeopathy had been suppressed by Imperial decree. The popularity of homeopathy reached a new height amongst the public and, as noted, was strongly supported by the nobility.

Yet all was not well in the State of Homeopathy!

Internecine discord

As previously alluded to, a new threat to the integrity of homeopathy had unfortunately raised its head – and this within the ranks of homeopathic doctors. The publication of *Chronic Disease* with its misunderstood *Psora Theory* had caused great controversy in the homeopathic world, and dismay and uncertainty among many of Hahnemann's following; now other polarities began to emerge. Whereas the popular swell of support from the public was pushing all before it, a division in homeopathic medical perspective threatened to adulterate and weaken the pioneering thrust at its source. With increasing numbers of doctors affiliating themselves in varying degrees to the homeopathic cause, a breed of medical homeopath was emerging, which whilst proclaiming its adherence to the principles of homeopathy, sought through compromise to combine homeopathic and allopathic methods of treatment – using one or the other system according to apparent needs. These 'half-homeopaths' were an anathema to Hahnemann – he labelled them the 'converted' and concentrated his innate mistrust on them and their prime proponent, Dr Moritz Müller of Leipzig. As early as 1823, he had castigated them with withering contempt in a letter to a Dr WE Wislicenus:

> The 'Converted' are only hybrids, amphibians, who are most of them still creeping about in the mud of the allopathic marsh and who only rarely venture to raise their head in freedom towards the ethereal truth.[12]

Apart from the division brought about by the 'hybrids', who attempted to be both allopath and homeopath (a more difficult feat in those days of barbaric allopathic methods than today), a further schism developed with the emergence of a 'low potency' group opposed to the use of the higher potencies. This limiting prejudice was doomed to become more invidious later in homeopathy's history.

Bönninghausen refers to both these delinquent groups in an article on the healing power of high potencies:

> High potencies have produced a division, especially among German homœopaths, which still exists and is in no way conducive to the progress of science.

> A war in our own camp has thus been caused, far worse and more dangerous than a war against an external foe – a war of *specifists* against the *Hahnemannians*, of the *materialists* against the *dynamists* – and in consequence the *amphibians* have lately arisen, who are neither fish nor fowl, neither homœopaths nor allopaths, and who frequently sacrifice their convictions to selfish considerations.[13]

Fortunately, the discord was largely centred in Leipzig and in consequence the 'Leipzig physicians' were not at all popular or respected in the homoeopathic circles of Germany. But it was in Leipzig, and because of the discord, that the next painful episode in Hahnemann's life would be enacted and in many ways he was to be the cause.

The Leipzig Hospital

Much to Hahnemann's delight at his jubilee, a gift of 1,250 *thaler* was made towards the erection of a homeopathic clinic in Leipzig. By 10 August 1832, through the efforts of the friends of homeopathy this had grown to 3,500 *thaler* (see Chapter 2). The same Moritz Müller, whom Hahnemann deemed an amphibian or hybridised allopath, now chairman of the association, informed Hahnemann that with these funds available, his committee had decided to purchase a house and proceed with the plan to open a homeopathic hospital. Hahnemann first expressed himself as being extremely gratified.[14] After all, it was his most ardent wish that homeopathy should possess its own hospital. He had written to the association as recently as May 1831:

> I ask you to apply all your energies (*nervos omnes intendas*) towards procuring for our homœopathy a clinic under the protection of a sovereign.[15]

However, despite these positive sentiments there can be no doubt that inwardly he nursed a great mistrust of the Leipzig physicians and deeply resented any who in the least swayed from the path of pure homeopathy. To him they were like worms eating away at the strength and health of the profession. In this state of brooding suspicion and sense that there were those within the fold who would betray and compromise his precious doctrine, it would take very little to rekindle the intolerant fires of his youth and provoke an explosion. Scarcely three weeks after expressing his approval, when all concerned thought that the Father of Homeopathy was amiably inclined to all that was being planned and that the launching of the hospital would be unmarred by dissension, Hahnemann suddenly lashed out with an uncompromising, aggressive attack upon the 'half-homœopaths of Leipzig' – in a letter which he made public by sending it to the Leipzig daily newspaper. What finally triggered the denunciation is uncertain – whether it was the suspicion that all the enthusiastic zeal of the influential, persuasive and intellectually agile Moritz Müller was actually directed towards appropriating for himself the position of chief physician of the hospital, the better to promote his 'false homeopathy'; or the fact that Dr Schweikert, a 'true homeopath,' whom Hahnemann favoured and nominated for the post was not appointed; or the unpalatable news that Müller, along with a Dr Schubert, was known to have recently treated a patient on her deathbed with leeches – any or all of these may have contributed – but most certainly fired by a festering hatred that had been eating at the old man's heart for some time and needed expression. Whatever the cause, the letter completed the rift in German homeopathy, creating a conflict which was never completely resolved and which inevitably led to the demise of the Leipzig homeopathic hospital after a mere ten years existence.

There could be no stepping back from the powerful invective that flowed from the old warrior's pen. In the letter of 23 October 1832, written in Köthen, after giving an exhaustive list of all the medical follies he so abhorred (blood-letting etc), he continues:

> . . . (these) are some of the quackeries by which, when used in conjunction with homœopathic prescriptions, we are able to recognise the crypto-homœopath, trying to make himself popular, as we recognise the lion by his claws. They swagger in the cradle of the homœopathic science (as they like to call Leipzig) where its founder first stepped forward as a teacher. But behold! I have never yet acknowledged you; away from me, ye medical —!

The editor of the daily paper censored the final word. Since Hahnemann would have recognised and desired the added thrust that alliteration provides, we can presume that the omitted word was 'mongrels'.

Hahnemann then writes:

> Either be honourable allopaths of the old fraternity, ignorant as yet of anything better, or pure homœopaths intent on curing your suffering brethren. Once more I exhort you, and this, for the last time, to abandon this course and to give those abroad a better example, one more worthy of imitation.

> But he who from this day forward hesitates to follow this faithful advice, to prove himself in word and deed a homœopath, let him never come again to Köthen while I behold the light of day, for he may look for no friendly reception.

> But if he will persist in that behaviour, then may – be meted out to you alone.

(The editor kindly spares us the pain of knowing what awful fate Hahnemann wished to befall deviant homeopaths!)

Hahnemann concludes the letter with the following:

> Hence I must solemnly protest against the employment of such a bastard-homœopath, whether as teacher or medical attendant. Let no one of this description enter upon the sacred offices of our divine art in this hospital – no one of this type!
>
> For should any false doctrines be taught under the honourable name of Homœopathy, or should patients be treated otherwise than by pure Homœopathy (with no trace of this allopathic muck), you may depend upon it that I shall raise my voice aloud honestly and to its utmost. In all the public papers far and near I shall warn a world weary of deceit against such treachery and degeneracy, which deserves to be branded and avoided. Today my paternal admonition sounds through this journal within the precincts of Leipzig, hoping for your improvement.
>
> (Signed) Samuel Hahnemann.[16]

Never did a tigress defend her cubs more fiercely than Hahnemann fought to protect the principles and purity of his beloved homeopathy.

In a formal reply to Hahnemann's letter on behalf of the Directors' Board of the Homœopathic Association, the ever-smooth Dr Moritz Müller was remarkably moderate and measured in his response, his carefully weighted arguments calculated to make Hahnemann appear prejudiced, unjust and dictatorial. His tone is placatory, condescending and self-righteous. He makes it clear that the association of the friends of homeopathy:

> . . . is absolutely independent of any individual – even the founder of Homœopathy himself – and – at no time in its career have the members of this association been required to practise exclusively in the homœopathic way.

One can imagine Hahnemann's ire when, further on, he read these patronising words of rebuke:

> The limitation of scientific views to the expressions of one person is called dogmatism, a form of despotism, by all cultured and scientific men, whilst intolerance of one's fellow believers is known as fanaticism. This form of excess, extinct even in religion (was he serious?), should be allowed no place, least of all in the science of healing – an experimental science incomplete even with homœopathy.[17]

How often the calm and considered words of the shallow deceiver sound more substantial, correct and trustworthy than those of the sincere idealist carried away by passion.

As a conciliatory gesture, since Müller and his association knew all too well that they needed Hahnemann and his 'pure' homeopaths on board in order for the venture to progress and survive, Müller added this overture to Hahnemann:

> ... the Board of Directors now invites you in deep respect to accept the title as President of the Association. By so doing you will restore unity between friends of homœopathy and its founder, without which, scarcely half can be accomplished that might be possible with united efforts.[17]

Unfortunately, this was not to be, Hahnemann's open attack had caused irreparable damage, estranging all the 'pure' homeopaths and distancing them from the activities of the so-called 'free' homeopaths, who were now identified with the Leipzig physicians and their new hospital. Its survival was doomed even before its doors opened. Failing to realise such a golden opportunity to establish an academic and clinical institution in the heartland of intellectual Germany was surely one of the saddest blows that homeopathy had to endure. The very goal that Hahnemann most desired, he sabotaged at its inception. Haehl comments on this unfortunate happening:

> It is the most painful fact in the whole history of Homœopathy that its founder, in clumsy and thoughtless haste, should deal the blow which stifled the movement's united enterprise as it was coming to life. By his sharp and unexpected attack in the Leipzig daily paper, Hahnemann had branded the Leipzig movement as 'pseudo-homœopathic' and unreliable, and this admonitory Cane mark deprived them almost entirely of their moral reputation outside Leipzig; and as an open declaration of war, it stirred up the homœopaths amongst themselves. All attempts made later to appease or redeem the situation – even by Hahnemann himself – could not retrieve this bad mistake.[18]

Hahnemann had robbed his colleagues of the credibility and support needed to ensure the development and survival of the hospital.

Set in his ways and inflexibly rigid in his ideology, Hahnemann failed to grant, within the homeopathic framework, the space, time and tolerance required for doctors, newly inclined towards its tenets, to bridge the difficult divide existing between one medical paradigm and another. He failed to recognise that in the transition from allopath to homeopath, as with many species in nature, the novitiate needs to experience a number of moults as old preconceptions and perspectives are shed or modified. He should have anticipated that some would always remain incompletely metamorphosed when compared with the high ideal he demanded.

In the event, Moritz Müller was appointed director of the hospital on 22 January 1833 and managed to retain the position until September of the same year when he resigned partly because of the attacks made upon him by the 'pure' homeopaths, but more especially because of his own inability to cope with the responsibility and requirements of his task. His unwillingness or inability to fully cross the divide between allopathy and homeopathy let him down when teaching students in the clinic. He was man enough to admit this and included this confession in his assessment of the institution made shortly before stepping down:

> I myself could not give complete lectures – only parts, because my skill and memory fail me when I have to indicate in difficult cases the most suitable remedy on the spot, because, in fact, I have not the gift of lecturing unprepared in a detailed and comparative manner about the selection of the remedy.[19]

This previously 'holier than thou' gentleman left the finances of the institution in a state of disorder. His position was temporarily filled by Dr Franz Hartmann, one of Hahnemann's most loyal students, until Dr Schweikert, Hahnemann's original nominee, was able to take the post on 1 November 1833. His appointment resulted in a return of interest in the hospital on the part of Hahnemann. So great was this that in June 1834, at 79 years of age, he made the journey to Leipzig from Köthen in order to inspect the hospital facilities and to discuss the way forward with Schweikert and close colleagues. In his customary autocratic manner and with a vigour and certainty of purpose remarkable in one of his years, he assumed control of the administration of the hospital and with a view to expelling the 'half-homeopaths' pushed for the dissolution of the Central Association of Homœopathic Physicians. This he bulldozed through arbitrarily, without consensus and in defiance of the statutes. Meekly, without remonstration, the members yielded to Hahnemann's bold assertiveness and forthwith the Central Association ceased to exist; the ground had been levelled for the hospital's new director. Schweikert proved himself worthy of the trust Hahnemann placed in him and ran the institution strictly according to the master's doctrines. His tenure in office proved of great advantage to the hospital both clinically and administratively, but he was handicapped by lack of finance. The dissolution of the Central Association had removed a vital source of revenue – the subscriptions paid by its members! Hahnemann's impulsiveness and unrelenting intolerance of the 'half-homeopaths' had once again undermined his enterprise and he was forced to appeal for contributions to all friends of homeopathy and the hospital.

Destiny

At this important juncture, in the early autumn of 1834 – when a seventy-nine-year-old widower, attended by his two highly-strung spinster daughters, was running a busy practice and at the same time trying to administrate a hospital from an impractical distance – a hospital which lacked both financial backing and professional interest – when, as always, he was the particular target of the envy and maliciousness of the German allopaths and apothecaries, but now could no longer depend upon a benevolent patron to protect him – at this critical moment – destiny stepped in and she did so with determined resolve and irresistible persuasion! A very attractive, young lady with blonde hair and blue eyes, elegantly dressed in gentleman's attire, departed from Paris in a mail coach, with Köthen as her destination.

* * * * *

The demise of the hospital

Before our history takes us away from Köthen, Leipzig and Germany, a few last words about the ill-fortuned Leipzig homeopathic hospital. Indeed, little remains to be said. The five directors who held office during the ten years of the hospital's existence proved unremarkable and incapable of taking it forward. Dr Schweikert, the most promising of all, once deprived of Hahnemann's force of will and protective presence, fell victim to merciless attacks from the 'friends of homeopathy' who undermined him with accusations of appropriating funds donated to the hospital, of reckless spending or excess thrift, and of failing to adequately instruct students. In August 1835, before this slander could be made public, Schweikert resigned his position. His assistant physician, the conscientious and sincere Dr Seidel, described the denunciations as being "extremely unjust, obscure, paradoxical and at times ridiculous."[20]

No less ridiculous was the situation that emerged from the chaos following Schweikert's departure. An allopathic conman, Dr Fickel by name (and fickle by nature), wormed his way into the homeopathic fold by presenting himself as a convert. Despite his lack of homeopathic education, he gained the confidence of his colleagues in the clinic by inventing all sorts of convincing facts and experiences. His deceit was so successful that it finally achieved for him the position of director or Chief Physician, a post he held for seven months, all with the sole motive of damaging homeopathy from within by exposing it as a sham. Eventually, his lack of training threatened to unmask him and taking fright he quickly tendered his resignation. Fortunately, little came of this peculiar man's bold effrontery and malicious intent.

That such a farce could have been enacted throws light on the level of homeopathy being practised at the Leipzig hospital at the time. It shows the degree to which homeopathy had been diluted by the 'allopathising' influence of the too broad-minded Dr Müller and his 'half-homeopaths'. It was also symptomatic of a serious lack of drive and ambition among the physicians attached to the hospital to passively permit such a mountebank to rise to a position of authority over them. The clinical success of the institute suffered accordingly and this added to the erosion of popular support. Although Hahnemann had been extremely impetuous and foolish in releasing his scurrilous letter to the press on the eve of the hospital's opening, his mistrust of all involved was vindicated by subsequent developments. With hindsight, it is doubtful that the hospital would have survived even if Hahnemann had remained silent. Even his belated interest in the hospital failed to stem the steady decay that finally led to its dissolution.

References

1. Bradford TL. *Life and Letters of Hahnemann*. Philadelphia PA: Boericke & Tafel; 1894. p187.
2. Haehl R. *Samuel Hahnemann His Life And Work*. Vol 1. London: Homoeopathic Publishing Company; 1922. p169.
3. Bradford TL. *The Lesser Writings of CMF von Boenninghausen*. Philadelphia PA: Boericke & Tafel; 1908. p6.
4. Bradford TL. *The Pioneers of Homœopathy*. Philadelphia PA: Boericke & Tafel; 1897. p183.
5. Cook TM. *Samuel Hahnemann – The Founder of Homoeopathic Medicine*. Northampton: Thorsons Publishers Limited; 1981. p150.
6. *Ibid.*, p151.
7. Bradford TL. *Life and Letters of Hahnemann*. Philadelphia PA: Boericke & Tafel; 1894. p213.
8. *Ibid.*, p212.
9. Haehl R. *Samuel Hahnemann His Life And Work*. Vol 1. London: Homoeopathic Publishing Company; 1922. p173.
10. *Ibid.*, p179.
11. *Ibid.*, p177.
12. *Ibid.*, p187.
13. Bradford TL. *The Lesser Writings of CMF von Boenninghausen*. Philadelphia PA: Boericke & Tafel; 1908. pp4–5.
14. Haehl R. *Samuel Hahnemann His Life And Work*. Vol 1. London: Homoeopathic Publishing Company; 1922. p189.
15. *Ibid.*, p205.
16. *Ibid.*, pp191–192.
17. *Ibid.*, pp193–194.
18. *Ibid.*, p206.
19. *Ibid.*, pp208–209.
20. *Ibid.*, p211.

8

PARIS – REJUVENATION AND DEPARTURE

Mélanie

After an arduous journey by coach, which in those days, traversing many difficult roads, must have taken all of fifteen days, the elegant young lady, whom we saw depart from Paris, finally arrived in Köthen on October 7th 1834. From the outset, her appearance, manner and dress caused a great stir in this small provincial German town, far removed from the salons of fashionable Paris. She was French, an aristocrat, her manner self-assured and assertive; she was young and beautiful, tall, lithe and graceful; but what most set the tongues wagging was the fact that she was dressed like a young man.

The town's folk were accustomed to seeing the constant parade of the noble and eminent, who came to seek a cure at the hands of Köthen's most famous inhabitant – the reclusive hermit, Dr Samuel Hahnemann – but the initial curiosity and gossip that this visitor's first appearance evoked were soon to be further titillated by rapidly unfolding events, of such a nature that memory of her would persist in the community long after her departure.

According to Haehl, the German homeopath Dr Gustav Puhlmann narrated many years later, in 1891:

> The older inhabitants of Köthen told me, many years ago, veritable shocking stories about the emancipated appearance of the young French girl who had come to Hahnemann as a patient, and who walked about the streets in man's attire. She was a keen horsewoman and swimmer and practised pistol shooting and hunted; she painted . . .

In the eyes of the prudish villagers, these masculine pursuits coupled to her manner of dress were indicative of an unrestrained temperament and moral laxity, and she was suspected of being a sexual siren set to prey on the vulnerability of respectable men.

Puhlmann added a tart observation of his own:

> Elderly vigorous men are easily inflamed with women of that temperament, especially if the latter are kindly disposed towards them.[1]

The young lady in question, Marie Mélanie d'Hervilly, had indeed come to consult Hahnemann about her health, but more pertinently to meet and converse with the writer of the *Organon*: the founder of homeopathy: the gentle art of healing. Her ailment, which she claimed had prevented her for the past two years from practising her profession, portrait painting and writing poetry, was diagnosed by Hahnemann, in the terminology of the time, as a type of *tic-douleureux* or neuralgic pain, which recurrently afflicted her in the right lower abdomen: in modern understanding probably an irritable bowel or spastic colon. Writing many years later when wishing to highlight her scientific bent, Mélanie downplayed the importance of the problem and emphasised that her primary motive in consulting Hahnemann was her interest in medical science. She gave him her age as thirty-two, but in fact she never admitted her true age, her good looks always permitting her to pass herself off as far younger than she was, and it is quite possible that she was already thirty-four or thirty-five when they met. In this we are given a small instance of her vanity and willingness to bend the truth to her own advantage. This willingness must be born in mind when considering the short history of her life entitled *Confidential notes on the life of Madame Hahnemann*, which she wrote in 1846 as part of her defence when accused of illegally practising homeopathy. One gains the impression that on a foundation of truth, Mélanie would, when the need arose, elaborate an exaggerated scenario to suit her ends. She was very conscious of her intellectual, artistic and physical assets and never too shy to blow her own trumpet.

> I was born with an extraordinary character which manifested itself in early childhood; I never played but was always thinking and, therefore, appeared sad without actually feeling so.[2]

Her father, Monsieur d'Hervilly, was descended from a noble French family. She informs us that he possessed a great intellect and provided her with an excellent education, stimulating in her a love of science and encouraging her innate flare for art and music. Their relationship was tender and loving and she respected him, but judged him weak and subordinate to her mother, who dominated their home. Her mother was a beautiful, flirtatious woman who loved to be courted and admired, and needed to be the centre of attraction. As Mélanie grew into the beauty of her own womanhood, her mother became jealous of her. Mélanie describes the unfolding of her charms:

> Meanwhile the child was growing into girlhood, the comeliness of youth was developing in a body which had been fairly well equipped by nature.[2]

Conscious of her mother's jealousy, Mélanie avoided the limelight and conducted herself in a scrupulously modest manner.

> All my efforts to appease my mother were useless; she would take me to dances against my wish, because I had been invited and she did not dare refuse, but the next morning she would punish me for the success I had achieved, being a good dancer; briefly, she conceived such animosity against me that it almost amounted to insanity.[2]

The situation in the home became intolerable and eventually dangerous when the mother in a frenzy of jealous hatred attacked the fifteen-year-old Mélanie with a knife. Her father at last stepped in and arranged that Mélanie should be placed in the care of her art teacher, Monsieur Guillion Lethière, and his wife.

In these happy circumstances, her artistic aptitude continued to be nurtured and she resolved to pursue art as a profession. She became a very successful portrait painter, the equivalent of a modern day photographer, and through her work gained entry to high society and the artistic world of Paris.

> I worked with pleasure, and the fruits of my talent soon became considerable; I was much in demand, and my other social talents enabled me to achieve success everywhere. Illustrious friends surrounded and protected me.[3]

These protectors were often older men with whom she found far greater affinity than with the many shallow-minded, young admirers who must have been drawn to the flame of such an attractive, talented woman.

> The serious nature of my character made me seek always the company of superior men who were almost all friends of my father, and who encouraged the studious young girl.[3]

One of the influential people with whom she formed a close friendship was M. Louis Gohier, who had briefly been President of the Executive Directory of the French Republic in 1799, whom Mélanie, in her characteristic desire for reflected glory and eminence, described as "the last President of the French Republic."

Probably a good example of Mélanie's carefully orchestrated presentation of her past is a document furnished by her purporting to be an extract from Gohier's will, but lacking both signature and date:

> Two women have inspired me with feelings bordering on adoration through their excellence, the one, my life-long companion, to whom I can only bring an offering of tears; the other is Mademoiselle Mélanie d'Hervilly. I should have been

proud had I been able to adopt her, but as I was so fortunate as to be a father, it was not admissible. I would have offered her my hand, if her inclination to art, the only passion which so happily dominated her, would have allowed her to accept it.

The document continues:

> As I wish to leave to Mademoiselle d'Hervilly a special token of the great esteem which her extraordinary merits and talents inspired in me, I beg of her ... that after my death she would unite my name to hers ... so that through the tie of mutual esteem my name shall be associated with her whom the rarest of talents will render celebrated.[4]

One cannot doubt that Mélanie's hand is implicit in this declaration of admiration and high esteem, but this self-promotive ruse, highlighting her chaste dedication to the arts and her moral and professional excellence, should not place in question their close relationship or the very real affection and regard that the old man felt for her, nor should it diminish our estimation of her true ability, gifts and charm, which were considerable. Whatever the truth of the matter, Mélanie henceforth styled herself: Mademoiselle d'Hervilly-Gohier.

She asserts that she developed an early interest in biology and when eight-years-old dissected birds to satisfy her curiosity:

> I constantly tormented my father with questions that he might explain to me the functions of the organs.[5]

This soon expanded into an attraction towards medicine and healing.

> I had extraordinary inspirations when I was near patients. At twelve years of age I saved the life of one of my father's friends who had been involuntarily poisoned by opium.[5]

This she says she achieved by ministering a "decoction of lettuce." She quite correctly declares that she had "unconsciously employed" homeopathy; the narcotic power of wild lettuce, *Lactuca virosa*, was known to the ancient Greeks, and the administration of a remedy capable of inducing an opiate-like drugged state to a patient suffering from opium intoxication was the application of the like-cures-like principle. By observation, she soon apprehended that allopathic medicine more often caused mischief than cure.

> Very frequently I noticed that the doctors did more harm than good to the patients. I used to question the physicians who treated my mother, and their answers were so ambiguous and absurd that my analytical mind was not unreasonably scandalised.[5]

Despite her considerable success as a society portrait painter, the distractions of life amongst the rich and famous and her many physical pursuits, her interest in medicine steadily grew and her exasperation, at not having the means or education to help those in distress, grew apace. At heart she was a committed feminist, an outspoken opponent of the restrictions and exclusions imposed on women by the patriarchal dominance that prevailed in Europe. She was particularly incensed by the limited opportunities available for women to develop and express their intellectual prowess, and that men had arrogated the professions for themselves. At that time, women were denied admission to medical schools. Through experience, she had come to the conclusion that a gifted woman, especially if virtuous, either became an object of envy and aversion to men, or was regarded as a toy, which they were proud to own. With these sentiments dominant in her, it is not surprising to find her in her early thirties, highly eligible in every sense of the word, yet still unmarried, 'celibate' and seeking the more accommodating company of older men.

Her own health had begun to decline because of frustration, stress and "grief caused by the loss of several of my friends"[5] and she could find no one capable of helping her. It was at this point that her need was answered. A French translation of the *Organon* found its way into her hands and a new perspective opened before her.

She writes:

> The *Organon* of Hahnemann's doctrine suddenly opened my eyes and the first glance showed that it contained the whole truth about medicine; the sun of true medical science had at last risen for me.[5]

With characteristic decisiveness, she resolved to travel to the very source of this wisdom, to meet Hahnemann face to face, sit at his feet as a student and find an answer to her pains. The friends with whom she shared this decision thought she was crazy and tried to dissuade her. But to no avail; it had become the entire focus of her being and propelled her towards distant Köthen.

At the destined meeting of these two singular individuals, we enter the rarefied dimension of high romance. It is certain that the strikingly beautiful, tall, young woman, who was ushered into the elderly physician's consulting room by one of his two daughters, had set aside her masculine attire for all the feminine finery of Parisian fashion. Neither her bearing nor her glamour would have daunted the seasoned veteran who bade her welcome. He was well versed in the niceties of sophisticated exchange and had long tended to the health of the nobility. She, however, would have been unprepared for the youthful vigour and vitality of the old man who rose to greet her.

We owe to Dr Philip Wilhelm Ludwig Griesselich a marvellously clear impression of the master in his late seventies. He wrote the following soon after visiting Hahnemann in Köthen:

> Hahnemann, now at the age of 77 years, showed in every action all the vigour of a young man. No trace of old age could be detected in his physical appearance except the white locks surrounding his temples, and the bald crown covered by a velvet cap. Small and sturdy of form, Hahnemann is lively and brisk; every movement is full of life. His eyes reveal his inquiring spirit; they flash with the fire of youth. His features are sharp and animated. Old age seems foreign to body and mind. His language is fiery and fluent. . . . His memory seems excellent; after long interludes he continues where he left of. . . . In earlier years Hahnemann had not been so communicative as he is now.[6]

His visitor relates that even at that advanced age, Hahnemann could easily be moved to heated outburst against those who persecuted homeopathy:

> . . . his words flow forth uninterruptedly, his manner becomes extremely animated, and an expression appears on his countenance, which the visitor admires in silence. Perspiration covers his brow; his cap has to come off and his head cooled with a handkerchief; the long pipe, his trusty companion, has gone out in the meanwhile and must be relighted by the taper that is at hand and kept burning all day. The white beer must not be forgotten![6]

Mélanie's description of that first meeting is brief:

> Dr Hahnemann was living with his two youngest daughters, who were unmarried, in a small and unpretentious house. His remarkable face inspired me with respect and astonishment. He talked for a long time and immediately conceived a great friendship for me.[5]

One can only imagine the intense chemistry that arose between them during this coming together of like minds. Here was the attraction of extreme opposites, both of age and gender, and the affinity of two individuals who shared intense passion for their convictions, felt persecuted by authority and were driven to bring about change. On the one hand, an old, but brilliant, highly articulate man, still possessed of unusual mental and physical vigour, without a companion for four years and only linked to the outer world, other than through his patients, by correspondence with a few colleagues – an existence fulfilling, yet essentially professional, and devoid of the warmth of a close relationship. On the other, a beautiful, intelligent, vivacious and ardent young woman, brimming over with curiosity and enthusiasm, hanging on his every word, who despite being a socialite has never found a man to meet her high ideals and who now finds herself in the presence of an exceptional being who emanates the determination and drive that her dear father lacked.

During that initial consultation, a spark jumped across the divide between circumstance and age and kindled a fire that rapidly engulfed them, overcoming any barriers that either might have initially felt. Whereas it is easy to understand the attraction that a man, even when advanced in years, may feel for a comely, young woman, it is less easy to grasp what can move a young woman to become emotionally and physically attracted to a very old man. Partly because of this, posterity has generally judged Mélanie harshly, denouncing her as a manipulative, seductive adventuress who captivated the heart of homeopathy's founder by stealth in order to gratify her own selfish ambitions. The observer, however, must allow for the complexity of two remarkable individuals, for the unerring, universal law of synchronicity and cosmic purpose and for an irresistible appeal, which was mutual, and, though undoubtedly having a physical component, rested primarily on a far deeper emotional, intellectual and spiritual foundation. In the magic of that first meeting they were caught in an autonomous, creative field moving them with compelling intent towards an unseen goal.

Within a matter of days they had decided to marry. Mélanie affirms that Hahnemann proposed to her:

> Hahnemann wished to marry me, and his friends who had learned to estimate my character at its true worth, did all they could to persuade me to accept his offer.[7]

In saying this, she is being rather disingenuous as there were no friends who could possibly have had the time or opportunity of assessing her, one way or another.

She avers that she hesitated before accepting the proposal:

> It was not the outlook of having to nurse a noble old man that frightened me, but the fear of losing him too soon and missing him so much that I might die of grief.[7]

Haehl, Hahnemann's biographer, when considering the proposal of marriage, grows hot under the collar, as have many generations of homeopaths:

> Is it likely that the old man will have courage and resolution enough seriously to propose marriage to so young a lady – unless she approaches him fairly obviously, unless, in the French phrase, 'she makes advances to him?'

> It was not Hahnemann who married her, the foreigner, but she who married him, the young woman marrying the old man. This is, in short, a confession of a clever woman's skilful calculation, and of her attainment of the goal she had set herself – namely the possession of this man.[8]

In his indignation, he invokes the perennial, patriarchal myth of innocent Adam and duplicitous Eve tempting her man towards his downfall. After repeatedly emphasising the ongoing clarity of Hahnemann's mind and his physical robustness, he still concludes that in the matter of Mélanie, Hahnemann was suddenly in his dotage, a helpless and hapless pawn in the hands of a conniving female. While it is true that the seductive power of a beautiful woman can never be underestimated and history records how many a wise man has had his brain addled by a *femme fatale*, was Mélanie such a woman? In the eyes of Hahnemann's two daughters, she most certainly was.

From the outset, they were suspicious of Mélanie's motives and hostile to her – and small wonder, given the circumstances. They had devoted themselves to caring for their father and supporting him in his life's work, both before and after their mother's death. They loved and venerated him and now, to their shock and utter disbelief, witnessed this man of immense stature and wisdom being beguiled by a scheming, dazzling dilettante, falling from the lofty pedestal on which they had placed him and becoming an infatuated, old fool. So it must have seemed to their anxious, filial eyes. Along with Rima Handley – who, in her well-researched book *A Homeopathic Love Story – The Story of Samuel and Mélanie Hahnemann*, consistently presents Mélanie in a sympathetic light – we can imagine the jealous sisters trying to eavesdrop on the conversations of the absorbed couple and at every opportunity walking in upon them under some or other pretext. By one ruse or another they must have tried to insinuate themselves between the pair in an attempt to disrupt and obstruct the alarming turn of events and hold their father to them. To this end, the younger daughter, Louise, played upon her uncertain health. Both she and Charlotte denigrated Mélanie to him, pointing to her free and easy ways as indicative of moral permissiveness. Their neediness and their fears for his and their future, together with his love for them, must have caused him great anguish.

Handley has translated from French the eighteen letters written by Mélanie to Hahnemann between October 1834 and January 1835. In these letters Mélanie professes her undying love for him:

> I can no longer live now without your good opinion and love.

> . . . you will always be my husband in my thoughts; no other man will ever lay a profane hand on me, no mouth other than yours will kiss my mouth. I give you my faith, and I swear to you eternal love and fidelity.

Hahnemann responds by making a passionate avowal of love written at the bottom of one of her letters:

I love you eternally, more than I have ever loved anyone in my life.[9]

In other letters Mélanie draws the attention of the concerned father to what she sees as the possessive and controlling behaviour of his daughters.

> Your daughters are foolish, the whole world knows it. You are not obliged to pay attention to the desires of fools. Louise has been ill for a long time and through this has established absolute domination over the affairs of the household, but she is well at present.[10]

> I forgive them [their antipathy] because it is an illness, but neither I nor your friends want you to be the victim of their madness any longer. Oh God, what would Europe say, which so admires Hahnemann, if she knew that the great doctor cannot have a consultation without the presence of his daughters?[11]

The daughters' influence, which had long held domestic sway over the 'great doctor,' was soon demolished by the combination of compelling pressure and warm coaxing exerted by Mélanie. Once Hahnemann's initial paternal concern and misgivings were overcome, she took firm control of affairs and the old man was swept along in the wake of her unswerving drive and determination. They were married on 18 January 1835 in the front room of Hahnemann's house in Köthen, less than four months after their first meeting. With remarkable expedition, Mélanie had overcome the not inconsiderable difficulties attached to marriage between a French Catholic and a German Lutheran. Once married, her driving aim was undoubtedly to return to Paris with her husband, but she realised that his uprooting would have to be achieved by degrees, particularly in view of the distraught condition of Charlotte and Louise, and his attachment to them. She therefore disclosed nothing of her intentions to Hahnemann, leading him to believe that they would remain in Köthen and that the time had now come for him to rest from his labours and enjoy his remaining years in her company. The emotionally fraught atmosphere and their open animosity to Mélanie meant that the sisters could no longer continue to live under the same roof as their new step-mother, therefore Mélanie arranged for Hahnemann to buy a neighbouring house for them.

Mélanie's next step in disentangling Samuel from his family was to have him draw up a new will in which it was stated that Mélanie would receive no portion whatever of Hahnemann's estate, either during his lifetime or at his death and that he would immediately assign all his property to his children and grandchildren. This was made public in an article published by Hahnemann's lawyer, Insensee, on 11 March 1835, in defence of slanderous gossip that was being circulated accusing the new Frau Hahnemann of being a fortune hunter. The promptings of Mélanie are visible in the lavish praise the lawyer heaps upon her in his affidavit, while asserting her independent wealth and drawing attention to how great a sacrifice she had made in dedicating her young, promising life to the comfort and happiness of an old man. But this first will was only the initial part of Mélanie's strategy, intended to ease Hahnemann's conscience regarding his family and to place her in a better light. On 2 June 1835, Hahnemann executed a second and final will. It confirmed the public declaration made three months earlier regarding the division of his property and possessions between his heirs:

> I declare that I have divided nearly the whole of my property among my children solely on the particular wish and desire of my wife, which is proof of her noble disinterestedness; to her, my children owe it, that they have received nearly all my own fortune, which I have acquired with so much labour and exertion, but which I could never quietly enjoy.[12]

But Hahnemann now emphasised that this disposition was not irrevocable; he annulled the clause barring his wife from all inheritance, and excluded from his general estate all the possessions that he would be taking to Paris. On his death, none of his heirs would have any claim upon the properties or possessions accrued during his future life with Mélanie; she would be the sole beneficiary of his future estate. A stern warning was included:

> But should any of my family, contrary to all expectations, not be satisfied with this my last will, and begin an action of law about it, he is to lose at once one-half of his whole inheritance.[12]

He further warned that should any of his children "in the least way annoy my beloved wife" they would forfeit their inheritance, which would be given to charity.

In the light of future developments, Hahnemann includes a curious and significant clause regarding his funeral and this injunction also contains an attendant threat of reprisal:

> My mortal remains shall be left to my dearly beloved wife, who is to have free choice of the place of interment and of the funeral arrangements, unfettered by anyone; but should one of my children or grandchildren dare to interfere with her directions, he is forthwith to be punished by losing one-half of his inheritance.[12]

At this point, it is apparent that Hahnemann was definitely contemplating retirement from practice, for he states in the will:

> I am now in my eighty-first year, and naturally desire to rest, and to give up my medical practice, which has become too burdensome to me.

Also by this time, Mélanie had persuaded him of the necessity of distancing himself from his past life, with all its tribulations, and to retire with her to Paris:

...where, far away from the country in which I have endured so much, I shall probably remain, and where I hope to find with my beloved wife that peace and happiness for which my desired marriage will be sufficient guarantee.[12]

It is notable that after meeting Mélanie, the first letter that Hahnemann wrote to his closest friend, Clemens von Bönninghausen, with whom he was usually in constant communication, was on 8 February 1835, when he had already been married for three weeks. Perhaps he felt somewhat shy about the considerable age difference between himself and his bride and wondered what Bönninghausen would think of his mentor, or possibly the rapid passage and intensity of events had so commanded his attention that he neglected to inform his friend of what was transpiring in his life. Whatever the reason for the delay, when he did at last write, he was at great pains to first explain how he intended to provide for his heirs and only after having done so, does he mention his recent marriage to

...a distinguished and excellent lady from Paris, who is held in great esteem there, of the purist morality, great learning, clear intelligence, and the best of hearts, who inspired me first with the most perfect love which she reciprocated in the fullest measure; she is handsome, tall and is 32 years of age.[13]

When news of the marriage of the famous octogenarian became general knowledge, it was a topic for gossip, ridicule and ribald comment. While mocking Hahnemann, his adversaries often at the same time took the opportunity to mock homeopathy. A particularly scurrilous article appeared in *Dorfgzeitung von Saxe-Menigen*, which down the years has become well known and now raises a smile rather than an outcry:

The renowned father of Homœopathy, Dr Hahnemann of Köthen, was married again on the 18th of January in his 80th year, to prove to the world how his system has been glorified in him. He married a young Catholic, the daughter of a Parisian nobleman. The young man is still vigorous and strong, and challenges all Allopaths: imitate me if you can! It is rumoured that several allopaths are inclined to consider homœopathy.[14]

This and similar snide attacks and derisory comments must have helped Mélanie move a usually obstinate, but highly sensitive, Hahnemann to make the decision to leave Köthen and Germany for good.

Even today, this marriage of a very elderly man to a lovely young woman raises many an eyebrow and the, often unspoken, question of whether they could have had a sexual relationship. Apart from Hahnemann's advanced age, there should be no reason to suspect otherwise – his health was excellent, he was physically active and sturdy of build, his faculties were unimpaired and his beautiful handwriting retained all the firmness and flourish of a young hand; besides, he was a passionate man and very aware of her beauty and her fine figure, which he frequently comments on. The speed with which their relationship quickened and ripened surely suggests more than just a consummation of cerebral ardour. Besides, Mélanie was a woman of the world and she knew that her beauty and sexual allure would give her power over him. Handley provides evidence of their physical intimacy in the second of Mélanie's letters to Hahnemann in which she teasingly expresses concern for his safety in the heat of her embrace:

> . . . an angel whom in my violent love I dare not even press too strongly on my burning heart for fear of inspiring him to transports too lively and funereal.[15]

Even Hahnemann's will leads us to the same conclusion – that this was a marriage in every sense of the word:

> Should my present wife bear me any children, then this child or children, as a matter of course, have the same claims on my property as the children of my first marriage.[12]

Paris

With the finalising of the will, Mélanie had succeeded in cutting all ties with the family. Hahnemann was hers and hers alone, and she took the reins of his life firmly in her capable hands. When they departed from Köthen in the early morning of 7 June 1835, it was never to return. While Mélanie had no doubt whatsoever about what lay ahead for her husband and herself, Hahnemann was still uncertain about future events, but happily willing to place himself under her direction. Despite his noting in his will that he might not return from Paris, we find him writing in a letter to his neighbour shortly before his departure:

> On this occasion I wish you and your family good health and well-being, and would ask you at the same time to remember my daughters who live opposite you, until I return.[16]

Writing to Bönninghausen, soon after his arrival in Paris, he gives the impression that he was merely accompanying Mélanie, who had affairs to attend to in the city, and would be returning to Köthen when these were concluded:

> I cannot avoid accompanying my dear Mélanie (without whom I cannot exist even for two hours) who has to settle her own financial affairs there. The most excellent French pupils also eagerly await me (particularly those belonging to the Soc. Hom. De Paris, who insist more upon purity than the large number of those belonging to the Soc. Hom. Gallicane who are distributed all over France), and I shall not withhold my good advice from them. Apart from that I intend to rest chiefly, and see very few patients.[16]

Paris – rejuvenation and departure

Hahnemann had a close professional friendship with Princess Louise Auguste, the daughter of King Frederich Wilhelm 111 and Queen Louise of Prussia. In February of that year, the princess had written to him from Düsseldorf:

> ... my surprise was not small when I read in the local paper the announcement of your marriage as I had not any idea of it and I send all good wishes for your welfare ...

In March, she wrote again asking him to let her know when he had returned from Paris, so that she could forward her 'journal' (progress report) to him, at a time when he would be in Köthen to receive it.

These communications indicate that Hahnemann had not yet made a firm decision about his future and was relying entirely on his "beloved wife" to plan the way forward. In this she did not fail him, or herself. She brought to the task her youthful vitality, her passionate enthusiasm, her burning, personal ambition and above all her nurturing care and love for homeopathy and its founder. It was as if her energy suffused him and so buoyed up his entire being that he was able to set aside the limitations of age and once again preside over the profession he had brought to life, but now at last in circumstances both harmonious and supportive, and with an adored companion beside him who cherished him with tender devotion and attended to his every need. With prudent foresight, Mélanie realised that their first need must be to obtain official authorisation for Hahnemann to practise medicine in France. In February, almost four months before their departure from Köthen, she persuaded him to apply to the Minister of Education and Public Health, Guizot, for a licence to practise. Through Mélanie's influence in high places this was granted on 12 August, but not without the opposition of the members of the French Academy of Medicine. With a broadness of vision and lack of prejudice rarely shown by Health Departments even to this day, Minister Guizot responded to their protestations with a telling admonishment:

> Hahnemann is a scholar of considerable merit. Science must be free for all. If Homœopathy is a chimera or a system without inward application, it will fall of itself. If, on the other hand, it is a measure of progress it will extend in spite of our preventive measures and that is just what the Academy should pre-eminently desire. For the Academy has the mission of furthering science and encouraging her discoveries.[17]

On 15 July, after a short stay at Mélanie's Paris apartment, they moved to more spacious accommodation at Number 7, Rue Madame, close to the Luxembourg Gardens. Hahnemann expressed his delight at the situation in a letter to Bönninghausen thus:

> We are living here in the purest air as if we were in the country; we are like a couple of doves and our love for one another daily increases (which seems almost impossible) for no husband could be happier on earth than I am . . .[18]

As much as he must have come to relish the thought of retirement and of at last relaxing into his last years without the pressures of practice and the responsibility of furthering the homeopathic cause, especially after so many years of unremitting industry and heroic effort against continuous opposition, these seductive murmurs were soon pushed aside. Beside him he now had a young, influential woman of immense energy and an enthusiasm for homeopathy that matched his own; his fame had preceded him and Parisian society waited eagerly for the ministrations of the great healer; French homeopathy embraced him with reverence and awe; and he now lived at the very centre of culture, enlightenment and the romantic movement. Every facet of his being was flattered and gratified by the attention, respect and adulation he received, and he was stimulated and motivated by his changed circumstances. There was a newfound spring in his step, a resurgence of his mental and physical powers, and in his correspondence, as if in wonderment, he repeatedly comments on his sense of energy and wellbeing.

In his address to the members of the Gallic Homœopathic Society, who had enthusiastically arranged a festival to celebrate his residence in France, and on the occasion made him their Honorary President for life, he responded to their homage with these words:

> I am deeply touched by the expressions of affection which I have received from all its members. I combine my zeal with theirs, and will support their endeavours for the furtherance of our divine science, because old age, which has never diminished its march, has not chilled my heart nor weakened my thoughts and homoeopathy will always remain the object of my heart.[19]

Writing to Bönninghausen in January 1836, he states:

> . . . many friends who saw me before assure me unasked that I never looked more sprightly and fresh than I am now; and I do feel well, thank God![18]

Mélanie, writing in August 1837, tells Dr Paul von Balogh, a member of the Society of Medicine of Lyon:

> Rest assured that the most thoughtful and tender cares are bestowed incessantly upon him. He is fresh and ruddy as a rose and as blithesome as a young bird; indeed, one might truthfully say that since he has been with me he becomes every year one year younger. May God give him health here with us![20]

Although we obviously do not have a photograph to confirm these observations, we do have a portrait of Hahnemann painted by Mélanie in 1835, which bears testimony to her artistic competence, and shows the Master wearing an amiable, benevolent expression on a countenance denoting sharp intelligence, remarkably unworn by the passage of time and events.

Given all these intoxicating excitements and his innate love of celebrity, which the French were so adept at glorifying (even striking a medal in his honour, wrought by the famed sculptor Pierre Jean David, and bearing his portrait), and his sense of rejuvenation, it must have taken very little cajoling on the part of Mélanie for Hahnemann to reconsider the matter of his retirement and agree to see patients again. So, after an interlude of only a few months, which could be considered somewhat of a honeymoon for the couple, Mélanie opened Hahnemann's Paris practice. What began in a small, modest way soon gathered impetus. The combination of his reputation and her wide circle of contacts among the wealthy and influential of Parisian high society ensured the success of the practice, which soon became extensive. With their finances augmented from this source, they were able to create a free, outpatient clinic for the poor. It was in serving these underprivileged people that Mélanie was able to at last fulfil her ambition of practising homeopathy.

At first, this was under the tutelage of her husband, but with her eager and receptive mind, her brilliant intellect, which Hahnemann never tired of praising, her intense application to the homeopathic materia medica, and her ongoing exposure to clinical conditions through sitting in with Hahnemann during his consultations with the wealthier patients, she soon became a confident prescriber in her own right. The poor were generally easier to treat than the affluent because they had not been exposed to the deleterious and expensive 'pernicious methods' of therapy applied by the French allopaths. Once she commenced treating patients independently, without the direct supervision of Hahnemann, she stepped outside the law, but while Hahnemann was alive, officialdom seemed to tolerate her activities and Mélanie built up a considerable practice of her own.

Writing to his intimate friend Baron von Gerdsdorff, to whose two sons he was godfather, Hahnemann describes his circumstances in June 1836:

> We live as if we were in the country, surrounded by most beautiful scenery, and are away from all the noise . . . (yet) the patients from Paris have easy access to me (also by carriage), as they are chiefly from the higher and highest classes, but I also give my help with pleasure to the poorest, as my excellent wife lends me a most helping hand, as she is a warm friend to our science. To sum up, I am so happy in my present position as I never was before during the whole of my life. I have a highly educated wife who loves me dearly. She is endowed with knowledge of the most varied kind, and has a kind disposition, great intelligence and refinement; I also love her as the most precious jewel of my earthly existence. Her incessant care is only for me, even to the most trifling details, so

that every wish of mine is fulfilled, no matter what it may be. I feel myself as strong and vigorous and free from infirmity as I was in my thirtieth and fortieth years.[21]

So vigorous indeed, that after a busy day in practice, this man of eighty and more years, accompanied by his wife or one of his students, took to doing something which he had never done while practising in Köthen, other than for the Duke and Duchess: when occasion demanded, he would now visit bedridden patients in the evening. For this purpose he had to purchase his own carriage – a considerable expense.

However, Mélanie's care for Hahnemann ensured that all was not work and that there was time for pleasure, socialising and entertainment. She introduced Hahnemann to the cultural delights of Paris, which had always been close to her heart. They regularly attended the opera, concerts and the theatre, often accompanied by Mélanie's father, a man of similar age to Samuel. Monday evenings between eight and half past ten were set-aside for homeopathic get-togethers in the tradition of his Leipzig years. In his spacious apartments, he would host an enthusiastic group of ardent colleagues with whom he would devote the time to informal homeopathic discussion. We can be sure that both the velvet cap and the smoking gown would be in place and that, as of old, his erudite discourse would be interrupted by intermittent puffs from his beloved long-pipe.

Reputation and high connections cannot sustain a medical practice, results are essential for its growth and survival, and these came in abundance. Homeopathy worked its magic for them. Soon the somewhat remote Luxembourg situation and the premises, as grand as they were in comparison to the simplicity of Köthen, proved inadequate to deal with the pressure of patients that threatened to inundate them. More space and a more central position in the city were required if the practice was to keep pace with the demands made upon it. In the spring of 1837, they removed to the busy and fashionable Rue de Milan, north of the Seine. In these major decisions one recognises the drive and ambition of the young woman. A man of Hahnemann's age and temperament would surely have been satisfied with far more modest and quieter working conditions.

No 1, Rue de Malan was palatial and its furnishings sumptuous. Mélanie spared no expense in setting up the practice, which was soon to become the most celebrated in Europe. Her personal finances were certainly not as prosperous as she would have had everyone believe, and Hahnemann's estate had already been allotted to his family, therefore considerable debt must have been incurred in creating this elegant establishment, on such a grand scale, designed to cater for the discerning taste of the French elite. A well-known American actress, Anna Cora Mowatt, visited the practice in

1839, and subsequently wrote an article describing her experience, under the *nom-de-plume* of Helen Berkley. She recounts the slow progress of the line of carriages, many bearing the coats of arms of the nobility, waiting to gain access to the spacious court before the 'palace-like mansion'; and she details the liveried domestics, the wide staircase, the opulent décor, the fine artworks, the children with their nurses, the fashionably dressed ladies and gentlemen waiting their turn, and not a vacant seat to be found.

While waiting in the quietness of a small, adjoining boudoir, Mrs Mowatt enters into conversation with the Countess de R, a young Italian married to a distinguished French count, who knows all there is to know about the Hahnemann's and is eager to share this with the American. The dialogue between the two reads like an unashamed, *curriculum vitae* extolling all the wondrous virtues and talents of Madame Hahnemann. Miss Mowatt must have struck up a friendship with Mélanie, and developed sympathy for her enterprise, because the effusive admiration for Mélanie expressed by Countess de R, and related in the American's narrative, could only have originated with Mélanie herself: a marketing ploy in which the actress was surely complicit. However, this said, the article gifts us with a precious glimpse of the Paris practice and when Mrs Mowatt is finally ushered into the inner sanctum, a chamber more simply decorated than the rest, we find the Master sitting in a comfortable armchair, capped, gowned and with pipe in hand, his deep set eyes glittering and full of animation.

Allowing for the self-promoting influence of Mélanie in the recounting of the consultation that followed, it is apparent that she played a large role in assisting Hahnemann in his work. Under his supervision and guidance, it was she who largely conducted the interview. While he sat in repose, she occupied the desk with gold pen in hand and note paper before her. read to Hahnemann from the doctor's letter of referral, asked a multiplicity of questions, made copious notes and brought the conversation back on track when Hahnemann and Mrs Mowatt digressed while talking of Germany. Finally, after conferring with the Master, it was she who wrote out the prescription, explained how it should be taken and provided the patient with a pamphlet listing substances which might prove detrimental to the action of the homeopathic remedies. This scenario explains how it was possible for Hahnemann to continue his work at such a pace, it was her energy that sustained him. Mélanie acted as his amanuensis, his interviewer, his assistant, his colleague, his second opinion, his practice manager and most of all as his protector, shielding him from all vexations, conflicts and administrative responsibilities and ensuring that he was not overtaxed and that she attended to his every need and comfort.

Many of Mélanie's critics have portrayed her as a slave driver, exploiting Hahnemann's genius for her own gain, pushing the old man into a hectic practice which would have burdened a far younger man, and robbing him of his well earned leisure years. It was also held against her that due to the many distractions she introduced into his life, and the intense schedule of work she imposed upon him, he produced no further literary works after leaving Köthen. In this latter criticism, is it not rather the critics themselves who would have imposed additional responsibilities to homeopathy upon Hahnemann – responsibilities, which he had surely already discharged in abundance? Careful consideration of the facts, and the comments of Hahnemann himself, provides a different interpretation of Hahnemann's Paris life.

In a letter to his dear friend Bönninghausen in September 1836, Hahnemann writes:

> . . . my hours of leisure are few. I am in the midst of a large practice which includes local personages of high rank, and I achieve the best results, and can therefore hardly protect myself from the onrush . . . here they know how to appreciate and how to remunerate a true physician, by which the costly living of this place is compensated. Through my activities our science has already acquired great honour here. Even if I were fifty to sixty years younger, I would never think of returning to Germany . . . I am in better health and happier than I ever was in my life, and I wish you the same. I only wish you were here, but no one else; therefore do not speak of this wish of mine to any other homœopath, because only you would be in the right place here . . .[22]

Hahnemann was evidently enjoying himself, gratified by having the eminent and famous seek his advice, by his popularity, his success and the financial rewards all this was bringing. In Germany, he had developed and expounded the homeopathic doctrine and science, now in his latter years and in his new country, the task was to be different: it was proof and persuasion by successful outcome – by curing the sick. Mélanie provided the energy and means. Together they were a powerful team. This letter also confirms how highly he esteemed Bönninghausen.

Just over eighteen months later in January 1838, again writing to Bönninghausen, he discusses his strategy in France. He relates that he has abandoned his previous hope of establishing a homeopathic hospital or clinic in Paris, because official and public prejudice against homeopathy would prevent this. He complains:

> Even the King himself is to be numbered among the staunch allopaths, and always carries about with him the blood-letting nozzle when in the country.

He largely ascribes this resistance to the mischief done to the homeopathic cause by the half-homeopaths before his arrival in the city, through their ignorance and incorrect practise. He continues:

> As I considered it worth while to change the prevailing opinion in the capital of France and win recognition as well as admiration for our system of treatment, seeing that Paris gives the tone almost to the rest of the world ... I endeavoured to begin this difficult task, but I found this could not be accomplished by writings – because here a great deal is written. No! We had to accomplish cures. Successful treatments must open the eyes of the public.[23]

He was as good as his word. It is not possible to statistically assess the effect of Hahnemann's Paris years on homeopathy in France, or further afield, but so many persons of note and influence from many parts of the world attended No 1, Rue de Milan during those busy years and so many of them benefitted from the experience, one cannot doubt that the results were positive and considerable, contributing to homeopathy's spread and popularity both in and beyond France. Nor were the common people neglected. Large numbers of the poor received free treatment from the Hahnemanns, especially from the hands of Mélanie, and this must have left a legacy among the general populace. Furthermore, during these years Hahnemann was not content to simply continue using the methods he had developed in Köthen and earlier. He continued to experiment using remedies in different ways, different potencies and different sequences. He also pondered the matter of the initial aggravation that the higher, centesimal potencies of the similar remedy sometimes initiated in sensitive subjects, and devised a new scale of remedy dilution and potentisation, the LM potency scale, to reduce or obviate this.

We can confidently conclude that he was not just a figurehead behind which Mélanie could safely practise, he was not just a passive dotard, submissive to her manipulation and exploitation, he was an active participant in a joint venture and retained to the end his own goals of further promoting homeopathy by achieving cures, and of improving and refining its methodology through practical experimentation. Nor did he discontinue teaching. An ever-increasing number of doctors requested permission to sit in with him as students and the busy Paris practice proved ideal for Hahnemann to tutor colleagues in a clinical setting.

The fame and success of the practice inevitably aroused a good deal of professional jealousy and resentment against Hahnemann and Mélanie and a rumour was circulated that he had become senile and was unfit to practise. Dr HV Malan, a Swiss doctor, who, during 1841–42, spent eighteen months as a personal pupil of Hahnemann in Paris (when his teacher was 86–87 years old), stoutly defended the Master in this regard:

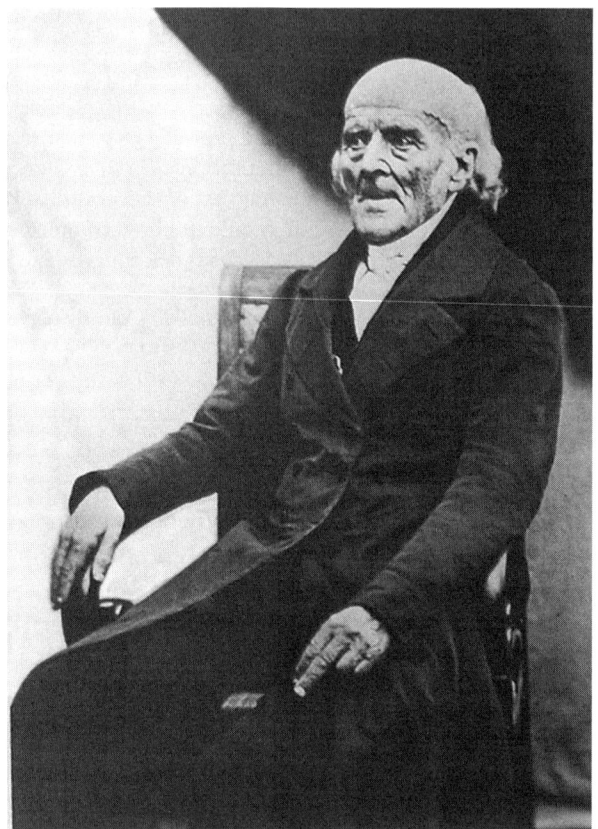

Figure 8.1 Photograph of Samuel Hahnemann aged 86, taken 30th September 1841 by H Foucault of Paris

According to the Rev T Everest, "It was a dark rainy day, with violent gusts of wind, Hahnemann was rather unwell that day"

Faculty of Homeopathy Collection

I should particularly like to point out that Hahnemann's intellectual powers show no sign of senility. On the contrary, I have witnessed some remarkable cures successfully accomplished by the very aged physician. He expounds his teaching with wonderful exactness and great erudition. He maintains throughout that pleasant modesty which was always characteristic of him.[24]

In addition to these endeavours, during these latter years he was anxious to revise and expand the last edition of the *Organon*.

He wrote to Bönninghausen about this project in June 1841. This document also provides evidence of the remarkable amount of clinical work he was still doing.

> My time has been too limited to enable me to answer your kind letter sooner. I am preparing the sixth edition of the *Organon*, to which I can only devote a few hours on Thursdays and Sundays, as the remainder of the week is occupied in treating patients . . . .[25]

In August 1842, he sent a dictated letter to an unknown German colleague, which apart from referring to the imminent appearance of the sixth edition, expresses in no uncertain terms his undying antipathy for the German half-homeopaths. To the last, they were anathema to him.

> Forgive me if since I left Germany I have never again troubled to waste one single word against my German slanderers and the distorters of our art. In a similar way I shall not think of them in my next edition (the sixth) of my *Organon* which will soon appear.

In his last communication to Bönninghausen, dated March 24, 1843, three months before his death, he informs his dearest friend that the work is complete and to his utter satisfaction:

> I . . . would like to draw your attention to a sixth edition of my *Organon*, which will soon, if God wills, at least appear in French, it will satisfy you in every way.[26]

Bönninghausen never had the opportunity of studying this last edition of the *Organon*. At the time of Hahnemann's death, the manuscript was, as yet, only a printed copy of the fifth German edition, extensively annotated in Hahnemann's tiny, meticulous handwriting "in the margins, between the lines and on pieces of paper stuck into and over the text."[27] Given the times, an immense amount of work was still required to achieve an accurate copy, faithfully detailing all the changes and additions to the text intended by the author. Despite many approaches and monetary offers made over the years by various homeopathic doctors, and particularly by the influential Homeopathic College of Pennsylvania (HCP), Mélanie refused to part with the manuscript during her lifetime. Trace of it was temporarily lost during the siege of Paris during the Franco-Prussian war of 1870–71, and again after the First World War, but it was eventually recovered by Richard Haehl and finally published in 1921. It is only in recent years that some of the more innovative concepts contained in this work have been adopted by sections of the profession e.g. the use of the LM potencies.

Hahnemann was aware of the dissatisfaction and complaints of the medical fraternity regarding Mélanie's obvious participation in his practice, and anticipating that she would at some time be subjected to attack from that quarter for practising without medical qualification, he wrote, in March 1841, to Dr Constantine Hering, the principal of the Academy of Allentown in Philadelphia (later the HCP):

> If I have been correctly informed, your Academy of Allentown grants diplomas to good homœopaths. If that is so, you would confer a favour on me if you would send one to my dear wife, Marie Mélanie Hahnemann, née d'Hervilly, for she is better acquainted with homœopathy, both theoretically and practically, than any of my followers, and I may say lives for our art.

In this letter he once again finds an opportunity to express his abhorrence of the 'traitors' within the ranks of the homeopaths and provides us with an endearing image of himself:

> The two little cameos will give you a fairly correct representation of my head. . . . The copper-plate engraving on the whole is a good likeness, only the artist has taken me in an unfortunate moment when I was probably vexed by the bad behaviour of the bastard homœopaths of Germany; there is no trace in it of the kind-heartedness seen in my features.[28]

In principle, Hering replied positively to this appeal, but the diploma did not materialise, and in 1842 Hahnemann, sensitive to the urgency of the matter, renewed his request:

> She has already treated 6000 poor patients, without my help, with such courage and skill that it made me confident of her success. She can now treat as well as I can. This is the reason why I desire this diploma for her. Time passes quickly and I would like to procure for her this title, all the more through you, because you have done so much for homœopathy.[29]

For reasons unknown, the diploma only arrived a considerable time after Hahnemann's death – the delay possibly due to reluctance on the part of Hering's academic committee to award a diploma to an unqualified person and thereby set an awkward precedent, even if she was the wife of the founder of homeopathy and strongly recommended by him. Hahnemann's fears for Mélanie were realised less than four years after his death on February 20, 1847, when she was prosecuted for illegally practising both medicine and pharmacy. The American diploma failed to protect her, being invalid in France, and she was found guilty on both counts, even though two sympathetic homeopathic physicians, Dr Croserio and Dr Deleau, gave evidence on her behalf, stating that she had worked under their supervision. She was fined 100 francs and debarred from practising. Needless to say, knowing her temperament, she continued to do so, but more discreetly.

During the Paris years, the Hahnemanns lived well and opulently; the fine mansion, the sumptuous apartments, the extensive household, the personal carriage and its horses, the regular visits to the opera and the theatre and the soirées held at No 1, Rue de Milan, all bespoke an elegant and comfortable lifestyle befitting the celebrity physician that Hahnemann had become. The high point of the social year was always the celebration of Hahnemann's birthday on April 10. The grand soirée held in 1838 in honour of Samuel's eighty-third was a particularly lavish affair, staged with all the flare and flamboyance dear to Mélanie's aristocratic heart. Remembering the grandiose style Hahnemann assumed when lecturing at the medical school in Leipzig, there can be no doubt that he was gratified by all the pomp and homage of the occasion, and a happy participant. The approach to the mansion was lined on both sides by the private carriages and hackney coaches of the beau monde; the first floor salon abuzz with their informed chatter and gossip as they awaited the entrance of their host and hostess.

> Hahnemann entered the room, a vigorous old man, looking more like sixty-three than eighty-three years of age. He came in on the arm of his wife, a lady who had the appearance of great intellectual power, and he welcomed his guests with a genial smile and a handshake.[30]

During and after the banquet, French and Italian poets and German musicians entertained the guests. The Parisian reporter, who provided the above description, notes the cosmopolitan nature of the assemblage, which numbered many Italians, English and Americans. The following day, out of curiosity, the reporter visited the Hahnemann residence and reported that the courtyard and the stairs were filled with poor people whom Hahnemann treated gratuitously, and he counted no less than fifteen persons in the ante-chambers.[30] It says much for the commitment and stamina of the couple that they were willing and able to see patients the day after such a socially demanding event.

As glamorous and extravagant as this birthday celebration was, it was, possibly surpassed by that which honoured the renowned doctor's jubilee in 1839, commemorating the sixtieth year since his graduation from the University of Erlangen. The only daughter to visit Hahnemann during his time in Paris was Amalie, his third daughter, who had always been the closest to him emotionally and before her marriage to Dr Suss, the most intimately involved in the clerical work incident to Hahnemann's practice. Unfortunately, Dr Suss died while she was pregnant with her only child, a son. He was to follow in his grandfather, Samuel's footsteps; after studying medicine, he became a homeopath and practised in London as Dr Leopold Suss-Hahnemann. After divorcing her second husband, Herr Liebe, Amalie joined her unmarried sisters in Köthen. More emotionally stable and independent than her two sisters and not daunted by travel or large cities, Amalie attended her father's jubilee and in writing to them left posterity a lively account of this important happening.

After the presentation of a silver-gilt cup to Hahnemann, the festivities began and continued through the day and far into the night:

> ... then one of the greatest cellists of Europe, (Max) Böhrer by name, ... enlivened the whole day until the evening, when the entire company was assembled. Among them were many ladies and gentlemen who brought beautiful flowers and excellent poems. Then we had the most beautiful music; the famous Klara Wieck (at the time 19 years old, already a piano virtuoso and later to marry Robert Schumann, the German composer) who is in Paris at present gave us the pleasure of her great talent. She, together with the violin-cellist mentioned above, entertained us so well that we were enchanted. Little father (*Fatti*) was so overjoyed and contented he looked like a blooming rose. The great salon, in which we were, was well illuminated, and handsomely decorated with beautiful oil paintings by little mother (*Mutti*).... Briefly it was a wonderful day. The festivities lasted until nearly three in the morning.[31]

It is sad testimony to the rift existing between Hahnemann and German homeopathy that on so momentous an occasion only one German physician was present, Dr Georg Heinrich Gottlieb Jahr (1800–1875), who resided in Paris. Dr Jahr started his professional life as a qualified teacher, became interested in homeopathy and subsequently worked with Hahnemann in Köthen, mostly in a literary capacity, completing for Hahnemann the compilation of the second, much enlarged, edition of *Chronic Diseases*. His homeopathic knowledge was so great that despite his lack of formal education, Hahnemann recommended him as personal physician to Princess Frederica of Prussia in Düsseldorf. This conspicuous position, always highly vulnerable to medical attack, convinced him that he must study medicine to achieve the necessary authority and clinical skills. He therefore resigned and enrolled at the university of Bonn. After qualifying, he moved to Paris, and there, Minister Guizot granted him permission to practise medicine without further examination, just as he had previously done for Hahnemann. Through his many written works on various aspects of homeopathic medicine, Jahr did much to propagate its growth. He always remained close to Hahnemann both in sentiment and in his unswerving adherence to 'pure' homeopathy.

Thus, the last years of Samuel Hahnemann in Paris, in the company of his beautiful and deeply beloved friend, partner and ever-supportive wife, Mélanie, whom he so admired and adored, seemed as though divinely bestowed in recognition and reward for his immense contribution to medical science. Every aspect of his multi-facetted nature was catered for. He found himself in the lap of luxury, surrounded by the sophisticated elegance and refinement of French culture and the beauty of its language, the central figure of a celebrated practice, the healing icon of both the aristocracy and the common populace and blessed to the very end with the health, strength and intellect to continue practising and honing his homeopathic expertise.

In a letter written to Baron von Brunnow in July 1841, just two years before his death, he gives testimony to the idyllic circumstances that prevailed during this last chapter of his life:

> After having been so misunderstood by my countrymen, I have happily found a haven of rest . . . where I can accomplish unhindered much that is useful and good through the only true art of healing. I have means, and am beloved by my wife who is a model of virtue and knowledge, such as I have not found before in any other woman in this world, and who does everything possible in order to satisfy my wishes and to prolong my life, health and cheerfulness . . . I am better and happier than I have been for many years and I enjoy life.

In closing he, once again, provides an endearing example of his vanity:

> My wife wishes to be kindly remembered to you. In order that you may be able to remember me better, I enclose a small portrait of myself[32]

However, the longest life, no matter how joyful and fulfilling, even one steeped in homeopathy, must finally come to a physical end. Shortly after his eighty-eighth birthday, in April 1843, Hahnemann was taken ill with bronchitis, a complaint that had inconvenienced him in the spring of previous years and which had always responded promptly to appropriate treatment. Probably his ever faithful long-pipe was a contributory cause in these recurrent chest infections. Expecting this bout to be no different from the others, he at first treated himself, but gradually his condition worsened. Days extended into weeks without remission. Finally, when it became apparent that his condition was becoming critical and that his life force was beginning to ebb away, Mélanie sought the help of a homeopathic colleague, Dr Chatran. But it was to no avail, the physical vehicle had finally run its course and the time to depart had arrived. Dr Croserio attended Hahnemann during his last days and wrote of his patient's "equanimity, patience and imperturbable goodness". He observed that although he had "a distinct presentiment of his approaching end, (yet) he never permitted an expression to escape him which could alarm his wife."[33]

When Mélanie, in despair at his increasing respiratory distress, exclaimed that surely Providence owed him exemption from suffering for having brought relief to so many, he answered:

> To me, why to me? Everyone in this world works according to the gifts and powers, which he has received from Providence. Providence owes me nothing. I owe all to Providence. Yes, everything.[34]

Samuel's last request to Mélanie was that the inscription on his tomb should read: *Non inutilis vixi* (I have not lived in vain). Three words that echo down the intervening years to the present time and are imprinted in the minds of all aspiring homeopaths.

After ten weeks of illness, Samuel Hahnemann died peacefully in his sleep in the early hours of the morning of July 2nd, 1843.

* * * * *

Epilogue

During the enactment of these final days, and those that followed, the bereaved widow's conduct was unusual in the extreme. She, who, during their life together, had always sought as much publicity as possible, now surrounded her dying husband with a protective barrier, which permitted entry to only a select few. A veil of secrecy descended over the events unfolding in No 1, Rue de Milan. So much so, that Dr Jahr, always close to Hahnemann, both in Köthen and later in Paris, first became aware of the urgency of the situation when Mélanie belatedly sent a note requesting him to call. When he entered the bedchamber, he found a weeping Mélanie stretched across the bed next to the cold body of her husband, who had been dead for some five hours. Although Amalie, on hearing of the seriousness of her father's illness, had hastened to Paris with her seventeen-year-old son Leopold, the two were refused access to his deathbed until the very last moment when Hahnemann had already lapsed into unconsciousness. This added hugely to the bitterness that the family already felt towards Mélanie.

The following day, the body was embalmed and having gained special permission from the police to retain the body for a period of fourteen days, Mélanie maintained a solitary vigil beside her deceased husband until the early morning of July 11th when, in persistent rain, a pathetically small group of mourners, comprising Mélanie, Amalie, Leopold, an apothecary friend, Lethière (nephew to Mélanie's art teacher) and a few servants of the household, slowly followed the hearse to the cemetery of Montmatre. There the coffin was deposited in an old vault that already contained the remains of M Gohier, Melanie's old admirer, and M Lethière, her art teacher and adoptive father.

Hahnemann's grandson Dr Leopold Suss-Hahnemann (who later settled on the Isle of Wight in England), drawing from his memories of the occasion, wrote in 1864:

> The great affection which the wife professed for her husband whilst he was alive, disappeared immediately after his death. The immortal Founder of Homœopathy was buried like the poorest of the poor, shortly after five o'clock in the morning; a very ordinary hearse conveyed the body, and we followed on foot . . .[35]

Mélanie made no public announcement of Hahnemann's death; contrary to custom she sent out no mourning cards and omitted to send notice of the funeral to relatives, friends and colleagues until the very last moment, and then failed to give the hour of the funeral service, which she arranged to take place at the impossible hour of five o'clock in the morning. And what is more, despite the protestations of Amalie, she disregarded Hahnemann's request that *Non inutilis vixi* be engraved on his tombstone.

In Haehl's words:

> It was as if Madame Hahnemann completely forgot her husband after depositing him at Montmatre. The grave was untended. No loving hand ever adorned it with fresh flowers – not even on the anniversaries – so that, according to unanimous accounts from Parisian homœopaths, it assumed an entirely neglected appearance and with time would probably have fallen into complete oblivion.[36]

As accomplished and unswerving as she had always been in successfully marketing Hahnemann and herself, creating and maintaining a prosperous, professional image, choreographing a scenario of conjugal bliss and being seen to scrupulously and selflessly attend to his every comfort and need, under the duress, grief or shock of his illness and death, she utterly failed to consider how posterity would view and judge her behaviour, which could only be considered bizarre. Indeed, so odd that it would seemingly confirm the Hahnemann family's conviction, one that would be shared by the homeopathic world and his biographer, Haehl, that she had never truly loved her husband, that she was conniving and duplicitous and that she had used him for her own selfish, ambitious ends; her husband, no sooner dead, forgotten. But such harsh and prejudiced conclusions must be subjected to scrutiny and Mélanie's actions analysed from a kinder perspective, for during the Master's life, she proved unfailing in her devotion and dedication to him, both personally and to his cause. Surely, there must be a less damaging explanation for her strange actions.

Her world had quite suddenly and without warning disintegrated about her. Hahnemann's health, strength and reason had shown no sign of faltering right up to the very commencement of his final illness. She would have had no call to think that time was running out and that Hahnemann would not continue in practice well into his nineties, given his remarkably resilient constitution and his passion for homeopathy. With his death, from a pinnacle of prestige and fame and all the attendant trappings of success, she, who vicariously thrived on Hahnemann's luminary status and the brilliant life it afforded them, was, at once, cast down into mediocrity and confronted by an uncertain, insecure future and almost certain, financial collapse.

Small wonder that this intense, assertive, yet highly, vulnerable woman froze, that she cloaked the events with secrecy, evidence of her own denial of what was transpiring and a desperate attempt to hold her life together, while she was distracted by grief and dread of what was to come. Grief there must have been; love comes in many forms; the Master was, despite his irascible, suspicious temperament, a beautiful soul and she received him into her care in his mellow years. To love him must have been easy and unavoidable. Her love for him would have had many shades: as daughter, wife, mother and sister homeopath, all magnified by his special uniqueness, his endearing nature, her admiration for his noble mind and his philosophy and cemented through the inevitable co-dependency that developed between them.

During the all-consuming intensity of her emotions and her concentrated focus upon the last hours of her beloved genius, whom she had treasured and cosseted for so many years, and who was now slipping away from her, she could not bear the least intrusion that might dilute or disturb the silent and sacred communion of those concluding days – not even the presence of Amalie and Leopold. When he was gone, she did not emerge from this inner retreat, but sought to prolong it by holding the body close to her for as long as possible. Although she had been granted permission to do so for up to fourteen days, on the seventh day some unfathomable, internal process resolved and she was able to move forward, but not into the glare of publicity, pomp and parade that would have descended upon her had she invited it. By intent or unconscious remissness, she ensured the privacy of her mourning and sealed it by the early hour of the interment. Nature, in sympathy, conspired with her, solemnly shrouding the funeral cortege and the ceremony in a pall of incessant rain.

Critics of Mélanie, like Haehl, were scandalised by her failure to publicise Hahnemann's death, by her choice of burial site and by her subsequent indifference to its upkeep – a neglect that was, however, not remedied by either French or German homeopaths. But, the site was not chosen to satisfy the homage of Hahnemann's public or any future generation. As mean and obscure as it may have seemed to those who desired a monumental tomb set among the illustrious of the past, to Mélanie, the humble, brick sarcophagus to which she consigned the coffin was hallowed and fitting for the final resting place of her beloved Master's mortal remains. It already contained the coffins of the two men she admired most, and one day her own would be laid at the side of Hahnemann. It would seem that with Hahnemann's death, she held his spiritual presence before her inner vision, a shift possibly achieved during her extended vigil, and the decaying, physical counterpart and its residing place held no further significance for her.

Be that as it may, the grave remained forgotten, unvisited and untended until an American homeopath, Dr Thomas Lindsley Bradford of Philadelphia, who later wrote the first biography of Hahnemann's life, initiated a search for the site in 1896. In the light of information given by Leopold Suss-Hahnemann, the correct grave was identified in June of the same year. The gravesite was purchased by the Hahnemann College of Philadelphia with a view to restoring it. Belatedly, French homeopaths woke up to their responsibility and proposed that a commemorative monument should be erected on the spot. However, it was finally decided that the site was unsuitable for such a project, and therefore by common resolution, on 24th May 1898, the bodies of Samuel and Mélanie were ceremoniously exhumed and transferred from Montmartre to the beautiful and famed cemetery, Père Lachaise, in Paris, the resting-place of many celebrated men of the arts, science and war. Two years later, on 21st July 1900, an imposing monument was erected and consecrated there, inscribed as Hahnemann had wished – a fitting tribute to a great man.

The remaining details of Mélanie's life lie outside the focus of this history and the interested reader wishing to know more about her fortunes should read the book by Rima Handley mentioned earlier. It is sufficient to relate here that she continued practising homeopathy to some degree throughout her life, even after her prosecution. In a bid to find a registered homeopath to shield her from further attacks, she unsuccessfully attempted on numerous occasions to coax Baron von Bönninghausen to settle in Paris, that he might practise homeopathy with her. He was not to be persuaded – not even after he was awarded the Knight's Cross of the Legion of Honour through her influence with the Emperor Napoleon. Her similar overtures to Constantine Hering in America were equally unsuccessful and the Association of French Homœopathic physicians studiously kept their distance from her; indeed, many of its members were highly antagonistic. Never at a loss to further her ambitions, she, therefore, travelled to Münster with the express purpose of arranging a marriage between Sophie Bohrer, a young woman whom she had adopted as a little girl of five shortly after Hahnemann's death, and Karl, the medically qualified son of Bönninghausen. Haehl refers to this strategy with his usual caustic view of her machinations:

> She did so with the same craftiness with which she had proceeded with Hahnemann, and pursued her idea, with the same assiduity which had always enabled her to overcome all difficulties.[37]

Needless to say, she was successful in her endeavour, and soon had her new son-in-law ensconced in her Paris practice, despite his initial ignorance of the French language. Although now linked to Bönninghausen by family ties, over the years, and despite his many solicitations and her many promises, she never released Hahnemann's clinical notes or the annotated fifth edition of the *Organon*. These were her last remaining treasures that she guarded to the very end. She died on 27th May 1878, at seventy-eight years of age after an attack of broncho-pneumonia and her coffin now lies at the feet of her Master in the Père Lachaise cemetery.

There existed a duality in Mélanie, which has always divided those who would appraise her, best expressed and seen in contrast through the histories of Haehl and Handley, both of whom approach her character strongly influenced by their own subjective feelings; the former viewing her with unadulterated suspicion, the latter with consistent magnanimity. Hahnemann's family would certainly have sided with Haehl, and Hahnemann with Handley. Possibly, the true Mélanie is to be found somewhere in the middle.

Her testimony about herself is always coloured by self-admiring superlatives and one sees her calculated input in so many of the documents that furnish her history. She knew, it being the custom of her social class, that her letters would be preserved. No matter how kind an interpretation one attempts to put on Mélanie's actions and however much one wishes to believe the sincerity and veracity of her utterances, one is invariably left with the feeling that she was also playing to an audience that she wished to impress and which one day would judge her, and that despite Hahnemann's unswerving belief in her and his constant adoration of her, which must have had justification. In serving him she was also serving her own love of celebrity and her own professional ambitions. In all fairness to her, this role-playing may have been because from the moment she walked into Samuel's life, his family viewed her with suspicion, as later would the entire homeopathic world. Hence, she may have continually felt obliged to vindicate herself to posterity and exaggerate her virtues – as she undoubtedly did at her prosecution.

Whatever her motives, she came into Hahnemann's life like a breath of revitalising energy, just as in modern times the appearance of Rudolph Nureyev re-ignited the career of the prima ballerina Margot Fonteyn. Just as the partnership of Rudolph and Margot brought a unique magic to ballet, so the partnership of Mélanie and Samuel benefitted homeopathy. Mélanie was essential to Hahnemann's destiny and to the destiny of homeopathy. The years in Paris afforded Hahnemann the opportunity to confirm, develop and evaluate his therapeutic methodology through clinical experimentation. She enriched his last years and brought him a happiness and contentment, which he could scarce comprehend; she came as a blessing from above – a reward for all his tribulations. As such, his homeopathic progeny owe her a deep debt of gratitude. In judging her, it must never be forgotten that when the Master's body was exhumed, and his remains exposed, a long tress of woman's hair was found entwined about the neck and she could not have known that anyone would ever discover this token of her love.

References

1 Haehl R. *Samuel Hahnemann His Life And Work*. Vol 2. London: Homoeopathic Publishing Company; 1922. p327.
2 *Ibid.*, p320.
3 *Ibid.*, p321.
4 *Ibid.*, p326.
5 *Ibid.*, p322.
6 *Ibid.*, pp256–257.
7 *Ibid.*, p323.
8 *Ibid.*, pp225–226.
9 Handley R. *A Homeopathic Love Story – The Story of Samuel and Mélanie Hahnemann*. Berkeley CA: North Atlantic Books; 1990. p9.
10 *Ibid.*, p7.
11 *Ibid.*, p8.
12 Haehl R. *Samuel Hahnemann His Life And Work*. Vol 2. London: Homoeopathic Publishing Company; 1922. p337.
13 *Ibid.*, p327.
14 *Ibid.*, p328.
15 Handley R. *A Homeopathic Love Story – The Story of Samuel and Mélanie Hahnemann*. Berkeley CA: North Atlantic Books; 1990. p11.
16 Haehl R. *Samuel Hahnemann His Life And Work*. Vol 2. London: Homoeopathic Publishing Company; 1922. p341.
17 *Ibid.*, p231.
18 *Ibid.*, p347.
19 Cook TM. *Samuel Hahnemann – The Founder of Homoeopathic Medicine*. Northampton: Thorsons Publishers Limited; 1981. pp170–171.
20 Bradford TL. *Life and Letters of Hahnemann*. Philadelphia PA: Boericke & Tafel; 1894. p368.
21 Haehl R. *Samuel Hahnemann His Life And Work*. Vol 2. London: Homoeopathic Publishing Company; 1922. p348.
22 *Ibid.*, p351.
23 *Ibid.*, p355.
24 *Ibid.*, p377.
25 *Ibid.*, p379.
26 *Ibid.*, p380.
27 Handley R. *A Homeopathic Love Story – The Story of Samuel and Mélanie Hahnemann*. Berkeley CA: North Atlantic Books; 1990. p205.

28 Haehl R. *Samuel Hahnemann His Life And Work*. Vol 2. London: Homoeopathic Publishing Company; 1922. p353.
29 *Ibid.*, p354.
30 *Ibid.*, p369.
31 *Ibid.*, p370.
32 *Ibid.*, p375.
33 *Ibid.*, p382.
34 *Ibid.*, p381.
35 *Ibid.*, p383.
36 *Ibid.*, p245.
37 *Ibid.*, p348.

9

OF PASSION AND POTENCY

The Father of Homeopathy in America – Constantine Hering

A very important figure in early homeopathic history was Dr Constantine Hering (1800–1880), a pioneering spirit who played a vital role in establishing homeopathy as a force in the USA. It was from him that Hahnemann, in 1841, had requested an American diploma on behalf of Mélanie, and to whom Mélanie appealed, after Hahnemann's death, to join her in homeopathic practice in Paris.

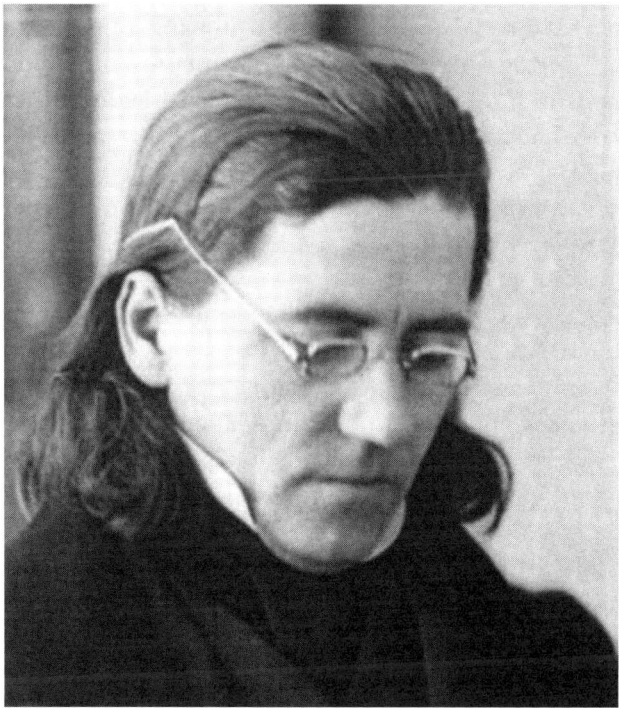

Figure 9.1 Constantine Hering (1800–1880) – The Father of American homeopathy.

He was born on 1st January 1800, and certainly for homeopathy the new century could not have started in a more propitious manner. His father was the assistant rector at Oschatz in the Electorate of Saxony. His early schooling revealed a studious nature, a particular flare for the classics and a remarkable proficiency in mathematics. In 1817, he attended the Surgical Academy of Dresden and after spending three years there, moved on to the University of Leipzig to study medicine. While still a junior student, he heard of the eccentric, medical heretic who was giving lectures on a strange, new method of treatment at the Medical Faculty. He would also undoubtedly have heard his professors and lecturers ridiculing both homeopathy and its founder. Nevertheless, either out of curiosity, or to fill an idle moment with entertainment, he attended some of these lectures, but remained on the periphery never introducing himself to the Master or seeking closer contact with the older students of Hahnemann's inner circle. Shortly afterwards, Hahnemann departed for Köthen and any influence Hahnemann's lectures might have had on the young Hering was cut short. Circumstances decreed that the two should never meet.

Enlisted to expose homeopathy

Although now at a distance, Hahnemann's growing influence and fame, or notoriety, in Leipzig and the increasing scepticism and animosity entertained towards him by the allopaths, encouraged Baumgärtner, a Leipzig publisher, who had a sharp nose for a good story and shared the allopaths wish to bring Hahnemann down, to approach the eminent surgeon Robbi, an outspoken critic of homeopathy, and propose that he write an article that would expose homeopathy as a fiction, and Hahnemann as a charlatan. Robbi, for all his distaste for homeopathy, could not be bothered to exert himself against what he considered a spurious doctrine, beneath his consideration or contempt, and pleading excess of work, recommended his promising young, assistant surgeon, Hering, for the task. Hering, pleased by his preceptor's confidence in him and flattered by the publisher's willingness to take up Robbi's recommendation, forthwith immersed himself in Hahnemann's published works, the better to understand Hahnemann's hypothesis and expose its flaws.

His perfectionist nature and mathematical mind made it necessary not only to subject homeopathy to theoretical analysis, but also to put it to the test by practical investigation. He reasoned that his starting point had to be the Cinchona (quinine) experiment, which had opened Hahnemann's eyes to the law of similars. He approached an apothecary acquaintance for a supply of the drug and when asked for what purpose he required it

Hering replied,

"For the purpose of proving it, in order the more thoroughly to attack the new folly (homeopathy)."

The apothecary raised an eyebrow and knowingly commented, while handing Hering the preparation, "Let it alone Hering; you are stepping on dangerous ground."[1]

Conversion

As far as Hering's allopathic convictions were concerned, these words proved to be true. His findings with cinchona reduplicated Hahnemann's original observations. He went further, doing more extensive provings and testing the results clinically. The results left him with no doubt about the truth of Hahnemann's teachings. As if to drive home this conclusion, very soon afterwards he developed a dissecting-wound of the hand – a condition that was much feared in those days, long before the advent of antibiotics. The associated infection could become so severe that only amputation would save the surgeon's life. He was at first treated by his allopathic teachers, but when the wound steadily deteriorated, one of his fellow students, who had studied with Hahnemann, sought advise on Hering's behalf and the recommended potentised remedy promptly did the trick. With this final proof, Hering's conversion to homeopathic science was complete.

Hahnemann's warning

Hering, unconscious of the possible danger to his progress in the medical school, intrepidly and rather naively, reported the results of his investigations to his superiors and to Baumgärtner and at the same time openly declared his belief in the homeopathic method. Interestingly, the publisher later also changed his allegiance and in fact proved a good friend to homeopathy by helping to spread the word through publishing homeopathic journals and books. Hering's defection to homeopathy changed the attitude of his Leipzig professors from pride in his abilities to bitter animosity. When he was certain of his new persuasion, Hering had contacted Hahnemann, explaining his situation, but Hahnemann's warning response, sent on 31 December 1824, came too late – the cat was already out of the bag:

> As you wish to take your medical examination next Spring, I would beg of you and advise you not to let the Leipzig allopaths know of your homœopathic views; least of all that worst of all allopaths, Clarus, if you do not wish that he should annoy you terribly at your examinations, or perhaps reject you altogether. But when once you have obtained your degree and have taken your place in your

future profession, then be no longer afraid of the obstacles which the Apothecaries Guild will be capable of placing in your path. . . . I trust you will be one of the few who are capable of practising the Divine science faithfully and with enthusiasm.[2]

As the future would prove, Hahnemann's trust was never better placed. Fortunately, Hering, finding his position at the Leipzig University untenable, left Saxony, and completed his medical studies at the University of Wurzburg in the Kingdom of Bavaria, graduating in 1826. His doctoral thesis left no doubt about his homeopathic convictions, it was entitled *De Medicina Futura* – On the Medicine of the Future. After achieving his Bavarian qualification, he returned to Saxony and sat a state-examination, which permitted him to practise medicine there. In this way, he managed to by-pass the notorious Dr Clarus.

Surinam

His first professional post was as science instructor and house physician to the Blochmann Educational Institute, which, with the backing of the Saxon Government, sent him and the scientific researcher, Weinhold, to Surinam (Dutch Guiana) on a botanical and zoological expedition. His wife accompanied him. He was to spend more than five years there (1827–1833). One of his major tasks was the collecting of plant and animal species for classification. The rich biodiversity of the fauna and flora of the Upper Amazon region provided a wealth of research material. His stay in South America was to prove of incalculable value to homeopathy, because, at this early point in its history, Hering discovered a remarkable remedy that would become of pivotal importance in the treatment of a wide range of ailments, both emotional and physical.

Lachesis

Soon after Hering's arrival, he heard of the reputation of the dreaded Surukuku – a huge snake, which lurked in the depths of the equatorial forest. The local inhabitants were terrified of it and many lurid tales of its vicious, aggressive nature, its ambushing skills and its deadly poison were related to him. Although the work he was doing for the Institute was unrelated to homeopathy, nonetheless, whilst in the field, he was always on the look out for unusual, new remedies, which might prove valuable. On hearing these exaggerated, apocryphal stories, his interest was fired. The fact that the snake possessed a rich folklore and elicited such reverential terror gave him a hint of its importance. He offered a handsome reward to anyone who would bring him a live specimen. This provided the necessary lure and some time later,

> ... one was brought to him in a bamboo box, and those who brought it immediately fled, and all his native servants with them. Hering stunned the snake with a blow to the head as the box opened, then, holding its head in a forked stick, he pressed its venom out of the poison bag upon sugar of milk.[3]

To ensure that he would capture the full medicinal power of the venom, Hering immediately set to work on preparing the lower attenuations (potencies) of the remedy. This he did by means of triturating the venom-saturated sugar of milk in a mortar and pestle for an hour. As we have previously described, this mixture then formed the basis for the following potencies in the process of serial dilution and trituration.

It was inevitable that during this lengthy procedure, Hering was continuously inhaling emanations from the highly toxic venom. The consequences were dramatic.

> The effect of handling the virus (venom) ... was to throw Hering into a fever with tossing delirium and mania – much to his wife's dismay. Towards morning he slept, and on waking his mind was clear. He drank a little water to moisten his throat, and the first question this indomitable prover asked was: 'What did I do and say?' His wife remembered vividly enough.[3]

They carefully documented the details of their experience and these provided the introduction to the proving of *Lachesis muta* – the Brazilian pit viper or bushmaster. Clarke completes the story by writing:

> The natives crept back one by one next day, and were astonished to find Hering and his wife alive.[3]

This magnificent creature, a denizen of the tropical and equatorial rainforests of South America, is the largest and longest of all the pit vipers, growing up to 3.3 metres. It is powerful and thick-bodied, possessing awesome, scimitar-like fangs, easily measuring 3 centimetres in length. It has a handsome reddish-brown skin marked along the back with black-brown rhomboidal spots. This disruptive colouring is ideal for concealing the snake amongst the dead leaves and dappled light of the forest floor. Here, like other heavy-bodied pit vipers, *Lachesis muta* lies in wait, relying on its superb camouflage to enable it to surprise prey and is therefore relatively easy to unwittingly step upon – with fatal results! Being immensely powerful, despite its bulk, it is able to strike with explosive, lightning-like speed. The sheer length of its fangs ensures that it can penetrate the flesh of its victim to an unusual depth and deliver a large dose of most virulent poison, sited to have maximum impact.

The pit vipers are the most evolved snakes on the planet. Common to all the Viperidae, they possess the most elaborate fangs in the snake world, far more intricate and refined than the Elapidae (e.g. the cobra and mamba). They are hollow and act like a hypodermic syringe when injecting poison into the tissues. In order to accommodate their great length when the snake's mouth is closed, the maxilla (upper jaw) to which they are attached, is hinged in such a way that the fangs are folded backwards along the palate, when not in use. When the snake gapes to strike, the fangs erect by swinging down and forward, enabling the viper to stab while striking. The appellation pit viper, which distinguishes *Lachesis* and its close relatives from other vipers, refers to highly sophisticated, sense organs, unique in the animal world which have evolved in the pit vipers (and in simpler form in the more primitive boas and pythons). These organs, situated between the eyes and nostrils on either side of the head, are specialised, heat-sensitive pits (thermo-receptors), which permit the snake to detect the infrared rays emitted by a heat source. This sense provides the pit viper with a formidable ability to locate and strike warm-blooded prey, such as birds and mammals, even in the almost pitch-black of a moonless jungle-night.

As we shall discuss later, nothing in life happens by chance or coincidence; every happening, however sublime or tragic, however uplifting or harrowing, occurs with purpose and positive intent, at the correct time, and at the right place. Chaos is merely perfection's veil. So it was with Hering and this particular snake; they were predestined to meet at that moment, on that day in 1828, in the sultry, oppressive heat of the jungle – a sacred and (to homeopathy and ailing humanity) a momentous event. When he seized it by the neck, milked its venom and captured its essence through potentisation, he materialised an atavistic, primordial energy of immense, yet subtle power. From time most ancient, the snake has been regarded with awe, reverence, fascination and horror – a universal symbol of extreme ambiguity – the duality of the divine and the diabolical. Above all, the snake was, and remains, a magical and religious embodiment of the primeval, autonomous life-force, which permeates all existence and consciousness, and taken to its highest form in the *ouroboros* motif, a snake swallowing its own tail, symbolises eternal renewal and divine self-sufficiency. To Jung it was a dramatic metaphor for the *integration and assimilation of the opposite* (the realisation of the shadow; the incorporation of our undeveloped or rejected aspects), essential to our individuation (spiritual attainment), which *proceeds from the clash of opposites*.

The ancient Greeks intuitively recognised the healing power of the snake and hence the symbol of *Asklepios*, the God of Medicine, became a staff round which a snake coiled – the serpent of life and death, mortality and immortality, wreathed around the tree of life.

While all snakes exemplify to a varying degree these arcane and chthonic aspects, none is more archetypal of all that a snake embodies than the magnificent Surukuku – not even the cobra! Why should this be?

Lachesis is the giant representative of the most highly evolved snake family, the Crotalinae, and dwells in the very centre of what may be termed the metabolic, reproductive and immunological heart of our planet, Gaia – the equatorial rainforests – and no region on earth is more evocative of this primordial image than the Amazon basin. Its vast extent, vitalised by the mighty river snaking through it, gives it primacy. Here speciation is at its most prodigious – it is Gaia's hothouse for the generation of diverse life forms – a paradise – a Garden of Eden – and deep within its steamy reaches lies the mighty Bushmaster. Of all the pit vipers, she is the only one that is oviparous – she lays eggs; all the others are ovoviviparous and bear live young. She is the progenitor, the source, the essence, the matriarch and the jungle is her shrine. She epitomises all that the snake represents in our myths, legends, beliefs and superstitions, and all that is visualised in our dreams, our delusions and our fears; her venom is charged with all that is sacred and profane within the human psyche!

We can be certain that in the remedy Lachesis, we possess the ultimate therapeutic representative of the snake kingdom and that although other snake venoms are important and more appropriate for certain clinical and emotional states, especially when we consider members of families other than the Viperidae, nonetheless, there is none that can depose Lachesis from her pre-eminent throne.

The influential American homeopath Dr James Tyler Kent (1849–1916) wrote:

> Lachesis seems to fit the whole human race, for the race is pretty well filled up with snake as to disposition and character and this venom only causes to appear (and therefore only cures) that which is (already) in man.

Not even a name is by chance. In his classification of the animal kingdom, the Swedish botanist Linnaeus, called the Surukuku, *Lachesis*, after one of the three fates of Greek mythology. Their names are not found in Homer, but are first given to us by Hesiod, who presented them as daughters of Zeus and Themis. Collectively, they were known as the Moira and were understood to have a defining influence upon the course of a person's life. They were, therefore, held in great awe and respect. Although vaguely conceived, they represent destiny or 'man's lot' and therefore our fate in the sense that our birth and death and the events, which transpire between these extremes are pre-determined or ordained. *Lachesis* is pre-eminent amongst the Moira. It is she who *assigns the lot* and thus determines a person's destiny; it is *Clotho* who *spins the thread of life* and it is *Atropos* who *cannot be stayed*, who finally severs it. Their relationship to their father Zeus is not without difficulty and conflict, for at times they seem to be independent of his will, or even above it. In a sense they represent the fundamental laws of the universe, which even Zeus may not transgress.

Once again, we are persuaded of this snake's fundamental importance in the treatment of the distressed and tormented psyche seemingly subject to an uncertain destiny, externally at the mercy of unseen, relentless, arbitrary forces, internally pushed and pulled by conflicting impulses and urges – the turbulent passions of the mind, body and soul. Into this maelstrom, when indicated by the nature of the contention, Lachesis can bring harmony and promote the sublimation of ungoverned passion towards serenity and bliss. Lachesis represents the primordial serpent force of the instinctive, primitive, animal will within all of us, which it is our destiny to wrestle with through many incarnations, until through transcendence we, like the snake shedding its skin, cast off the layers of ego-self which veil the true-self and emerge as the resplendent beings we really are.

The rest of the Hering/Lachesis story is provided by Catherine Coulter in an essay contained in her exceptional set of books, *Portraits of Homœopathic Remedies*, in which she presents comprehensive, psychological studies of many of the major homeopathic archetypes, including Lachesis. In a footnote she informs us that:

> The seven-foot snake is now preserved in the Philadelphia Academy of natural Sciences, entered in the ledger as item #7039 and listed as *Lachesis muta*, collected in Surinam by Dr Hering.

She continues:

> For several decades thereafter, most (surely all) of the homeopathic Lachesis remedies in the world was made from Hering's single milking of this one snake until, in 1868, the homœopathic pharmacists in America decided that they could not go on diluting the substance ad infinitum and ordered a second Bushmaster to be shipped up from Brazil. When the animal arrived, it caused a sensation in the homœopathic world: *Lachesis 11 arrives in America* was the headline in the homœopathic journals. Photographs of the snake from different angles were displayed, and its habits and physical dimensions were described as lovingly as if it was a film star!

She then adds

> (Homeopathic) Lachesis was recognised as one of the most useful and frequently indicated polychrests (remedies of many uses).[4]

As a member of the research team sent to Surinam, Hering was not permitted to publish homeopathic material. When circumstances permitted, he resigned from his post and became the personal physician of the governor of Surinam's capital, Paramaribo, which afforded him time to do research for the homeopathic materia medica. In 1833, he returned to Saxony for a short stay, before leaving once more for America. Having German friends in Philadelphia, he made this his first destination and it proved a permanent one. He soon became involved in homeopathic education there and this lead in 1848 to the founding of the Homœopathic Medical College of Pennsylvania, which became the foremost teaching institute for homeopathy in the world.

Hering's Law of Direction of Cure

Hering is particularly known to homeopathic students for his *Law of Direction of Disease Progression*, and its converse, the *Law of Direction of Cure* – the latter often simply called: Hering's *Law of Cure*. This stipulates that *disease progresses* (makes deeper inroads into the constitution of the patient) through a hierarchy of tissues and organs of ever-greater importance – *from superficial* (e.g. skin, mucous membranes, connective tissues) *to deeper seated and more vital organs* (e.g. liver, heart, endocrine and nervous systems) and at its deepest impinges upon *the mind and emotions*. This can be best understood by considering the frequently seen progression of allergic disease (atopy) from an initial manifestation on the skin, *eczema*, later extending to the mucous membranes, producing *allergic rhinitis* (hay fever) and finally reaching the bronchi of the lungs, causing *asthma*. The converse of this follows the 'law of direction of cure': the focus of the disease expression, during curative response, moving in the reverse direction, from deeper and more vital organs to more superficial organs and structures, finally often externalising on the mucous membranes or skin. In the atopic patient, therefore, it is a clear indication of curative reaction when the illness changes its emphasis from asthma to hay fever and then with further progress from hay fever to eczema. The final curative change will be the resolving of the skin condition. The mind, encompassing the emotions, intellect and memory, stands at the pinnacle of the hierarchy of 'organs.' Therefore, no matter what improvement is witnessed in the presenting symptoms of a case, if the emotional condition of the patient has worsened then the rule of the direction of cure is being transgressed and the outcome of treatment is proving unfavourable. Likewise, if certain superficial symptoms have increased under treatment, yet symptoms related to deeper causes show a positive shift, particularly in the mental state, the physician can be certain that the direction of cure is also positive.

In addition to the shift to deeper and more important organs as disease progresses, and the reverse during its cure, Hering noted that *disease moves from below upwards* as its becomes more severe, and conversely, that during cure the condition recedes from above downwards. Again using eczema as an example, as the skin disease increases in severity, an initial presentation on the hands and/or feet will spread upwards along the limbs and eventually involve the trunk. The external head must be considered in the same light as the limbs: a cradle cap or eczema of the scalp which spreads down onto the face and behind the ears is worsening, moving from the periphery towards the centre (the same as from below upwards when considering the arms and legs) and the reverse of this constitutes improvement. No matter how severe the eczema may become on the hands and feet, the associated clearing of the face and trunk indicate a positive change towards cure.

Finally, Hering, as had other homeopaths before him, drew attention to the fact that during the process of cure more recent symptoms would disappear only to be replaced by older symptoms from the patient's past, which in turn would resolve and be followed by even more remote symptoms, sometimes even dating from the patient's childhood or prenatal life. This phenomenon was incorporated in his law of cure and stated that: *symptoms clear in the reverse order of their appearance.*

CASE 9.1 Example of Hering's Law

A good example of Hering's law is the case of a middle-aged patient who attended my father William Lilley because of debility, excessive thirst and the constant need to pass large amounts of urine. Diagnosed with diabetes, he had managed at first to keep his condition under control by means of diet, but now required oral medication or possibly insulin therapy. Because of a quite intuitive hunch that his present condition was the end result of previous ailments he had suffered, he preferred to try an alternative approach. His story revealed that as a youngster he had suffered from recurrent crops of boils, some of which could be described as carbuncles. These had been strenuously treated with powerful antibiotics. He had a large number of scars as evidence of boils that had burst or been lanced. Although the antibiotics eventually brought each crop to an end, they did not prevent the next attack, and left him with lack of energy and chronic, intermittent diarrhoea. When he reached puberty, the boils seemed to clear spontaneously, but within a year of the last attack, he started to show signs of asthma, which eventually reached such proportions that he required chronic medication. The attacks were often precipitated by emotional stress and the onset of damp, rainy weather. With the passing of years, he showed steady improvement and eventually was able to reduce his medication, and in his mid-thirties the asthma cleared, although he remained very inclined to chest infections during winter. A good-health period took him into his forties when, after a business failure and the breakup of his twenty-year marriage due to his wife's infidelity, he developed the symptoms of diabetes. He then received homeopathic and dietary treatment for the presenting symptoms of diabetes, which had fortunately not been complicated by drug therapy, and over the period of a year the symptoms gradually subsided. Within eighteen months the diabetes had cleared, but he began to experience warning symptoms of asthma, especially when tense or the weather threatened rain. This condition was treated homeopathically and never reached the intensity it had in his youth. The asthma progressively lessened and eventually petered out, but shortly after its complete disappearance, he started to develop boils, especially on his buttocks and the back of his neck, areas which had troubled him as a young boy. Needless to relate, this condition of the skin responded promptly to further treatment and never returned. The cure was complete!

This case exemplifies the progression of disease from an organ of lesser importance, the skin, to an organ of greater importance, the lungs, and finally to an even deeper organ, the pancreas, and also the rule that symptoms clear (recede) in the reverse order of their appearance (onset).

We can express the positive direction of cure in the following criteria (the reverse of these criteria constitutes disease progression):

- From within outward – from organs more deep-seated and vital to life to organs or structures more superficial and less vital.
- From above downwards (from the centre to the circumference).
- From the mental sphere to the physical sphere.
- From symptoms of recent occurrence to symptoms of past, even remote. occurrence i.e. symptoms clear in the reverse order of their appearance.

Mental symptoms also show a hierarchy of importance. To understand this, it is of value to consider the response of a rat to threat. Confronted by a human or other large predator, the rat will flee. This can be equated with anxiety, fear and phobia. If cornered, no matter the size of the predator, the rat will respond to being trapped by aggression and retaliation – it will attack and bite. This can be equated with anger and rage. If resistance is futile, or attempted and failed, the rat freezes and may feign death. This can be equated with depression. The sequence gives us a hierarchy of response to the challenges and stresses of life, which humans mirror – the most superficial being fear and the deepest being depression. When, under treatment, a patient moves from a state of depression into one of anger, it is, therefore, a sign of improvement and parallels Hering's law of curative direction. Furthermore, we must understand that beneath anger, rage and aggression, supporting and energising them, lies deep-rooted fear. When anger dissipates, the underlying fear is laid bare and witnessed as the initial cause of both anger and depression.

Hering's law proves invaluable in clinical practice. It enables the physician to evaluate response to medication and monitor progress with a clear understanding of what is unfolding. If physical symptoms show improvement or even disappear, but the patient's emotional state deteriorates, it is clear that suppression has been caused, not cure, and that the patient's response to treatment is negative not positive. If, however, the mental deterioration reported by the family is found on analysis to be a change from passive, introverted indolence and sadness to one of frustration, indignation and anger, then the direction is positive, despite the family's discomfiture.

Other parallels to the law of direction of cure are to be found. In *Chronic Diseases*, Hahnemann postulates a continuum of disease, which commences with the *Psoric* miasm and then progresses through the *Sycotic* miasm to the *Syphilitic* miasm. During chronic treatment bringing positive directional response, this miasmatic sequence will be reversed, the syphilitic picture weakening and giving way to a sycotic presentation, which in turn fades away to reveal the original underlying psoric condition. During a curative process, the miasmatic disease expression is seen to move from one of depth and complexity towards one that is superficial and of greater simplicity.

When the selection of remedies in a given case necessitates the sequential choice of elements of decreasing atomic weight, this will also be a sign of positive direction. For example a patient initially requiring Tellurium (*syphilitic*) may, with improvement, present clear indications for the use of Selenium (*sycotic*) and eventually with further progress produce the picture of Sulphur (*psoric*). These three elements are found together geologically and lie next to one another on the periodic table of elements, Tellurium having the greatest atomic weight and Sulphur the least, with Selenium in between.

Hering's influence

Hering was the fountainhead of American homeopathy. He brought a passion, vigour and originality of thought that enthused others. Like Bönninghausen, he had an encyclopaedic knowledge of the materia medica and apart from his busy practice, devoted his considerable energies to spreading the word, teaching medical colleagues and furthering homeopathic research through the conducting of provings. On 10th April (always a significant date for homeopaths) 1844, the American Institute of Homœopathy was founded and Constantine Hering was elected its first president. This was fully two years before the allopathic American Medical Association was founded, largely as a defensive response to the advantage gained by the Institute. The political climate in the USA was, at the time, both liberal and competitive, which favoured the rapid dissemination of the new method of healing. In fact, the orthodoxy found themselves very much in the back seat as far as popularity with the public was concerned. Homeopathy thrived, and dispensaries, clinics and hospitals sprang up throughout the USA.

Hering was less conservative than Hahnemann in the matter of potency. Whereas Hahnemann was always concerned, even to a limiting degree, about the risk of excessive, initial aggravations from potencies higher than the 30 centesimal, Hering was interested in pushing these boundaries and experimenting with ever-higher potencies. He kept in touch with homeopathic developments in Germany and corresponded with those closest to Hahnemann, especially with Stapf and Gross the co-editors of *Archiv für die homöopathische Heilkunst*, who, contrary to the Master's views on the subject, were eager to develop the potencies beyond the 30th. Through them, Hering came in contact with Caspar Julius Jenichen and his 'superhigh' potencies.

* * * * *

Caspar Julius Jenichen – Manually attained high potencies

Caspar Jenichen (1787–1849) was an almost mythological figure. He was variously described as an equerry, a farrier, or as a *stallmeister* (horse trainer). Of the three, farrier was his most likely occupation, because in those days the job of farrier, which included horseshoeing, hoof trimming, forging and repairing tools and the fabrication of metal artefacts, was practically synonymous with that of blacksmith and Jenichen had the physique of one who plied that trade. A human counterpart of *Hephaistos*, the Greek God of Blacksmiths and Fire prophetically invoked by Paracelsus as the divinity able to strip away the dross cloaking the medicinal power of potential remedies, Jenichen was a veritable oak of a man, prodigiously powerful with great breadth of shoulder and strong, muscular arms, ideally fashioned for holding and restraining horses, wielding a hammer and for feats of endurance and strength, which he was to put to good use in the service of homeopathy – for above all, he was a passionate and zealous, amateur homeopath.

The horse homeopath

It is not surprising that with his enthusiasm for homeopathy, which amounted to religious fervour, Jenichen should have started treating ailing horses in his care. Through private study, Jenichen had acquired an extensive knowledge of the action of homeopathic remedies and soon achieved a number of significant cures, which resulted in him being consulted by various horse owners, as if he was a qualified veterinary surgeon. Never lacking in confidence, he began to treat human patients and in no time had a regular following and was able to lay his hammer to rest. His successes spurred him on. He was a large man with a vision as wide as his proverbial shoulders and a drive and passion of similar proportions.

Potencies higher than the 30th centesimal

He only had the lower potencies (up to the 30th centesimal) at his disposal and having no doubt that the higher potencies would possess even greater healing power, he determined to achieve these by his own industry. Understanding the process of potentisation, it will be realised how concentrated, time-consuming and arduous a task it is to attain the 30th centesimal potency by serial dilution and succussion from the mother substance. Each step involves a separate bottle charged with distilled water or alcohol, into which is added the appropriate number of drops (1 drop in 99) taken from the previous potency. The bottle is then subjected to vigorous succussion, usually ten sharp strokes against a firm but yielding surface. It is feasible, and in fact desirable, and practised by the best homeopathic pharmacies, to raise the potency of each remedy not only to the 30th attenuation, but also to the 200th by this manual method. However, beyond this level of potency it becomes a practical impossibility to progress further without a mechanical device to replace the hand and arm of the potentiser.

That is, unless your name is Casper Jenichen!

Of passion and potency

The story goes, that one day, Jenichen, found the bottle of his 30th potency of Plumbum aceticum empty due to a shrunken, loose cork that had permitted the contents to evaporate. He decided that instead of discarding the bottle he would determine whether it still contained any medicinal virtue by putting it to the test, and accordingly added the requisite quantity of alcohol to the bottle and potentised the 'remedy' in the traditional way up to the 200th. Soon afterwards, he was given the opportunity of using the remedy when a man suffering from chronic, offensive foot-sweat consulted him. Much to his delight, the remedy acted both positively and promptly. This so impressed him that he conjectured that possibly the best starting point for the higher potencies he intended creating would be the 29th potency, which had been permitted to evaporate to dryness. At first he used this method only on mineral remedies, but it is almost certain that he must have proceeded to use it on plant and animal preparations as well.

As innovative as this method of preparation was, he followed it up with a potentisation process even more unique and controversial. Although he knew of the high potencies being produced by the Russian General von Korsakoff (whom we shall consider later) using a single bottle, emptied and recharged after each step of dilution and succussion, Jenichen tackled the Herculean task that lay before him in a different way. He used as the vehicle for his dilutions 70 to 80% alcohol up to the 800th potency and beyond that the water from Lake Schwerin in the Mecklenberg lake district of Northern Germany, noted for its purity. The proportions he used were: for dilutions up to 200th – 6 drops in 294 of the vehicle (alcohol); from the 200th to the 800th – 1 drop to 300 (alcohol); for dilutions higher than the 800th – 2 drops to 12,000 drops (lake water). For potentising, he used bottles of such a size that the dilution filled them only to one third – this to ensure that on each stroke of succussion the contents would impact on the surfaces of the bottle with maximum friction and effect – hence, for the lower potencies he used smaller bottles, and much larger bottles for the highest potencies which contained a greater volume of vehicle. He also employed a different number of strokes according to potency: from 200th to 300th – 10 strokes per potency; from 300th to 800th – 12 strokes per potency; from 800th to 40,000th – 30 strokes per potency.

In preparing the 200th potency, Jenichen would start the process with the evaporated bottle of the 29th potency of the remedy to which he added 300 drops of alcohol. This was succussed for 10 strokes; he would then take 6 drops of this 30th centesimal potency and place it in the first of eight bottles each containing 294 drops of alcohol. He gave this bottle 250 succussions without stopping, and considered that he had potentised it up the scale by 25 potencies – ten succussions counting as one degree of potency. He would then rest for a moment while transferring 6 drops from the succussed bottle to the second of his eight prepared bottles. When feeling sufficiently recovered, he then gave the second bottle 250 strokes, which according to his thinking raised it another 25 potencies, and so he proceeded through the remaining six bottles finally achieving, through eight steps of dilution and succussion, his 200th potency ($8 \times 25 = 200$). Calculated by the standard Hahnemannian method of potentising, despite all Jenichen's efforts, this was merely the 38th centesimal potency. Jenichen and those who later used his remedies asserted otherwise. All depended on whether succussion alone, without, or with very little, serial dilution, had the power to raise the potency of a remedy.

After the 200th potency, he pressed on to the 800th in the same manner, but now with 1 drop transferred to 300 drops of alcohol at each step and the number of strokes increased to 12, and finally he broke into the unchartered sphere lying beyond the 800th, transferring the virtue of the remedy by means of 2 drops into 12,000 drops of lake water and lifting each potency by means of 30 mighty strokes. The lowest dilution he produced in this way was the 200th, the highest remains uncertain, but probably 'his' 60,000th centesimal potency ($10^{-120,000}$) or 60M was the limit – a considerable achievement for one remedy, let alone the great number that he exposed to the might of his arm.

He started to use these remedies on his patients, animal and human, and was soon convinced that the remedies prepared by his method were far superior to any others available. Being both large of frame and large of mouth, the stalwart farrier-cum-homeopath soon ensured that news of these exceptional Jenichen remedies was broadcast far and wide. Being the editor of the major homeopathic journal in Germany, rumours soon came to the ears of Dr Gustav Gross, who felt obliged to investigate the matter further on behalf of the profession and his readers. He induced Dr Johann Stapf, his co-editor to conduct clinical experiments with the new potencies. Stapf was impressed with their efficacy and passed favourable word on to Hering in America, who asked for samples to be sent to him. A farcical element raised its head in these affairs when Gross, in a sympathetic paper on the subject, failed to hail Jenichen as the brilliant inventor of an entirely unique method of potentisation, merely referring to him as the one who prepared the remedies. Jenichen, as sensitive as he was passionate, was infuriated at the omission and undoubtedly influenced by the refined sensibilities and habits of the aristocratic, equestrian world in which he moved, challenged Gross to a duel. Gross declined him satisfaction and Jenichen in retaliation refused to release details of how he achieved his potencies.

However, Hering, whose interest had been whetted by use of the remedies, now corresponded directly with the piqued, erstwhile blacksmith and by tactfully catering for his injured pride so mollified Jenichen that he divulged his 'secret' on the strict understanding that Hering would tell no one. Hering honoured this confidence until well after Jenichen's death.

The *British Journal* of January, 1880 (31 years after Jenichen's death) carried an editorial on Jenichen's mode of manufacturing the so-called high potencies.

> Drs Gross and Stapf were the first patrons of these novelties – not that Jenichen was the first introducer of high potencies ... Von Korsakoff preceded him.... The novelty of Jenichen's high potencies was there mode of preparation, which he kept a dead secret, and secrecy also was a novelty in homœopathic pharmacy; if these gentlemen knew Jenichen's method, at all events they did not reveal it. Dr C Hering certainly knew it, and after the death of Gross and Stapf – if not before – was the only one who possessed the secret. Hering was frequently appealed to, to reveal the secret, but his answer was, "If any one wishes to know how Jenichen's preparations are made, let him apply to Jenichen; I know it, and that is sufficient for my purpose."[5]

The demon potentiser

Not only did these three closest disciples of Hahnemann use and report favourably on the first high potencies produced by Jenichen, they also encouraged him to continue this work and spurred him on to ever-greater efforts both in the number of remedies he developed and also the rarefied levels of potency he strove for. Hering's approval meant much to Jenichen and fired him to set his potency sights higher and higher, reaching up into the intangible realm of 'nothingness' in which the origin of everything is found. For him the act of potentisation was a spiritual one transferred from the ritual of the smithy, with its metamorphosis of iron into steel through the tempering power of fire, violence and determination, to the ritual of the laboratory with its metamorphosis of matter into energy through the dynamising power of sweat, toil and dedication. For the task he stripped himself to the waist and performed the succussion in the standing or sitting position, or by changing from the one to the other as discomfort demanded. He held the bottle in his fist in a slanting direction, always from left to right,

> ... and gave the strokes perpendicularly with all his force, so that the fluid in the bottle made a noise like the jingling of silver coins. At first the violent muscular action caused, after three day's work, so much pain in the arm, that he was forced to discontinue it and rest for a week.[6]

Once his muscles had accustomed themselves to the unusual and sustained nature of the labour, he was able to pursue his violent exertions for prolonged periods on consecutive days without ill effect. To get the immense amount of work done, he established an extremely exacting routine. He commenced succussing at 10.00 p.m. and would continue, without break, other than that demanded by nature, in this demanding and intense labour until 3 in the morning; and this night after night.

One can well imagine the remarkable scene: a man of Herculean proportions, his face depicting intense focus, every muscle of his naked torso standing out in relief and highlighted by the flickering light of the lamps set about him, his magnificent physique rippling and sheaned with sweat as his tightly clenched fist holding a precious glass vial, rises and falls with unfailing, metronomic rhythm, his incessant toil made audible and punctuated by his heavy, measured breathing, the impact of his hand against leather and the tinkling of the liquid in the tube. This image repeated on the walls of his chamber in eerie, gargantuan form, the elongated, looming shadows seemingly depicting some demented being about some mysterious or nefarious act; a subject worthy of an el Greco. Evidence of Stapf's deep involvement in this enterprise was the full-sized portrait of the half-naked Jenichen, admirably reflecting his muscularity and showing him gripping the 'magic vessel,' that graced a wall in his house.[7]

In the pursuit of the most powerful homeopathic potency, Jenichen's efforts convinced him that the release of innate, individualised energy latent in all substances could be achieved by succussion alone, without further dilution, once the initial imprinting of the medium (alcohol, water) had been achieved by the classic method of potentisation up to the 6th decimal or 3rd centesimal potency. This became his new starting point (rather than the dried-out 29th potency) to which he then gave a more or less enormous amount of succussions, depending on the potency desired. He was certain that the singular efficacy of his remedies was due to the sustained and intense exposure of the potency to violent friction and the magnetic power of his own enthusiasm and force of will.

In the face of the almost universal disapproval of the rank and file, low-potency homeopaths, Gross, Stapf and particularly Hering continued to support Jenichen, always urging him to further endeavour in extending the limits of potency. In fact, holding him in high esteem, Jenichen attributed to Hering's enthusiastic encouragement and backing much of his own ability to persist in his sacrificial labours:

> The triumph I hope for (the efficacy of his high potencies) does not belong to me, but to Hering's (exhortation): *"Every year higher"*.[8]

Bönninghausen was prepared to use Jenichen's remedies and through experience became convinced of their efficacy. He therefore defended them and their creator in an article published in the journal *Allgemeine Homöopathische Zeitung* after Jenichen's death. While regretting the fact that mystery still shrouded the exact method of preparation of the remedies and recognising that suspicions abounded that the Jenichen's potentising technique seriously deviated from that of Hahnemann, he chided the dissenters:

> In spite of so many and weighty voices which give all praise to these preparations they have even refused to make any experiments with them, merely because they have not this knowledge (the method of preparation).[8]

He added that though willing to excuse those who were resistant because of inflexible, scientific scruples, he condemned the many, indeed, the *very* many, who rejected the remedies not because of strict adherence to principles, but because of inherent prejudice against the use of any high potencies (i.e. members of the low potency brigade).

In a letter to the Baron, dated 18 November 1845, which gives some indication of the degree of familiarity existing between them, Jenichen describes the arduous and demanding nature of his self-appointed responsibility and his unswerving commitment to it:

> I wish that the preparation of the high potencies, especially the highest, might not be so troublesome and did not take so much time. The excessively tedious uniformity is also a burdensome addition. And yet, we are not allowed while potentising to think of anything else (on account of counting the strokes); if we would secure uniform preparations, it would not be at all strange if the enthusiasm should give out long before the time. But the certain knowledge that I am making medicinal preparations for the whole sick world, which will gradually spread, and that these preparations are such that no other person can prepare them thus – it is this that keeps up my courage and continually vivifies anew my bodily powers; and I do not therefore, deserve any particular praise for I do nothing but my duty.[8]

As Bönninghausen suggests, the reader cannot doubt that these are the words of an honourable man "as given in a familiar letter." Nor was it a vain statement that only he could fulfil this unusual responsibility for it is inconceivable that anyone else would ever again willingly expose themselves to such obsessive and protracted toil – and so far no one has!

While Hahnemann cautiously sanctioned the Korsakovian potencies, he strongly repudiated Jenichen's work. However, much later, during the Paris years, Hahnemann, instead of becoming more fixed and less venturesome in his prescribing, as one could well anticipate in a man of his age, to the contrary, showed all the curiosity and innovativeness of a young man and critically tested his own earlier prejudices and dictums in practice. So, we find Dr Malan, who spent time with Hahnemann in his final years, writing in the periodical *Organon*:

> I frequently saw Hahnemann prescribe very high dilutions. One of the most remarkable cures had been brought about by one single dose of a very high potency; as far as I know, this remedy came from Jenichen. I have often heard him say that the 30th potency should by no means form a fixed limit for medicinal dilutions[9]

There can be no doubt that Hahnemann, like Hering and Jenichen, also suspected that agitation (succussion/trituration) alone in some way affected potency. Hence, his varying recommendations over the years regarding the number of strokes to be employed for raising potency and the fear he entertained that excessive succussing might render a high potency more likely to create initial aggravation. In a note to paragraph §280 in the fifth edition of the *Organon*, Hahnemann writes:

> Moreover, the homœopathic medicine is potentised at every division and diminution by trituration or succussion. This was such a development of the latent powers of medicines never dreamed of before my time, that in later years I have been compelled by convincing experience to reduce the ten succussions, previously prescribed after each dilution, to two. 10 Years later, in *Chronic Diseases*, (1837), he once again advocates ten succussions rather than the limit of two, but is enabled to do so because of distributing the dose over 15, 20, or 30 days and more, now no potency in a vial is too strong if prepared each time with ten succussions.[11]

Towards the end of his life, Hahnemann devised the LM (50 millesimal) potency range with the specific purpose of producing potencies that were both gentle and curatively powerful, yet possible to prepare in high potency by practical, manual means (see below). In the preparation of these potencies succussion assumed an even greater role in the process of dynamisation than it did in the centesimal attenuations. In the sixth edition of the *Organon*, Hahnemann gives detailed instructions as to their manufacture, along with copious explanatory footnotes. In these he emphasises the primary role of succussion. In footnote §269b he states:

> Succussing the solution (of a medicinal substance) develops the medicinal powers lying hidden in the medicinal substance and discloses these powers more and more. The dynamisation spiritises the material substance, if one may use that expression.[15]

In footnote §270f when speaking of the dynamising potential of a single globule (100 of which weigh a single grain) in 100 drops of wine spirit which gives a ratio of dilutant to medicine equal to 50,000:1, he affirms:

> In this much higher ratio of the dilution medium to the medicine, *many* successions of the vial filled to two thirds with wine spirit can bring about a far greater development of power.[12]

This greater emphasis on succussion is reflected in the number of strokes he advocates with each step:

> Give the tightly corked vial 100 strong succussions with the hand against a hard but elastic body.[13]

A great jump when compared to the previously recommended 2 or 10 strokes for the centesimal potencies. In this he displays his awareness that continued succussion increasingly releases or potentiates the healing power of a potency – otherwise 10 strokes would surely suffice!

This concept is born out in his further comment under footnote §270f:

> With a ratio of the dilution medium to the medicine as low as 100:1 very many impacts by means of a powerful machine, as it were, are forced in. As a result, medicines arise that, especially in the higher degrees of dynamisation, almost instantaneously but with stormy – indeed dangerous – intensity, impinge on patients (especially delicate ones) without bringing about an enduring, gentle counter-action of the life principle.[14]

Although this is expressed in exaggerated terms and in the light of experience proves alarmist and inaccurate, since high potencies prepared from such dilution ratios (100:1) do not necessarily provoke aggravations, severe or otherwise, and certainly prove curative when correctly selected, nonetheless, Hahnemann again draws attention to what Jenichen postulated, and with which Hering tacitly concurred: that (in Hahnemann's own words) succussion develops the medicinal powers lying hidden in the medicinal substance and discloses these powers more and more. Jenichen could certainly be likened to a powerful machine, but his dilution ratio of medium (lake water) to medicine (12,000:2) for the highest potencies, was an approach more in line with the Master's choice for the LM potencies (50,000:1). Jenichen's bottles were only filled to one third allowing for more turbulence and friction and, therefore, having possibly greater potentising effect.

A final word from Bönninghausen about Jenichen's potencies was given when writing about his own preference for the high potencies (especially the 200th):

> We have even had a number of cases in which the usual potency with us, the 200, did not suffice and the cure was only effected through Jenichen's high potencies.[15]

This commendation, coming from a very correct and observant researcher, carries a lot of weight, as did Hering's continued interest in Jenichen and his willingness to keep his potentising method secret, something he would never have done had he had any doubts about its validity.

Unfortunately, the story did not end well for poor Jenichen.

His compulsive, intense nature, which ceaselessly drove him forward with little, if any, heed for rest, health or sanity, finally broke him down. For years he had slaved like Sisyphus at a task without end, which stretched before him into the interminable distance, for though he achieved so much there always remained the next potency, the next remedy and the next night's ordeal. Even this man of indomitable strength and relentless will began to falter, but only when he had reached deep into his fifties. The years of punishing labour, always executed in the same fixed position, whether standing or sitting, and demanding an ever-repeated swing of arm, shoulder and lower back, caused such wear and tear on his spine that the nerves into his legs were impinged, causing him great pain, restricting his movement and eventually making it impossible for him to continue. When he could no longer take the 'magic vessel' in his grasp, make the liquid 'sing' and infuse its contents with healing power, all that he lived for was denied, his ardent spirit was trapped and for him there was no recourse other than to put a pistol to his head. He died in his sixty-second year.

The homeopathic world did not mourn his passing; many probably sighed with relief. Dr RE Dudgeon, who possessed a very dry sense of humour, rather cruelly commented:

> Fortunately Jenichen shot himself when he reached the 60,000th potency or there would be no telling what heights he might have reached.[16]

It was also on many unsympathetic lips that the deluded Jenichen, a high potency fanatic, had finally succumbed to a single, strong dose of crude lead.

This redoubtable man of horses, homeopathy and high potencies, left a large legacy of specially prepared remedies and willed an amount of 12,000 thalers for the foundation of a homeopathic dispensary in the northern German town of Wismar, to be conducted by a physician who would exclusively practise with his remedies. Stapf duly appointed Dr Rentsch of Potsdam to the position and Bönninghausen let word be known that these remedies would be made available at a reasonable price to any who wished to obtain them.

William Lilley – Super-succussion potentisation

Jenichen was soon forgotten and many homeopaths today have either never heard of him or only recall him as a rather comic or misguided figure, an image cultivated by his detractors, even by one as eminent as Dudgeon. However, my father, William Lilley, who, after emigrating from England in 1949, practised homeopathy and chiropractic in Pretoria, South Africa, became very interested in Jenichen's history and work. They certainly shared the same all absorbing passion for homeopathy and both were remarkable individuals, though in quite different ways. Like Hahnemann before him, my father believed that to be certain of the quality of the remedies he prescribed it was necessary that he dispense his own remedies. His original stock of remedies, which he brought with him from England, had been obtained from Dudley Everett of Nelson's homeopathic pharmacy in Duke Street, London (see Chapters 18–20). Dudley was sadly killed in the Trident air crash of 1972 that claimed the lives of many prominent British homeopaths. Over the years, many of the high potencies became depleted and some, as experienced by Jenichen, suffered evaporation. These he replaced by ordering new stock from overseas. However, most often he still had lower potencies of the remedy required on his dispensary shelf and in the late 1950's, he pondered the possibility of running these up to the higher potencies using Jenichen's method of continuous succussion, but aided by modern, mechanical means rather than strength of arm.

In making the decision to experiment along these lines, my father was strongly influenced by the fact that the chief supporters of Jenichen's remedies were all drawn from the ranks of Hahnemann's closest and most steadfast disciples: men who were held in high regard by the Master, were familiar with high potency prescribing and considered by their peers to be outstanding exponents of the homeopathic method. According to the testimony of these prominent physicians, the Jenichen potencies were particularly effective. Was this really so? Could a 30th or lower potency achieved by the classic method of serial dilution and succussion be further lifted into the higher realms of dynamisation by continuous succussion alone?

As always, the best way to approach such an uncertainty is to put it personally to the test. My father determined to do so. He designed a potentising machine with a central piston driven vertically up and down by an electric motor, set to deliver high revolutions per minute. On either side of the piston, he attached clips to which two potentising bottles could be firmly secured, slanted at forty-five degrees to the vertical, similar to the grip adopted by Jenichen. This configuration balanced the machine and permitted the simultaneous potentisation of two remedies, a great saving in time and labour. His starting point was the 30th or 200th CH potency (CH = manually-produced, centesimal potency according to the method of Hahnemann). His medium was 90% alcohol; his dilution ratio was 1 part of potentised medicine to 99 of the vehicle; the bottle was two-thirds full;

the number of piston excursions per lift of a single potency was set at 10; and the duration time of succussion determined by the desired lift of potency and the revolutions per minute of the machine. As with the eight bottles of Jenichen, key potencies were removed during the process e.g. every 100th up to 1000th (M), and every thousandth up to 10M, 50M and CM (100,000th). Each time a potency was preserved, the bottle containing it would be removed from the apparatus and put into stock. One part of this potency would be added to a fresh bottle containing 99 parts of alcohol, which after 10 hand succussions would be clipped into place ready for the next period of continuous succussion. It was only at these points of change that dilution and hand succussion were employed. In this way even the 'CM' and 'MM' potencies (1,000,000th) could be reached within a practical period of time.

Viewing the SS machine in action, one is impressed by the degree of agitation generated within the liquid charge by the explosive, rapid, short excursions of the piston. The angle of the vial setting ensures that the contents are exposed to maximum friction and impact and form a swiftly, spinning vortex of liquid, which is constantly and violently disrupted. Due to the extreme kinetic energy generated, an appreciable rise in the temperature of the vial results. Subtleties are often born from cataclysmic events and this process provides an instance of such a transformation.

Although these potencies cannot be considered equivalent to either the Hahnemannian centesimal potencies (CH) or the Korsakovian (K) potencies (see below) because of their lack of serial dilution, and must be regarded as part of an independent range generated through a different protocol, they can be compared clinically and they passed the test with flying colours. That they should not be confused with either CH or K potencies, my father designated them SS or super-succussion potencies and utilised them in his practice alongside the conventionally prepared remedies through the nineteen-sixties until his death in 1972. I joined him in practice at the end of 1966, fresh from training at the Royal London Homeopathic Hospital and with the Dean, Margery Blackie's, frequent passionate injunction, "Give him (or her) a 10M" still resounding in my ears. I was soon introduced to these Lilley SS potencies and any vague scepticism I might have felt was soon dissipated by their very positive action. Although I eventually obtained for my dispensary an excellent Korsikovian machine from Helios Laboratories of Tunbridge Wells, England in 2001, many of the old super-succussion remedies still remain prescribing favourites.

General von Korsakoff: single bottle potentisation

The conjunction of passion and potency found another exemplar in General Iseman von Korsakoff (1788–1853), a noble Russian landowner living in the vicinity of Moscow. He, like Jenichen, was an enthusiastic amateur homeopath, who very soon after being introduced to the concepts of homeopathy pondered how it would be possible to simplify and expedite the process of dynamisation so that higher potencies could be attained without the use of thousands upon thousands of vials or bottles. Although medically unqualified, he proved himself a serious student and practitioner of homeopathy and it was due to his influence that homeopathy gained a sure footing in Russia.

He conjectured that when the glass vial used to prepare the first centesimal potency was emptied of its fluid contents by inverting it, sufficient liquid would adhere to the inner surface of the glass to provide the one part necessary to prepare the next potency. Ninety-nine parts of diluent, could then be added to the emptied vial before succussing it by means of ten strokes. After succussion, the vial would be emptied again and the residual liquid used as the basis for the next attenuation, and so on. In this manner one vial and pure water could be used for the entire potentising process, except when key potencies were to be preserved, in which case the vial would be charged with nine parts of high concentration alcohol/water mix instead of water and then succussed and put into stock. A new vial would receive one part of this preserved potency and nine parts of pure water and then, after succussion, with this as the starting point, the potentising process would proceed as before, until the next key potency was reached. Korsakoff achieved the 1,500th dynamisation by this means, sometime before Jenichen commenced his labours.

Korsakoff thought that the material division or attenuation of a medicine actually ceased at the sixth centesimal dilution [10^{-12} or 12X] and that after that the medicinal power of the remedy was entirely dynamic or spiritual. When this energetic level had been attained, he postulated that one medicated globule placed in a bottle containing a thousand unmedicated globules had the power to medicate the whole. In 1832, he published an article in Stapf's *Archiv für die homöopathische Heilkunst* entitled *Experiences on the Propagation of the Medicinal Power of Homœopathic Remedies, with Ideas on the Mode of Propagation* in which he elucidated his concepts.

Before publishing Korsakoff's article, Stapf first brought its contents to Hahnemann's attention, because the same edition contains a letter from the Master commenting on Korsakoff's observations and method of potentisation. Knowing Hahnemann's uncompromising attitude to any deviation from his tenets, it is surprising how considered and moderate his comments were:

> I must say these procedures seem to show chiefly how high one can go with the potentised attenuation of medicines without their action on the human health becoming *nil*. For this, these experiments are of inestimable value; but for the Homœopathic treatment of patients it is expedient in the preparation of all kinds of medicines to remain stationary at the decillionth (10^{-60} or 30CH) attenuation and potency, in order that Homœopathic practitioners may be able to promise themselves uniform results in their cures.[17]

He offers no criticism of the proposed methodology and hence would seem to give it his tacit approval. In this letter, Hahnemann once again reveals his extremely conservative approach to the matter of potency, lagging well behind many of his best disciples. It was only in the Paris years that he ventured beyond the 30th, and even then only infrequently.

A letter, which later came to light amongst Korsakoff's papers, reveals the respect that Hahnemann felt for the enterprising Russian general:

> I admire the zeal with which you devote yourself to the beneficial healing art, not only in order to have help for your family and neighbours, but also to penetrate the secrets of nature, as proved by your valuable notes.... With my utmost power I try above all things to find out what will be of most use to my fellow-men ... and I am convinced that you are also of this opinion. Continue an activity which satisfies a feeling heart and do not relax.[18]

In addition to his professional affairs, Korsakoff conducted a busy homeopathic practice. Between 1829 and 1834, his practice journal records details of 11,725 cases that received treatment. He was also deeply committed to the promotion of homeopathy in Russia and devoted considerable energy to spreading the word.

> He was an active and efficient propagandist, and his literary productions bear the stamp of an eminently original and thoughtful mind.[21]

Writing in 1897, Bradford gives credit to Korsakoff for the development of the first high potencies (those beyond the 30th):

> As originator of the high potencies, he did great service to the cause of science, and it cannot be denied that he proved the efficacy of certain substances in a degree of attenuation far beyond all conceivable limits. Future times, perhaps, will know better how to appreciate such discoveries, which, hitherto, it must be owned, have promoted discord and contention to a far greater extent than they have produced conviction.[21]

Here he alludes to the sometimes-bitter conflict that arose between the protagonists of the low potencies and those of the high potencies, a conflict, which began in Hahnemann's time and sadly divided and substantially weakened the homeopathic cause in the late 1800s and the early part of the 1900s. Today, modern homeopaths consider the scale of potencies, from low to high, much as a pianist does his keyboard, each potency possessing its unique importance in the spectrum of healing. The deft and able practitioner uses all potencies according to the task in hand.

Korsakovian machine

Future times did indeed come to value Korsakoff's pioneer observations and the technicological era was able to bring them to fruition and provide the profession with truly reliable high potencies. Although Korsakoff himself still used manual succussion during his single vial process, his method lent itself to mechanisation. Based on the principle that the potentising vehicle, when emptied of its charge will always contain sufficient residual liquid adhering to its surface from the previous potency to medicate the next, potentising machines have been designed to reproduce the action of the Korsakoff procedure. The amount of liquid retained in the chosen vehicle can be accurately estimated and becomes the 'one-part' required for medication. On the basis of this, the 'ninety-nine-parts' of diluent is determined and its accurately measured delivery at each potentising step built into the design. The length of the succussing 'arm' of the apparatus can measure that of the average human forearm and the end to which the vehicle is fixed made to strike a firm but elastic pad a predetermined number of times (usually ten), thus reproducing mechanically, as close as possible, the action of manual succussion. After succussion, the liquid charge is ejected by compressed air and the vehicle rapidly recharged with distilled water (serial dilution). The entire procedure is controlled by a computer set to notate and lift the potency step by step to the desired level (key potency). As with the manual procedure, key potencies are preserved in high percentage alcohol.

Fluxion Machines

Korsakoff was not the only pioneer engaged in the quest to find a mechanical means of attaining the realm of the high potency. Many ingenious, machines of varying complexity were designed, among which were those of Boericke, Fincke, Skinner, Swan and Kent. Based on the one vial system, water was used as the succussing force, either by 'continuous flow' through a narrow necked tube (Fincke) or a perforated screen (Swan) or by 'discontinuous flow' through injection into a glass container under pressure

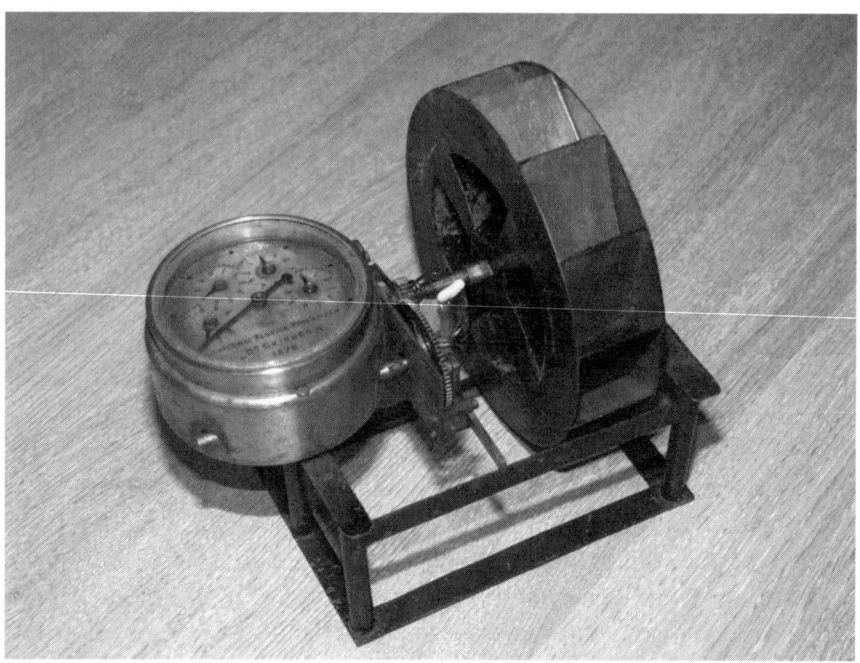

Figure 9.2 The Skinner Potentiser
Faculty of Homeopathy Collection

followed by ejection or 'dumping'. The latter, known as a Skinner Potentiser, is shown in Figure 9.2.

Swan was convinced that the water passing through his apparatus "caused a perturbation even more violent than succussion."[19]

These devices were called 'fluxion' machines and produced high potencies, but could not be standardised. Debate at the time centred on how much the remedies they produced represented true centesimal potencies rather than on their efficacy, because they were generally found to be therapeutically active. This would seem to confirm Korsakoff's and my father's conclusion that at a certain point in potentising, possibly as low as 6X, and certainly by 23X (Avagadro's number) further serial dilution of the attenuating medium yields precedence to succussion because the healing power it contains is no longer in any way dependent on matter: it is dynamic and no longer subject to material division. While each of the fluxion machines mentioned above enjoyed its day, and had a limited following, none of them are in operation today.

The 50-millesimal (LM) Potencies: Hahnemann's hand-made high potencies

Hahnemann always remained mistrustful of potencies above the 30th, believing that even when correctly selected they could produce initial, healing aggravations before bringing relief. Although he did occasionally prescribe higher potencies during his last years, this was the exception and certainly not the rule, and he always recommended that his followers should adopt a 30th potency ceiling in their prescribing, in order to avoid the risk of such reactions and to maintain a therapeutic standard. After all, he had stated in the second aphorism of his *Organon*:

> . . . the highest ideal of cure is rapid, gentle and permanent restoration of the health . . . in the shortest, most reliable, and most harmless way.

This prejudice against the high potencies is another example of an unexpected bee that flew into this brilliant but eccentric man's cap and got stuck there – along with warm coffee and Chinese tea. It was contrary to his usual, considered approach to every aspect of homeopathic practice, in which his conclusions were always based upon practical, personal observation and experience. In this matter, he, who had scarcely ever prescribed at this level, remained hesitant about their use, while Bönninghausen and Hering, convinced of the higher potencies' superiority in treating chronic disease, used them by preference and without concern. Perhaps this fear of aggravation was residual from his earlier experience when working with his original dilutions, or stemmed from the experiences of high potency prescribing colleagues and their patients. Be that as it may, his anxiety persisted and was coupled to an urgency to resolve the difficulty of achieving a high potency without the use of elaborate machinery. In Paris, his desire for a potency scale that could be manufactured by hand, reach deeply into the constitution and yet prove gentle, but efficient in action, was fulfilled when he conceived the LM potencies – and only a mind such as his could have done so.

The preparation of these potencies differs considerably from the centesimal method. The designation LM (50-millesimal i.e. 50,000) refers to the diluting sequence, which employs a ratio of 1 to 50,000 instead of the 1 to 100 of the centigrade scale. The other name for the LM scale is the tongue-twisting *quinquagesimillesimal* (Latin: *quinquagesimus* – 50th; *millesimus* – thousandth), thankfully shortened to Q. However, the term LM is more commonly used.

The starting point for the preparation of all LM potencies is the 3C triturate of the remedy, whether the mother substance is in liquid or solid form. The 3C of a solid substance (e.g. quartz, plant material) is produced by the usual method of three one-hour triturations, each step progressively lifting the potency from the mother substance to the one-hundredth, the one-thousandth and finally the one-millionth potency (3C). If the starting substance is a liquid (e.g. petroleum, venoms, etc) 1ml of the liquid is added to 99gm of lactose powder (1 to 100 dilution) and triturated for one hour to produce the 1C potency. Then, as for the solids, one part of the 1C added to ninety-nine parts of lactose and triturated for one hour yields the 2C potency and from this the 3C potency is prepared in a similar manner.

Hahnemann chose to use the 3C trituration as the basis for his LMs rather than the dilution because he was convinced that dynamisation through trituration developed the inner healing power of a remedy far more efficiently and to a far greater degree than the parallel process of liquid dilution and succussion. Each trituration process was done in three steps and the exact method is meticulously described in the sixth edition of the *Organon*. Using the centesimal scale of dilution, he would take 100 grains of pure lactose and divide it into three equal portions. The first portion he placed in a glazed porcelain mortar, the bottom of which had been roughened by rubbing it with fine, moist sand. To this he added one grain of the powdered medicinal substance. After mixing this with a metal spatula, he proceeded to triturate (grind) the mixture *rather strongly* for 6 to 7 minutes, using a porcelain pestle that had also been previously dulled. This done, 3 to 4 minutes were taken to thoroughly scrape the compressed powder from the bottom of the mortar and the pestle, *to make it homogenous*. This operation was followed by a further 6 to 7 minute period of strong grinding, followed in turn by another 3 to 4 minutes of scraping. When finished, the second portion of lactose was added and the entire painstaking procedure repeated, and yet again for the third and final portion, a process which altogether consumed a full hour and raised the potency of the triturated powder by one centesimal degree. Two more hours of trituration would be required to reach the 3C potency.

He was now ready to commence the preparation of the LM potencies. He dissolved 1 grain of the 3C powder in 500 drops of alcohol/water (90% alcohol: distilled water: 1:4). A single drop of this mixture was placed in a glass vial. To this 100 drops of 95% alcohol was added and the tightly corked vial given 100 strong succussions *with the hand against a hard but elastic body* (the vial size was such that when charged it was two-thirds full allowing for thorough succussion). This liquid was the LM1 potency and was put into stock. One drop from the LM1 stock bottle was used to medicate 500 sugar globules (poppy-seed size). These were spread on blotting paper, and when completely dry, stored in a glass vial marked LM1, ready to be dispensed to patients.

To obtain the LM2 potency, one LM1 globule was placed in a new vial with one drop of water to dissolve it. To this 100 drops of alcohol was added and the vial succussed 100 times, thus producing the LM2 potency for stock. One drop from the LM2 stock bottle was used to medicate 500 sugar globules, which after drying were stored in a glass vial marked LM2. In this manner by unit progression the LM30 was eventually reached, each step producing its respective LM stock bottle in liquid form and its prescribing bottle of medicated globules.

With the ratio of dilutant to medicine being 50,000 to 1, Hahnemann felt that increasing the number of succussion strokes to 100 (from the 2 or 10, he advised for centesimal potencies) would bring about a far greater development of healing power, while ensuring gentleness of action.

> By means of this mechanical processing ... a given medicinal substance, which in its crude state is only matter, is subtilised and transformed by these higher and higher dynamisations to become a spirit-like medicinal power. The medicated globule becomes the *carrier* of this invisible power ... even when it is used dry, but far more so when it is dissolved in water.[20]

Hence, in his later life, Hahnemann preferred not to give his patients dry medication. He would dissolve the dry carrier in water, vigorously stirring the mixture, and administer the medicine by teaspoon doses. LMs are, therefore, prescribed for the patient in liquid form, and not as globules or pillules. A single, medicated globule of the selected potency (e.g. LM1) is placed in a bottle and then dissolved in 100ml of distilled water, containing 15 drops of medicinal alcohol to act as preservative. The bottle must have sufficient empty space at the top to enable the patient to succuss the medicine before use. This is the patient's stock bottle for home use. In order to take a dose, the patient first succusses the bottle by means of 8 firm strokes against the palm of the hand then takes one teaspoon of the contents and stirs it vigorously into 100ml of water (preferably filtered water) in a cup. Once fully stirred, the patient takes a single teaspoon dose from the cup. The rest of the liquid is discarded.

Hahnemann reasoned that after a dose of the correct remedy, there will be a degree of positive shift in the health of the patient, no matter how small, and that the next dose of the same remedy needs to be adjusted to this change towards improved health – it must keep pace with the shift – and this could be achieved by succussing the remedy before each dose, thus giving a subtle lift to the potency. If patients were oversensitive or undersensitive to the action of the LM remedy, the number of succussions before administration could be altered – less strokes for the oversensitive and more strokes for the undersensitive. In the markedly hypersensitive, apart from reducing the number of succussion strokes, it was possible to double-up on the diluting process by taking a teaspoon from the first cup and adding it to a second cup of 100ml water before administration and in more extreme cases even using a third or fourth cup. Another method of reducing the risk of aggravation was by increasing the amount of diluting fluid in the patient's stock bottle e.g. one globule of the selected LM potency in 150ml or 200ml (rather than the standard 100ml).

The dosage of LM potencies is generally more frequent than for centesimal potencies. In chronic cases a daily dose is usual. When the patient's LM1 stock bottle is finished, the next potency, LM2, is given, and then the LM3, and so forth, while ever the chosen remedy remains indicated. Although the scale has been taken as high as LM30, it is very rare for a patient to require that level of potency, usually the expected response has been achieved by LM10. Though more commonly used for chronic conditions, some LM prescribers will also use LMs for acute prescribing, in which case a teaspoon dose may be taken as frequently as every hour, each dose being preceded by a vigorous stirring of the contents of the cup. Since doses follow one another at fairly close intervals e.g. every 1–2 hours, they can all be taken from the same cup; it is not necessary to discard the contents after each dose.

The annotated fifth edition of the *Organon*, which Hahnemann was so anxious to have published before his death, as the sixth and final edition, was not released for publication to the homeopathic profession by Melanie or her heirs, until 1920, when Richard Haehl, with the financial assistance of William Boericke, salvaged the original manuscript from the revolution-torn Ruhr area of Germany. The first English translation was published in 1921. This lapse of almost eighty years had a huge impact on the unfolding of homeopathic methodology, and still has, to this very day. Central to the practical application of the homeopathic principles expounded in the sixth edition was the use of the LM potency, which superseded the centesimal scale of previous editions. This switch in Hahnemann's thinking was unknown to his contemporaries, and, therefore, without the Master at the helm, the outstanding physicians and teachers who followed him remained on the same centesimal trajectory he had first developed. The only difference being the height to which some pushed the potency level. By the time the sixth edition was finally published, expertise in the use of the centesimal scale had been refined, developed and firmly established.

Some of the greatest names in the homeopathic teaching tradition were centesimal exponents and achieved remarkable results. Skilful use of the centesimal keyboard was found to successfully obviate or moderate healing aggravations. In the early 1900s, homeopathy, in both the United States and Britain, was dominated by the influential figure of James Tyler Kent, who died in 1916, five years before the publication of the sixth edition. His legacy of high potency prescribing still holds considerable sway. Hence, the LM scale remained almost totally disregarded, despite the Master's advice, until it was rediscovered in the 1950s. Its use has since become particularly popular in India where the majority of LM practitioners are to be found. Many practitioners in the West, who habitually prescribe decimal and centesimal potencies for their patients, reserve the use of LM potencies for hypersensitive subjects, especially those suffering from atopy (allergic states e.g. eczema, hay-fever, asthma), who are more likely to produce marked or prolonged aggravations as part of their healing response.

Passion and potency have proved constant bedfellows and so it is with the LM exponents; and supporting their faith and enthusiasm stand the last written words of the Master. They proclaim that these potencies act more quickly than those of the centesimal or decimal scale; that they penetrate more deeply into the constitution, some claiming that they can impinge even upon the spiritual domain; that they act more efficiently in combating disease suppression, which is so rife in modern medicine; and, most especially, that they are more gentle in their effect, and if aggravations should arise, they soon abate, and, if not, can be more easily managed: a list of superlatives, which cannot pass unheeded. As with all passions, but especially those pertaining to healing, this passion for potency must be evaluated through practice and experience: the dispassionate arbiters.

References

1. Bradford TL. *The Pioneers of Homœopathy*. Philadelphia PA: Boericke & Tafel; 1897. p345.
2. Haehl R. *Samuel Hahnemann His Life And Work*. Vol 2. London: Homoeopathic Publishing Company; 1922. p509.
3. Clarke HC. *A Dictionary of Practical Materia Medica*. Vol 2. London: Homoeopathic Publishing Company; 1955. p211.
4. Coulter CR. *Portraits of Homœopathic Medicines – Psychophysical Analyses of Selected Constitutional Types*. Vol 1. Berkeley CA: North Atlantic Books; 1986. pp301–302.
5. Bradford TL. *The Pioneers of Homœopathy*. Philadelphia PA: Boericke & Tafel; 1897. p399.
6. *Ibid.*, p396.
7. *Ibid.*, p394.
8. *Ibid.*, pp131–133.
9. Haehl R. *Samuel Hahnemann His Life And Work*. Vol 1. London: Homoeopathic Publishing Company; 1922. p328.

10 *Ibid.*, p325.
11 *Ibid.*, p326.
12 O'Reilly WB. *Organon of the Medical Art – Samuel Hahnemann, M.D.* Washington DC: Birdcage Books; 1997. p237.
13 *Ibid.*, p239.
14 *Ibid.*, pp240–241.
15 Bradford TL. *The Lesser Writings of CMF von Boenninghausen.* Philadelphia PA: Boericke & Tafel; 1908. p136.
16 Dudgeon RE. *Theory and Practice of Homœopathy.* London: Leath and Ross; 1854. p355.
17 Bradford TL. *Life of Hahnemann.* Philadelphia PA: Boericke & Tafel; 1894. pp459–460.
18 Bradford TL. *The Pioneers of Homœopathy.* Philadelphia PA: Boericke & Tafel; 1897. pp420–421.
19 Winston J. A brief history of potentizing machines. *British Homoeopathic Journal* 1989; 78(2): 65.
20 O'Reilly WB. *Organon of the Medical Art – Samuel Hahnemann, M.D.* Washington DC: Birdcage Books; 1997. pp241–242.

10

PRIDE, PREJUDICE AND POLITICS

Homeopathy under attack

The hostility and antagonism that homeopathy has engendered amongst the rank and file of conventional doctors presents a curious phenomenon, which is as intense today as it has ever been in the past. The reasons for this are complex, undoubtedly political as much as ideological, and provide a sad insight into the general, modern perspective of life and its values. This perspective has been moulded by the concepts of Newtonian science, which exercise a powerful and insidious influence upon us no matter what religion, belief system or philosophy we ascribe to. Daily, we are surrounded by evidence and facts that validate the truth of these concepts and persuade us, despite our inner promptings and hopes, that we are bound by, subject to, and the product of, the inflexible laws of chemistry and physics extending into the biological realm of living forms; that the world we inhabit is three dimensional, concrete and finite; and that no matter our aspirations, our abilities and even our genius, there is no higher purpose to our life experience than achieving utilitarian excellence and propagating our genes. We are assured that there are no hidden dimensions other than the farthest reaches of space and the inscrutable mysteries of the ultramicroscopic; and even these are ever more vulnerable to our probing curiosity. Most devastating to our deepest sensibilities, if we are swayed by the cult of technology and materialism, is the certainty that we exist in a godless environment, ruled by inexorable, merciless, mechanical laws, devoid of intelligence, purposeful design and sentiment, and that we ourselves, despite our exquisite sensitivity, high intelligence and creative brilliance, are a temporary assembly of atoms: mortal, expendable and ultimately insignificant. These stark, cold, scientific observations and conclusions are brandished before us by the most respected and vocal champions of science.

Stephen Jay Gould

Stephen Jay Gould (1941–2002), the renowned neo-Darwinist, palaeontologist, evolutionary biologist and science historian, who was at the same time one of the most influential writers of popular science, leaves us in no doubt about modern scientific philosophy:

> Evolution has no purpose. Individuals struggle to increase the representation of their genes in future generations, and that is all. Evolution has no direction; it does not lead inevitably to higher things.

And critically, because his words reflect science's materialistic thinking, including that of medical science, he states:

> Matter is the ground of all existence – mind, spirit and God as well, are just words that express the wondrous results of neuronal complexity.

Gould is best known for his theory of *punctuated equilibrium*. This theory proposes that the fossil record reveals an evolutionary process characterised by long periods of 'species stasis,' a state of stability or equilibrium during which species remain unchanged, and that these periods of prolonged quiescence are punctuated by sudden, relatively short-lived, intervals of immense and dramatic change. Gould concluded that this was the reason why palaeontologists have failed to find the smooth, structured sequence of intermediate forms, which would be consistent with Darwin's theory of gradual and continuous transition, based on the steady accretion of random, genetic mutations; now known as *phyletic gradualism*.

This conclusion, however, exposes to question Gould's assertion that all evolution is arbitrary, random and without purposeful design. If evolution occurs in successful, great bursts, lasting a relatively short time, this would necessitate the perfect synchronisation of vast numbers of genetic mutations, each calculated to immediately increase the chances of survival during an unknown and as yet indeterminate future – the next phase of stasis. Such multiple and collective alterations, bestowing adaptive advantages to species prior to the circumstances requiring them, indicate a symphonic, harmonious and orchestrated response requiring a composer with vision and design: a creative intelligence.

Gould was a passionate advocate of evolutionary, scientific theory and often aroused the ire of the fundamentalist creationists, to whom he was anathema. To resolve the conflict between science and religion, he proposed the principle of non-overlapping magisteria (NOMA); a *magisterium* being an independent domain of concepts and teachings within which meaningful discussion and debate can take place with the possibility of consensus and resolution because of a commonality of thought and precepts. By this means he sought to separate and distance what he considered to be two highly incompatible (non-overlapping) foes, as one would oil from water; the magisterium of science holding sway over the facts and theories of the empirical realm while the magisterium of religion governed the sphere of ultimate meaning, morality and worship – and never the twain shall meet! He expected that the respective magisteria, while viewing one-another through binoculars from their remote (non-overlapping) standpoints, should exercise goodwill towards each other. This surgical solution to dissension is typical of the pragmatic, reductionist mindset of science, which has yet to comprehend the unity of all things. The same tendency to compartmentalise was evidenced medically in the analysis of Gould's death from cancer. In 1982, at 41, he was diagnosed with peritoneal mesothelioma, a very aggressive form of cancer affecting the abdominal lining and most frequently found in those who have been exposed to asbestos toxicity. Fortunately the cancer was detected early and treatment by radiation, chemotherapy and surgery over a difficult period of two years proved successful. He became a beacon of hope and comfort for many cancer sufferers. However, 20 years later, in 2002, Gould died of metastatic adenocarcinoma of the lung, which had spread to the brain. The two cancers were viewed by medical science as being unrelated. When regarded superficially, this conclusion is accurate, both their site and structure support the independent origin of the two malignancies, but when considered at a deeper level, the existence of an underlying susceptibility of the constitution must link the two, and, furthermore, the aggressively suppressive nature of the therapy required to force the initial malignancy into remission must have increased that susceptibility.

Richard Dawkins

Richard Dawkins, the ethologist (animal behaviourist) and evolutionary biologist, who is one of the leading and most vehement advocates of science-based atheism and a militant critic of creationism (the religious belief that the universe, animate life and humanity were created by a deity, without recourse to evolution) disagrees with Gould's proposed principle of NOMA. He discounts it as a political gesture, a peace offering designed to lure ambivalent minds into the scientific fold, and as specious, since the religionist's belief in miracles directly impinges on the scientific magisterium. Needless to say, Dawkins' acerbic diatribes against religious faith (and any scientific perspective other than his own) and his arguments against the existence of God, or a cosmic intelligence, propounded in his polemic book *The God Delusion*, represent a major impingement on the religious magisteria.

An intellectually fulfilled atheist

In the first chapter of *The Blind Watchmaker*, Dawkins, who has been voted one of the world's three top intellectuals, explains his choice of title for the book by quoting and commenting on a famous passage from the 1802 treatise, *Natural Theology – or Evidence of the Existence and Attributes of the Deity Collected from the Appearances of Nature*, by the Christian apologist and philosopher, William Paley (1743–1805). Paley expounds on the fact that if while walking on a heath one found a watch lying on the ground, the very precision and intricacy of its design would force us to conclude:

> . . . that the watch must have had a maker . . . who formed it for a purpose . . . who comprehended its construction and designed its use.

He continues:

> . . . every indication of contrivance, every manifestation of design, which existed in the watch, exists in the works of nature . . . and that in a degree which exceeds all computation.

Paley's compelling conclusion is that nature must have had a creator – a designer – a watchmaker – just as the watch had. However, Richard Dawkins even when surveying the majesty and magnificence of the creation, concludes quite differently, and is at pains to dissuade us from what he considers to be Paley's misconception:

> All appearances to the contrary, the only watchmaker in nature is the blind force of physics, albeit deployed in a very special way. A true watchmaker has foresight . . . a future purpose in his mind's eye. Natural selection, the blind, unconscious, automatic process which Darwin discovered, and which we now know is the explanation for the existence and apparently purposeful form of all life, has no purpose in mind. It has no mind and no mind's eye. It does not plan for the future. It has no vision, no foresight, no sight at all. It is the *blind* watchmaker.[1]

He further muses:

> . . . although atheism might have been *logically* tenable before Darwin, Darwin made it possibly to be an intellectually fulfilled atheist.[1]

At least, Dawkins limits his sense of fulfilment to intellectual satisfaction. The contemplation of a creation brought into being by blind, fortuitous events, even when on the grandest scale and with the most wondrous consequences, must leave one ultimately without balm for suffering, without solace at the death of a loved one, with scant motivation for pursuing a spiritual path and with the conviction that in the final issue, life, with all its strivings and sacrifices, is transient and futile; hardly a fulfilling or uplifting scenario. Surely, to find in atheism a source of fulfilment, either emotional or intellectual, and to desire to impose such a glacial cult on others, must require the erasure or numbing of something infinitely precious and sacred within us, present from our earliest years, which enriches our lives with a sense of the magical and the sublime, and inspires the genius of the poet, artist and composer: the intuitive awareness of a different and higher order of existence that lies concealed behind that which it projects as manifest and tangible.

Mythos and *logos*

Gould, an amiable, plump, teddy bear of a man, a secular Jew, who described himself as an atheistically inclined agnostic, believed that natural selection provides the explanation for all the phenomena in the natural world, but, nonetheless, also felt that science was not competent to pass judgement on the existence of God, because the terrain in which it operated was physical, not metaphysical. He, unlike Dawkins, was not ardently opposed to or contemptuous of religion. Hence, his proposed concept of separate magisteria, which provided a 'live and let live' solution for the irreconcilable differences existing between science and religious philosophy. This concept is reminiscent of the easy tolerance with which the ancients regarded the coexistence of the temporal and the spiritual. The people of the past, like many primitive, indigenous communities today, possessed an intuitive perception of reality, including a psychic awareness of the spiritual realm. They were comfortable with both the mystic, spiritual aspects of existence and the external, practical necessities of everyday life. They did not find these different views incongruous, or in conflict, or confuse one with the other; mysticism gave meaning and purpose to life – practical skills were essential for survival. The rich, mythological tradition (*mythos*) of ancient and classical Greece provided metaphoric insight into the deepest regions of the human unconscious, but was not understood by the enlightened seer to represent rational thinking (*logos*). Related in parable form, the myth delivered a moral tale making universal and eternal truths intelligible and significant to the listener. The most profound wisdom, which otherwise might remain obscure and difficult to comprehend, is oft best conveyed through stories that teach.

In those early times, both *mythos* and *logos* were understood to be indispensable to a balanced understanding of life, but, as Gould wished to have formally recognised, they were also understood to be distinct from one another, each applicable to its own domain. This distinction, based on difference not division, was a natural one and either faith or fact could be happily and appropriately invoked according to necessity, and there was certainly ground where the two came together in morally motivated action. It was not necessary to renounce one or the other, or to make one dominant over the other; both were essential. The unseen dimension was not limited by the rules of the objective, natural world, and thinking in myth was not confused with rational thinking, for to make metaphorical or mystic stories the basis for practical policy would court disaster.

Rudolph Steiner

In the late eighteen hundreds, a young Austrian philosopher and esotericist, Rudolph Steiner (1861–1925), sought to find a synthesis between *mythos* and *logos* – between mysticism and science. Steiner had been deeply involved with the Theosophical movement founded by Madame Blavatsky, but when the leading lights of this organisation, Annie Besant and Charles Leadbeater, promoted the young Indian boy, Jiddu Krishnamurti, as a messianic, spiritual teacher (a role later emphatically disavowed by Krishnamurti), Steiner broke away from the order and subsequently founded the philosophical system of Anthroposophy.

He was convinced that for humanity to progress fully on all levels, spiritually, culturally, educationally and medically, the division or polarisation between science and faith must be recognised as artificial and dispelled. No longer must we separate perception and thinking as they are complementary and together are essential to gaining understanding of life and the cosmos. He postulated that being in essence spiritual, the human being is capable through inner development of accessing and directly experiencing an objective, intellectually comprehensible spiritual world, and to a degree equivalent to the clarity, precision and verifiability with which the natural world can be observed and evaluated by science. To achieve this, faculties of perceptive imagination, inspiration and intuition need to be cultivated, faculties which have largely atrophied and become dormant due to humanity's increasing reliance on the intellect and sensory experience. This increasing intellectualisation of the consciousness has led to excessive focus on objective reality and loss of contact with spiritual reality. The return of full psychic awareness, which is inherent in all of us, even when suspended through persistent disuse, permits the consciousness to realise our own nature and that of the inner and outer worlds, which are found to be interpenetrating and indivisibly one. Steiner, furthermore, stipulated that essential to this process of inner and outer illumination is the parallel unfolding of the searcher's spiritual morality.

Steiner, like Hahnemann before him, remains far ahead of his time – the realisation of a 'science of spirit' is dwindling rather than gaining strength, the gulf between *logos* and *mythos* widens and as the lines of battle are drawn, that most gentle yet powerful, scientific yet spiritual, system of healing, homeopathy, finds itself in the firing line.

Religious fundamentalism

In modern times, particularly in the West, the remarkable advances of science and technology have swayed the human mind away from the esoteric and fixed it increasingly, and even exclusively, upon the material, sense-perceptible world as the only justifiable reality. *Logos*, in the form of scientific rationalism, often pushed to extreme reductionism, has assumed primacy, and, in the estimation of its adherents, has become the arbiter of truth. In response to this powerful shift to secular modernism, with its attendant dogmatic repudiation of faith, a worldwide religious fundamentalism has arisen. Challenged by the might of empiricism, fundamentalists within various religions present the basic tenets of their sacred scriptures as incontestable fact, asserting that the *mythos* of their faith is in fact *logos*. Such doctrinal dogmatism has not only contributed to the widening gulf between scientific and religious thinking, but has created increasing division within and between religions. Passions have become politicised and radicalised, and militant groups have emerged willing to use religion to mask their subversive reasons for violence and murder.

Scientific fundamentalism

Most recently, partly in response to the swell in American Christian fundamental sentiment after the September 11th terrorist attacks in 2001, which gained political expression through the largely unpopular Bush Administration, on the scientific side of the gulf, an atheistic form of secular fundamentalism has arisen among intellectuals who claim the absolute incompatibility between religion and science. With the same fixation upon a literal interpretation of sacred texts as their religious counterparts, the fundamental atheists, with Dawkins at their fore, ignore the allegorical meaning of scripture and subject it to the hard and fast criteria of scientific and historic analysis, and, not surprisingly, find it wanting. Likewise, in judging religion, they focus on the worst possible examples of religious bigotry and fanaticism, and the atrocities committed in religion's name. In consequence, they see religion as the root of all modern evils, a hindrance to scientific education and a crucible for division and extremism. Lost to their view are the transcendental majesty and sublime truths central to the spiritual teachings of most faiths. To them, everything that makes us human, including our altruism and capacity for self-sacrifice, is the result of environmental pressure, genetic mutations and natural selection – even love evolves from the need to survive and propagate. Characteristic of these atheists is their smug arrogance, proselytising fervour, superficial knowledge of that which they desecrate and a profile of exclusivity and extremism similar to that of the hidebound, religious fundamentalists they so abhor.

These self-styled 'New Atheists,' amongst whom, Dawkins, Christopher Hitchens and Sam Harris are, or were, dominant personalities, object to the pejorative term *fundamentalist atheist*, arguing that such an appellation is a distortion of the defined meaning of fundamentalism (the unshakable, resolute belief in the prescribed tenets of a religion, philosophy or doctrine), because atheism has no beliefs intrinsic to it, nor, for that matter, non-beliefs, since the proponents of science invite change through expanding knowledge and are willing to lend an ear to, and incorporate into their system, new evidence-based facts. However, no matter how they wriggle under the label '*fundamentalist*' and protest their open-mindedness and that their passion is misconstrued, to the observer it is apparent that their strict, unswerving and vehement adherence to the science of the observable, fundamentally excludes all knowledge and experience that proves inaccessible to the inflexible, scientific method they propound. Despite their self-righteousness, they represent an extreme element in scientific thought, which analogous to religious forms of fundamentalism, expresses not just a belief in the scientific model of reality, which alone would not make them fundamentalists, but also the adamant certainty that the only dimension of existence is the physical world, that the only truth is that which is revealed by their scientific method and that all policy should be governed by these dictums. In this they resemble Islamic fundamentalists, who would have Sharia law imposed at every level of society.

Their uncompromising views pressurise more accommodating scientific minds to adopt a harder line when deciding policy regarding systems and methods that in the least deviate from what they regard as scientific. The repercussions of this are ominous, particularly when applied to the world of medicine where vested interests can give them added impetus and support towards establishing a medical oligarchy. Apart from the possibility of demolishing a child's belief in fairies or their parent's belief in the Exodus, in Christ, or the Prophet, the push of the scientific atheists, and others like them, to arbitrate for society what is true and what is false, endangers the public's right to choose the form of medical therapy it desires. Tolerance has given way to open hostility and the desire to eradicate any form of medicine that does not conform to the conventional model, even when practised by qualified medical practitioners.

Homeopathy – a target

Spanning the divide between the two extremist viewpoints and the magisteria of science and religion, like the colossus at Rhodes, homeopathy becomes a target for both factions. Homeopathy personifies, more than any other form of medical therapy, the marriage of the spiritual and the physical, embodied in the form of its immeasurable, infinitesimal potencies: the homeopathic vehicle for healing. Yet, for those who dictate orthodox, medical policy, homeopathy, above all other forms of alternative medicine, is a thorn in the flesh, its very existence an irritation and a reproof. That so many practise it and so many have faith in it and give testimony to its efficacy counts for nothing.

Against a backdrop of millions of individuals only able to function efficiently while under the influence of psychotropic (mood-altering) drugs; an entire spectrum of incurable chronic diseases that are creeping into ever-younger age groups; the rapidly increasing incidence of cancer; widespread chronic viral conditions; opportunistic organisms which rapidly mutate; antibiotic resistant bacterial strains; the emergence of superbugs in the hospital milieu; the constant problem of iatrogenic (drug-caused) disease; the escalating cost of modern drugs; and a great number of disillusioned physicians and patients, the antipathy of the gurus of conventional medicine towards homeopathy has intensified. In circumstances that clamour for medical leaders to recognise and acknowledge the limitations of science-based, mechanistic medicine in the face of the complexity and multifaceted nature of human disease, and when there is a burning need to add, to the truly remarkable achievements of modern medicine, alternative approaches and modes of therapy, they complacently assert that the homeopathic model is biologically implausible, absurd and undeserving of investigation.

Champions of 'scientific medicine'

Edzard Ernst, who qualified as a physician in Germany in 1978 and was the only Professor of Complementary Medicine in the world, working at the University of Exeter in England, until his early retirement in 2011. He was, somewhat paradoxically, one of the most vociferous and influential of homeopathy's critics. Ernst was a modern day Dr Claris, ubiquitous and energetic in evidencing his aggressive contempt for homeopathy and its adherents. He became known as 'the scourge of alternative medicine' because of his unflagging efforts to discredit therapies such as homeopathy, acupuncture and reflexology. Like Dawkins his criticisms were extreme, highly prejudiced, uninformed and one dimensional, being based on the narrow parameters of orthodox methodology. In an article written to other physicians by Ernst and Michael Baum, Professor Emeritus of Surgery and visiting Professor of Medical Humanities at University College, London, entitled *Should We maintain an Open Mind about Homeopathy?* and published in the *American Journal of Medicine*, the two authors uncompromisingly slate homeopathy. Their language and thoughts betray the bigotry lying behind a façade of scientific rectitude:

> Homeopathy is among the worst examples of faith-based medicine. . . . These axioms (of homeopathy) are not only out of line with scientific facts but also directly opposed to them. If homeopathy is correct, much of physics, chemistry and pharmacology must be incorrect. To have an open mind about homeopathy . . . is therefore not an option. We think that a belief in homeopathy exceeds the tolerance of an open mind. We should start from the premise that homeopathy cannot work and that positive evidence reflects publication bias or design flaws until proved otherwise. . . .

How sclerotic a perspective is displayed in these few words and how obstructive to the expansion of medical knowledge. The argument is equivalent to stating that if the theory of quantum mechanics is correct then much of Newtonian physics is incorrect. We now know that both are correct in their sphere of action and are complementary to one another and not exclusive: a relationship, which should exist between conventional and homeopathic medicine. Contrary to the understanding of Ernst and Baum, homeopathic practice relies upon clearly defined, objective principles and is not faith-based.

The article continues by them lauding their myopia, and asserting that homeopathy refutes all scientific progress:

> The true sceptic therefore takes pride in closed mindedness when presented with absurd assertions that contravene the laws of thermodynamics or deny progress in all branches of physics, chemistry, physiology and medicine.[2]

Michael Baum, an oncologist specialising in the treatment of breast cancer, who, by virtue of his modality is about as far removed as one can get from the province of primary health care and the intimate physician/patient relationship of family practice and the concept of 'cure', has described homeopathy as a "cruel deception."[3] Baum, whose destructive scepticism is expressive of the narrow, scientific viewpoint common to medical critics of homeopathy, characterised by preconceived prejudice and absence of personal experience, would have homeopathy, banned from the British National Health Service (NHS), despite the fact that a considerable number of medical colleagues actively practise homeopathy. He and thirteen other scientists (shades of the 13 against Hahnemann) wrote to the chief executives of all the acute and primary care trusts in Britain expressing concern and criticism that "unproven or disproved treatments are being encouraged for general use in the NHS."

This was followed by the customary gratuitous expression of righteous open-mindedness:

> While medical practice must remain open to new discoveries for which there is convincing evidence, including any branded as 'alternative', it would be highly irresponsible to embrace any medicine as though it were a matter of principle.[4]

Their argument is that money used to supply free homeopathic treatment through the NHS is wasted and would be better employed in the service of conventional medicine. The result would be homeopathy only for those who could afford to receive it privately, and for those less affluent, the undemocratic removal of the right to have free access to their therapy of choice, even when registered, trained professionals are available to provide the service and monitor response. This autocratic attitude is an unfortunate tendency too frequently seen in medicine both within and outside the consulting room.

Charles, the Prince of Wales, has long been a protagonist and promoter of alternative medicine. Ever since Queen Adelaide called upon the homeopathic services of Dr Stapf in 1835, the British Royal Family have had an interest in homeopathy and favoured it with their patronage. This is taken much amiss by physicians of the Ernst/Baum mould since it endorses a system of medicine they wish to expose as sham and would like to see eradicated. In June 2004, Prince Charles delivered a keynote speech to a joint cancer symposium in which he recommended a collaborative approach to cancer research through which the efficacy and value of alternative therapies could be investigated. The Prince of Wales did not promote any specific alternative treatments to cancer, but mentioned, by way of example, how anecdotal reports of the value of carrot juice, coffee enemas and the Gerson diet could be looked into. This open-minded and considered recommendation to leave no stones unturned in the fight against cancer stirred the indignation of Professor Baum and to such a degree that he was moved to make an excessive and extraordinary response in an open letter to Prince Charles, which was published in the *British Medical Journal* of July 10, 2004, and entitled *An open letter to the Prince of Wales: with respect, your highness, you've got it wrong.* Taking a hefty mallet to a proverbial nut, Baum sought to smash the kernel of care and concern it contained. He rebuked the prince for supporting alternative therapies and therefore (in his opinion) misusing his power and misleading the public. His letter is redolent with rectitude, condescension and bigotry. His conceit can best be savoured by reading these pretentious words, which are quite devoid of the respect he invokes in his title:

> The power of my authority comes with a knowledge built on 40 years of study and 25 years of active involvement in cancer research.... Your power and authority rest on an accident of birth.... It is in the nature of your world to be surrounded by sycophants (including members of the medical establishment hungry for their mention in the Queen's birthday honours list) who constantly reinforce what they assume are your prejudices. Sir, they patronise you! Allow me this chastisement.[5]

Two implacable enemies of homeopathy came together when Richard Dawkins interviewed Michael Baum on the matter of alternative and complementary medicine in 2008. This was filmed for Channel 4's *The Enemies of Reason*. Baum unctuously extolled the "scrupulous honesty" of the randomised control trials (RCT) conducted by scientific medicine in testing the efficacy of modern drugs, and decried the value of anecdotal evidence in the assessment of therapeutic success, emphasising the deceptive role of the placebo effect and the phenomenon of spontaneous remission. In distinguishing between complementary and alternative medicine, which he referred to as 'slippery' terms, his argument proved equally slippery. While he correctly welcomed any patently beneficial complementary adjunct to main-line therapy, and mentioned art therapy as his particular passion, he argued that there was no such thing as alternative medicine since, by definition it did not work, for if it did, it would already be used by the orthodoxy, and would not be alternative i.e. if a system of medicine (homeopathy) is an alternative to a system which works (scientific medicine), it cannot work.

His interviewer had no problem with this obfuscation.

Despite telling the audience that only scientific medicine works, when referring to his own discipline Baum described it as "trying to cure cancer." Trying is never a powerful word, nor a word that promotes confidence that what is being tried will work. And 'cure', in the light of modern medicine's achievements in cancer therapy, still remains a hope; unfortunately, even today, it is more accurate to speak of remission than of cure. For anyone working in the sphere of 'trying', and much of modern medicine's endeavours are of this order, it would be wise to seek alternatives. But, how can a scientist possibly unearth any alternative if he believes that only his paradigm works and additionally, in the case of medicine, if his hallowed benchmark of efficacy is the RCT, which is only appropriate for that paradigm? Prince Charles' plea was that all avenues should be explored and tested, but Professor Baum, although professing to be open to anything proven, will certainly not deign to investigate that which he has already decided is absurd and implausible. In the early 1600s, Galileo was the victim of a similar mind-set. Baum would seem to expect practitioners of alternative forms of therapy to conduct the vastly expensive trials necessary to provide conventional medicine with evidence of efficacy (according to its rules) when surely aware of the lack of financial resources, such as research grants, to do so.

When asked about reports of the successful homeopathic RCTs that have been done, he discounted any positive outcome as being the result of either selective bias in the interpretation of the results, or flaws in the trial design. His answers were carefully worded and, to the uninformed, delivered with authority, magnanimity and immaculate argument. The influence of such champions of the scientific method cannot be underestimated. Their yardstick is rigidly Newtonian and the evidence-based proof of efficacy they demand has to conform to the inappropriate protocols used to assay chemical drugs. Through their activities and the influence of the multinational drug companies, homeopathy in the United Kingdom has become severely threatened. The title 'homeopathy' has become so weighted with orthodox opprobrium that politics has dictated that it should be subsumed under the wider definition of 'integrative medicine.' Thus, in 2010, over 150 years after its founding, the Royal London Homoeopathic Hospital (RLHH), a well known landmark in Central London and a visible presence of homeopathy within the NHS, was renamed the Royal London Hospital for Integrated Medicine (RHIM).

Religious paranoia

At the other, thankfully harmless, pole, radical elements among ultra-conservative Christians regard homeopathy's energy remedies as potential vehicles, not for healing, but for satanic influence. They fear that behind the caring, empathetic guise of the attentive, unwitting homeopathic physician lurks a demonic force capable of subverting the dematerialised medicine to its own ends: the eternal damnation of the patient's soul. Even evidence of the good wrought by homeopathy, especially when contrary to medical expectation and hope-fulfilling, is viewed with the deepest suspicion and seen as indicative of the seductive, wily ways of Satan, luring the innocent into his clutches. This religious paranoia, not evidenced by the adherents of Judaism or Islam, first manifested in the 'bible-belt' of the Southern States of America and spread widely in the world of Christian fundamentalists. In the late nineteen seventies the superstition arrived in Pretoria, South Africa and resulted in a number of 'born-again' Christian patients, and even families long associated with the Lilley homeopathic practice, leaving the fold. It must be noted, however, that many sharing their religious persuasion remained staunchly committed to homeopathic treatment. This episode reached comic proportions when a rumour was circulated that it was my custom to enter my dispensary at midnight (probably at full moon) to place evil spells on the remedies.

Comparing therapeutic methods

Richard Dawkins has not hesitated to give comment on medical matters. In a foreword to John Diamond's *Snake Oil*, a book devoted to disparaging alternative medicine, he asserts that alternative medicine is harmful, if only because it distracts patients from more successful conventional treatments, and gives people false hopes. And in his own book *A Devil's Chaplain* he, in echoing Baum, categorically states: "There is no alternative medicine – there is only medicine that works and medicine that doesn't work."[6] In the eyes of Dawkins and orthodox, medical science only conventional medicine works. But, what do they mean by 'works?' When conventional medicine works, are we convinced that this working is satisfactory, beneficial, gentle, harmless and the best that can be achieved? Is it bringing about a permanent resolution of the clinical problem – is it promoting a curative response from the body – or is it acting merely by suppression, inhibition and control – if the latter, should we be satisfied – should we not try to do better; seek an alternative – and if we do, may not the answer lie outside the limited paradigm of conventional, chemical medicine? Working and curing are not necessarily the same thing!

To the homeopath, cure does not mean merely the disappearance of symptoms, but the full and permanent restoration of the state of health and a feeling of on-going wellbeing, experienced both emotionally and physically. To achieve this, a high degree of similarity must exist between the symptoms experienced by the patient and the symptoms the chosen remedy can cause when used in a proving trial on healthy subjects. When this obtains, the remedy works by stimulating and maintaining a progressive healing response initiated by the body's own systems of defence and repair. But this is not necessarily the *modus operandi* of other therapeutic systems.

Ways in which medicinal substances can 'work'

If we compare the various ways in which medicinal substances can 'work', we find that there are fundamentally four methods of employing remedies:

1. **With no regard for matching the remedy and the disease**
This was prevalent in Hahnemann's time, when venesection, leeches, blistering, purging and emetics were used; methods, which obviously could not cure and could certainly harm. We might argue that such crude forms of treatment were arbitrary and totally without method, however, they did have a definite purpose in mind and that was to balance the essential humours of the body. As barbaric and injurious as these methods were, the intent, nonetheless, was to externalise or throw the morbid force outwards and away from the threatened internal economy by establishing a vent, much as one does in lancing a boil. Although the methods chosen were futile, harmful and often proved fatal, there was still virtue in this concept. Such thinking supported the heroic use of mercury in the treatment of syphilis, which sought through salivation, sweating, diuresis and purgation to bring about a healing catharsis, but resulted in toxic mercurialisation with all its dreadful consequences. In modern times, the action of conventional medicine is largely the reverse of this, either suppressing, or compensating for, the manifestations of malfunction, resulting in the implosion of the disease potential, which eventually leads to further disturbance of homeostasis (balanced function); the disease process is masked, perpetuated and potentiated.

2. **By supplementation, substitution or replacement therapy**
An example is the treatment of diabetes by means of insulin and underactive thyroid by administering thyroid hormone. While being essential in the presence of serious or complete organ failure, replacement therapy does not cure, it can only maintain and support. Unfortunately, such therapy may be chosen prematurely at the first signs of a functional weakness. One of the earliest signs of an underactive thyroid is raised values of thyroid

stimulating hormone (TSH), a hormone secreted by the pituitary gland in response to negative feedback due to reduced levels of thyroid hormone, *thyroxin*, in the blood. This is an attempt by the body to stimulate the faltering gland to secrete more thyroxin. The simplistic response of orthodox medicine to this under-activity is to administer a pharmaceutical preparation of the hormone to the patient in material and measured doses sufficient to artificially restore the normal level of thyroxin. The pituitary gland is foxed into believing the bogus, positive feedback and reduces its production of TSH. In doing so, the self-healing response of the body is curtailed and the condition of hypothyroidism (underactive thyroid) is firmly established, leaving the patient with a life-long dependency on the drug substitute. The underlying cause of the slowed thyroid function remains frequently unaddressed and will then continue to express itself in some way, emotionally and physically. Likewise, except in cases of definite malnutrition and deficiency, the use of various supplements (vitamins, trace elements, tonics, etc) often provides whitewashing for a constitutional condition of mal-assimilation and dysfunction, which will persist unchecked despite any temporary improvement that may be experienced.

Modern medicine has developed a highly mechanistic approach to the body and its diseases. This has resulted in protocols of therapy which centre on balancing and maintaining a normal biochemical profile and are often aimed at simply topping up that which is low or lacking, much as we would do in servicing a car. The extent to which such an approach can obscure rational, medical thinking is witnessed in the treatment of menopausal women. Since the 1960s, the most popular treatment for the so-called 'change of life' has become hormone replacement therapy (HRT): the administration of synthetic or 'natural' oestrogen (prepared from the urine of pregnant mares) and more recently with the addition of synthetic progesterone or progestogen, by tablet, cream, implant, patch or loaded intrauterine device (IUD). The combination misleads the body into thinking it is still pre-menopausal and the symptoms of change are suppressed.

The advent of HRT was hailed by the orthodoxy as a panacea for all the changes and ailments associated with the menopause. Indeed, apart from its suppression of hot flushes, night sweats, vaginal dryness, loss of libido and osteoporosis, it was vaunted as a 'female fountain of youth,' capable of holding at bay the ravages of the ageing process. It provided a quick fix for the previously stubborn and debilitating complaints that afflict a certain proportion of women as their reproductive life comes to a close. Instead of considering the unique psychosomatic, and hence also physiological, state of each individual, and guiding the body to achieve its own natural homeostasis, the cause of HRT has been promoted with great vigour and conviction and with an enthusiasm reminiscent of the fanaticism of the medieval blood-letter. Many a woman has excited the ire of her physician by declining the use of the sacred nostrum. A mythology emerged, in which menopause, no longer regarded as a normal transition phase, became an inevitable illness of the older woman brought about by the diminished output of a critical hormone by an aging body. At the outset, HRT had at least been reserved for women who manifested symptoms of hormonal deficiency; now many physicians regard it as a necessity for any woman approaching mid-life, recommended as a prophylactic against a variety of threats to future health and a means to pushing back the signs of encroaching age.

Success in the suppression or removal of patient's symptoms through substitution therapy is impressive for both the patient and the physician. The reaction to such therapy is generally prompt, and, as long as the remedy is taken, the symptoms remain at bay. Frequently, however, because the cause of the deficiency is not being addressed, the body's own contribution becomes further weakened as it becomes increasingly dependent on the supportive substance, which has then to be given in increasingly stronger dosage. But, in the language of the clinician, as emphasised by Baum and Dawkins, this therapy 'works', and according to Baum's argument an alternative, by definition, will not work. He is gravely mistaken, because the alternative, which is imperative, since we cannot be satisfied that simple substitution constitutes cure or that it is the best that can be achieved, requires a change of approach: alternative but also different! Unless the organ failure is extreme or total, the alternative homeopathic approach would not be by substitution in the first place, but would be directed to coaxing the refractory organ into improved performance. And, this would be achieved not by treating the failing organ, as if it were independent of its owner, as is done in conventional therapy, but by selecting a primary remedy that acts on the unique, psychosomatic picture of the patient through the closest possible similarity, and, if necessary, supported by secondary remedies which act directly upon the organ in a stimulatory way, e.g. Fucus vesiculosis (from sea kelp) in low potency for hypothyroidism.

Modern, chemical medicine is now able through HRT to manipulate a woman's hormonal profile and thereby modify or subdue the external manifestations of menopause, and more ominously through the use of the contraceptive 'Pill' to hormonally suppress fertility – but at what risk to health? HRT and the Pill can be considered together because although oral contraception is not strictly substitutive both medications depend on the introduction of synthetic female hormones into the physiological system.

These regimes are undoubtedly effective, but are they intrinsically safe and since the 100 million women or more, who are currently on the combined oral contraceptive pill (COCP), excrete from their urine and faeces, in addition to their natural oestrogens, (estrone, E1 and estradiol, E2), synthetic ethinylestradiol (EE2) into water-treatment plants and rivers, how safe are they for the greater environment? It has been estimated that only 76% of synthetic EE2 is removed by water purification and that it is far more potent than either E1 or E2 in inducing hormonal disruption in wild fish populations, affecting sexual development and reproduction.[7,8] More significant than the hormonal disturbance these substances can cause in fish is the fact that the synthetic EE2 proves more potently disruptive than the natural oestrogens.

A characteristic of the medical minds of Hahnemann's time was the ostrich-like ability to refute all evidence of harm resulting from their drastic therapeutic regimes. The apothecaries became the bitterest opponents of all that Hahnemann stood for. Not out of any concern for ailing humanity, but because of the threat that the homeopathic, minimal dose posed to their vested interests. Today, the complacent eye of medicine tends to downplay the serious side effects potential in the use of HRT (and hormonal contraception) and the push of the drug houses is directed to maintaining and expanding its applications. Surrounded by present day statistics of what amounts to an epidemic of breast and uterine cancer and warnings of the increased risk posed by HRT in this regard, as also its implication in adverse psychological changes (anxiety, irritability, depression), hypertension, thrombosis, liver and gall bladder disease and sundry other PMT-like symptoms (breast congestion and tenderness, weight gain, water retention, bloatedness, headaches, etc) medical science appears untroubled and is reluctant to consider an alternative.

It does not take a scientifically trained mind to recognise the overt dangers of venesection and the other barbarisms of medieval medicine, however, neither should it require great physiological insight to suspect that the administration of synthetic or non-species specific hormones must hold serious, inherent danger. Yet, minds steeped in the remarkable knowledge of modern, medical science remain generally unperturbed that millions upon millions of women are on the Pill or are taking HRT. This nonchalance flies in the face of the exquisitely sensitive and critically, delicate axis of balance existing between pituitary, ovarian and adrenal function, which responds appropriately to every nuance of need and notion; the disruptive effect that indiscriminate dosing and timing of such hormones must cause; and knowledge of the hormone dependency of many breast and uterine cancers. The medical world should be particularly concerned about the accumulative effect of generations upon generations of hormonal contraception. If alive today, both Paracelsus and Hahnemann would not have minced their words when criticising many aspects of present day allopathic medicine and despite the impressive technical advances that have been made and the benefits which these bestow, they would have looked in vain for signs that medicine is even willing to search for *a system of curative medicine*. There is a complacency and conceit in conventional medicine, which underlies its proponents' animosity towards alternative forms of therapy.

3. **By combating the manifestations of disease by an opposing force (*contraria contrariis curentur*)**

This involves treating by means of *opposites*. This is the method most frequently used by orthodox medicine and *the* method that has earned it the accolades and support of the general public. It has also fed the orthodox belief that its approach to disease is incontestably superior to all others and, indeed, that the use of other means of treatment is irresponsible and even negligent. Such is the degree of its apparent success that the orthodoxy, with complacent confidence, has claimed for itself alone, the title of 'rational medicine.' Viewed superficially, the results achieved by using *opposites* are highly impressive. Persuasive evidence and examples abound: antihypertensive drugs for the treatment of raised blood-pressure; bronchodilators for asthma; antihistamines for allergic conditions; diuretics for oedema; anti-inflammatories for inflammation; analgesics for pain, steroidal and immunosuppressive drugs for auto-immune diseases; laxatives for constipation, sedatives for insomnia, antidepressants for depression and antibiotics for infection and so the list goes on: an impressive array of medical and pharmaceutical achievement.

Without doubt, therapeutic knowledge of the use of drugs applied in this way is essential to medical practice and proves indispensable in the treatment of emergencies, life threatening conditions, organ failure and overwhelming infections in which the body is faced by insurmountable odds, and in cases where illness has progressed to a point where the assistance of chemical medicine is required, even if only as a stopgap. In such crises, one can only marvel at the resources that Western, medical technology possesses. But, does such therapy constitute *cure*? Is this evidence of a *curative* system of medicine? Do the results represent an in-depth constitutional change towards a state of ongoing health? Patently no! Though often life saving, capable of adjusting blood chemistry and eradicating infection, etc., *opposites* act only on a superficial level and are palliative and suppressive in their effect. Suppression of the symptoms and signs of any disease must lead to an increase in the overall disease potential. Even in infections where specific pathogens are eliminated by suitable antibiotics (too often only temporarily), the original weakness which permitted the infection remains, antibody formation is still inadequate, the immune response tardy, often even more compromised than it was before, and the balance of the body's own protective organisms (e.g. bowel flora) is disturbed. The vulnerability of the body is increased not diminished. In addition, due to indiscriminate and excessive use of antibiotics, resistant strains and so-called *superbugs* are becoming ever more prevalent: nature's response to chemical warfare! When infecting organisms challenge the body, it must be wiser, whenever possible, to rouse and support the patient's own defence mechanisms. Success must leave the body strengthened and better able to defend itself in the future. In taking over the protective responsibilities of the body, antibiotics defeat this essential objective.

No matter how conservatively administered, the use of *opposites* must be fraught with toxic side effects because the chemical force required to bring about change of function and suppress the patient's symptoms must be at least equivalent to the force of the disease. In consequence, intrinsic to the process and its seemingly successful outcome, is the compounding of the forces of drug disease and natural disease in an unholy alliance that can only lead to a further deterioration of health. This will eventually manifest emotionally, intellectually, or physically, either in the individual being treated or in their progeny. These detrimental consequences may appear so much later, and in so different a form, that the cause and effect relationship is invariably missed, and if suspected would prove difficult, if not impossible, to prove.

We may look back to Hahnemann's time and marvel at the drastic methods employed by his medical contemporaries in their attempts to eliminate disease. We may wonder at their failure to comprehend the futility of their extreme measures and the injury and suffering they were inflicting upon their patients. We may be perplexed by the incredulity and hostility with which they reacted to the possibility of an alternative approach as gentle and plausible as that posed by homeopathy and we may excuse, or at least explain, all of this as being evidence of the ignorance of the age they lived in. But was this not the age, not only of Hahnemann, but also of other towering intellectual and creative geniuses such as Goethe, Roussouw, Kant and Beethoven? Were the medical minds of that past era so different from those that are the custodians of our health today? Methods have fortunately changed and the vast expansion in medical scientific knowledge has proved of great benefit to humanity, but on a subtler level little has changed in the intervening centuries. The remarkable clinical expertise that has been developed in diagnosing the effects of disease and the impressive skill in manipulating these effects through modern drugs and technology has not been attended by greater insight into the essential nature and cause of disease or the development of a logical, structured system of healing. Conventional medicine can speak with justifiable pride of prevention, suppression, inhibition, substitution, palliation and even remission. The achievement of these objectives has largely become the goal of research and therapy, and, unfortunately, often a substitute for achieving an even greater and more urgent goal: *the ability to heal*. As seen in the Dawkins/Baum interview, resistance to influences from outside the faith is as obdurate as ever. Modern techniques used to combat disease harbour dangers more subtle than those obvious in bleeding or blistering a patient, but, nonetheless, can prove insidiously deleterious. Cloaked in the sophisticated mantle of accepted science, remedies are employed in opposition to disease, which in their suppressive effects can be as swashbuckling as those of a previous era and in the long term far more potent and persistent.

Randomised control trials (RCTs) are extolled as the gold standard for evaluating drug efficacy. They are well designed for testing drugs formulated to act by *contraria contrariis curentur* (opposing a clinical condition), but not appropriate to test remedies that act by *similia similibus curentur* (curing through similarity). Despite Baum's testimony regarding the "scrupulously honest" nature of RCTs, their results and conclusions need to be considered with a degree of circumspection because billion dollar markets are involved in their outcome and the considerable sums of money needed to conduct such trials are largely sponsored by the drug companies that develop the drugs being tested. The observer must ask the question: is medical science truly immune from the manipulation, duplicity and corruption that contaminates so many aspects of human affairs? As important as determining efficacy is the determining of safety and it is in this area that the need for circumspection is of greatest importance. There should be no compromise regarding safety, other than when the dangers from the disease outweigh the toxicity of the required medication. But safety is less easy to determine than efficacy; often drugs have accumulative effects which only become manifest over time and sometimes so remotely that the relationship is missed. Remedies that act by opposition, and hence suppression, are all potentially toxic since their efficacy depends on their chemical action which counteracts natural, though diseased, processes, and the processes thus suppressed must implode.

The RCT may be the gold standard for evaluating conventional drug efficacy, but it cannot be regarded as the gold standard for determining safety, and besides, safety is a relative, even nebulous, value dependent on accepted criteria. When those with vested interest and those representative of a system of medicine that lacks a curative methodology and must rely on sub-toxic doses of drugs to achieve results, set the criteria and parameters of acceptable toxicity, leniency and compromise are inevitable. The anecdotal evidence of patients, so minimised in assessing the efficacy of homeopathic clinical response, should alert the concerned physician in practice to the untoward effects of many of the drugs in common use and stimulate an interest towards finding an alternative. The alternative will often be found in the fourth method of treatment.

4. **By administering a medicinal substance capable of imitating the symptoms of the patient** (as when applying the homeopathic law of similars).
   Experience proves that this method acts *curatively*.

   Why should this be?

   To understand this phenomenon, two vital postulates must be made:

- *The symptoms of disease are the expression of nature's healing power.*
- *Only the body itself can heal.*

The symptoms of disease are the expression of nature's healing power

It was Hippocrates who first proposed this key concept. In any disease, the body, not the disease (other than provocatively), is producing the presenting clinical picture through its innately 'intelligent' efforts to maintain its state of health. By provocatively, we understand that specific organisms initiate certain illnesses (e.g. viral, bacterial and fungal infections) and that such specific infections produce, and are characterised by, common symptoms (generic symptoms). These symptoms, although generic to the type of infection, still constitute the body's defensive reaction and reveal not only clues to the nature of the infection but also, and more especially, insight into the nature of the patient's constitution. For even the most common generic symptoms and signs of the most common epidemic diseases will bear the characteristic impress and modifying influence of the patient's personal response to illness. It is these modified symptoms, which aid the homeopath in selecting the most similar remedy for the patient.

Similarly, in proving a remedy (pathogenetic trial) which shares toxic characteristics with other substances, symptoms will be elicited which are common (generic) to the particular group (even when they are derived from different kingdoms: mineral, plant or animal), such as dizziness, various pains (especially of the abdomen and head), nausea, vomiting and diarrhoea. However, a remedy tested in this way will also produce, in addition to such generic symptoms, certain highly characteristic, often unique and peculiar symptoms, which clearly differentiate it from the others as a curative force and guide the homeopath in selecting it for the appropriate patient. As previously noted, it is the symptoms, which are most characteristic, unique, rare and even strange or peculiar that differentiate the remedy from all others and which must be matched to the equally unique symptoms of the patient, particularly if they pertain to the mental or emotional state.

Generic versus unique symptoms

The differentiation between generic and unique symptoms is critical to successful homeopathic prescribing. As previously related, in 1831, Hahnemann successfully treated cases of cholera with his new system of medicine. However, although Camphor proved the most frequently indicated remedy for that particular epidemic, Hahnemann did not treat all his patients with a single remedy, based simply on the diagnosis of cholera. He carefully sought for differentiating symptoms in each patient and matched these to the differentiating symptoms of remedies known to cause cholera-like states. His most successful remedies were Camphor, Cuprum and Veratrum album.

There are five major remedies that, as a group, share symptoms common to cases of cholera, but each has certain characteristics that are dominant and help differentiate it from the others:

- Antimonium tartaricum (tartar emetic) – the *drowsiness*, faintness, trembling and a thickly coated white tongue.
- Arsenicum album (white oxide of arsenic) – the *prostration*, dehydration, *restlessness*, *anxiety* and toxic infectious signs.
- Camphora (camphor tree) – the *minimal discharges*, *severe collapse*, *coldness* and nausea.
- Veratrum album (white hellebore) – the *copiousness of all the discharges* (diarrhoea, vomiting, sweat, salivation) and the aching of the body.
- Cuprum metallicum (copper) – the *cyanotic blueness*, *violent cramps in the limbs*, commencing in the toes and fingers and spreading upwards.

When these differentiating symptoms form the basis for remedy selection, the remedy will prove most similar in its action to the disease/patient complex and therefore capable of stimulating the most powerful immune response. Needless to say, other supportive measures, such as ensuring adequate hydration, are also essential.

To summarise and emphasise these important points: regardless of the similarities discerned in the common or generic symptoms of any disease syndrome or any remedy proving, careful analysis will reveal unique, singular or peculiar symptoms which enable one to differentiate the particular case or remedy from all others. It is these highly personal and unique characteristics, which lend a unique difference and colour to each patient and to each remedy, especially if mental or emotional, which must be matched in order to bring about a cure. In homeopathy, these unique symptoms, which are the very hallmark of a remedy and by association the very hallmark of the patient requiring the remedy, are dubbed *strange, rare and peculiar* (SRP) and are given highest value in any case analysis.

CASE 10.1   Measles – an example

To understand the homeopathic approach more fully, we should consider the simple example of two young sisters who at the same time have gone down with measles: a condition that can cause serious complications and is wonderfully responsive to correct homeopathic treatment. Both manifest the typical generic symptoms and signs of measles: the rash, Koplik spots and catarrhal inflammation. The diagnosis is therefore apparent. It is worth noting here that contrary to a common misconception, the conventional diagnosis of a case of acute illness or chronic disease *is* important to the homeopath. It indicates the group of remedies most likely to contain the required remedy; it provides knowledge of the symptoms common to the disease and therefore not unique to the patient; and it informs regarding the possible course, complications and prognosis of the patient's condition. It can also give warning that additional supportive measures, even surgery, may be required to deal responsibly with a particular case. However, the homeopath does not select the remedy on the basis of the diagnosis. He views the totality of the case and gives priority attention to those symptoms that are characteristic of the patient rather than characteristic of the disease. He looks for those symptoms that render the case distinctive, because it is in those singular, personal and often peculiar symptoms (out of context, out of character and out of proportion) that he can discern the action of the patient's healing response – a response that he must imitate in his selection of the *curative* remedy.

The first young lady is very weepy, emotional and clingy, filled with self-pity, and wants her mother with her all the time. In fact her mother's presence alone is not sufficient, she needs her physical contact and wants to be held, cuddled and caressed. She cannot bear to be alone. Despite her fever, which is not particularly high, and her very dry mouth, she is not at all thirsty. At night, although extremely photophobic due to conjunctivitis, she wants a nightlight because she is so afraid of the dark. Her tongue is coated white and she complains that everything tastes bitter. Her catarrhal stage soon tends to secondary infection with the production of fairly profuse yellow-green nasal discharge and she has an associated inflammation of the middle ear. She is sensitive to heat and lack of fresh air and therefore prefers to have the windows open, as she feels worse if the room becomes stuffy. Her physical symptoms and her emotional dependency become worse as evening twilight approaches. She sleeps on her back with her arms stretched out above her head. She enjoys all the fuss that is made of her and is quite unconcerned about falling behind in her schoolwork; in fact the longer she can protract her convalescence and receive loving concern and attention the happier she will be.

Her sister is not in the least weepy or clingy, but is irritable and impatient and resents any interference, even being examined, and wants to be alone. She lies curled up on her side with her back to the room as if to keep people out of her space. When she communicates, she is very demanding and critical and never satisfied, wanting this and wanting that and then rejecting it when given. Her mouth is even drier than her sister's, so much so that her lips become dry and cracked, her tongue is also coated white and her taste is nauseatingly bitter, however, unlike her sister, she is very thirsty and avidly drinks large quantities of cold water, but only at long intervals. She is not afraid of the dark and complains of a severe bursting headache, which is increased by the least movement. Both her headache and her inflamed eyes are better in the dark, which she prefers and insists upon. Like her sister, she is intolerant of becoming hot and will kick her covers off, wants the windows thrown open and benefits from cool, open air. Although her temperature only rose slowly over a few days, it is now much higher than her sister's. At the height of her fever, she is liable to become delirious, and, imagining that she is no longer at home, may repeatedly demand to be taken home. Or, she may worry about her school and pester her parents to see that she is kept up to date with her homework. Unlike her sister, she is eager, even anxious, to recover and get back to school so that she can catch up. She does not readily develop thick catarrhs and her infection tends to descend onto her chest, producing a very dry, painful cough and even pneumonia rather than an ear infection.

Two cases of measles and yet so different when viewed in their totality. The differing response to a common viral challenge provides an invaluable window through which the homeopath is able to view the underlying constitutional and emotional states of the two patients – and how poles apart these sisters are. Whereas orthodox medicine has no remedies for measles (other than measles prophylaxis) and can only offer symptom suppression and antibiotic cover for secondary infection, homeopathy is able to tailor the appropriate treatment by accurately matching a particular remedy picture to the individualising symptoms thrown up by the patient's defensive response to the measles viral challenge.

In the first case, the required remedy is **Pulsatilla pratensis**, the meadow anemone, a small plant that produces a beautiful flower with purple petals and a bright, golden centre, which always grows in the company of others and belongs to the Ranunculaceae family. The second child would receive **Bryonia alba**, the white bryony, a creeper, with most tenacious tendrils, that erupts each growing season from a very substantial and stable tap root and belongs to the Cucurbitaceae family.

When we fathom those momentous words of Hippocrates, written so many years ago, "The symptoms of disease are the expression of nature's healing power", words which are still at variance with general, medical thinking, we can fully understand why *the remedy capable of curing must be the remedy capable of causing* a response must similar to that which nature has already chosen in its attempt to achieve health; and the necessity of applying the Law of Similars, in order to affect a cure, becomes obvious.

Only the body itself can heal

The second postulate, which must be added to Hippocrates' profound observation, is the inescapable fact that *only the body itself can heal* and displays the innate 'knowledge' of how this can be achieved through the symptoms it produces in its defensive and healing response to challenge. Our responsibility is clear: we must respect nature, model our treatment on her example; move with her (*similia similibus curentur*) and not against her (*contraria contrariis curentur*). Only when natural cure is impossible should this rule be transgressed. Unfortunately, it is a rule more often honoured in the breach than in the observance.

Even in the simple matter of fever, we so often err through interference. The natural reaction to the presence of fever is to bring down the temperature by the administration of an anti-fever remedy (anti-pyrexial). A conventional physician attending our young measles patients would most likely have prescribed such a remedy, especially for the second child. In doing so, the most vital and fundamental response of the body to an infective challenge is undermined. The beneficial effect of raised body temperature is at least twofold: it accelerates the mobilisation, proliferation and activity of the protective, white blood cells in the blood and it impedes and slows viral and bacterial replication. Both are central to cure. By hindering the activity of the immune system, anti-pyrexials must contribute to the development of complications. Worse still, they are toxic and given when the body is under duress and needs to react to the very best of its capacity. Their use is often motivated by the fear of pyrexial convulsions which are not of themselves harmful and which must not be confused with epilepsy.

In keeping with the frenetic rhythms of modern life, dependence on high technology and the power of almost instant communication, most people are geared for 'quick-fix' medicine. High levels of stress, flight from the least discomfort and ignorance or lack of faith in the body's capacity to heal itself compound to produce the current press-button, drug consciousness of Western society. In a shrinking world, fraught with wide-scale war, tribulation, and environmental deterioration, the intrusive pressures on the psyche are pervasive, inducing escalating levels of stress, anxiety, fear, anger and depression, all of which contribute to the development of disease. More than ever before, it has become essential to protect one's internal and external environment against the threat of such impingement. This cannot be achieved by atheism, and it cannot be achieved by tranquilisers, sedatives and antidepressants. It requires spiritual, emotional and physical attunement to the natural forces that prevail in all dimensions.

In the physical domain, we need to know that the human organism is the product of millions of years of natural selection, survival of the fittest and adaptation to the environment. *Homo sapiens* is a highly successful species possessing admirably, sophisticated systems of homeostatic defence and repair. Although inherited, emotional and environmental influences may impair the perfection of these functions, nevertheless, these systems always perform to their optimal best (i.e. the best possible under the circumstances). When treatment is called for, it should be selected to work in harmony with the natural, healing processes of life and not attempt to suppress, modify or supersede them.

If we acknowledge and respect the superior, innate wisdom of the body to defend itself appropriately and to the best of its ability in any given state of disease, and if we accept the disease manifestations, especially those which are most differentiating, as being the direct expression of the body's healing processes, then we must select in order to cure, a remedy capable of harmoniously synchronising its curative action with that of the body: the most *Similar Remedy!*

The process of cure induced by the correct remedy chosen through similarity brings about changes that reflect the multidimensional nature of the human being. In chronic constitutional states, sometimes after an initial increase in superficial symptoms, a gradual transformation takes place. Not only does this involve diminution in the severity of symptoms, their final dissipation and the restoration of the clinical state, it also gently induces a more subtle, deeper, silent metamorphosis – like the grass growing, like a blossom opening and like falling in love. At first the change may be imperceptible and immeasurable, yet, as it grows in strength, it brings a buoyancy of being, a beneficial change of perspective, and synchronistically things start to fall into place: fortune smiles unexpectedly and events take on a positive bias. True healing is multifaceted and embraces all dimensions of expression.

The homeopath can confront the likes of Dawkins, Ernst and Baum – and with Hamlet confidently state:

> There are more things in heaven and earth . . . than are dreamt of in your philosophy.[9]

References

1. Dawkins R. *The Blind Watchmaker*. London: Penguin Books Ltd; 1991. pp4–6.
2. Baum M, Ernst E. Should we maintain an open mind about homeopathy? *Am J Med*. 2009; 122(11): 973–4.

3   Janes H, The Lifestyle 50: The top fifty people who influence the way we eat, exercise and think about ourselves. *The Times*; September 6, 2008.
4   Baum M, Ernst E, Colquhoun D *et al*. Full text of a letter from Michael Baum and 13 other scientists. *Sense About Science*; May 19, 2006. Available online at: www.senseaboutscience.org.
5   Baum M. An open letter to the Prince of Wales: With respect, your Highness, you've got it wrong. *Br Med J*. 2004; 329:118.
6   Dawkins R. *A Devil's Chaplain*. Boston MA: Houghton Mifflin; 2003. p58.
7   Johnson AC, Williams RJ, Simpson R. What difference might sewage treatment performance make to endocrine disruption in rivers? *Environmental Pollution* 2007; 147(1): 194–202.
8   Johnson AC, Williams RJ. A model to estimate influent and effluent concentrations of estradiol, estrone, and ethinylestradiol at sewage treatment works. *Environmental Science Technology* 2004; 38(13): 3649–58.
9   Shakespeare W. Hamlet: Act 1. Scene 5.

11

QUANTUM MEDICINE

Disease is a natural process

We have asked the question: What exactly do Baum and Dawkins mean by the word 'cure' and 'works'? To this we may add two further questions:

- What is conventional medicine testing with its randomised control trials (RCTs) – palliative effect or curative effect?
- What does the homeopath imply when speaking of 'cure' and 'healing'?

All of these can be slippery words; used casually without careful consideration. To cure or heal is to bring about restoration of health. In the young, and those not suffering from a condition of permanently impaired function or structural damage, this restoration of health should be complete and permanent and experienced both emotionally and physically. It should also achieve the removal of the constitutional predisposition or vulnerability, which lead to the development of the clinical condition. In addition, and as Hahnemann so often reiterated, every effort should be made to remove all external hindrances to recovery together with attention to correct diet and regular exercise. This is the ideal of cure, and whether or not fully realised in any individual case of disease, for every case is multifaceted, it is the goal for which a curative system of medicine must aim, and which it must be capable of attaining.

- In contrast to this goal, may we speak of cure when pain, such as intense migraine is removed by the action of a drug?
- Have we cured chronic tonsillitis when we surgically remove the tonsils, or a growth when we excise it?
- Can we confidently consider it a cure when we bring down and control blood pressure by chemical means?

Obviously not!

The problem that originally gave rise to the condition is still present and even if thwarted in expressing itself through drug action or surgery, its energy still prevails. Like a cork that has bobbed up on the surface, suppression carries it deeper and deeper into the depths gaining potential energy as it descends. Even when this increased potential seems dormant, it is dynamically at work and must sooner or later gain expression, even in future generations. Through suppression, the disease energy may shift from one body system to another, so masking the relationship between the new condition and the initial problem. It is not uncommon to find a patient suffering from gouty arthritis controlled by uricosuric drugs, which reduce uric acid levels in the blood, developing hypertension or cardio-vascular disease. The disease energy is displaced sideways and not cured. While drugs and/or surgery may be essential in any given case, e.g. when disease has reached a certain level of severity, or is a threat to life, we must not complacently think that the submerging of the clinical evidence of underlying pathology constitutes 'cure', and more important still, the pride in our undoubted success in achieving control and palliation (the successful 'working' of drugs) must never persuade us away from seeking an **alternative that cures**.

Disease should never be construed as contrary to nature, it is as much part of nature as are the tides, the seasons and the crops. Disease, like health, is part of nature's creative, impersonal energy, akin to the fall of the magnificent buffalo beneath the fangs and claws of the feline predator. It is an affront to our sensibilities, a threat to our security and can rob us of those most dear, but it is not unnatural. It is the playing out of eternal laws without malice; it seeks atonement, not punishment. It is only rendered unnatural when it is turned in upon itself and forced to implode. This is the blessing, for the conclusion to be drawn from such insight is that disease is essentially benign and compensatory; subject to mitigation and absolution through the application of curative laws that honour the natural healing power of illness and its chosen direction; that work with the process instead of against it, and achieve a healing consummation.

Nature produces the symptoms and signs of disease to create a physical, external or localised outlet for a generalised, internal problem produced by a disturbance of the energy field of the body. Even a cancer serves this purpose, for nature would rather have a malignancy than a psychosis (insanity). When the attempt of the body to externalise the problem is thwarted, the healing energy is introverted, prevented from achieving its purpose and the disturbance it sought to expel is confined to a deeper and more damaging level of expression. It is correct to speak of a natural morbid force, which cannot be eradicated by opposition, only by dissipation.

This energy, although described as morbid is in fact beneficial and needs to be assisted in achieving its curative goal. To understand how this can be achieved it is useful to invoke *mythos* rather than *logos*, for a parable can simplify and give a clarity that even a child can comprehend. Because it is remedying chaos, the externalising force of natural healing can appear chaotic; like a wild horse running free; left to its own devices, it can either kill or cure. Erecting a brick wall in its path, darting or shooting the horse will not help – another horse appears, wilder and more chaotic, and running on more difficult terrain. The horse knows where it must go, but needs a restraining hand to slow its pace and guide it round or over obstacles. To marshal its energy and take it harmlessly over the healing line, we need to ride beside it on a horse going in the same direction [the similar remedy] and at the correct speed [the correct potency]. In this way we can ally our knowledge to the healing wisdom of nature and bring about a curative resolution.

The Healing Power of the Infinitesimal Dose

> **The first law or principle of homeopathy,** the *Law of Similars*, which is central to its efficacy, states that *a remedy can cure the symptoms that it can cause.*
>
> **The second law of homeopathy,** the *Law of the Infinitesimal Dose* states that *when a homeopathic potency is prescribed according to the Law of Similars, its curative power increases in direct ratio to its degree of potentisation.*

What do we understand by *curative power*, for it must be contrasted with therapeutic or pharmacological power?

Curative power is the ability of a remedy to stimulate or enhance an appropriate curative or healing response in a sensitive individual. The patient demonstrating symptoms similar to those within the causative capacity of the remedy is sensitive, indeed hypersensitive, to this curative power. In this phenomenon lies the secret of cure!

The mode of action of the homeopathic remedy is indirect with regard to the disease state [clinical diagnosis] and direct with regard to the restorative systems of the body. Its ability to bring about physiological change does not stem from any pharmacological action (except in the case of very low potencies) but from its capacity to stimulate self-healing and this capacity depends entirely on the successful remedy's ability to evoke a defensive response most similar to that which the patient is already demonstrating. The similar remedy provides the appropriate stimulus to bring the healing process to a successful conclusion, but it is the body that achieves the healing.

Since the curative power of a remedy increases progressively with each step of serial dilution with succussion (or trituration in lower potencies), we must conclude that the positive effect of the remedy is due to the progressive release of its healing energy through the process of potentisation and does not depend on the presence of residual molecules or atoms. The homeopathic remedy owes its efficacy to subatomic influences and is energy based.

As mentioned earlier, it has been mathematically calculated that after 23 steps of serial dilution on the decimal scale (10^{-23}), a point known as the *Avogadro Constant* is reached after which any further dilution will be devoid of any molecules or atoms of the diluted substance. Yet, the most powerfully acting potencies used in homeopathic practice, the so-called high potencies, the 30th centesimal (10^{-60}) and above, have been diluted far beyond the *Avogadro Constant* and remain not only therapeutically effective, but far more profound in their action. A healing energy has been released, which is totally independent of matter.

Serial dilution with succussion is a process of dematerialisation and the progressive release and imprinting of the carrier substance with a specific energy pattern derived from the potentised substance. This is not pseudoscience. We may not know the exact science of what transpires in the process of potentisation and we may never know how the energy pattern of a potentised substance can be indelibly inscribed and carried forward in lactose, distilled water or absolute alcohol, but we do know from the combined experience of homeopathic physicians, pharmacists and countless numbers of patients over 200 years of practical application that this is exactly what happens.

The fact that homeopathic remedies, other than the very lowest potencies, contain no remaining physical trace of the remedial substance from which they are derived has made them the target of disbelief and ridicule. Conventional medical thinking, being limited to the Newtonian model, cannot conceive that such remedies could possibly have any therapeutic effect, and as exemplified in the dismissive attitude of Ernst and Baum, largely regards homeopathy as an elaborate hoax and its practitioners as charlatans. From this obdurate medical standpoint, it is implausible that a remedy devoid of medicinal atoms is capable of eliciting a healing response. It would seem that the homeopathic dose is utterly insubstantial, a mere nothingness, and quite incapable of influencing the human or animal organism for good or ill. Materially speaking, these potentised remedies are insubstantial, even ethereal, but *it is in this insubstantiality that their success lies.*

Subjective plane of existence

To understand this, we need to consider the human state at its deepest level. In orthodox, medical training the student is generally taught a very objective, materialistic form of medicine in which the body is regarded as a rather sophisticated mechanism. This mind-set evolves from the outset, encouraged by the sequence of tuition, proceeding from chemistry and physics to anatomy, physiology, biochemistry, pathology and finally embracing clinical medicine. It is further crystallised when the ailing human is scrutinised through the all-seeing eyes of medical technology (X-rays, scans, scopes, and laboratory tests), and when witnessing the remarkable and often life-saving changes induced by chemical drugs and the dramatic results of modern surgery. It is understandable that this impressive array of medical achievement not only convinces the graduate of the correctness of conventional medicine's therapeutic principles, but also induces the tendency, despite their own human qualities, to think of the patient as a clinical entity, an object for analysis, calibration and adjustment. In the search for a cause, everything is weighed and measured, and according to findings a diagnosis is made and a protocol of treatment devised. Even emotional symptoms, such as depression, may be considered the result of chemical imbalance. The medicine then practised is in danger of being reduced to removing excess, supplying for deficiency, killing pathogens and suppressing symptoms – and, in achieving these things, of being deemed adequate and satisfactory.

However, no matter how important, even vital, the objective level of investigation may be, it can only appraise the lowest level of human experience and evaluate effects; the affect lies beyond reach. It is essential to add to the assay of body functions, a scrutiny of the inner nature of the patient, for it is here that many answers lie. To grasp the prime importance of this conclusion, we need only consider our own hidden aspects, our doubts, our fears, our aspirations, our longings, our desires, our creativity and our ego-based suffering. At once we appreciate that we are so much more than the physical body, so much more than a sophisticated mechanism and so much more than a product of neuronal complexity, no matter what the atheists and evolutionists tell us.

We are profound and complex beings, a conflicting blend of the sublime and the perverse, with physical, intellectual, emotional and spiritual facets.

We dwell and experience on all these levels, but in the deepest and most enduring sense on a subjective dimension far beyond the reach of the most searching technology and the effects of molecular medicine. These all pertain to the objective world while, in our essence, we are creatures of a subjective plane and the human mechanism we see in the mirror is merely bearing witness to processes taking place on a much deeper and higher dimension, including that from which disease emanates.

Disease is dynamic

The deepest aspects of human experience transpire on an intellectual, emotional and spiritual plane: a dynamic, immaterial, invisible dimension that is energetic. Disease is a human experience of the deepest form and only its effects are visible. In response to the trials and tribulations of life, energy waves generated at a dynamic, causative level flow to the cells, tissues and organs and, if perturbed and persistent, will manifest in altered function and eventually physical pathology. The unseen, causative level of disease is sited in the sphere of our emotions where all that is hallowed and haunted contend. Behind every change in matter lies a changed energy pattern. The very nature of matter is congealed energy. The manifestations of disease always have an energetic or dynamic cause, which is a dysfunctional response to human experience. In this sequence, the patient is always primary; the disease is always secondary. Since the patient thinks, feels, experiences and suffers on a subjective plane, it must be upon this energy level that the cause of disease is sought and found, and it is on this level that the indicated remedy must be able to act in order to effect a cure. Once this is understood, it becomes at once apparent, that *only* a remedy that is immaterial and infinitesimal [dynamic] can *cure* disease, because the cause of all disease lies on an immaterial plane.

The cause of disease is dynamic, therefore the cure of disease has to be dynamic and the remedy chosen has to be in dynamic (potentised) form.

With this concept, we move beyond objective, molecular, conventional medicine into the realm of subjective, imponderable, homeopathic medicine.

Quantum physics

To understand the implications of this requires a major change in our conceptual framework, since we are inclined to regard as nonsense anything that does not conform to the rational edifices that we have constructed. Heavily influenced by the dogma and prejudice of rational science, conventional medicine has been unable to change its Newtonian perspective. For 200 years the 'airy nothings' of homeopathy have attracted its suspicion and scorn and still continue to do so. In the days of Hahnemann and before Max Planck, Albert Einstein and Niels Bohr this was not surprising, but given our present knowledge of quantum physics and the interchangeableness of matter and energy and all that science has revealed about the weird and unpredictable, counterintuitive realm beyond the atom, it is strange that this incomprehension and prejudice should still prove so inveterate.

The process of potentisation takes us out of the world of Newtonian physics, to which the large-scale world about us, and conventional, Western medicine, belongs, and we enter the world of the quantum, the invisible world of elementary particles, which is also the world of causation. We know today that the Newtonian model is valid for objects consisting of large numbers of atoms. Newtonian physics does not work in the realm of the very small.[1] Here, classical physics has to be replaced by quantum theory. It is odd that despite the obvious quantum nature of the homeopathic potency, the opponents of homeopathy persist in their Newtonian arguments against the possibility of its efficacy.

An encoded medicinal signal

In seeking for an explanation of how the curative power of a remedy can be encoded during the process of serial dilution and succussion, and conveyed by a carrier substance in infinitesimal form, it is useful to enter into the unseen dimension of energy waves and to employ the analogy of telecommunication. Whilst this analogy does not provide scientific proof, it assists our understanding of the process of serial potentisation and the sensitivity of the patient to the action of the potency.

A basic audio-visual telecommunication system consists of three elements:

- A transmitter that takes information and converts it into an encoded signal which can be modulated in frequency and amplitude.
- A transmission medium that carries the encoded signal.
- A tuned receiver that receives the signal and decodes it back into useable information.

In the process of potentisation (transmission), the unique, energy pattern of the curative properties of a medicinal substance (information) is converted by serial dilution and succussion, or trituration, into an 'encoded signal', which is imprinted on, and carried forward by, the carrier substance (transmission medium) and progressively taken to a higher frequency and amplified (modulated) by each step of potentisation. The patient, whose defence system has produced in response to disease a similar mental and physical symptom pattern to that of the medicinal substance, is the 'tuned receiver', hypersensitive to the signal with which it resonates, and able to '*decode*' the medicinal image (usable information) and respond to it curatively. The healing response of the body is enhanced.

When conventional doctors scoff at the possibility of the invisible, immeasurably small doses of the homeopathic remedy having any power to treat disease, their attitude resembles the disbelief of the untutored mind when told that invisible waves carry the information responsible for the image displayed on a TV screen. In both instances, the critical information making the phenomenon possible is imperceptibly held within the respective transmission medium and is 'downloaded' by a tuned receiver.

In the case of homeopathy, the imprinting of the medicinal image or encoded signal is achieved by the first step of potentisation. Further steps 'modulate,' or potentiate, the signal, taking it to ever finer and higher levels of vibration. The higher frequencies reached in the highest potencies give the remedy power to influence the entire organism, not only physically, but even to the furthest reaches of the ego-self. This power is not the mindless, robust strength of a molecular drug but a subtle, persuasive, informed energy, which through similarity of expression aligns its healing activity with that of the animating and regulating vital force of the body.

Understanding the quantum nature of the homeopathic remedy gives us a clearer perspective of the qualities of the homeopathic potency and the process of homeopathic cure. Physicists delving into the subatomic world in pursuit of the ultimate stuff of the universe find matter dissolving into energy and that subatomic particles are in fact energy. Subatomic activity is therefore the interaction of energy upon energy and in relationship to the world of matter this is the sphere of creation and causation. The animate being, in physical terms, is a vast assembly of atoms maintained in equilibrium (homeostasis) by subatomic reactions of energy upon energy and the cause of health and disease lies on this level of interaction. Energy manifests in either particle or waveform. Waves are frequencies and in health the totality of energy upon energy reactions in the organism creates a specific frequency, which is as unique as our fingerprints. Deviations from this ordered frequency constitute disease and are portrayed by the systems of the body, firstly through altered function and emotional disturbances, and finally through structural change – all of which are carried forward constitutionally and through heredity.

The totality of symptoms in any case of disease is the image of an altered quantum state.

The similar homeopathic remedy selected for this image, and given in quantum form, matches the disturbed frequency of the patient, and being dynamic is able to act on the causative level restoring health through a specific action upon the body's self-healing ability.

Anyone incredulous of the power contained in the infinitesimal dose has only to give a quantum of Sulphur 10M ($10^{-20,000}$) to a few cases of eczema to have the centrifugal energy of Sulphur revealed to them. The experience leaves both patient and physician with a healthy respect for quantum medicine.

Clinical trials and the quantum remedy

Unable, or unwilling, to consider the critical difference existing between the phenomena of quantum science and the laws of classical physics, and to appreciate the critical differences that separate a system of medicine based upon *similarity, harmony and cure* from one based upon *difference, control and opposition*, advocates of conventional medicine, constantly demand that the therapeutic value of homeopathy's quantum remedies must be evaluated by the same scientific procedures used to demonstrate the efficacy of molecular drugs. When dismissing homeopathy and justifying their contempt for it, homeopathy's opponents invariably declare: "Homeopathy has never been proven scientifically!" Medically qualified colleagues who have successfully practised homeopathy for years have given testimony based on anecdotal evidence, clinical notes and expert opinion. Sadly, this has been met with disdain and discounted. Stubborn resistance to the quantum concept that infinitesimally small doses of the similar remedy possess healing power persists. If the underlying conceit was supported by evidence of 'scientific medicine' curing chronic disease and mastering the ever-increasing threat of resistant organisms and viral epidemics, one could understand this complacency and indifference, but given the ever increasing incidence of chronic disease in increasingly younger age groups, the problem of iatrogenic (drug induced) disease due to the toxicity of modern drugs, and the prohibitive cost of medical treatment, it is sadly misplaced. The foundation upon which orthodox medical pride is based is the very impressive, but, nonetheless, synthetic manipulations of high technology.

The gold standard by which drug efficacy is weighed and judged is the *randomised clinical trial* (RCT), so vaunted by Professor Baum, which is ideally run double-blind and placebo-controlled. In such a trial design, neither the participating individuals nor the trial supervisors know which participants are receiving the experimental drug and which are receiving a placebo (blank dose). In this way, the effects of expectation (placebo effect) can be neutralised and a truer measure of drug efficacy evaluated. Critics of homeopathy assert that if homeopathic remedies were subjected to such trials, and found measurably more effective than placebo, then many barriers to the acceptance of homeopathy would fall. Unfortunately, homeopathic trials cannot realistically be conducted according to RCT protocols.

The first obstacle lies in the very nature of homeopathy. Allopathic RCTs test the efficacy of a drug to bring about a desired chemico-physiological change of measurable significance in a selected group of patients diagnosed with the same disorder. A positive meta-analysis (the combined statistics from a number of studies) is an indicator of the efficacy of the substance to affect this. It is a qualitative measure of toxicity, which can be quantitatively adapted to the clinical situation for which the substance proves effective. The RCTs, from which the results of the meta-analysis derive, pertain to the lowest level of existence, the chemico-physical; they have circumscribed focus; the variables influencing their outcome are minimal; their parameters are Newtonian; being run blind and placebo-controlled, the influence of the observer is avoided; and their central objective is the control or suppression of symptoms. As discussed, homeopathy pertains to the entire being at all levels; variables are multiple; its science is quantum based (hence the observer/participant is essential to the outcome); and its focus is cure. The allopathic RCT is concerned with pharmacological efficacy; homeopathy depends on curative efficacy. The two sciences stand poles apart. The inappropriateness of RCT evaluation of homeopathy would seem obvious. Yet hidebound critics, like the ugly sisters of Cinderella fame, insist that the elegant dancing shoe of homeopathy must be forced onto the gumboot foot of conventional trials, even if unusual, RCT designs are required to accommodate the special requirements of homeopathy.[2]

The second difficulty stems from the difference in diagnostic and therapeutic perspectives. Conventional medicine, on the basis of diagnosis, assigns the patient to a specific disease category and a specific schedule of therapy and this relationship supplies the frame in which the RCT is conducted. Homeopathy, while taking cognisance of the diagnosis, rejects the possibility of assigning a patient to a specific diagnostic category for the purpose of selecting a remedy. The remedy selection, as in the cholera and measles examples given earlier, is based upon the often-subtle differences existing in the picture exhibited by different individuals suffering from the same general diagnosis. Modern medicine, in reducing the patient to a diagnosis, focuses upon the resemblance among patients. Homeopathy seeks those symptoms and characteristics that reveal the patient as unique and different and tailors the therapy accordingly. The criteria for the selection of the required remedy in the two systems differ significantly. To allopathy, the clinical diagnosis is primary and defining, to homeopathy, the diagnosis is secondary and the individualising symptoms are defining. This incongruence is one of the major difficulties that RCT poses when, in deference to the dominant school, attempts are made to bend homeopathy to the inapposite protocols that such trials demand.

In supervising an RCT, allopathy assembles together what is regarded as a homogenous group of patients suffering from the same disease. To the homeopath, all such groups are distinctly heterogenous, despite their shared diagnosis. The inherited influences, the life experience, the circumstances and the emotional characteristics, as well as those unique symptoms so important to homeopathic diagnosis, will differ throughout the group. This poses the third difficulty: if one honours the individuality of each patient in a trial group, and to do so is essential for *cure*, then logically all trialists cannot require the same remedy. The choice of a single drug illustrates the dehumanised nature of the trial, which is simply based on a drug versus disease scenario – a scenario, unfortunately, too often re-enacted in the consulting room. It is quite possible that for ten cases of asthma ten different remedies will be required. Furthermore, any single case of asthma may require a sequence of remedies to affect a cure as well as supportive short-acting remedies and possibly the facilitating influence of a homeopathic vaccine (nosode). Behind the generic profile of any case of disease lies a unique mosaic of different elements of which, for example, asthma is only the most demanding. An RCT, regardless of how unusual its design may be, cannot accommodate so many variables.

Finally, homeopathic treatment is both a curative process and a quantum event and therefore cannot be run 'blind.' When a homeopathic physician faces a patient suffering from a chronic complaint with the purpose of bringing about a cure, the interaction that unfolds is very like a game of chess and the final cure is equivalent to a checkmate. Although, unlike chess, the homeopathic checkmate can in a small minority of cases be brought about by a single, well-chosen piece (remedy), nonetheless, even in such straightforward cases, each move (frequency of dose and indicated potency) has to be strategised. More generally, however, it is no single move or piece that brings success, but a series of remedies used in sequence or sometimes in concert. As the homeopathic therapy proceeds the presenting symptomatic picture changes and often requires a corresponding change of potency or remedy. For this the active participation of the physician is essential. An 'entanglement' between physician, remedy and patient is inevitable and essential to the healing process. The RCT design is too rigid, artificial and divorced from 'real life' conditions to cater for or measure the results of such subtle, therapeutic manoeuvring.

It is an adage of many philosophies that 'we create our own reality.' The revelations of quantum mechanics substantiate this ancient wisdom. They reveal that consciousness influences matter. The implications of this are profound. To influence is to change, modify or direct and from this we may infer that not only do we influence our reality, but in some degree we actually *create* it.[3] Subatomic particles are discrete packets of energy with wave-like properties and possess the conjugate variables of position and momentum. Contrary to the laws of classical mechanics, we can never make simultaneous predictions regarding these conjugates: we can either know the momentum of a particle or its position, but not both. To know one is to render the other indeterminate (*Heisenberg's Uncertainty Principle*). We *have to choose* whether the particle has position or momentum. In making this choice we bring into being something that has position, or, conversely, something that has momentum. In fact, whether energy is witnessed as a particle or as a wave depends on the intent of the observer. This phenomenon has caused quantum physicists to ponder the questions expressed by Zukav:

- Did any particle exist at all before we thought about them and measured them?
- Did we create the particles with which we are experimenting?[3]

John A Wheeler, an esteemed physicist at Princeton, has written:

> May the universe in some strange way be 'brought into being' by the participation of those who participate? . . . The vital act is the act of participation. 'Participator' is the incontrovertible new concept given by quantum mechanics. It strikes down the term 'observer' of classical theory, the man who stands safely behind the thick glass wall and watches what goes on without taking part. It can't be done, quantum mechanics says.[4]

It cannot be done says homeopathy!

This must be singularly true for the homeopathic therapeutic experience. The 'participator' in this case is not only the physician, but also the patient. There has to be a significant relationship and sincere exchange between the two for healing to take place. *Entanglement is essential!* The relationship builds up over time to bring about a trust and intimacy that can permit the physician access to that which is painful, private or hidden, often facets of life, unknown, forgotten, banished from memory or so harrowing that they have never been granted residence there. These are not immediately accessible or available to either participant and have to emerge during the process of extended therapy. Within all patients, even those currently suffering from some acute manifestation of inner disorder, there exists a disease state (or disease potential) that has evolved along time-lines of experience – personal, familial, racial, human and (as will be discussed in a future chapter) karmic – laid down in layers, as observed in the annular lines of a great tree or in the strata of the earth: an indelible register of all that has gone before; a structure upon which the unique ego-self rests. Some layers are yielding, others are seemingly impenetrable, hindering progress and producing the emotional and physical vulnerabilities, which continually add to the disease continuum. These influences play a role even in acute conditions and modify response to challenge and remedy action. To plumb these depths in search of the most similar remedy requires patience, knowledge, experience, skill and intuitive sensitivity on the part of the physician, and the informed and committed participation and perseverance of the patient.

To think that one can evaluate the efficacy of a curative remedy by freezing this multifaceted, symphonic event into the static frame of a randomised, placebo-controlled, double-blind trial, devoid of a 'participator' and with a patient reduced to an insentient object, is the fantasy of child-like minds so pragmatic and empirical that only the physical, large-scale dimensions of life and the universe are perceived and granted significance. Such thinking represents a barren, scientific paradigm that ignores the richness and variety of human idiosyncrasy and is destitute of concepts such as individuation, numinosity and immortality.

In evaluating the efficacy of a molecular drug, the format of robust RTC evaluation is undeniably apt and essential, though still vulnerable to bias, manipulation and misinterpretation. It is not testing curative action, but simply evaluating the chemical ability of a drug to bring about a specified effect. RCTs are neither apt nor essential for homeopathic remedies. Once the Law of Similars is understood and accepted as an incontrovertible, fundamental law of nature, on the basis of provings and their clinical application, RCTs to test the efficacy of a specific, proven remedy in a clinical situation becomes unnecessary, since a remedy accurately selected through similarity will be effective – to the degree that it is similar and to the degree that the condition of the patient's constitution permits. In 'real-life' there are always variables and always the entanglement of physician, remedy and patient, which cannot be accommodated by RCTs, no matter their design.

Homeopathy is a holistic system of medicine that embraces the life experience of the individual and its evidence-base is perforce built upon 'real' human (and animal) experience derived from remedy provings, case studies, anecdotal evidence, medical tradition, clinical use and expert opinion; an incomparable body of knowledge, which stands proud in the face of orthodox scepticism.

Given the inappropriate design of RCTs, it is not surprising that the results of the many RCT trials that have been conducted for the purpose of developing a homeopathic evidence-base acceptable to the orthodoxy, although often favourable, have generally proved inconclusive. This is inevitable. The parameters and protocols are dictated by the science of molecular medicine, and imposed on homeopathy, the science of quantum medicine; two different branches of medicine; two different frames of reference. This imposition is the equivalent of classical physics demanding that quantum physics should prove its validity in Newtonian terms. It is not possible; they are different aspects of reality!

Extra-remedial influences

A consideration of the quantum aspects of homeopathy cannot be complete without mention of the so-called *placebo effect*. The Allopathic explanation for any positive response to homeopathic treatment, is that homeopathy is no more than a placebo and that the improvement is due to the placebo effect. A placebo is an inactive substance, such as distilled water or a lactose pill, usually given as a control in an experiment. The placebo effect is the benefit a patient feels from taking such a substance due to the strong expectation that it will prove beneficial. Homeopathy's detractors particularly favour the placebo explanation for homeopathy's success and growing popularity because of the imponderable doses that are prescribed.

Expectancy and conditioning can certainly elicit or contribute to a positive therapeutic response to any medication or therapy. However, the orthodoxy insinuate that homeopathy depends on this and is particularly likely to promote it because of the searching nature of the extended homeopathic consultation during which the homeopathic physician displays a deeper interest, warmth, caring attention, empathy and confident encouragement than is customary in conventional, medical consultations. It is curious that qualities, which can only be regarded as exemplary, are, by inference, here associated with fraudulent deception.

In practice, whether homeopathic or conventional, the placebo effect on its own proves transient and unreliable. Because successful homeopathic treatment depends on a high degree of accuracy in remedy selection, the complexity of a chronic condition may at first result in an inadequate degree of patient-remedy similarity (acute conditions are far easier to match because the demanding symptoms and signs are usually clearly defined). In such cases, the expectation-response may provide an initial improvement, but this soon peters out. Only when the correct remedy is given will progress prove reliable and ongoing. When the placebo effect is coupled to remedy-response, it provides a wonderful kick-start to treatment and is not to be sneered at.

Suggesting that the placebo effect explains the therapeutic benefit derived from homeopathic treatment, highlights the ignorance and often-bitter prejudice of certain scientists. Do they truly believe that homeopaths only treat cases of self-limiting disease and conditions likely to resolve in spontaneous remission? From the time of Hahnemann's impressive results with typhoid and cholera, homeopaths around the world have successfully tackled the worst that disease has to offer; conditions for which reliance on placebo effect and spontaneous remission would be absurd. Even in advanced conditions, when cure is out of the question, homeopathy can provide relief, preserve dignity, and reduce the need for supportive drug therapy.

The first port of call for most patients seeking medical advice still remains the orthodox physician, hence, the majority of patients visiting homeopaths will have already received conventional treatment for their ailments and decide to try homeopathy because they are dissatisfied with the results and are seeking an alternative. Since the placebo effect is a factor in all forms of therapy, the subsequent improvement experienced by such patients when treated homeopathically cannot be simply discounted as an example of this phenomenon. And why is it that a patient who failed to experience 'spontaneous remission' while receiving orthodox treatment, and in fact proved stubbornly resistant to such a blessing, should do so when treated homeopathically? How is it possible that medical minds can smugly explain away homeopathic therapeutic success in this way? In homeopathic paediatric and veterinary practice, the foolishness of the placebo explanation is most apparent. What degree of expectation-effect can seriously be anticipated in infants and animals? Or, are we willing to accept that the parents, family and owners are also participants in a quantum event, their consciousness and concern contributing to the healing process?

The paradigm of healing to which homeopathy belongs takes us into a hidden, mysterious dimension of which the subatomic world of the quantum is only a part. Here energy and consciousness hold sway and the hard facts of classical physics, chemistry and objective reality are no longer relevant. Here we are closer to Reality, the sphere of causation, and we are in the presence of agencies of a higher order, which are in constant interaction with the physical plane. The placebo effect is the simplest example of these subtle influences; love is one of the most profound.

In keeping with scientific method, most modern pathogenetic trials (provings) of homeopathic remedies have been conducted according to RCT protocols. Neither the trialists (provers) nor the supervisors of the trial know what substance is being tested and a certain percentage of trialists only receive placebo. This would seem to protect the experiment from the placebo effect and ensure the validity of the symptoms collated from the trialists. In the event, provings frequently explode the concept of discreteness and mind-body duality. A placebo prover, singularly susceptible to the frequency of the trial-substance, may develop the most florid symptoms of all – symptoms that can only be attributable to the effect of the substance. The quantum dimension is a dimension of energy fields that are interpenetrating. The prover, whether on placebo or remedy, is inextricably entangled in the experiment and subject to the influence of the quantum dose. This phenomenon is even more likely to occur when the trial introduces the crossover technique in which provers on placebo and those on the trial-substance are interchanged during the experiment. The healing effect of the homeopathic quantum dose, unlike the crude effects of orthodox drugs, persists in the system for a prolonged period and will still be active after the switch to placebo; this carryover effect nullifies the intent of the crossover. Furthermore, quantum science informs us that while ever there is a mind that knows the identity and origin of the trial-substance (the director or designer of the proving), that mind is not only an observer but also a participant in the trial and will inevitably influence the outcome. No pathogenetic trial of a remedy in quantum form can be run blind!

Whichever way we turn, we are confronted by the presiding unity of all realms of the Creation and the inappropriateness and futility of attempting to conduct homeopathic trials designed according to the paradigm of orthodox medicine. In yielding to this uninformed demand of the dominant school, homeopathic researchers disavow the very science upon which their system is based and the results of such distorted trials can only at best provide evidence of the most common and superficial patient-symptom-remedy relationship; insufficient proof for the doubting Thomas's of the orthodox school.

A healer of the sick needs to embrace the placebo effect with respect and reverence, promote it and take it at the flood, for it is evidence of the power of consciousness and self-healing, and a hint of other extra-remedial influences with which the healer needs to be aligned, not least of all, the gift of healing, which is common to us all. In quantum healing there exists, in addition to the placebo effect, a critical entanglement between physician, remedy, patient – and the entire Cosmos!

Once again the words of Paracelsus echo down the centuries to us:

> If Providence has determined otherwise than you physicians intend, you will not be able to cure the patient by any remedy. But if the hour of Providence has struck, you will succeed in curing him. . . . Only when the hour of recovery strikes for the patient, does God send him to the physician, not before. All those who go to him before go to him in vain. . . . God has created remedies against diseases, and He has also created the physician; but He holds them back until the hour predestined for the patient. Only when the time has been fulfilled, and not before, does the course of nature and art set in.[5]

Predestination is operative in the physician-patient relationship and through synchronicity brings the two together at the chosen time, linking what is healing in the physician to that which is to be healed in the patient. The curative event is the confluence (entanglement) of cosmic grace, unseen healing from spirit, the physician's gift of healing, the receptivity and participation of the patient, the influence of loved ones and a healing environment – all facilitated by the action of the similar remedy.

* * * * *

Practical aspects of the quantum nature of the homeopathic remedy

Once the attenuation of a homeopathic remedy has exceeded the *Avogadro constant* we can be certain that we are dealing with a remedial frequency and not a remedial substance. We have completely entered the domain of quantum physics. It can be postulated that once the first decimal potency has been achieved, and certainly by the sixth, residual atoms or molecules of the starter mother-substance are superfluous to the quantum process of serial potentisation, and that the efficacy of even the lowest potencies is energy based rather than matter based. By further attenuation, the frequency of this energy is exponentially amplified or intensified, rendering it more and more curatively potent.

In practice, it is found that the lower frequencies of the lower potencies 'transmit' over a wider, but more superficial, band or spectrum and are less intense and profound in their effect. The higher potencies, 30C–200C and above, transmit over a narrower, more sharply focussed band, and are far more powerful and deep acting. The low potencies are well suited to treating patients at the physical level, for acute conditions, especially when localised to a certain tissue or organ, or where the function of a specific organ or system requires balancing. Because they draw less energy from the patient in achieving their effect, they are preferred when the vital energy of the patient is depleted due to the sapping effect of prolonged illness or through old age. Low potency remedies are generally prescribed at more frequent intervals (even 2 to 3 times per day) and are often used to provide supportive therapy while the deeper acting constitutional remedy is prescribed in higher potency and less frequently.

The degree of similarity required in prescribing remedies weighted to the lower end of the potency spectrum is less critical than for higher potencies and it is not always essential that the finer, emotional symptoms should be matched. For instance, the plant *Ceanothus americanus* (red root) has such a specific affinity for the spleen that the homeopathic remedy Ceanothus proves beneficial in the treatment of almost all cases in which the spleen is especially affected and may be given in low potency as much as 3 times a day over a prolonged period to promote and regulate splenic function. The qualification 'almost' must be given because there are always exceptions, especially in medicine. But, if the 'splenic' patient also experiences a deep-seated pain in the upper, left abdomen or under the lower ribs on the same side, the 'almost' falls away. And if, in addition, the patient is dispirited and apathetic, with little inclination for work, and fears this increasing incapacity, then Ceanothus can be prescribed with the greatest confidence of success. Hence, even though lower potencies can prove beneficial and even healing when prescribed simply on the basis of purely physical or pathological indications or for their organ and tissue affinity, nevertheless, as with higher potencies, the greater the similarity existing between the symptoms of the remedy and the complete picture of the patient, the deeper the remedy will work and the more certain it is that it will bring relief. Indeed, when the characteristic homeopathic Ceanothus pain and mental disposition accompany splenic involvement, such a clear-cut similarity would justify the physician prescribing a higher potency from the outset.

In bruising of the soft tissues inflicted by a blow from a blunt object, the call for the use of the herb Arnica montana (leopard's bane) is such that hardly any thought need be given in its selection. Likewise, the use of Calendula officinalis (pot marigold) in lacerations, and Hypericum perforatum (St John's wort) in penetrating wounds, such as inflicted by a needle. Low potencies of these remedies administered fairly frequently, e.g. initially every 1–2 hrs and then less and less frequently with improvement, can be given with complete confidence in the absence of any confirmation other than the type of injury sustained. If, however, the patient has been involved in a severe motor accident in which the car rolled and multiple contusions have been sustained and the patient is in such a state of shock that they resist assistance, declaring that they are fine and not in need of help, then the condition of injury has permeated the whole constitution, emotionally and physically. The entire patient is in the 'Arnica state' not only the injured part. Although the lower potencies of Arnica will still give wonderful relief and bring about healing, the more penetrating and profound action of a higher potency is called for, confirmed by the highly characteristic Arnica symptom 'says there is nothing the matter with him,' even when grievously injured or ill. My own preferred potency in such a case would be the 10M ($10^{-20,000}$) given every half hour for three doses and then at longer intervals as the patient emerges from the state of shock. If the patient is concussed, Arnica becomes even more essential as it has the capacity to heal contusion of the brain, reduce cerebral oedema (swelling) and prevent or stop haemorrhage. The long-term after-effects of concussion can be prevented. Needless to say, such a patient also requires careful monitoring in case indications for surgery should develop.

Indications for low potencies

To summarise, the lower frequency of the lower potencies suits them for use when problems are focused at a more physical level, when the condition to be treated is more superficial and circumscribed (localised), when similarity is not as clear-cut and when selection is largely based on physical signs and symptoms.

Other reasons for using a lower potency in preference to a higher potency:

- When the vital force of the patient is weak: the action of the low potency requires less energy from the constitution to bring about its effect; it coaxes the weakened constitution more gently towards cure; it usually needs to be given more frequently.
- For the elderly in whom the available energy needed to induce a curative reaction is low.
- For the hypersensitive individual e.g. atopic (allergic) patient suffering from eczema, urticaria (hives), hay-fever or asthma: the constitution is already in a state of high alert; the immune response is exaggerated; the less searching and less confrontational effect of the lower potency may be desirable to avoid an initial aggravation, which could be provoked

because of the remedy's capacity to elicit a reaction so similar to that which is already excessive in the patient. This may be an indication for rather using an LM potency.
- In cases where the disease has already progressed from the stage of dysfunction into structural change and definite pathology: the lower potency can prove more immediately supportive and less aggressive in mobilising accumulated toxins and breaking down diseased tissues; an initial, gentle stimulation of healing can be applied to the more severely compromised system and then gradually increased by carefully moving up the scale of potencies as progress takes place.
- When a degree of organ failure is present e.g. hypothyroidism (underactive thyroid): the remedy required to stimulate function is given in low potency 2–3 times per day.
- When a physiological effect is essential and the physician wishes to avoid the use of harsh drugs: e.g. in early heart failure when the action of the myocardium (heart muscle) is weakened and cardiac oedema (water in the tissues) is present; heart remedies such as Strophanthus hispidus (kombe seed) or Adonis vernalis (pheasant's eye) may be indicated in low potency (3X or 6X), or even in mother tincture (Ø) to provide both a healing and supportive effect – strengthening the heart's action and dispersing accumulated fluid; in addition a remedy suited to the entire mental and physical state of the patient (constitutional remedy) will be given in higher potency.
- When similar acting remedies are combined in a mixture to produce a complex remedy that targets a specific clinical indication e.g. cystitis (bladder infection), or a specific organ.
- The Schüssler Tissue Salt range of remedies: in 1872 Dr Wilhelm Schüssler grouped together twelve inorganic salts, which he deemed essential for healthy physiology and presented them to the profession as *An Abridged Homeopathic Therapeutics*; they became the so-called Twelve Tissue Salt Remedies – forming a valuable mini materia medica of homeopathic remedies with very clearly defined clinical indications that have made the group popular for domestic use; these remedies are usually prescribed in the sixth decimal potency (6X).

Indications for High Potencies

In contrast, the higher potencies (30C [10^{-60}] or above) transmit over a less diffuse band and at a higher frequency. They are far more intensely focused and penetrate to the deepest mental and emotional levels of the psyche. For full efficacy of action, remedies in high potency require far greater accuracy of selection (a high degree of similarity) and are given less frequently. They are less forgiving of error. In skilled hands they are used for both acute and chronic states. In life threatening conditions or severe collapse, even when the vital force is desperately low, a high potency of the indicated remedy (e.g. Carbo vegetablis 10M [vegetable carbon or charcoal] or Camphor 10M, may be required every 5 to 10 minutes to save life; all the remaining available energy is summoned to pull the patient back from the edge. Once the pulse strengthens and the body warms, the potency and dose frequency must be reduced to conserve energy, while still urging the body towards recovery. When the dire condition has lifted, another remedy in moderate potency, selected for the cause of the collapse and the presenting symptoms, will usually be indicated. Fortunately in acute and severe conditions, the prescribing symptoms on which the remedy needs to be selected are far clearer than in the majority of chronic cases.

When the energy (vital force) of the patient is adequate or strong, when there is a high degree of similarity between the patient and the remedy and when there are no conditions obtaining, which indicate that it would be wiser to use a low potency first (e.g. hypersensitive subjects, marked pathology, the elderly), then the homeopathic high potency comes into its own.

Source of homeopathic remedies

Homeopathic remedies are derived from a very wide range of sources. Any energy or substance – however imponderable (X-ray) or weighty (lead), however nebulous (hydrogen) or gross (a slab of marble), however simple (an element) or complex (a plant or animal), however natural (spring water) or synthetic (latex) – may be used to produce a homeopathic potency.

Over 3000 remedies have become available over the years, and the number is constantly being augmented. Of these, some 1250 are in common use, and a far smaller group of remedies, varying from 100 to 250, comprise the therapeutic core of most homeopathic practices.

The remedy sources may be categorised as follows:

- *Mineral*: More or less 30% of all remedies.
- *Botanical*: Approximately 60% of remedies are of plant origin.
- *Animal* (including insects): About 5% (but in recent years, increasing quite rapidly in number because of widening interest and research).

- *Biological*:
  - *Nosodes*:
    - Pathological material of plant, animal or human origin
    - Cultures of pathogens or commensal micro-organisms (bowel flora)
  - *Sarcodes*: Healthy human or animal tissues, organs or secretions (including venoms)
- *Imponderables*: Prepared from a carrier medium that has been exposed to an energy source e.g. electricity, magnetic field, X-ray, micro-wave, sun and moon rays, colour remedies, sound.
- *Allergodes*: Prepared from various allergens (a source material known to cause allergic reaction), e.g. house dust, pollens, animal hair, feathers, synthetics, and food allergens such as eggs, milk, gluten, chocolate, etc.
- *Tautodes* (also known as *tautopathic remedies*): Made from allopathic drugs and used to overcome dependency or to antidote the deleterious effects of the specific drug e.g. cortisone, penicillin, aspirin, methylphenidate (*Ritalin*), citalopram (*Cypramil*). This group also includes environmental contaminants;
  - Industrial chemicals: volatiles, solvents, paints, polish, detergents, disinfectants.
  - Insecticides: e.g. organophosphates, specific commercial products to which the patient has been exposed.

The last two categories, allergodes and tautodes, contain remedies that are antidotal to substances that are capable of eliciting allergic reaction, drugs that have toxic potential and contaminants that are patently toxic. In certain cases these adjunct remedies can prove helpful either in desensitising a patient against a specific allergen, or assisting the body to fend off the side effects of allopathic chemical drugs, or to help rid the body of toxic contaminants and the long-term, suppressive effects of specific drugs that have been administered.

When remedies prepared from allergens and pathogens (the causative agents of a disease process), or the products of a disease are given, the method of therapy is termed *isopathy*. Although these *isopathic* remedies are given in potency, and are therefore essentially homeopathic, they are selected for their associated role in the specific disease and not for their similarity to the patient's unique emotional and physical features (constitution). This distinction in nomenclature is made because in *isopathic* therapy the remedy chosen is selected for being the same as the disease (treating 'same with same'), whereas in homeopathy the selection is based on similarity (treating 'like with like').

When remedies derived from allopathic drugs or environmental contaminants are administered in potency in order to counteract the respective substance's effect, or toxic influence, the method of therapy is referred to as *tautopathy*.

Nosodes

A group of remedies, which are invariably administered in higher potency are the *Nosodes* (usually 30C or 200C). These are remedies derived from pathological material of plant, animal or human origin: diseased tissue, or the products of disease processes – excretions, discharges and effusions. Remedies prepared from cultures of pathogens (organisms that cause disease, such as viruses, bacteria and fungi) and other micro-organisms, commensal or mutualistic, (e.g. bowel flora) are also defined as nosodes.

Examples of remedies derived from nosode source material include the following:

- *Plant nosodes* derived from plant infestations:
  - Secale cornutum: rye infected with the fungus *Claviceps purpurea*, known as rye ergot.
  - Ustilago maydis: a fungal disease of maize (*Zea mays*), known as corn smut.
  - Solanum tuberosum aegrotans: prepared from diseased potatoes infected with the oomycete, *Phytophthora infestans*, which was implicated in the Irish potato famine of 1845.
- *Animal nosodes* derived from pathological excretions:
  - Ambra grisea: a physiological or pathological excretion from the gut of the sperm whale (*Physeter macrocephalus*), consisting of a collection of faeces round the indigestible parts of the giant squid, which is the whale's major prey; voided by the whale the buoyant mass floats to shore and is used as an exceptional, perfume fixative.
- *Bowel nosodes*: Prepared from organisms shown to be proliferating in stool cultures derived from patients responding positively to specific homeopathic remedies given for specific disease patterns. The relationship between bowel organism, disease pattern and associated, successful remedy or remedies provides the indication for the use of a bowel nosode.

  Bowel nosodes may be prescribed:
  - On the indications derived from the disease pattern of such patients.
  - As constitutional remedies in their own right, based on their own specific homeopathic emotional and physical profile (derived from clinical experience).
  - To augment the action of their associated remedies.

- According to miasmatic indications (certain of the bowel nosodes show particular affinity for miasmatic patterns of disease).
- *Micro-organism nosodes*: Organisms (viral, bacterial or fungal) derived from pathological samples, or from cultures, provide a valuable group of nosodes. When a patient has never enjoyed good health since a certain infection, e.g. since glandular fever (mono), measles or pneumonia, or when a patient is prone to recurrent infections by a specific organism e.g. *Escherichia coli* urinary infections, treatment with a nosode of the responsible organism can prove critical to success.
- *Miasmatic nosodes*: The five primary nosodes linked to the five chronic miasms:
  - *Psoric* nosode, Psorinum, prepared from the contents of the scabies vesicle.
  - *Sycotic* nosode, Medorrhinum, prepared from a gonorrhoeal urethral discharge or culture of *Neisseria gonorrhoea*.
  - *Syphilitic* nosode, Syphilinum or Lueticum, from the exudate of a syphilitic lesion containing the infective organism *Treponema pallidum*.
  - *Tubercular* nosode, Tuberculinum, Tuberculinum bovinum, Bacillinum, prepared from tubercular infected tissue or culture of *Mycobacterium tuberculosis* or *Mycobacterium bovis*.
  - *Cancer* nosode, *Carcinosin*, prepared from cancerous tissue – the most important being cancer of the breast.
- *Diseased tissue nosodes*: e.g. Atheroma derived from arteriosclerotic material from diseased arteries; Osteo-arthritic nosode (OAN) derived from osteophytes.
- *Autonosodes*: These are prepared from the patient's own body fluids, discharges or exudates from infected lesions. Such nosodes are of particular value as adjuncts to constitutional prescribing when response is slow or disappointing. When a case of recurrent boils, abscesses or carbuncles proves resistant to treatment, a nosode may be prepared from pus expressed from such a lesion and given to the patient in potency to quicken response. Similarly, a chronic ear or vaginal discharge may be used as the source for a patient-specific nosode.

An important autonosode is the Autohaem nosode prepared from the patient's own blood. After being centrifuged, the serum is run up by serial dilution and succussion to the 30th or 200th centesimal potency. This adjunct therapy is of particular value in the treatment of sufferers from autoimmune diseases (e.g. rheumatoid arthritis, lupus erythematosis, multiple sclerosis and diabetes) and for chronic viral infections due to organisms that escape the immune response of the patient through rapid mutation, as seen in chronic viral fatigue patients (ME) and HIV/AIDS. In the latter cases a fresh nosode needs to be prepared every six weeks or so, depending on response, in order to keep pace with viral mutation. In the autoimmune diseases the preparation of the autohaem nosode captures and potentises the self-damaging antibodies responsible for the disease changes. The nosode used in conjunction with a constitutionally selected remedy will aid curative response.

It will be immediately apparent that the use of nosodes to stimulate the body's resistance to certain specific clinical conditions or infections resembles conventional medicine's use of immunisation and is an example of 'same cures same'; this parallel is conveniently ignored by those sceptical of the similar principle. However, there is also a great difference between conventional immunisation and homeopathy. In immunisation, a crude disease product is engrafted onto the body, and, though bestowing immunity, its effect is harsh and fraught with potential hazards, while the action of the homeopathic nosode, being in potentised form, is gentle and without harm.

It must be stressed that the method of preparation of homeopathic nosodes from infected tissues or cultures ensures that the organisms are destroyed in the process, thus obviating any risk of the spread of infection.

Sarcodes

Similar to the nosodes are the *Sarcodes*, remedies prepared from healthy human or animal tissues, organs and natural secretions (e.g. chemical messengers, enzymes, hormones, venoms). Sarcodes derived from organs and body chemicals are used to regulate the metabolic functions to which they are related. The potency required is determined by whether the function is excessive or deficient. In hyperthyroidism (overactive thyroid) the sarcode, Thyroidinum, is indicated in higher potency to quieten the thyroid, while in hypothyroidism (underactive thyroid) the same remedy is given in low potency in order to stimulate the organ. Sarcodes of this type are never prescribed singly, but always in conjunction with a constitutional remedy; their role is supportive. Sarcodes, however, prepared from the venom or secretions of animals are numbered among the most important homeopathic remedies and match some of the major archetypal patterns of the human psyche e.g. Lachesis muta (bushmaster) and Sepia officinalis (common cuttlefish ink).

As can now be appreciated, the homeopathic potency scale is like a piano keyboard; all the notes are important, from the mother tincture (herb) or mother-substance (mineral and animal), through the lower potencies, to the very highest. Each has its own special sphere of action and influence. Some physicians prefer to play the lower notes (as did Hahnemann), others swear by the higher notes and some even have a favourite note, which they feel resonates best for them. But, the most versatile cover the entire keyboard, led in their selection by the demands of the clinical situation, the full picture of the case and the dynamic capacity of the remedy.

Stability, storage and sensitivity

The indelible imprinting of the encoded, energy pattern upon the carrier medium is an important factor in potentisation. This quantum phenomenon accounts for the remarkable truth that if homeopathy had been available to Tutankhamen and his medicine chest of favourite remedies placed beside him in his coffin – over 3,000 years later, an out-of-line archaeologist, suffering from an Allium cepa-like cold, would have benefitted from surreptitiously taking a few doses of the ancient remedy as he recovered it from the young Pharaoh's tomb. Whereas chemical, molecular medicines have a limited shelf life, homeopathic remedies, if well looked after, remain potent indefinitely. However, being in quantum form, they are singularly vulnerable to the impingement of energy radiation. A remedy in a clear, glass vial, carelessly left on a windowsill and exposed to the rays of the sun will soon have its encoded, energy pattern distorted or erased; an amber glass bottle will prove far more resistant, but direct exposure to the sun should, nevertheless, always be avoided. Similarly, in order to retain their potency, homeopathic remedies should be kept away from the immediate vicinity of electronic devices that receive or transmit energy waves: mobile phones, computers, TV sets, micro-wave ovens, etc. X-ray scans at airports, although of low intensity, will also harm remedies; this would seem to be accumulative, each exposure *de-potentising* the remedy further; after a number of flights the remedy should be discarded as unreliable. Plastic containers should always be avoided because they steadily exude toxic material, which interacts chemically with homeopathic mother tinctures and potencies.[6]

Homeopathic remedies are ideally stored in well-sealed amber glass bottles in a cool, dark place. Even mother tinctures retain their efficacy for an indefinite time if kept in this way. Freshly prepared mother tinctures may be supersaturated and therefore, after a long period of storage at low temperature, become cloudy or produce a layer of sediment at the bottom of the container. This is not an indication of deterioration. The tincture should simply be filtered until all insoluble material has been removed. The clear filtrate will still possess the full medicinal activity of the fresh product. Another cause of sedimentation is loss of alcohol through evaporation. This will be confirmed by a drop in the fluid level and indicates a poorly sealed container. Such a mother tincture should be discarded.

Once in potentised form, heat *per se* does not seem to harm remedies. From personal experience on a safari trip to Botswana, remedies that were left in the 'cubbyhole' of a 4×4 vehicle at a temperature of 44°C, on returning to civilisation, still proved effective. Nevertheless, such exposure is harsh and should be avoided. A remedy secured in a pocket and exposed to body temperature for a long time remains undisturbed, but if it should share a pocket or handbag with a mobile phone it will inevitably deteriorate.

The well-sealed or well-stoppered injunction is important because homeopathic remedies are susceptible to deterioration if exposed to strong aromatic substances e.g. soaps, perfumes, camphor etc. Domestically, remedies should always be stored in drawers or cupboards that do not contain any strong smelling substances or chemicals.

The quantum paradox of unique and extended durability, coupled to extreme sensitivity to subtle forces and emanations, influences the care required in dispensing, medicating, handling and administering homeopathic remedies. The most common vehicle used is the lactose tablet, pillule, or much tinier granule. Conventionally, the number constituting a dose is given as: two tablets or two to four pillules, depending on their size; and 12 to 20 granules. This latitude of number is possible because of the immaterial nature of the dose, which just needs to be sufficient to convey the coded signal to the recipient. In dispensing (medicating) these solid forms, the liquid potency in alcohol is added to a measured volume of the lactose vehicle in a glass container, the number of drops being determined by the amount to be medicated. A gentle shaking of the container ensures that the medicating drops thoroughly and evenly coat all the contents. On smelling a freshly prepared remedy, the faint and not unpleasant odour of the alcohol used in medicating it will be detected. This gradually becomes fainter as the remedy penetrates and permeates the porous lactose vehicle. Eventually, when completely dry, little or no alcohol odour is detectable. The encapsulation of the remedy carrier within the protective lactose sheath contributes further to the permanence of the captured potency. It will be understood from this description of the medication technique, and the fact that the remedies are intangible energy, that strict safeguards against cross contamination from one remedy to another have to be observed and that the medicating area must be scrupulously prepared and maintained and devoid of any possible contaminants. The same fastidiousness must extend to the dress and habit of the dispenser. Indeed, although it may be idealistic and, in the event, unrealistic to expect the presiding emotional and dynamic ambience of the laboratory or dispensary and those working within them to be at all times harmonious and altruistic, nevertheless, any discord or purely acquisitive motivation must impinge on the purity and efficacy of remedies, which can only be described as ethereal and spirit-like.

Correct usage

Tablets, pillules or granules should not be touched with the hand as any impurities, such as chemicals and body exudates may interfere with their efficacy. The dose should be tapped into the cap of the container and from there onto or under the tongue. Alternatively, a clean, dry spoon may be used. Homeopathic remedies are ideally absorbed through the mucous membrane of the mouth and particularly from beneath the tongue. For optimum uptake, the nerve endings and highly sensitive taste receptors of the mucous membrane must be alert and not refractory due to recent contact with strongly aromatic substances such as peppermint, menthol, eucalyptus or garlic. In this sense, think of the experienced wine taster wishing to fully savour and distinguish the piquant subtleties in the flavour of an excellent wine. He must be certain that he has not previously taken anything into the mouth that might occupy or dull his acuity of taste and smell. Before tasting a second wine, the mouth is rinsed with water to remove any lingering memory of the previous one. It is just as important for the homeopathic patient to avoid strong tasting things before taking a remedy. Coffee falls into this category. However, contrary to a common misconception, a cup of coffee taken at a time remote to the dose of medication will not interfere with either its absorption or efficacy. Where practicalities and time constraints pose difficulties for a patient, a good rule of thumb is to take the medication before a meal rather than afterwards, before brushing the teeth rather than afterwards, and to permit a short interval before either eating or brushing the teeth.

Due to their immaterial, quantum nature, homeopathic remedies may be administered by *olfaction*: inhaling the vapour from the liquid remedy through the nose (or less frequently by snuffing the powder form). Because it avoids the vagaries of oral activity and condition, Hahnemann thought highly of this method, which he introduced to the profession in 1827 and utilised in his practice until his death. On the continent, the use of homeopathic suppositories, which also circumvents the uncertainties of oral and gastric absorption, is popular.

References

1. Zukav G. *The Dancing Wu Li Masters*. London: Rider; 1994. p46.
2. Kayne SB (ed). *Homeopathic Practice*. London: Pharmaceutical Press; 2008. p38.
3. Zukav G. *The Dancing Wu Li Masters*. London: Rider; 1994. p54.
4. Wheeler JA, Thorne KS, Misner C. *Gravitation*, San Francisco CA; 1973. p1273.
5. Jacobi J. *Paracelsus: Selected Writings*. London: Routledge & Kegan Paul Ltd; 1951. pp155–156.
6. Cook TM. *Homeopathic Medicine Today*. New Canaan CT: Keats Publishing; 1989. p66.

* * * * *

> By following the enduring legacy of Samuel Hahnemann, we have been able to observe the critical early development of homeopathy and gain understanding of the basic principles upon which this science of healing is based. With this knowledge in place, it is time to change our perspective and consider a form of healing even more ancient than those which gave birth to modern homeopathy: the science of spiritual healing. Once again, it is possible for us to gain insight into a mysterious dimension of healing through relating the life-story of a remarkable man: William Henry Lilley – my father.

Part two

THE SCIENCE OF SPIRIT

The remarkable history of William Lilley

Note

All photographs have been obtained by scanning original prints from the Lilley family archives and are presented without enhancement.

12

THE GIFT OF HEALING

Mother and son

A small boy and a young woman, warmly wrapped against the bitter cold of an icy, West Yorkshire winter afternoon, stood patiently waiting at the bus stop in the small village of Oulton. It had been snowing on and off during the previous few days and along the path and on the road before them dirty grey sludge lay piled and furrowed, dark, thick and ugly, adding

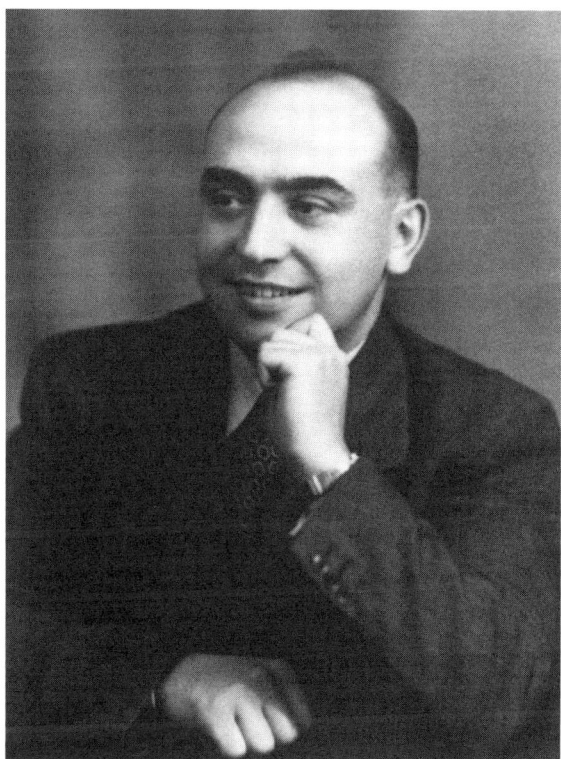

Figure 12.1 William Henry Lilley (1914–1972)

a chill emphasis to the bleakness of the day. Snow had little chance of remaining pristine in the grimy environs of industrial Leeds where the surrounding countryside was poxed and scarred with the pitheads and slagheaps of collieries and the air heavy with the emission of coal fumes and dust. Although early afternoon, the heavy ceiling of cloud made it seem much later. The mother and son were alone, and, as if warned by some premonition of delay, no one joined them while they waited. It was 1924, and the bus service probably more vulnerable to the effects of heavy snowfall and bad weather than today. As time passed, and the expected transport failed to appear, the mother grew anxious. She had timed the bus-trip to get them to the neighbouring village of Kippax shortly before the start of the Spiritualist séance she wished to attend. As a gifted psychic medium, Sarah Ellen Lilley, known to all as Sally, had made the trip many times before, for she was one of the central figures in the sittings that were held regularly in a cosy room above the village pub. She knew that any further loss of time would result in them arriving too late.

The sharp wind freshened, adding to the redness of their cheeks, and bringing with it an increasing flurry of snowflakes that clung to the scarf she had bound over her curly black hair and tied under her chin, and speckled with white the dark, plaid flat-cap the lad wore; a small replica of his father, who, before light, had set out that morning for his shift at the local mine. Suddenly, stirred by some inner prompting, possibly the silent influence of her Chinese guide, Li Chu, Sally decided to tarry at the bus stop no longer, but to set off on foot towards Kippax with her son, William Henry junior, in tow. It was not a conscious decision, because had she applied her serious consideration to the situation, given the prevailing weather, a ten year old beside her, ice, sludge, mud and snow underfoot, the distance to be covered and the lateness of the hour, it was not possible for them to reach their destination in time. At first she stuck to the main road hoping that the bus would still come, but before long, the area being well known to her from childhood, she turned off and by lane, stile and path sought to at least reduce the walking distance. Written into the memory of the child, and related many years later, apart from the snow and the nipping air, was how he had marvelled at the spirit-like vapour rising from the surface of the river Ayre. Unheeding, the mother pressed on, unwittingly moved by predestination as natural as a wave seeking the shore. Awareness of their surroundings, the ground beneath their feet, the damp chill and their efforts faded away. They spoke not a word and as if cocooned and cradled by some unseen influence seemed transported in silence through space and time. When their perceptions returned, they were already in the High Street approaching the pub.

Upstairs, the ladies of the circle were still arriving, shedding their scarves, gloves and protective outer garments in the séance room warmed by a cheery fire dancing in the ancient hearth. Sally and her, young 'Billy' had miraculously arrived with time to spare. This was the first time that William had ever attended a séance. He was no stranger to the other-worldliness of his mother. More gentle and sensitive than either of his two older brothers or his miner father, he was closer to his mother and did not find it strange that she was able to see and converse with spirit beings or that people visited their home for advice, for spirit healing and to have their palms or tea leaves read. After all, psychic powers were a tradition in his mother's family. His grandfather, Joseph Palfreyman, had been a clairvoyant psychic, like his father before him, and augmented his miner's pay packet by practising herbalism. Joseph was quite a character in the village, known for his talking jackdaw that accompanied him to the local pub of an evening, eagerly supped beer from a hollow in the wooden counter, and, clinging to his shoulder on their walk home afterwards, was more unsteady on its feet than its master.

On that fated Wednesday afternoon, William accompanied her only because Sally had been unable to find anyone to look after him on his return from school. The ladies present all made a great fuss of the young boy and spoilt him with tea and biscuits, but soon it was time for the more serious matter of the séance to begin. These sittings were held every month at the same venue and were always attended by the same sitters. Admission to the circle was carefully controlled and could only be achieved after all the members were in accord that the person seeking to join possessed qualities which would enable them to conform with the spiritual aspirations of the group; for the introduction of a discordant note would disturb the essential harmony of the circle. Invariably, prospective new members would be introduced by one or other of the established sitters and were, therefore, well known to them. However, the final decision of whether they should be admitted lay with the spirit inspirers, for whom Li Chu was the spokesman.

The common bond that initially drew these ladies together in their desire to lift the veil of death was often the loss of someone close through illness or tragedy. In 1924, due to the Great War of 1914–1918, after which in many British villages it seemed as if an entire generation of young men had been wiped out, it was more often than not the loss of a father, brother or son in action. Sally Lilley, who was born in 1888, and on that afternoon in Kippax was thirty-six years of age, had manifested psychic awareness from an early age, being conscious, both clairvoyantly (psychic vision) and clairaudiently (psychic hearing), of spirit children, who were her playmates and confidantes. In the Palfreyman household, this was regarded as perfectly normal, natural and healthy. Against a relaxed Methodist Christian background, the family believed implicitly in the intimate interaction of the world of spirit and the world of everyday life. They understood, in their simple and relatively uneducated way, that those who had 'passed on', their nearest and dearest, were not removed to some remote nebulous Heaven or Hell, but resided in a spirit 'afterlife,' which interpenetrated the material world, and given the right circumstances, or need, could manifest to the sensitive beholder and communicate with them.

Sarah Ellen Lilley

Joseph soon perceived that his daughter's psychic senses were far greater than his own, and although she never attended a 'development circle' to advance her abilities, his interest and encouragement fostered their unfolding. It was he who predicted that she would one day bear a son destined to perform great healing works. Shortly after she passed puberty, her personal 'guide' or inspirer, Li Chu, a Chinese gentleman versed in philosophy and healing, first made himself known to her and remained with her throughout her long life. She died in 1980, at the age of ninety-two. She was short in stature, no taller than four foot eleven inches, and after producing her three sons lost her narrow waist and developed the solid frame of a strong, active, Yorkshire miner's wife; more muscular than obese. She had an ample bosom, which was a great comfort to me as a child, particularly during the time my mother and I stayed with her in Woodlesford, when we were evacuated 'up-North' during the World War 11 rocket blitz of London. I still remember snuggling up to her on cold, dismal winter days, and feeling so safe. She had black, curly hair, which later became 'pepper and salt', but never completely white, and warm, twinkling brown eyes. For me she was like a gypsy fortune-teller, and when I grew to know her well in later years, possessed an insight into people and events typical of the proverbial wise, old woman, or crone. Indeed, she was affectionately known as the village witch; the sometime midwife; a lass to be consulted when there was family distress or illness; who could see and converse with spirits; contact and receive messages and advice from wise beings and departed loved ones; read your palm, your cards and your tea leaves; see into the future; 'lay on hands'; and give good counsel. Sarah Ellen Lilley was, to say the least, well known and respected in the mining community.

I was always impressed by the strength of her forearms, developed, apart from hard domestic work, through the hours of massage she would give those who sought her help for their various aches and pains, especially for their 'lumbago', or lower backache. Even when she was seventy-two, I know she was not past shovelling her miner-widow's coal allowance into her coal-bunker unaided. She was, besides, an excellent baker, and I have watched her for hours kneading dough with all the expertise she could apply to kneading an ailing back. Her hands were small and powerful and yet, when administering treatment, gentle and tender. Whenever she applied them to a painful spot, her palms would redden and become wonderfully warm, their contact bringing comfort and relief. Those hands wrought magic, they painlessly removed my loose teeth when I was terrified to have anyone else come near me, and much to my delight deftly and mysteriously conjured pennies and half-pennies from my nose or ears as a reward for my bravery. In her teens she entered 'service' in a grand home outside Leeds and it was there, 'downstairs', that she learnt the craft of good baking. During the Great War, she, like many women, volunteered to work in the gunpowder mills. Many years later, she told me about how many of the young women she knew during that time had become seriously ill from working with the toxic powder, suffering severe headaches and developing a yellow discolouration of the skin, and of others who had been killed or maimed by explosions.

The séance

In the centre of the séance room was a low table around which the required number of chairs had been arranged in a circle. Here, the ladies took their seats, all the while chatting and catching up on family doings and village gossip. The atmosphere was friendly and relaxed, all helped by the warmth and glow from the fire. William was given a comfortable chair to one side of the circle and told to be a good boy, to mind his 'Ps and Qs', and sit quietly while his Mummy and the good ladies said prayers, sang a few hymns and talked with the friendly spirits. The main purpose of these spiritualist sittings held above the village pub was to extend healing to people known to the sitters or to those whose names had been given to the circle by villagers who knew of the meetings and believed in spiritual healing; to make contact with deceased loved ones and the personal guides of the sitters; and to receive guidance in dealing with the demands and difficulties of life. Often unsought advice would come through for relatives or friends, or unexpected contact would be made with spirits wishing to use the circle to make contact with individuals quite unknown to any of the sitters. Although there were other 'sensitives' in the circle, of varying psychic ability, it was Sally and her guide Li Chu, who presided over affairs.

With William an intrigued observer, the séance began. Although not regarded by the sitters as a formal religious gathering, but rather as a coming together in spirit, the séance was conducted from a Protestant Christian perspective with due reverence and respect for the powers that were being invoked and a solemnity appropriate to the seriousness of the occasion and its high objectives. First the ladies joined hands, creating the circle, bonding the sitters and focussing the spiritual energy necessary for spirit communication and the transmission of healing. After a prayer of invocation delivered by Sally, the ladies discussed and identified the people to whom healing should be extended, one of whom was a member of the circle. When this had been done to everyone's satisfaction, the ladies once again joined hands, and, by way of totally surrendering themselves to the wishes of Divinity, sang their favourite hymn, *Lead, Kindly Light*, which commences thus:

> Lead, Kindly Light, amidst th'encircling gloom,
> Lead Thou me on!
> The night is dark, and I am far from home,
> Lead Thou me on!
> Keep Thou my feet; I do not ask to see
> The distant scene; one step enough for me.

The words of the hymn capture the need for the incarnated soul to transcend the pride and pleasures of the ego-self, to trust implicitly, hearken to and follow unquestioningly, as a child, the guiding light of spirit, which constantly prompts and cues us through the uncertain gloom of unfolding life events. They express the need to live trustingly in the blessedness of the moment, and to know that at the end of our earthly journey, those we have loved and lost await us in the peace of the spirit world.

White Hawk

On that bitter, Yorkshire afternoon, in a room above a village pub, drawn by the earnest sincerity of a small band of village housewives, the universal light of which they sang focussed upon a young boy and in touching him blessed him with the gift of healing. Hardly had they closed with: "To rest forever after earthly strife in the calm light of everlasting life", than William, with eyes closed, as if in sleep, rose to his feet and with a noble and imperious gesture of his arm threw across his shoulder an unseen robe or cloak, much as a senator of old might have done before addressing his distinguished peers. Then, much to the amazement of all those present, in a voice lower in pitch than his own, the boy boldly spoke to them in an unknown language. This was not the unintelligible gibberish of a person 'speaking in tongues', but clearly articulated and structured speech, delivered in measured tones and with remarkable authority, especially when heard issuing from the lips of so young a person. His entire being, small as it then was, emanated maturity, confidence and composure; all shared in his bearing, which was erect and imposing. Although his eyes remained closed, his audience knew he was surveying them as his hidden glance encompassed the room. He continued to speak for what seemed later to have been some time, but considering the circumstances was probably quite brief. Since they could not understand what he imparted, the sitters could only conclude that the inspiring spirit who had taken possession of the lad was actually communicating with 'others' who were present, but unseen. Only at the end of this discourse did he speak a few words of heavily-accented English, informing the circle that he was White Hawk, the appointed 'gate-keeper', or spirit protector of the young medium, and that this visitation was the beginning of important healing work that William was destined to perform. With a final injunction that Sally should assist the development of her son's mediumship, followed by a few words in his own language, which, judging by the intonation and stance that accompanied them, was a short prayer or blessing bestowed upon the group, their visitor resumed his seat and seemed to enter into a state of deep meditation. As White Hawk's animating influence withdrew, the boy's features and posture slackened, his breathing deepened, and he appeared to be peacefully sleeping. The circle remained silent and still, fully understanding the momentous nature of what had transpired and sensitive that the transition from the 'next world' to this should be gentle and undisturbed. After drawing a deep breath followed by an audible sigh, William opened his eyes with surprise and embarrassment to find all eyes upon him. He thought he had in some way disgraced himself by falling asleep. When questioned, he had no recollection of what had taken place during his 'absence'.

Much as Hamlet, after the appearance of his father's ghost on the battlements, enjoined Horatio and the watch to hold what they had seen and heard secret, so my grandmother cautioned her fellow-sitters to share that afternoon's revelation with no one. William was scarcely out of his boyhood, much work lay ahead to confirm and develop the remarkable mediumship that had been displayed and Sally had no desire for her youngest son to become a curiosity. A few weeks later, she returned to Kippax accompanied by a very reluctant and apprehensive William. On this occasion, all the energy of the circle was concentrated upon assisting his entrancement. Not surprisingly, although his mother had been at pains to explain to him that a kind spirit wished to use him in sleep as a channel for communicating knowledge from the beyond; that he was very special to have been chosen for this role; and that he would come to no harm; the youngster was so frightened and overwhelmed by what was expected of him that he could scarcely bear to close his eyes, let alone fall sleep. This second afternoon sitting proved a great disappointment to all, but not to Sally. She realised that the first séance had been successful expressly because William had been completely relaxed and unaware of what was about to happen. It was only stage fright that stood in the way of further progress. By the time of the third séance, Sally's explanations and reassurances had prevailed, and, despite an initial anxiety, William again slipped easily into trance and was controlled by the same presiding spirit. During these first trance experiences, spread at intervals over the following months, very little communication took place. On the spirit side, however, there was considerable activity as spirit scientists devoted the time to preparing the young instrument psychologically and physiologically for the arduous trance-work that lay ahead and perfecting the process of entrancement to a point of seamlessness.

The Great Ramesôye

During the fourth successful séance, this had developed to such a degree that after the initial overshadowing by White Hawk, without the trance state being in any sense interrupted or disturbed, the sitters became aware that the North American Indian had departed and that they were in the presence of someone else – a personage, whom they would later learn, came from a far higher sphere. This illustrious being, speaking through the ten-year old medium without trace of a Yorkshire accent, made his presence known, announcing himself, after blessing the sitters, as the Ramesôye, an Egyptian doctor who had resided in the spirit world for the past 2000 years. He spoke English and expressed himself with immense dignity, strength and compassion, employing a turn of phrase that was both poetic and of another age. He graciously thanked the circle for their critical contribution to the development of the young medium, who was destined to become a great psychic healer and physician and told them that William's initial preparation for the important work that lay ahead was now complete. Before taking leave of them, he spoke directly to Sally advising her that her son's further development should be continued at home and no longer through attending the Kippax circle. The energy of the group was no longer required for what still remained to be achieved and the familiar, relaxed home environment would prove ideal and more practical for this purpose.

In accordance with the Ramesôye's advice, regular sittings for William were commenced in the Lilley home in Oulton with the help of a few close friends, and in particular a devoted fellow Spiritualist, Mrs Westmoreland. I never heard this lady referred to by any other more familiar name, even though she was such an important and diligent participant in the final stages of my father's mediumistic development.

At that time, it was the custom, born of financial necessity, for young boys from the mining communities to leave school at the age of thirteen, sadly often younger still, and descend, like their fathers and grandfathers before them, into the stygian depths of the coal mines, exposing their young lungs under effort to the ruinous effects of coal dust and their tender bodies to the dangers intrinsic to working underground. By the time my father reached that age, both his older brothers, Tom and Jesse, were already down the mines pushing or pulling heavily laden trams or bogies along rail tracks, filled with the coal that their elders had hewn from the coalface. At this juncture, a vital decision had to be made about William's future. Despite the disapproval of the rest of the family, Sally, supported by Mrs Westmoreland, was adamant that "our young Billy" was not for the mines. She won the day, and during his teens Billy worked as a store assistant, thus providing his essential contribution to the family finances, earning money that he could never call his own. It was a difficult time for him because his brothers and his erstwhile school friends thought him soft, a 'sissy' and a 'mummy's boy.' Years later he would speak to me of the pain he endured during that period of his life, being a young boy in such a tight-knit community, estranged from both family and fellows through ever widening differences in behaviour and interests, which set him apart and isolated him. This isolation was intensified by the unique changes that were being wrought within him, which brought a precocious seriousness and depth to his disposition during years that are usually the most carefree and light-hearted. It would not be long, however, before two important people would enter his life and he would never feel alone again. The first was a deceased Hindu doctor and the second was my mother.

Psychic development

After the Ramesôye's appearance and advice, the intensity of the training increased, made possible because the sittings could be conducted at home, even nightly if need be, and could last as long as was required. Longer and deeper periods of trance were achieved, essential for both the lecturing and healing work that was envisaged. The transition both in and out of trance was refined to the point of being scarcely detectable, other than to the most attentive observer and those who knew the medium well. In this way, four critical, formative and preparative years, coinciding with William's passage through puberty, passed under the tutelage, direction and presiding influence of the Ramesôye. He was scarcely fifteen when he had so matured as a full-trance medium that his inspirers from Spirit could communicate with him and overshadow him at any time, no matter the circumstances. This was to prove of great value in the trials to come. Commensurate with his ability to yield effortlessly to the trance state had come the development of clairvoyant and clairaudient powers: the ability to see those who resided in the realm of spirit and to hear their discourse. Out-of-the-body experiences began to take place. At first these caused him a great deal of alarm, but White Hawk, reassured him, explaining the sensations he felt during the projection and the unusual visions that appeared. Shortly after falling asleep, or less frequently during the course of the night, he would suddenly be conscious of floating out of his body and hovering above it. In the gentle half-light, his vision and awareness seemed to extend in all directions, unlimited by the restraints of physical eyes. He would contemplate his sleeping body on the bed beneath him and see the 'etheric cord', which during life connects body and soul and is capable of infinite extension. These preliminary phenomena were later followed by periods of flying over vast landscapes and seeing impressive and remarkable architecture quite different to anything he had ever seen before, even in books. During these experiences of 'astral travel', he was always conscious of others being with him, seen only peripherally, but ever-present. Much later, he would meet with them face to face whilst in 'astral projection', his beloved guides and inspirers, and others whom he recognised as friends from past lives. Often he would accompany them to the 'Halls of Learning' where teachings were given by exalted beings. On returning to the body, he would experience a sensation of falling or being drawn downwards and at times a feeling, very frightening when it first happened, as if he was passing through an electrical force field accompanied by rapidly flashing lights and a fine vibration of very high frequency, which caressed him as he descended.

These phenomena were intrinsic to the psychic development that William was undergoing, and are not uncommon amongst sensitive individuals, but they also proved highly instructive. From an early age, he was made aware, at the deepest level possible, of his spiritual and eternal nature. He knew conclusively that the body, while being a tabernacle for the soul and an instrument upon which the soul can play, does not constitute either the identity or the essence of a person, even though in its configuration of feature, form and function it might bear witness to the nature and disposition of its inhabitant. He possessed the precious knowledge that there is no such thing as death, that each night as we enter sleep we 'pass-on' or 'die' to the physical world. We enter a finer world, more real and immediate than that of earth, in which we are not in a state of suspended animation, but find ourselves in our natural milieu and according to our spiritual unfoldment are interactive with this environment and with those we meet. He soon learnt that for the beleaguered soul, the sleep state, in which the soul to a variable degree, dependent on its level of enlightenment, remains awake and aware, provides not only respite from the struggles and sufferings of physical life, but also the care, advise, encouragement and love of spirit beings who are intimately involved in our affairs. No one is ever isolated, forsaken or alone – no one is ever forgotten. And, every morning after sleep, just as we 'died' the previous evening, we are 'born' into a new day. Indeed, if we are able to live powerfully, with utter focus, in the moment, in 'the Now,' no matter what has transpired over the years since our emergence from our mother's womb, even the most heinous crimes, each morning constitutes the first day of our lives, a fresh beginning in which we have the potential to rise from the ashes of the past as resplendent as the mythical phoenix.

With most of us the return into the body, which involves a descent from a state of high frequency to a grosser vibratory level, distorts or erases the memory of what has been experienced during the sleep state, but the effect is to some degree unconsciously retained and glimpses of happenings and meetings may be recalled. Advice given and insights imparted unconsciously modify our behaviour and decision-making, and may even convey a sense of anticipatory foreknowledge and preparedness for oncoming events. Attunement to these possibilities, and an urgent desire to penetrate the mist between the objective world and the Reality concealed behind it, will always be rewarded by an expansion of consciousness, which brings a closer proximity to the spiritual dimension. Old wisdom informs us that if we should knock, the door will be opened, and if we should ask, the question will be answered. Caught up in the swirl of life events, very few of us ever knock or ask, and if we should, our gesture is often too perfunctory and short-lived to achieve response.

Lejan Tari Singh

The young medium was now ready to commence his education in the art of healing, and hence the time had come for him to make acquaintance with his guiding spirit. The one entrusted by the higher spiritual masters with the task of leading William forward into the mysteries that lay before him, to inspire him and to tutor him, and to be his constant companion through his extraordinary life's journey was Lejan Tari Singh, a Hindu medical doctor, a Brahman, who had trained in both Calcutta and London and who 'passed on' in 1914, the year of William's birth. In those early years, my father saw his spirit mentor just as clearly as we, whose faculties are limited to the earth plane, can see those about us. He heard his voice, however, not in his head, as we who hear with our physical ears would expect, but in his solar plexus – in the pit of his stomach (which we will later learn relates to the energy vortex of the third chakra). He described the doctor as short of stature and dark-skinned, with handsome features, thick black hair and strongly marked eyebrows. His most salient feature was the beauty and intensity of his eyes, which though penetrating were softened by their warmth, tenderness and understanding.

A bond was established between teacher and disciple, which over the years, as William reached manhood and re-attained his spiritual maturity, would deepen to one of twin souls motivated by the same drive to spread the message of the eternal, imperishable nature of the human spirit; the spiritual significance of this physical life; the understanding and mastery of the subtle forces which pervade and order the creation; and the art of spiritual and natural healing. But this was yet to come; at first it was a relationship of pupil and master. There was so much for William to learn. He was a young, village lad, son of unsophisticated mining stock, spoke with a broad Yorkshire accent, had received only limited schooling and was untutored in the niceties of refined, social behaviour. Given this starting material and the elevated goal, even the most erudite and ambitious Pygmalion might have been daunted by the transformative task that lay ahead. But, a human being is not just the product of inherited characteristics, circumstances and conditioning. There is an endowment that is transcendent to outer appearances and qualities, derived from previous life experiences, achievements and accomplishments, a level of spiritual and intellectual development, which antedates birth into this life and will express itself despite the hindrances of racial, familial and genetic legacy. Working in concert with Dr Letari, as Lejan Tari Singh became affectionately known, were a team of doctors and skilled experts, each of whom had a particular role to play in William's education, development and healing work.

> Just as it took five years to perfect trance mediumship – the ability to leave the body at any time, quickly, effectively, without fuss or theatricality – so was another five-year term needed to make him an equally successful diagnostician.[1]

Medical education

From the very outset of William's training, Dr Letari concentrated on educating him in every branch of medical science, other than surgery and obstetrics, and imparting all the diagnostic and clinical skills necessary for him to be able to examine patients, interpret symptoms and signs and practise medicine in his own right, independent of his psychic gifts. In Britain, this was quite unique in the annals of what was generally referred to as 'divine healing', 'spiritual healing' or 'faith healing.' Invariably, the healer had little or no medical knowledge and was a sensitive, but largely passive instrument or channel for the healing power, which was transmitted from a higher source through the medium to the patient, by the 'laying on of hands.' In William's case, in addition to full trance mediumship and the use of hand passes specific to the demands of each case, nature's remedies always supported the spiritual therapy. Initially, these were herbal, therefore, William needed to become familiar with the herbs of the field.

Herbal lore

To this end, Dr Letari took William into the Yorkshire countryside and there, especially among the abundance of the hedgerows, he focused his pupil's eye on the common herbs which were to be found growing there. He learnt to identify plants that had long been part of European herbal folklore, used since early times in the healing of the sick, such as dandelion, chamomile, daisy and stinging nettle. William would see a blue light playing upon the herb in question and hear in his solar plexus the voice of Dr Letari giving him both its common and scientific name, pointing out its distinguishing characteristics and telling him of its uses. What started out as a game, filled with all the excitement and suspense of a nature trail, became by repetition the serious acquisition of herbal lore.

Both the inner and outer worlds of Billy Lilley were expanding at a remarkable rate. It was not by chance that this child, born in an obscure Yorkshire village, should have been given this special role. He was chosen before his birth and came replete, like Mozart, with all the potential; all that was required was tutorship. No coercion, persuasion or incentive was required of this willing and enthusiastic healer in training; he embraced the experience with all the vigour and determination at his disposal.

The next stage of his tuition lay in gathering and preparing the herbs he would require. Apart from the hands-on experience this afforded him, it was a necessity, for he did not have money to buy herbs from the local herbalist. Under instruction, he first identified a particular plant and then collected samples, which he cleaned and cut. The plant material was then boiled in order to extract the virtue. These tinctures he bottled, catalogued and stored in conditions, which would preserve them without deterioration. It was his introduction to what would become his particular interest: homeopharmaceutics – the formulation and manufacture of homeopathic remedies.

Baptism of a healer

However, providence was not willing to wait upon these developments before launching Billy's healing career. The challenge set for this momentous occasion was life threatening. He was still only fifteen when the 13-year-old son of Mrs Westmoreland, who had been suffering for the previous two years from chronic nephritis, then known as Bright's disease, started to deteriorate rapidly. The orthodox treatment of the 1920s could not arrest this decline. The parents were informed that his kidneys were failing and that there was no hope of saving him. As an important participant in the family circle, Mrs Westmoreland had witnessed William's progress; she had met and spoken with Dr Letari; and she knew that her friend's son was destined to become a great healer; therefore, it was natural that she should appeal to Sally for help when her son's condition became desperate. Alarmed by the urgency of the youth's condition, Sally was soon at his bedside, accompanied by William.

It was "Sally's young Billy" who, after taking a seat beside the bed, fell asleep, and then, with his eyes closed, got to his feet and without a word gently laid his hands on his half-comatose friend's head, lightly cupping his temples. He remained poised like that for what seemed an age. Time stood still and a powerful hush descended upon the room, strangely accentuated by the metronomic ticking of the clock on the mantelpiece and the heavy, oppressed breathing of the patient. Then, with an assuredness that belied his age, William drew down the blankets and began to slowly and repeatedly run his hands over his friend's body from the top of his head down to the soles of his feet. It was as if he was drawing off toxins from the boy's body, because on reaching the tips of the toes, William's hands continued downwards and then with a final upward movement and flick of the wrists, seemed to throw off some invisible contagion, much as one would cast off drops of fluid from the finger tips. After he had performed this a number of times, he turned his attention to the kidneys. The hand movements over the abdomen were graceful and dexterous following a specific pattern repeated many times, touching the skin with the lightness of a feather, each pass concluded by the throwing off gesture. Finally the treatment ended with a number of head to toe movements executed as before. The psychic healing had taken all of fifteen minutes. William then pronounced some words in a foreign tongue, resumed his seat and lapsed into a sleep from which he soon awoke with a deep sigh.

During the night that followed, the patient became very restless, developed a fever and a heavy sweat and the parents feared the worst, but by daybreak he was more aware of his surroundings, seemed less swollen and was definitely passing more urine. That evening further treatment was given, and this was repeated the following evening. By the third day it was clearly apparent that he had turned a corner and was emerging from his critical state. Although he was very weak, his face was far less swollen, he was urinating more and his urine contained less protein, he had become very thirsty and his thoughts were clear. Within three weeks his kidney function had improved markedly and his symptoms had cleared. He went on to make a complete and permanent recovery.

We do not know how the physicians reacted when faced by this unexpected turnabout in their patient's moribund condition, but if it was anything like that of modern-day professionals, their conclusion would have been that his recovery was due to an inexplicable, spontaneous remission and definitely not due to the ministrations of a village lad. In science caution is essential, but un-inquisitive scepticism and prejudice so often contracts our vision and renders us blind to marvels. This was not so in the mining villages around Leeds. Word spread like wildfire. There was a young lad in Oulton who possessed healing power. Within days a 38 year-old woman came to him suffering from chronic oedema, generally known as dropsy. She had been receiving medical attention for the past two years. In an attempt to rid her of the excess fluid, her doctors had treated first her kidneys and then her thyroid with little success. At intervals during the following two months she received spiritual healing through the mediumship of William and by the end of that time her cure was complete. Again the word went forth and the flow of patients continued to increase. His successes multiplied and word of him spread, at first locally then further afield. Patients usually came to him at his home in Oulton, but often he would visit those who were too sick or infirm to make the journey. He did not charge for his services and this added to the pressure he was placed under. Over time, the cases he saw covered the entire spectrum of human suffering from the superficial and often psychosomatic to the most severe and destructive. Treatment was tailored to the demands of the case, sometimes mostly herbal, sometimes both herbal and spiritual healing and oft times in the more serious cases almost entirely through the 'laying on of hands.' And all the time William's knowledge was growing. From the very beginning, he was never just an attuned instrument used by others; with every patient he was informed by the voice in the pit of his stomach as to the cause of the disease, its characteristic presentation and its cure. Just as in the identification of herbs, the blue light was his pointer, highlighting enlarged tonsils with their infected follicles, pinpointing the ulcer on a cornea and drawing his attention to the thickened, rolled edges of a skin cancer – the spiritual light always attended by the voice, which explained to him the significance of what the light focused on.

My mother

In 1930, when William was sixteen, he met Nancy Overton, a very attractive girl of the same age with blonde hair, blue eyes and a slim, athletic figure, who lived in the neighbouring village of Methley. She came from a similar background to William being the daughter of a miner, but her parents, Cyril and his wife May, were better educated and rather more refined than the Lilleys. It was she who taught Bill, as she always called him, to stand up when a lady entered the room, to open doors for her and how to lay a table. Her Yorkshire accent was far gentler than his, and she soon set about changing his vowel sounds and getting him to stop dropping his 'aitches'. However, of greater concern to her, coming from a strict Methodist upbringing, were the stories that she had heard about him being a Spiritualist, talking to spirits, going into trance and healing people by touching them. It sounded like hocus-pocus or black magic to her, and smacked of the Devil. But her heart was smitten, and in giving him a chance, while she sought to change his ways, she was inevitably and constantly exposed to the gratitude and testimony of the many villagers and others he had helped. She began to realise that "her Bill" was a truly unusual young man with remarkable gifts. Despite his local reputation, he remained diffident and unassuming. Nothing in his temperament or behaviour made her doubt his kindness, his sincerity and his determination to heal the sick. She was touched by the stories he told her of his experiences and his vision of life after death, a perspective that far outreached the limited, superstitious, doctrinal beliefs of the church and the dire picture it painted of original sin and the fiery torments of Hell. The weight of evidence she was exposed to transformed her thinking; the process quickened by her love for him and the fact that his entire nature was so perfectly in accord with the path he was walking.

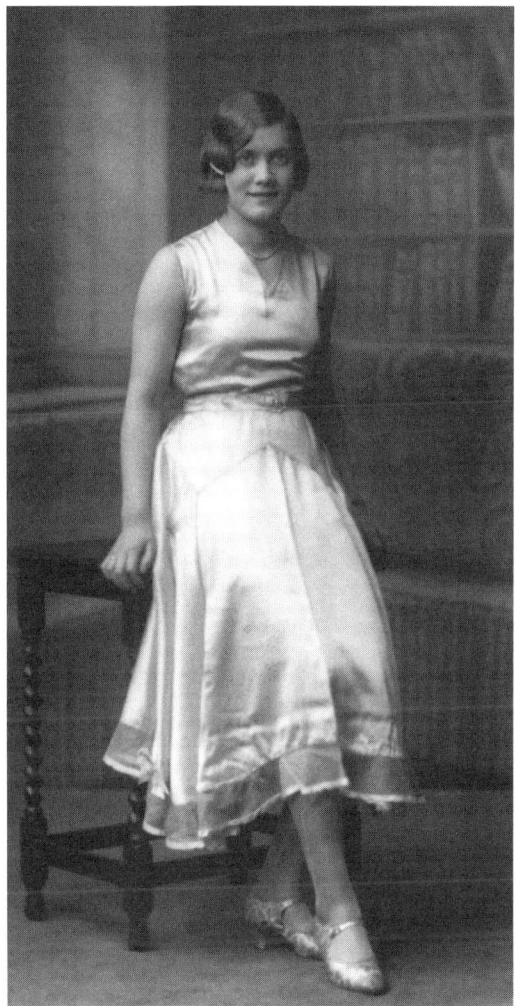

Figure 12.2 Nancy – my Mother – at 16 years old

Eventually, came the evening when for the first time she made acquaintance with the beautiful spirit who inspired William, Dr Letari. Before her eyes, she witnessed the transformation of the youth she now knew so well into another being with different facial expressions, different posture, different gestures, who spoke with a gentle Indian accent, utterly devoid of Yorkshire overtones and who above all addressed her with the wisdom and words of a sage. She knew she was in the presence of a superior being who radiated power, composure and empathy. It was a meeting she would always cherish. By then, she and Bill were deeply committed to one another. "The Doctor," as we most often referred to him in later years, welcomed her as a daughter and gave her insights into the very unusual and special life that lay ahead for William and herself. He emphasised the important supportive role she was destined to fill – a role crucial to William's success. At this sitting, the first of innumerable private and family sittings conducted during my father's life, he gave her the spiritual name that she was known by in the world of spirit; a name she carried from life to life. He never addressed her by any other.

A team

Their courtship years coincided with the Great Depression of the early 1930's, which particularly hit the north of England where the heavy industries such as coal mining, steel and textiles were situated. Times were extremely difficult and unemployment soared. Money was tight and I recall my father telling me how he would often only have sufficient money to buy a single Woodbine cigarette at a time. However, both he and my mother were fortunate enough to be employed. Nancy worked as a seamstress during the day at Joseph May and Sons, the clothiers and tailors on Holbeck Lane in Leeds and William worked night shifts, 5.30 p.m. to 5.30 a.m., at the Yorkshire Copper Works on Pontefract Road, at last earning a modest, but independent income. This difference in their working hours, which made the short periods they could be together even more precious, did provide one practical advantage. When he emerged from the factory in the morning, in winter before first light and often in the cold and dreary wet, though weary from the physical exertion of drawing and turning heavy copper and brass tubes throughout the night hours, William would make off into the countryside to collect the herbs he needed. These he would leave with Nancy, to whom he had taught the process of cutting, cleaning and curing herbs. In the evening, on her return from the textile factory, she would attend to this work assisted by her mother, who by now was fully committed to the young man who was obviously going to be her daughter's partner through life.

Marriage

In 1936, the year of King George V's death and the abdication of King Edward VIII, Cyril Overton, my maternal grandfather died of a heart attack while lying on his sofa in the lounge to which he had retired to ease a bout of "indigestion", which had halted him in his tracks while gardening. He was only 46 years of age, but had worked underground since childhood, at the coalface, often in dangerous 'wet mines,' standing in icy water for hour upon hour, always at the mercy of rotting timbers and corroding metal supports. He was by all accounts a gentleman, and, unlike my paternal uncles, sadly out of place in the rough, tough world of the collieries. Pressure of circumstances had forced him into a mould for which he was ill-suited and this undoubtedly contributed to the depressions that afflicted him over many years. This sudden event moved the young couple to bring their marriage forward, a decision they had delayed because of the difficult times. It now made good sense to pool their resources and move in with Nancy's mother at her home at 4 Appleyard Buildings in the village of Methley, West Yorkshire. They married on 1st August 1936; William was 22 and Nancy 21.

Non-stop industry and 'time-out'

This was a time of hard physical labour and intense preparation, both mentally and spiritually. It is a tribute to his vitality and inner drive that William was capable of achieving so much in so short a time; working long, strenuous hours at the factory, collecting herbs, studying with his spirit guides, administering healing and addressing Spiritualist groups while entranced by Dr Letari, and still finding time for his family. To top all this, his great love of music, lead him to join the Yorkshire Copper Works Brass Band in which he played the cornet. This was a serious commitment because the band, which was first formed in the early 1930s, was sponsored by the industry and was highly competitive, participating in many brass band championships each year. Band practice was held three afternoons a week and each practice session lasted two hours. As demanding as this was, he found playing the cornet very relaxing, for it provided much needed 'time-out', and he was proud of his prowess with the instrument. By the time he left the band, he had advanced to solo cornet.

The cures he affected lead to ever more patients approaching him for help; soon it was no longer practical for him to continue the time-consuming search for herbs along the local hedgerows. Besides, his expanding knowledge and experience, and the diversity of conditions that challenged him, demanded the need for a wider range of herbs than were accessible to him in this way. It became necessary for him to purchase the remedies he required from the local herbalist. The funds to do so came largely out of his own pocket since he was still not charging for treatments. Fortunately, he was assisted by the donations of the few grateful patients, who were suffering less from the dire, financial times.

The first press report

There was an onward driving force in the affairs of my father that never tarried. News of his healing work had thus far spread only by word of mouth, through the testimony of those whom he had helped. In May 1938, a wider audience was suddenly made aware of William's gift when *The Greater World*, a Spiritualist newspaper, founded to promulgate evidence of 'survival after death' and 'spirit return', featured him in a leading article. William, who was now 24, had been invited to attend the second anniversary service of the Castleford Spiritualist Church by a close friend and staunch Spiritualist, Mr W Brown, who lead a development circle at Normanton, which William had first attended some three years before. Brown had subsequently interested himself in William's work and had been a source of both spiritual and material support to him. During the service, Mrs H Ward, a seasoned clairvoyant and president of the congregation, noticed from the platform that the 'psychic aura' surrounding the young man in the audience was remarkably strong. After the meeting, Brown introduced William to Mrs Ward, explaining that the young man wished to become a member. She welcomed him with open arms.

During the next healing circle, held every Friday night under the guidance of Mrs Ward, Dr Letari 'came through' and after giving a prayer in Hindustani, which brought in a "wonderful influx of spiritual power", proceeded to make diagnoses and give treatment to patients who were present. This proved a revelation to Mrs Ward. As she expressed it:

> . . . by means of their X-ray vision, the seat of the patient's trouble is immediately located.[2]

At such sittings, diagnoses of cancer and tuberculosis were made and subsequently corroborated medically. Mrs Ward was enthused by what she had witnessed, and when Mr JB Nilan, a *Greater World* missionary, took services at the Castleford Church, she seized the opportunity to introduce him to the young medium she had taken under her wing. This led to an interview with William that resulted in the full-page article that later appeared in the periodical. When asked how his healing work had begun, William told of the two cases already described and in addition spoke of a case of diverticulitis which proved intractable to orthodox therapy, but responded well to herbal therapy over a period of six months. He also gave an example of spiritual diagnosis made by Dr Letari. The man in question was in the terminal stages of an undetermined disease. His son approached William for help. William visited him and in trance diagnosed cancer of the prostate with secondaries to the lumbo-sacral area of the spine. The patient's disease was too far advanced for successful treatment, either spiritual or material, and the very next day he was taken to the Leeds General Infirmary where he died shortly afterwards. Post mortem examination proved Dr Letari's diagnosis to be correct. William went on to speak of his inspirers and how they were able to make diagnoses and determine treatment through *psychometry*. All that was required for this 'psychic reading' was something the patient kept close to them. From this object, often a garment or an item, such as a comb, which carried an energy pattern derived from its owner, the guides were able to analyse the patient's emotional and physical state.

> I have had handkerchiefs from all over the country sent to me. All I need with the handkerchief is the patient's age. I can then give a full diagnosis and prescribe treatment. Many of the patients cured by my guides I have never seen personally.[2]

When asked about his own personal psychic powers as distinct from those demonstrated by his guides when he was entranced, he explained:

> During the first two years of my mediumship, I was clairvoyant, but I have almost lost this gift because, as my guides inform me, the power is needed for healing.[2]

What he failed to mention was the fact that his clairaudient ability, the faculty by which he could hear the words of his guides, had increased over the years rather than diminishing, and this sensitivity he retained for the rest of his life.

On request, William passed a number of recent testimonials he had received from grateful patients to the paper for inclusion in their article. Among them was one he particularly treasured because it came from Mrs Westmoreland, his development helper and the mother of his first patient. She and her husband wrote from Oulton:

> We are writing to you in appreciation of the wonderful recovery of our boy. It really seems too good to be true that our boy, after suffering for the past two years from nephritis, should be now in good health. To you and your inspirers we are deeply indebted for the happiness you have brought to our home, and we pray that you may be allowed to carry on your good work for many years to come.[2]

The article, which was entitled *Accurate Diagnoses By Castleford Healer's Guides*, concluded by informing its readers that when Mrs Ward visited the *Greater World* sanctuary to take the week-end service, she had personally vouched for Mr Lilley and spoke highly of his mediumship. A small, recent portrait photograph of a well-dressed William appeared at the top of the page with the caption, *William Henry Lilley*, beneath it.

Diagnostic ability tested

This article had far reaching consequences. Within months it transported William from village life to the nearby city of Leeds and made it possible for him to resign from the Copper Works and devote the rest of his life to diagnosing and healing. A Leeds businessman, who had been a committed Spiritualist for 35 years, read the story and knew from his previous experience with psychic phenomena that, if accurate, the report revealed a level of mediumship that was both extraordinary and rare, and deserved investigation. He approached a number of friends who shared his interest in the paranormal and they decided to approach the young medium with the purpose of putting his gifts to the test. Many years later, when my father related these early experiences to me, which he did many times, as I never tired of questioning him and always wanted him to tell the story again, he told me how anxious he was when he received the invitation to demonstrate his mediumship. Would he be able to go into trance, would Dr Letari be able to come through, would his guides be able to diagnose to the satisfaction of his examiners? No matter the experience, no matter the previous success, no matter the trust – at such times of trial how natural it was for him to be only twenty-four years of age, a young man untried in the ways of the world, unsophisticated and daunted at the prospect of exposing himself and his precious gift to the scrutiny of influential business men. In the event, he and his inspirers passed the test with flying colours. The group had gathered together a number of articles belonging to individuals suffering from a diversity of ailments, none of whom were present.

> The ability, then made apparent, to diagnose distant patients merely from an article supplied, made a tremendous impression.[3]

Arthur Richards

The businessman, a metal merchant, recognised the imperative need to foster William's remarkable gift and make it available to a wider public. For this, substantial sponsorship, expertise and assistance would be required. Through his work and his membership of the Freemasons, he was acquainted with a certain Arthur Charles Richards, or ACR, as he was known to business colleagues, the 42 year old chairman and managing director of a prosperous concern manufacturing piston rings in Hunslet, Leeds. This was an industry of prime importance in 1938, when the storm clouds of imminent conflict hung over Europe. Apart from his wealth and business acumen, Richards was not a natural choice for what the businessman had in mind. He was essentially a pragmatic, successful and materialistic man of the industrial world, and in his rise to fortune had never given thought to the existence of dimensions other than the physical, or perturbed himself with questions about the ultimate reason for life and the possibility of continued existence after death. Nonetheless, as it turned out, the businessman could not have chosen a better person with whom to share the excitement resulting from his recent experience of William's mediumship and his urgent desire to find a means of promoting him. Having reached the top in his profession and with the infrastructure and personnel in place for the continued success and smooth running of his affairs even in his absence, Arthur Richards had been searching in vain for a new challenge or philanthropic interest. Despite Richards' initial scepticism, the intensity of his friend's enthusiasm awakened his curiosity, and he immediately expressed a desire to meet Lilley.[3] In doing so, he was about to profoundly change his own life and that of William.

Medical proof

Characteristic of the man, Richards was not satisfied to simply accept the testimony of others, he needed to put the medium to the test himself lest he become involved in something that might prove spurious and an embarrassment. He concluded that the best way to proceed was to involve the medical profession in testing Lilley's diagnostic abilities.

> With Lilley's approval, he invited two well-known Leeds doctors to meet the medium, bringing with them complete diagnoses of three of their patients. These were contained in sealed envelopes and were seen neither by the medium nor his guide. The sole source of help available to the medium were three articles, one belonging to each patient – a bandage, a penknife and a comb.[3]

What followed astounded Richards and confirmed what he had been told by his friend. William was a psychic prodigy. The clinical diagnoses of the absent patients corresponded accurately with those of the doctors, but in addition Dr Letari provided in each case more detail regarding the true causation of the pathology and supplied symptoms that the patients were experiencing, which had not been noted in the case details, and explained their significance. In evaluating the cases, he laid stress upon the importance of both the emotional and physical symptoms in recognising and understanding the unique nature of the patient's condition rather than limiting the diagnosis to the common symptoms of a clinical condition or a Latin name. He spoke strongly against the common medical practice of assigning patients to specific disease categories and tailoring treatment according to diagnostic criteria instead of considering those symptoms and signs, which delineate the patient's unique individuality in order to determine the correct therapy.

In diagnosing one of the patients, Dr Letari, the spirit doctor, was in adamant disagreement with his living colleague. After holding the bandage that the doctor had provided, he diagnosed the presence of a serious growth with complications and added the following symptoms: pressure to the head; visual weakness; nervous debility; gastric acidity; and pain extending from the centre of the abdomen below the stomach to the spine. Asked where the growth was located, the spirit doctor answered that it was a malignant growth seated in the liver with a secondary growth in the lung. The doctor, limited by the diagnostic procedures available to him in the 1930s, told Dr Letari that X-ray had revealed a growth in the chest, but not in the liver, though he conceded that X-ray would not necessarily detect a liver tumour. Dr Letari insisted that the lung was not the primary seat of the condition and that although the lungs were certainly not healthy, the prime cause lay in the liver with secondary invasion of the chest. He added that if the doctor should "follow the advice of my mediator the condition of the growth will be eased, if not cured. I will show you the power of the spirit." The doctor replied, saying he would "think about it."[4]

Dr Letari then spoke for a while on the topic of cancer. Although speaking in 1938, his observations remain pertinent today. He warned that orthodox medical science cannot cure cancer. It may suppress and control, but cannot cure. He stressed that cancer is the end result of previous changes in the state of health, either emotionally or physically, and often both. Even constipation and chronic inflammation could be forerunners of malignancy. These warning symptoms and signs must be recognised by 'material doctors' at their onset and treated curatively and not by suppression, if cancer is to be prevented. The process of healing is then relatively easy. Unfortunately, most material doctors fail to detect and heal the pre-cancerous phase and by the time malignancy is discovered it is already too late.

At this point, the doctor who had submitted the case for diagnosis reiterated his conviction that the patient had carcinoma of the bronchus, but admitted that no method of curing such a case was known. Dr Letari disagreed with him on both counts. He reiterated that the seat of the trouble was the liver and went on to say that he would like to meet the patient and administer spiritual healing because the material world was unable to understand the process necessary to effect a cure. In order to resolve either malignancy or advanced tuberculosis the combination of spiritual and material healing was essential. Orthodox medicine was not curative medicine, because it lacked the essential spiritual element. With Paracelsian-like insight he stated: "There must be an understanding between God and yourself."[5] He concluded by saying he would welcome the opportunity to prove what the doctors of the Spirit could do. "In this case I can help. Will you consider the suggestion?" The earth doctor repeated his earlier promise to think it over. But Dr Letari's offer was not taken up. Within a few weeks, the patient 'died.' Post mortem upheld the spirit doctor's verdict that the cause of the problem was in the liver.[5]

Prior to considering the patient suffering from cancer, Dr Letari had already dealt with the other two cases, which were less serious – the first, an abscess to the neck and the second, a psychological case presenting with emotional problems. He emphasised that clinical diagnosis is always of secondary importance to the consideration of the past history and complete symptomatic picture of any patient. Without giving a name to the illness of either, since disease is essentially nameless, names only pertaining to the consequences of disease, he enumerated the symptoms experienced by each patient and highlighted the significance of a severe accident that the 'penknife' case had experienced some years before, and the presence of gynaecological problems, including a retroverted uterus, and sciatica due to spinal trouble in the emotionally labile 'comb' case. In both instances, these detailed pictures so accurately described the patients known to them that the doctors were left with no other conclusion but that, by some mysterious means, the young medium sat before them, in an apparently entranced state, was able at a distance to miraculously fathom a patient's state of health through focussing on an object which had been in their possession. They were deeply impressed. As an afterthought, and somewhat irrelevant after all that had been revealed, one of the doctors asked about a condition that had not been mentioned – the carbuncle on the back of the neck of the 'penknife' case. Dr Letari smiled and replied that it was superficial, not serious, and connected to the deeper symptoms he had given.

The doctors had nothing more to say. The experience had taken them into unknown territory outside their comfort zone and far beyond their medical understanding. They needed time to reflect on what they had witnessed. Whether this would make any difference to their future lives or their philosophy we will never know, but one would like to think that such revelations would someday have born fruit for their patients and themselves.

However, before the sitting was concluded, Richards had a last test for William. This time on behalf of a friend he had known for many years and whose condition was well known to him. He had brought with him one of her handkerchiefs. He was curious to know what Dr Letari would make of the woman's case.

Richards later related how Dr Letari's observations tallied perfectly with all the information he had been given and the conclusions of her doctors. On completing the diagnosis, Dr Letari offered to personally extend treatment to her. On this note, the momentous séance came to an end.

Unlike the doctor with his cancer patient, Richard's friend gladly accepted the offer of help. She had been ill for many years and was now confined to bed. The least effort precipitated attacks of angina. The condition was compounded by severe nervous tension and anxiety, which at its worst caused a generalised tremor of the body that would shake the bed.

Richards reported the visit of Dr Letari to this patient as follows:

> When the medium called on her, it was in the presence of four witnesses – the woman's husband, our friend the metal merchant, myself and one other. Lilley passed quickly into a trance. The patient was told to close the eyes and relax. The guide made a few passes over the body, immediately the nervous tension was arrested: the woman became as quiet as a sleeping child. The husband was amazed.[6]

After he had completed the 'laying on of hands,' Dr Letari announced that the woman would be completely cured within the space of three to four months. His prognosis proved correct.

Tubercular meningitis

There is perfect order in the affairs of humanity, both collectively and personally; nothing happens by chance; events which we sense as meaningful, but explain away as coincidence, are most often due to what Jung termed: synchronicity – the hand of destiny. This was evidenced as the governing dynamic in the life of William Lilley moved forward with the inexorable intent of enlisting Arthur Charles Richards in its objectives. As if to erase any vestige of wavering on the part of Richards, providence now provided him with final, conclusive proof of the immense power of spirit – a power capable of achieving the seemingly impossible. A friend of Richards was lying desperately ill in hospital. She had been diagnosed with tubercular meningitis, a frightening diagnosis even in these days, which if survived often leaves permanent damage to the nervous system. Only supportive therapy could be given. Richards brought Dr Letari three of her handkerchiefs, thinking, understandably, that for such a critical condition more than one would prove of greater assistance. The woman had been placed in isolation; therefore the healing had to be transmitted from afar by what is known as 'absent healing.' Holding the handkerchiefs while sensing their energy pattern, the guide stated that death was very close, but he would nevertheless do all in his power to help.

The following day, after a harrowing night during which the patient hovered on the brink of death, she had visibly rallied and the following evening, when a relapse was feared, instead of deteriorating, her condition held. Over the following days, her health slowly but steadily improved, and by the end of the week a blood test showed no trace of tuberculosis. Her improvement was so contrary to expectation that the doctors began to question whether she had ever had meningitis. They were perplexed. Soon afterwards, she was discharged from hospital with total absence of any residual consequences from her severe illness.

The House of the Ramasôye

Richard's life would never be the same; he had changed within the space of weeks from a pragmatic agnostic into a committed Spiritualist. He embraced the healing and teaching mission of the Ramasôye with all the vigour and drive that had brought him business success. To this end, he brought to bear not only his considerable financial means and those of certain business associates, but also his own personal participation in the work and the use of premises at his factory in Hunslet. Arthur Keith Desmond, who chronicled the early years of my father's healing work, dramatically described the scenario that had suddenly been created almost within the blink of an eyelid.

> Facilities were provided whereby in future Lilley could devote the whole of his time to healing. He gave up his work at the copper mills. Part of Richards's contribution was the provision of a healing centre. It was to be accommodated in his own premises at Hunslet. Piston rings would continue to be made on one floor; health would be restored on another. Strange amalgam, but it 'worked.' They said he was mad. They shook their heads. To mix business and religion (Spiritualism) was to court disaster – for the business. So they averred. But Richards looked neither to the right hand nor the left. He went straight ahead with his plans. And that was the beginning of The House of the Ramesôye.[7]

References

1   Desmond AK. *The Gift of Healing – The Story of Lilley the Healer*. London: Spiritualist Press; 1943. p12.

2   Anon. Accurate Diagnoses by Castleford Healer's Guides. *The Greater World*; May 14th 1938. p233.
3   Desmond AK. *The Gift of Healing – The Story of Lilley the Healer*. London: Spiritualist Press; 1943. p16.
4   *Ibid.*, p17.
5   *Ibid.*, p18.
6   *Ibid.*, p21.
7   *Ibid.*, p22.

13

THE SANCTUARY

Black Bull Street, Hunslet

On January 29, 1939, the Sanctuary, as it came to be known, opened its doors to its first patients. From the start it was not a trickle, but rather a flood of humanity that found its way into this most unlikely of havens set amongst the grime and gloom of industrial Hunslet, one of the least prepossessing areas of Leeds; a zone of soot, smoke and toiling machines, as far removed from a place of comfort and care as can be imagined. The address was 20, Black Bull Street, Leeds, 10.

This was the factory site of the Aero Piston Ring Company, of which Richards was the managing director, a hive of industrial activity, shortly to become a strategic asset in the defence of Britain, turning out piston rings for aircraft, tanks and other vehicles of war. The creation of the Sanctuary necessitated drastic changes to the administrative section of the building. On October 12, 1940, *The Greater World* presented a front-page article on the Sanctuary and its team of workers under the title *Business Man's Inspiration Over Spiritual Healing*:

> The ground floor of Mr Richards' factory is taken up with machinery, but running round part of the building is a gallery, out of which there are a number of rooms. These were occupied by managers and secretaries, but with the goodwill of all concerned, parts of the floor below were partitioned off for office purposes and the rooms above were converted into a beautiful Sanctuary, consulting and healing rooms. It is most interesting to go through the building, and to see how every corner has been utilised . . .[1]

Because of its situation, the main treatment or healing room became known as the 'Upper Room.' At one end was an altar draped with rich-blue, velvet curtains trimmed with gold braid and graced with silver candlesticks and a matching vase of flowers, giving the room an air of sanctity, appropriate to its purpose.

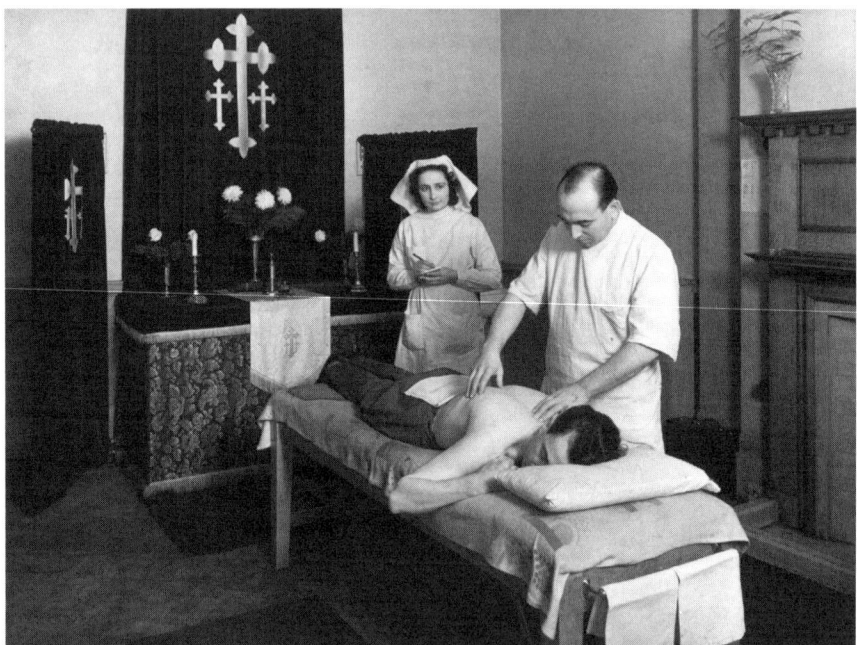

Figure 13.1 Dr Letari giving treatment at the Leeds Sanctuary (1938)

Consecration

It was in this special room that 16 people gathered on the memorable day when the Sanctuary was consecrated. On this occasion it was the Ramasôye who first 'came through' and bestowed his blessing:

> I dedicate this Sanctuary to God, that all who might pass through these portals at all times shall feel the blessing of the Spirit, that those who shall enter therein – the crippled in body or of mind – shall be uplifted in radiant health.
>
> In this small tabernacle of truth, two worlds are joined together in holy communion. The age of miracles is not past. Within each one of you is your own truth, and light, and power, and by your own seeking you can unfold that which will enable you to perceive that which is of God.[2]

The majestic language flowed on. He spoke of the need for understanding (knowledge) and faith (trust) in the pursuit of light (enlightenment) and stressed the vital principle, so often forgotten: "knock and it shall be opened" – i.e. the need for the disciple to initiate and drive the process of spiritual enlightenment and unfolding.

> And so you will realise that you must come to us before we can come to you.

Furthermore, he bade them come with the openness and susceptibility that is born of child-like innocence and a mind uncluttered by the hubris and materialistic values, prejudices and scepticism of the intellect. From such commitment and surrender, and the setting aside of the distorting filters of the ego-self (ego-personality), on-going attunement to the ways of Spirit rather than of humanity can be achieved, ensuring that by word and deed the aspirant is a vehicle for the divine plan.

> I say unto you that if you come as little children then it is that surely you can be blessed with the Spirit, and at all times will you dwell under the shadow of the spirit. Accordingly is it written that you shall do and speak as He would wish you to.[3]

He encouraged them to continue with the work of Spirit with confidence and pride, enriching the lives of others despite the enmity, prejudice and ridicule that opposed them.

> You know the happiness that you create; you know the love that you give to your brother or your sister: then, my children, go forward in this great fight, and, as I have told you before: 'Great things have I done but even greater things shall ye do'.[3]

The Ramesôye explained that behind the affairs of humanity, the creative influence and power of the spirit world presides and moves, working with patience over time to prepare and inspire initiates on the physical plane to fulfil their destiny through doing its bidding. This healing Sanctuary, "a creation of ourselves who are spirit," was evidence of this long term planning, to promote a healing wisdom, which would extend beyond time. Its walls were hallowed, sanctified by spirit to be a temple of love, bestowing truth and understanding upon those who passed through its portals and bringing about the healing of mind, body and soul.

The Ramesôye brought his benediction to a close using the masculine terms for the Universal Intelligence traditionally used by the faith of those present.

> I know the Lord our God has passed this way, and that his holiness and his Godliness is left in this room. So be it that here shall be always peace and love to one another. So, my children, I leave you. Farewell and God bless you all.[3]

After this "great person," as Dr Letari spoke of him, had departed, the doctor himself came through to say that he was "highly privileged" to be able to serve divinity in this Sanctuary of spiritual light. White Hawk, William's 'gatekeeper,' then brought the ceremony to a close with a prayer of thanksgiving. This dedication extended far beyond the Upper Room in the factory in Black Bull Street, which could only provide a temporary abode for the Sanctuary, to the future sites of the spiritual work of healing that was at the heart and soul of the mission initiated on the icy road to Kippax, fourteen years before. It encompassed all that lay ahead for the young medium and his inspirers.

A healing clinic

During the first weeks of the Sanctuary's use, patients received healing in small groups while they sat on chairs arranged in a circle in the centre of the room. Dr Letari would move from patient to patient applying both laying on of hands and more specific hand passes directed to affected areas, hardly touching the body at all, or, if so, with feather-like lightness. Helpers, like Arthur Richards, were needed as a source of energy and to give assistance. The helper would stand in front of the seated patient and hold their extended hands while treatment was being administered. Later, group healing of this sort was practised less frequently being replaced by private or family sittings, which permitted confidentiality and greater intimacy. This necessitated an adjoining room being pressed into service to accommodate patients waiting to receive treatment.

From its inception, the Sanctuary, under the personal guidance and instruction of Dr Letari, developed into a well-run professional clinic. During the healing sessions, a secretary was always present to record in shorthand all the comments of the doctor regarding the treatment and diagnosis of the patient and the advice given about diet, exercise and lifestyle. These notes were typed onto record sheets and alphabetically filed with all the patient details. All staff members were uniformed in white, and my father and his helpers wore the traditional long-white doctor's coats of the time, which were collarless and buttoned on the right from neck to shoulder and from beneath the arm down their entire length. Soon, an examination couch replaced the chairs in the treatment room, and later, a Zenith chiropractic couch was also installed; now a treasured heirloom, its ornately scrolled metalwork testimony to its age. Other essential pieces of diagnostic equipment became necessary and were acquired, such as: a stethoscope, a sphygmomanometer [for measuring blood pressure], an otoscope and an ophthalmoscope. Dr Letari instructed my father in their use.

To the laying-on-of-hands and transmission of healing energy through psychic means, Dr Letari added massage, percussion therapy and both chiropractic and osteopathic manipulative techniques. Initially, it was the doctor who administered these therapies, but in accord with his insistence that William was not just an instrument, but must master all modes of healing in his own right, Dr Letari tutored him in these physical disciplines until he was adept. The years of physical labour at the Copper Works, which had developed his strength of arm and his practical skills, together with an inherent sturdiness inherited from his mother, and his excellent sense of rhythm, honed by playing in the brass band, suited him for the work. The technique of percussion therapy applied by the doctor, and later by William, was a miracle to behold. Both hands were used with the precision and tempo of a drummer, the outer edge of the curled small fingers providing the instruments. The speed of movement can only be likened to that of the classical pianist playing a virtuoso work like Rimsky-Korsakov's *The Flight of the Bumble Bee*, a piece of music dear to my father's ear from having played it many times on the cornet. The hands were a blur as they directed their percussive energy to the site of treatment, usually the musculature along the spine from the base of the neck and the shoulders to the buttocks or concentrating on an acupressure point, organ dermatome or energy meridian. Despite the speed of impact, the depth and force of each blow was wonderfully controlled, stimulating, vibrating, stretching and loosening the underlying tissues without inflicting pain. In fact, to receive such treatment was sheer tactile pleasure, which, when sustained, induced profound relaxation and a desire to sleep. It could reduce minor spinal subluxations and provided ideal preparatory therapy when manipulation was called for. Within moments, a definite erythema, or flushing of the skin, would appear with a marked increase in local temperature. After such treatment, this outer glow was accompanied by an inner soothing warmth and sense of tranquillity. Remedies in ointment or gel form applied topically to the stimulated area, while still suffused with blood, acted more promptly and with greater efficacy (e.g. Rhus toxicodendron and Bryonia for musculo-skeletal conditions).

Homeopathic scholar

In the years prior to the meeting with Richards and the establishment of the Sanctuary, Dr Letari had already commenced teaching his young 'mediator,' as he always spoke of my father, the science of homeopathy, which he regarded as the most vital of all the disciplines essential and central to healing the sick. The doctor built this knowledge on the foundation of herbal medicine, which he had already laid. William managed to scrape together sufficient money from his limited funds to buy two pillars of homeopathic education: Clarke's *A Dictionary of Clinical Materia Medica* in three volumes and Kent's *Materia Medica*. Now, with the backing of Richards, he was able to purchase further textbooks on the subject, and he systematically began assembling a homeopathic library, which he expanded throughout his life. He obtained four of the major foundation works of the homeopathic materia medica: Hahnemann's *Materia Medica Pura* and *Chronic Diseases*, *Allen's Encyclopaedia* in ten volumes and *Hering's Guiding Symptoms*, also in ten volumes. These are vast compendiums of proving symptoms, which have stood the test of time and form the basis for all modern works. To these, he soon added the materia medica of Nash, Cowperthwaite, Farrington, Dunham and Hughes; the repertories of Bönninghausen and Kent; works on homeopathic theory: various editions of the *Organon*; the two *Lectures on Homoeopathic Philosophy*, one by Kent and the other by Close and the recently published, *The Principles And Art Of Cure By Homoeopathy* (1936) by HA Roberts – a book he highly valued.

He was neither a collector nor an accumulator; he was a consumer. I have his original copies of Clarke, their battered, bent and dog-eared state not due to age, but to the repetitious intensity with which he addressed them. That he read and studied them from cover to cover is clear from the extensive underlining of the text throughout in either pencil, or blue and red ink, depending on how he valued a line or paragraph, and the numerous annotations added from his personal experience. Passages of particular significance were highlighted by multiple lines and often by exclamation marks, inverted commas, asterisks and even margin lines or brackets, providing familiar signposts for frequent revisits. Looking at these books today, one is immediately impressed by the voracious appetite for knowledge displayed in their worn and weary pages, accentuated by the application of the underscoring without recourse to a ruler; waving, irregular lines employed with dash, enthusiasm and emphasis. He was a psychic who became a scholar, and through both gifts developed into an ardent homeopath. I recall the many beach holidays we spent as a family, when, enjoying time away from a busy practice, he would relax in his deckchair reading a book on homeopathy. He never read novels or magazines; a book by one of the masters always lay next to his bed, bristling with bookmarks.

Nor did he neglect the study of the basic medical sciences and the developments within contemporary orthodox medicine. His library reveals that he delved into anatomy, physiology, bacteriology, clinical diagnosis, internal medicine, gynaecology, abnormal psychology and psychiatry. His mind was curious, scholastically adventurous and intrepid. Like Isaac Newton, he wanted to know everything about everything, especially when pertaining to spiritual philosophy, human behaviour, understanding disease and investigating therapeutic measures. Undeterred by lack of formal education, he fearlessly strode forward to do combat with sickness on all levels, whether spiritual, emotional or physical. But, as he explained to me many years later, when I marvelled at the heights he had reached from such limited and humble beginnings: always, in times of doubt or concern, the voice of the beloved doctor would come to him from within with words of wisdom, advice and encouragement. He was never alone, never without support, and always had someone to consult – someone he trusted implicitly. He then always repeated what both he and Dr Letari had told me many times before: that the close relationship between spirit guide and physical medium, as evidenced in such a tangible form with them, was not unique, not exceptional, other than in the degree of its development and outward expression; that each one of us is never alone; that there are always unseen companions with us – those who are appointed to walk our earthly path beside us – our personal spirit guides – our 'guardian angels' – embracing and supporting us with their love – prompting us, alerting us, urging and inspiring us – and so often laughing and weeping with us. Our deafness, our blindness and our insensitivity to these subtle, beneficent influences that eternally enfold us, stem from the veils of conceit with which the false-self or ego-self cloaks the spiritual senses and lures us away from the contemplation of Reality to become seduced and mesmerised by the addictive distractions of the physical plane. Hence, the importance of the Ramesôye's words: "And so you will realise that you must come to us before we can come to you."

These words must be understood in the light of the above. Those of Spirit are always with us, their uplifting influence never leaves us, but just as we are always surrounded by unseen frequencies of sound and image but are unable to access them until we, of our own volition, switch on the radio or television and tune in, so we cannot fully partake of the richness of our dual existence as spirit and mortal beings unless we are willing to tune ourselves into the vast creative power that envelops and permeates us. This adjustment involves a conscious desire, a change of perspective and a determined commitment, which, as with all pursuits, if it is to bear fruit, must be vested with intent, focus, persistence and energy – only then will our eyes be opened, our ears unstopped and our senses attuned to the promptings and inspiration flowing from the spirit world.

The dispensary

With the therapeutic shift from the simple use of herbs to the far more complex art of homeopathic prescribing, a development that increased rapidly after the launching of the Sanctuary, it became necessary to create a dispensary. This was achieved by making yet another room available – this time on the ground floor. It was equipped with all the working surfaces, cupboards and shelving necessary for dispensing and storing remedies. Dr Letari was particularly exacting regarding the layout, lighting and hygiene of this tiny factory within a factory. A wide range of homeopathic remedies, ranging from mother tincture to the highest potencies, were ordered from A Nelson & Co's homeopathic pharmacy situated in Duke Street, London. To these were added the Schüssler range of twelve biochemic tissue salts, and the Bach flower remedies. Herbs, although now secondary in importance to the homeopathic potencies, were still stocked and dispensed in both dry and tincture form. Various herbal lotions and ointments were manufactured for topical use in the treatment of a variety of conditions such as injuries, burns, skin diseases, haemorrhoids, etc.

At the centre of this vital arsenal worked William Henry Lilley senior, newly retired from the coal mines; his pure white hair vying with the white of his laboratory coat, and both highlighting the fresh, cherubic pinkness of his skin, a quality retained despite being in his fifties and his long years spent underground; surely testimony to his abstemious habits, since, contrary to the times and his environment, both alcohol and tobacco were foreign to him. Pop Lilley, or simply "Pop," as he was known to all, had been enlisted when the pressure for prescriptions and their dispatch became too heavy for William and his small staff to handle. My grandfather took to the dispensary work as if it was his natural vocation. Taught by his son, in no time at all, he had mastered the concept of potencies, unerringly knew where every medicine was to be found, and became adept at hand potentising, dispensing pillules and granules and making ointments. He was an extremely fastidious man, probably his compensation for a lifetime spent in soot and grime. The exacting methods of correct homeopathic dispensing suited his taste for the meticulous and immaculate. As a young boy, I would spend hours observing him at work with his beloved remedies, fascinated how, perched on a small laboratory ladder, his miner's hands could reach behind the rows of small bottles he had arranged, like soldiers, in strict order of precedence, low potencies in front, high potencies at the back, and miraculously fish out a CM potency without the least disturbing its neighbours. His hands were so steady and sure, it was hard to believe that but a short while before he had earned his living wielding pick and shovel. My young eye was ever-captivated by the exquisite skill and infinite care with which he could coax a single drop of medicine from a small bottle between its loosened cork and the glass rim. The drop would hang there for a delicious moment before falling onto the white pills below and then, if called upon, I would see another slowly gather, swell, and then, as I held my breath, gently quiver before it too became independent and made the plunge; all the while, as grandpa's thumbs and forefingers wrought this magic, the remaining fingers of both his hands would be elegantly raised and spread like those of a society lady sipping her coffee from the finest china. It was he, and not my father, who first made me familiar with the names of the commonly used remedies, especially those occupying the lower shelves; the ones I could reach and bring to him.

The *Yorkshire Evening News*

But in 1939, my open-eyed wonderment was yet to come; at that time I was, as my grandmother told me, "still only a tiny star in the sky." During the early months of that fateful year, Black Bull Street was a hive of activity as all these developments were taking place. Even the ominous news coming out of Europe did nothing to weaken the endeavour of those involved or cause them to have misgivings about the future. The rate of growth of the healing centre was so remarkable that it soon drew the attention of the *Yorkshire Evening News*. A reporter was sent to interview William Lilley and this resulted in the first tabloid press report on my father's work. The article appeared on Friday, June 2, 1939.

> Sick people are flocking in hundreds to a spiritual healing sanctuary in a Leeds engineering works, where it is claimed that remarkable cures are being made of people who have been 'given up' by medical men. Today I went to the sanctuary, which is at 20 Black Bull Street, Leeds, saw the patients, the methods used and heard of their results.[4]

The reporter then went on to give details of the interview he had with Mr Tom Bailey, while his 25 year-old son, Jim, lay on the examination couch receiving "the ministrations of the healer, Mr William Henry Lilley." Jim had experienced an extreme fall some five years before, which had caused severe concussion of his brain. Since then, he had been suffering from nervous debility and mental illusions. Visits to specialists, neurologists, osteopaths and other therapists had brought no relief. The head injury had rendered Jim incapable of performing simple tasks. Bailey told the reporter:

> "Four weeks ago I brought him here, and after one treatment the improvement was absolutely wonderful. Since then he has done even better. This morning before we came here Jim went round to the garage, reversed the car out and brought it round to the door as well as, if not better, than I could have done it myself."

When asked how much the treatments had cost him so far, he replied:

> "The cost? Not a halfpenny. They won't take anything from me."

The reporter continued:

> This I was told, is the story told by many people who come to the sanctuary. And it is declared that some of them are people whom doctors have given up as incurable.
>
> The man behind it all, Mr Lilley, is a small, stocky, dark fellow of 25, who told me that he has been practising spiritual healing since he was 14 years old.
>
> "I want to make one thing clear – I am no different from anybody else, except that I happen to be a good medium for the healing power of the spirit world. We do not hold séances and manifestations. We believe that we are doing the work that should be done by churches of all denominations.
>
> A part of my work is diagnosis – by handling a handkerchief or some similar piece of clothing or article from the person who is ill. When I take it in my hands I can feel vibrations running up my arms and 'clairaudiently' I hear the voice of the spirit doctor telling me what to say. He also tells me what is the right course of treatment. I have diagnosed without that, however. Only last week a man in Leeds telephoned about his wife who was in London for treatment by a specialist and I was able to give my diagnosis."

William realised that this report in a leading Yorkshire evening paper would in all probability lead to an inundation of patients at a time when the Sanctuary was already stretched to its limit. He therefore told the interviewer:

> "We cannot deal with any more patients here for the time being, but that is no reason why people should not benefit from the spiritual healing power, which can best be described as the tincture of life."

He went on to explain about 'absent healing,' which was such an important element in the healing work of the Sanctuary. His words were recorded in the newspaper report:

> "If someone is ill, he should send us his name and address and age. Then we will put him on our 'absent healing' list. Then it is up to him. He should relax and make himself receptive either between nine and 10 in the morning or between nine and 10 at night or both.
>
> There is no need to come to see us at all, and they will be included in our prayers. We have between 4,000 and 5,000 patients on our absent healing list, and in addition we are doing between 300 and 400 diagnoses each week. Patients from all parts of the world have sent handkerchiefs and similar objects for diagnosis, and we are glad that we have been able to help many of them."[4]

This I was able to verify when many years later, in the course of my own practice, I came in contact with a number of my father's South African patients dating from that time, who had received their initial treatment from him by way of absent healing, and who gratefully spoke to me of the lasting benefit they had experienced. During the period of treatment, each patient would receive correspondence from my father explaining their diagnosis, the objectives of the treatment and how and when to make themselves receptive to healing. Advice would be given regarding the best diet for their condition, often accompanied by suggestions regarding their circumstances, and sometimes, when appropriate, words of counselling, frequently relevant to matters they had not divulged in their request for help, showing knowledge of facts only known to the patient or those close to them.

The article concluded by confirming the philanthropic nature of the services offered at the Sanctuary:

> Two or three Leeds business men were so convinced of the value of the healing work, and the real need that exists for such a sanctuary, that they are meeting out of their own pockets the whole cost of maintaining the sanctuary, and providing the simple remedies which are given to patients who are in need. The result is that the treatment is free and available to everyone.[4]

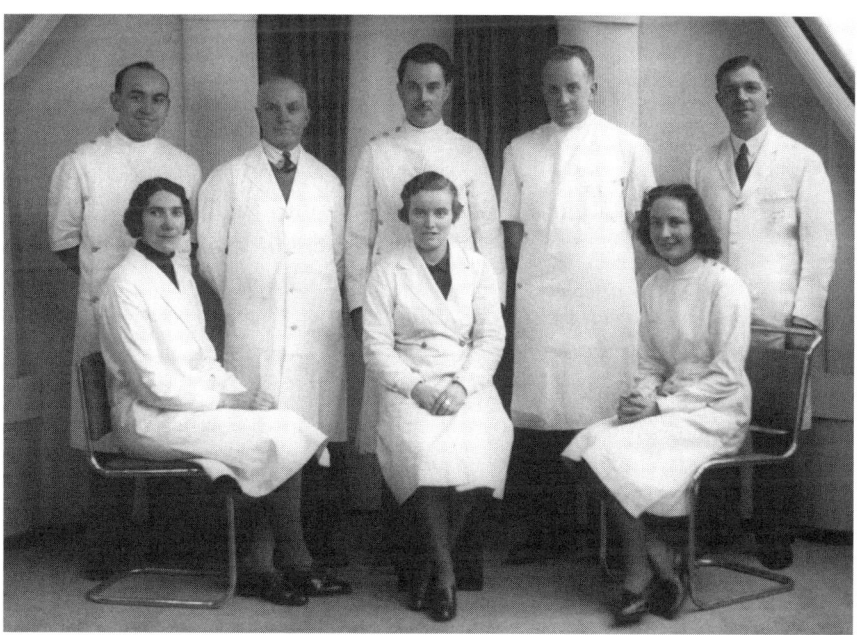

Figure 13.2 Staff at the Sanctuary, Leeds, 1939
Standing: William – William Henry Lilley (senior) – G Usher – A Halstead – Arthur Richards
Sitting: Miss Wilson – Annie Naylor – Joyce Curry

This newspaper article was soon followed by another, this time in the *Armley and Wortley News*, June 9, under the title: *A Hunslet Spirit 'Doctor.'* This was a shorter version of that carried by the *Yorkshire Evening News*, but my father was now described as "Mr Lilley, this exponent of medical science" rather than as a small, stocky, dark fellow.

Added, was an inventory of the Sanctuary staff:

> Mr Lilley's staff includes three doctors, five lady assistants, one receptionist and one dispenser in a highly equipped laboratory. Mr Lilley has taken 10 years to develop his powers and he is entirely vegetarian.[5]

These details, while evidencing journalistic idealism, certainly did the cause no harm. The three helpers, made up of my two uncles: Tom Lilley (William's eldest brother) and Wilfred Overton (my mother's older brother), together with a very close friend of Wilfred's, Arnold Halstead, had suddenly become doctors. The truly well equipped dispensary had become a laboratory and overnight my father had become a vegetarian, which for a young man who for the rest of his life would enjoy roast beef and Yorkshire pudding was purely wishful thinking.

The *Psychic News*

More important for the Sanctuary and William's future was the article that appeared the following day, 10 June, in the *Psychic News*, the influential and widely read weekly Spiritualist newspaper, which was founded in 1932 by Maurice Barbanell, Hannen Swaffer, a Fleet Street journalist, and Arthur Findlay, who was to become an important figure in the history of Spiritualism and psychic research. The details of the *Yorkshire Evening News* report were reproduced verbatim under the heading: *Doctors Fail, But Psychic Healers Cure – This 25-Year-Old Medium Now Has 5,000 Patients*. This was to be the first of many articles featuring William Lilley that would appear in the *Psychic News* over the following ten years during which the editorial staff followed my father's healing career in Britain. It would later lead to a meeting between William and Maurice Barbanell, who apart from being the editor of *Psychic News*, was the full-trance medium of the greatly loved spirit guide and teacher, Silver Birch, and the forging of a supportive friendship between the two.

The Sanctuary day

From the above details, some idea of the magnitude of what had been established in the space of a few months and the explosive nature of the public response can be gleaned. The day began early and often extended well into the evening hours. The five "lady assistants" spoken of comprised personal secretaries to William and Arthur Richards, two typists and a housekeeper. During the morning, the diagnosis and direct treatment of patients visiting the Sanctuary took place. This necessitated an almost constant state of trance for William, broken only for the mid-morning cup of tea and a cigarette (as incongruous as that now seems – but this was the age of the iconic Humphrey Bogart, spats, hats, braces, sleeve-bands and the inevitable cigarette – a world so brilliantly captured by the contemporary Scots artist Jack Vettriano – and William was no exception). The midday break involved a light lunch and often a relaxing interlude of table tennis. The afternoon would frequently commence with more live patients, but by mid-afternoon the team would begin the immense task of dealing with the vast correspondence that the Sanctuary generated. For William this would

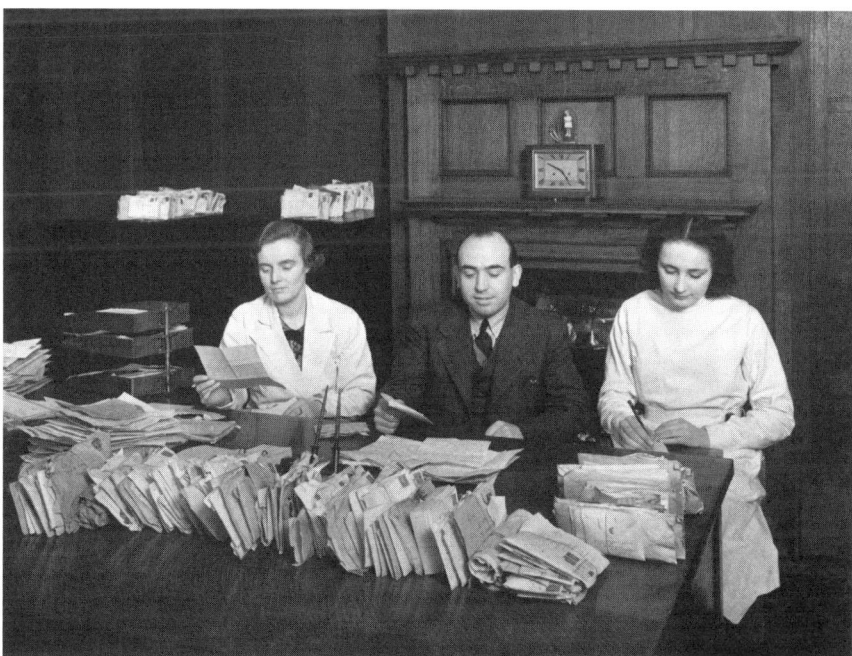

Figure 13.3 William and secretary, Annie Naylor, and nurse, Joyce Curry, dealing with correspondence and diagnosis, 1939. The bulky envelopes contain items for psychometric reading

involve further full-trance states for deep psychometric analysis of objects sent in by patients, or consciously working clairaudiently with his spirit guides.

Parallel to the essential psychic element of the afternoon shifts must be added the dictation of hundreds of letters to distant patients, all taken down in shorthand, since wire and tape recorders still lay in the future; a mammoth work which usually kept William, Richards and the secretarial staff busy until late in the evening; my mother saw very little of my father during these intensely busy times. On more than one occasion, the urgency of the cases needing treatment resulted in him spending almost twenty-four hours in and out of trance. Although William was astrally projected (out of his body) throughout this time, the strain experienced by the physical vehicle and its psychic centres during such prolonged periods of trance was considerable and would exact its toll.

The letters that poured in came from patients all over the world, but especially from the countries of what was then the British Empire and among these a significant majority were from the Southern African region: South Africa, South West Africa (later Namibia), Northern and Southern Rhodesia (later Zambia and Zimbabwe respectively). I knew this because I

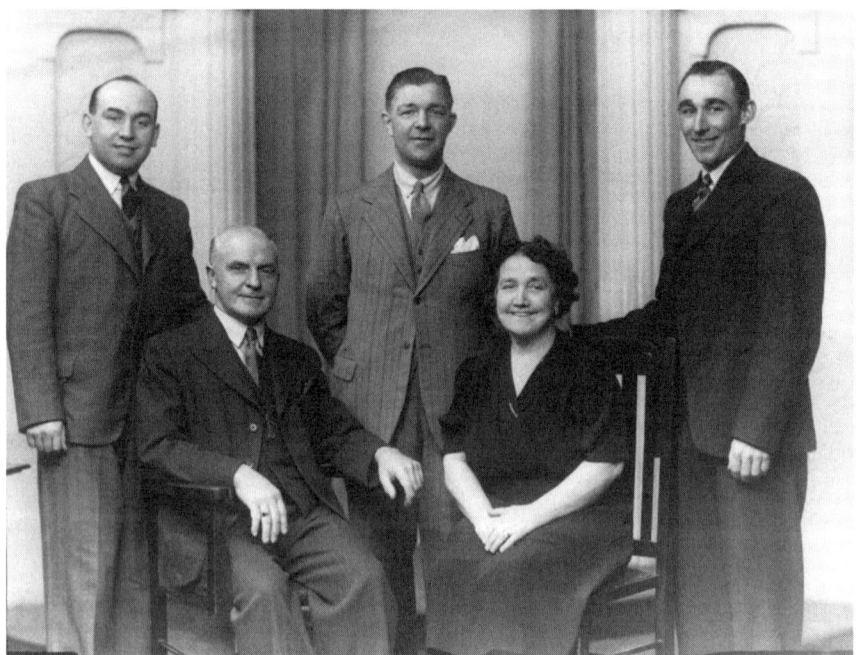

Figure 13.4 Opening of the Sanctuary, 1938
William – WHL (senior) – Arthur Richards – Sarah Ellen Lilley – Thomas Lilley

regularly and assiduously rifled the numerous waste paper baskets in search of stamps for my collection.

It will be realised from the nature and magnitude of the task and the need to extend absent healing to many thousands of patients that although Dr Letari was pre-eminent among my father's guides, a team of spirit doctors participated in the healing work. Dr Moy, Dr John and Dr Cerise are names known to me although I never met them. Knowing of these unseen, silent, dedicated beings, who healed so many through their compassionate ministrations, and transposing this awareness into our own lives, it is empowering to know that in all our endeavours, if they be wholesome and creative, there are always gifted beings close at hand who will prompt and inspire us. This process can be keened by our acknowledgement of their presence and our reaching out to them for assistance.

The mentor

Apart from the financial support that Richards provided, he was also personally involved in every aspect of the Sanctuary's smooth running. He helped with the healing sessions, was responsible for staff selection and management and controlled the administration of the Sanctuary. Through his years of experience as chairman and managing director of a successful engineering firm, he was perfectly suited for the role he played in creating a smart, efficient, well-run clinic, in marketing it and in promoting spiritual healing.

On another level, he was an important mentor to my father. An educated, polished, charming and influential man who moved confidently in the best circles, and a Freemason, Richards introduced William to a world with which he was quite unfamiliar. In acquiring social and business skills, William displayed the same eagerness and aptitude to learn and to adapt that he had shown under the guidance and tuition of his spirit inspirers. What they had achieved at the deepest level, Richards set about creating at an interpersonal and cultural level. The pupil proved so apt that it was not long before he equalled his master and eventually surpassed him. It began with designing an impressive signature and extended to the manners of good society, dress sense, the writing and answering of personal and business letters, professional terminology, managing subordinates, dealing with accountants, bankers, and the bureaucracy, business strategy, chairing meetings, correct speech and the art of public speaking; finally Richards introduced William to Freemasonry. The transformation from unseasoned, unschooled village youth to accomplished gentleman was so swift that it seemed Richards imparted nothing new, but rather released that which was inherent. William possessed an innate drive for excellence. If my father had a motto it was stated quite clearly on the inside cover of volume one of Clarke's, *A Dictionary of Clinical Materia Medica*, which he gave me on the occasion of my medical graduation. It reads:

> My son, may this book serve you well as it has served me, and remember above all: 'Only the Best is Good Enough!' – love Dad.

Words that echo down the years and in many ways sum up my memory of him.

This high aspiration found expression in his speech, his manners, his habits and his dealings with people. Later, when he had the means to do so, it would also be reflected in the clothes he wore. But in the 1940s, despite his celebrity, William was still a salaried man, working for the Sanctuary, which was a charitable organisation.

War!

Against a backdrop of heightened tension in Europe, and the increasing threat of war, work at the Sanctuary continued apace. For those involved, absorbed as they were in coping with the pressure of patients, the posturing and psychopathic raving of Hitler in Germany seemed distant and of secondary importance to their healing mission. Then, on the 1st of September 1939, Germany attacked Poland and two days later France and Britain declared war on Germany. With only a meagre volunteer force with which to face a highly professional German army, in October, the British government introduced conscription, announcing that all men aged between 18 and 41 who were not working in 'reserved occupations' [such as miners, farmers and utility workers] would be liable for military service. Apart from Pop Lilley, who was too old, and Richards, who was exempt, because his engineering firm was vital to the war effort, all the male personnel of the Sanctuary were eligible for mobilisation. The first group to be 'called-up' were those aged between 20 and 23. The next would be William's. Dr Letari had no doubt about the necessary course of action, the work of the Sanctuary must go on, his 'mediator' must appeal to the military tribunal for exemption on the grounds of the spiritual nature of his occupation and its importance to the nation. A healer could not become a potential slayer!

Conscientious objector

My father was aghast, the thought of becoming a conscientious objector when Britain was threatened by a bloodthirsty warmonger at the head of an enemy that had before, within the space of his lifetime, sought to bring Europe to its knees, was abhorrent to him. For the first time he rebelled against the advice of his beloved spirit mentor. As a boy, when spared the rigours of a miner's life through the intercession of his mother and Mrs Westmoreland, he had endured for a number of years the belittling remarks and sneers of others, and now he was being asked to yet again expose himself to further ignominy. All the past hurt of the sensitive adolescent and the memories it brought swept over him and he baulked at the thought. Could he brand himself a coward and brave being shown the 'white feather'? Could he withstand what he anticipated would be the sceptical and unsympathetic inquisition of the tribunal? In the face of his fears, Dr Letari remained adamant, but reassuring. He would be with William every step of the way and encouraged him: "Do not fear, all will be well." Nothing could endanger what had been set in motion from a higher plane.

Military Tribunal

During the many months of the 'phoney war,' which extended well into 1940, the Sanctuary established and confirmed itself as a centre for spiritual healing. The initial response to its opening was not only sustained, but increased both at home and abroad. On 10 May 1940, the strange calm of poised inactivity that had hung over Europe was finally broken by the German invasion of France, and the war began in earnest. A month later, on 4 June, the last day of the evacuation of British troops from the beaches of Dunkirk, William appeared before the military tribunal. The *Yorkshire Evening News* reported the event under the heading, *Leeds Objector Says He Is Healer, Not Killer; Tells of Sanctuary In Factory*:

> A 26-years-old Leeds objector, William Henry Lilley of Stainburn Mount, Moortown, Leeds, told the Conscientious Objectors' Tribunal at Leeds, to-day, that he was a 'divine healer,' who had been curing invalids since he was 15 years old.[6]

The article went on to relate that Mr AC Richards had appeared on Lilley's behalf and had vouched that he had been in daily contact with him for more than a year during which time the Sanctuary had been in existence at his factory. Richards spoke of the large number of patients seen weekly at the clinic and added:

> Many thousands scattered throughout the world are also receiving absent treatment and diagnosis – a great gift which Mr Lilley gives freely without thought of personal reward.

Under questioning, William was reported as saying that: he objected to military service because he could not destroy life. He was willing to help the country provided that killing was eliminated from his duties. Judge Stewart said that the Court would take William at his word and registered him for non-combatant services.

Mr EC Behrens (appearing for the tribunal) said:

> Mr Richards comes here with a mass of evidence as to this man's peculiar ability in a special direction. That has nothing to do with this tribunal at all. There is no reservation on the occupation of healers. It is his conscience we are concerned with, not his work.[6]

On the same evening, the *Yorkshire Evening Post*, in its report of the hearing gave a closing quip delivered by the judge who said that he did not suppose this method of healing would be one which would be set up in an RAMC (Royal Army Medical Corps) clinic![6]

As he had feared, William's conscientious objection made him the butt of vilification. He was mortified, more especially because much of the scorn and malicious comments that were visited upon him came from friends and relations. He never informed me who among the members of our family were guilty of this cruelty, but when speaking to me of these events many years later it was evident that he had been hurt to the quick.

Appellate Tribunal

Much had been achieved, but not enough. Dr Letari was not satisfied. Although his medium had been exempt from combatant service, if he was called up to serve as a non-combatant, which was very likely, given the besieged state of the land, then the work of the House of Divinity, the name now given to the Sanctuary, would grind to a halt. That could not be permitted. William's ordeal was not over, he must appeal against the ruling of the tribunal. His heart quailed. He knew that to achieve complete exemption his motives and character would be subjected to far more intense scrutiny. Dr Letari assured William that when the appeal was heard he would control him and address the tribunal.

The day for the hearing was set for April 3, 1941 at City Library, Manchester before a judge, Sir Miles Mitchell (a previous Lord Mayor of Manchester) and one other member.

My father was first to be called. He could well remember the questions asked and the answers he gave because during this part of the appeal he was not entranced. He was asked to explain the work that he did and particularly the process of absent healing, a concept that clearly perplexed the members. William told the tribunal that he had first become aware of his powers when he was ten years old and that his mother was similarly gifted. He informed them that everyone possessed the power of healing; it was not unique to him, but few were aware of it and even fewer could access it; hence there was a great need for such therapeutic help. He then explained how by psychometry he was able to diagnose a person's state of health from a handkerchief and determine the treatment they required even when the patient was residing in a distant country. All individuals differed from one another, even with regard to their fingerprints; duplication was never found. Likewise, each and every person radiated or transmitted vibrations peculiar to themselves. The handkerchief received with a request for diagnosis, held the vibrations of the sender, and it was from such vibrations that the patient was diagnosed and spiritually contacted.

The panel wondered why a spiritual healer should need to prescribe herbal remedies when he possessed such a powerful gift. William answered: "We are definitely spiritual healers, but the herbs of the field are God's gift, and we must make use of them."[7]

Richards was called to give evidence. He gave the tribunal members the patient statistics and stressed how many of the sick came to the Sanctuary after having unsuccessfully tried orthodox treatment. He confirmed what William had already told them, that the only fee charged was a nominal sum, introduced as recently as three months before, to cover the cost of medicines. He explained that Lilley had no thought of personal reward and he (Richards) counted it 'a great privilege to have supported him "with all my heart and soul and pocket." Richards was asked if Lilley should continue with his present work in the national interest and whether he regarded it as of national importance. He replied that he considered it of world importance. At this point one of the members interjected, suggesting that we should deal with this country first.[7]

When my father was recalled, Dr Letari, as he had promised, took full control of his mediator and answered all the questions posed. One wonders if the members of the tribunal noticed the change of manner, expression, accent and use of language in the young man appearing before them.

Unwittingly, they were witness to a marvel taking place before their very eyes – the full trance control of a physical vehicle, temporarily vacated by its owner, by a spirit being from a higher plane of existence, with the express purpose of persuading them to further the noble aims of unseen healers. With the advent of Lejan Tari Singh, the level of exchange between jury and defendant was lifted from the dock to the pulpit.

In his role as William Lilley, Dr Letari was asked by his interrogators whether it was not possible for him to continue to render the service of absent healing if he were in the army.

Dr Letari responded with an emphatic "No!" and then proceeded to elucidate the profound nature of the work that was being done through the Sanctuary; a work that was in essence a war against the human condition that leads to such catastrophic conflicts as that which now seized Europe.

> While we know that the Germans cause all this destruction, we cannot blind ourselves to the fact that such destruction was taking place in man's heart years ago, and this war is the manifestation of these conditions.[7]

He insisted that a wider perspective was essential when addressing the forces of adversity. While physical preparedness, defence and retaliation were critical for survival in a world beset by greed, envy and hatred, a parallel and subtler campaign against warped human thinking and feeling was imperative. War was symptomatic of a distorted or diseased state of the mind, which, though evidenced between nations, and more starkly conspicuous in the aggressor, originated in the hearts and homes of individuals on either side of the battle-line.

Of equal importance to defence by weapon and assault was the counselling of and ministering to the besieged, both spiritually and physically – therapy essential to the preservation of morale and the allaying of fear, stress and grief. This was the work of the Sanctuary, lead by its principal. Central to understanding both life and death was the certainty of a continuity of existence, unbounded by either.

> We must therefore look at it (the conflict) from an entirely different angle. There are men and women all over the world who have been suffering, not because of war, but because of some condition of disease – diseases not only of the body, but also of the mind. To those who suffer in this way I can bring light; I can bring the understanding that life does not end here.[8]

He went on to explain the perfect unbroken confluence existing between the physical and spiritual realms, which made spirit visitation a natural phenomenon, and spirit influence upon the living not only possible, but universal. He spoke of the continuity of life extending beyond the grave and how important the certainty of immortality is to those who suffer on the earth plane. Furthermore, he explained that even when spiritual healing was administered, success was not always possible:

> We cannot always heal the body or the mind in this material life, but if we do not, we at least have the satisfaction that comes of giving them an understanding of spiritual existence.[8]

He spoke of the need for treatment and counselling at a personal, one-on-one level regardless of absent healing being extended. While both forms of healing were of great value, for many the physical presence, touch and word of the healer was essential.

> I know that we pass to another life – a spirit life. This material existence is but an experience to give us a realisation of the future. Therefore, I help not only those who visit the Sanctuary, but those at a distance who have been cast aside, seemingly forgotten, with nothing to look forward to, nothing to live for. Those are the people to whom I give a realisation of the after-life.[8]

No written words can fully capture the power of the spoken word, nor, under circumstances such as these, conjure up the immense influence that is exerted when spirit directly addresses the divinity residing within us all regardless of the peculiarities and eccentricities of the ego-self that obscures it. We do not know what preconceptions or assumptions the members of the tribunal carried into the Manchester City Library with them on that day, but we do know that they were swept off their feet and that after a few minutes of conferring together, they unanimously pronounced that William Henry Lilley, the spiritual healer, be granted unconditional exemption from all military service because his work was of national importance.

On the next day, Friday, April 4, 1941, *The Manchester Guardian* carried a brief description of the hearing at the head of its list of appeals allowed by the Northern Appellate Tribunal. Under the heading, *A Healer*, the article reported that the tribunal had given unconditional exemption to a Leeds man described as a divine healer, whom Leeds tribunal had registered for non-combatant work in the Army.[9]

The Sanctuary in Hull

Three weeks later, April 26, the *Psychic News*, prompted by this unprecedented happening, devoted another full-page report to the history and work of Lilley and the Sanctuary. The article headline read: *Army Tribunal Gives Spirit Healer Complete Exemption*. The paper also reported the opening of a branch of the Sanctuary in Hull, during October 1940. This intrepid step had been decided upon soon after the first tribunal hearing and fully six months before the outcome of the appeal was known. Having no doubt that the result would be favourable, Dr Letari had pressed on with preparations for the clinic's opening, while calming the understandable anxieties of Richards and his fellow benefactors. Although the sanctuary in Leeds was doing great and valuable work, he knew that within a short time there would be an even greater call for help from Hull and it was with this in mind that he had urged his medium to create another sanctuary there.

Hull on the Yorkshire coast of North East England was a major and recurrent target of the Nazi German strategic bombing campaign. It was an important port and industrial centre and an easy target for the Luftwaffe bombers. It suffered heavy bombing raids between May 1941 and July 1943, so much so that half the population were rendered homeless due to bomb destruction or damage. Much of the city centre was destroyed and heavy damage was inflicted on residential areas, industry, the railways and the docks. The blitz of Hull was second only to that of London in intensity.

It was into this beleaguered city and port haunted by air-raid sirens, the drone of bombers and the death and devastation wrought by the multiple impacts of high explosive and incendiary bombs that Dr Letari and William came to speak words of comfort, 'lay-on-hands' and administer small, white homeopathic pills for trauma and stress. At first their visits were limited to once a week, but with increased need for assistance this was doubled. The address of the subsidiary Sanctuary was No 7 Chariot Street, Hull – a distance of some 60 miles (96 km) from Leeds; even in these days a considerable journey to travel back and forth.

> Here was an extensive building replete with cubicles, medical apparatus, and all the equipment that experience in Leeds to date had found to be necessary. They took the whole three-storeyed building on a seven years' lease. Contiguous was a health food store . . . where patients who were put on diet could obtain the prescribed foods. The whole was very beautiful.[10]

As ideal as these premises were and as noble and altruistic as the work was, nevertheless, the Sanctuary was at the mercy of an enemy that had Hull fixed in its sights. In May 1941, the Germans were preparing to launch their attack on the Eastern Front and regarded Hull as a potential, key supply port for Russia. Their intention was its utter destruction. On the dread nights of the 8th and 9th of May, two of the heaviest air raids of the Hull blitz shook the populace. The Sanctuary received a direct hit and was totally demolished. Fortunately, the raids were at night and my father was in Leeds. Undaunted, within a week of this setback, Richards and William had opened new premises at No 100 Park Avenue and found a small shop in the centre of the city from which they could continue to carry on the health food service. The last of the heavy raids on Hull was on 18 July 1941 and although raids continued sporadically until the end of the war, the Hull Sanctuary survived and kept its doors open.

My birth

It was into this frenetic and at times harrowing scenario that I was born on 2 August 1940 in Moortown, Leeds. Although my father always tried to protect my mother as much as possible from direct involvement in the many adversities he encountered throughout his career as a healer and homeopath, nonetheless, their relationship was so close and her intelligence and interest in his work such that she was unavoidably party to all that he went through. She had absolute trust in the wisdom of Dr Letari, but fully understood that despite his overshadowing and guiding presence in our lives, events on the earth plane had to play out according to a universal plan, and could be painful. Her pregnancy was fraught with the stresses of impending war, its outbreak, unfamiliar circumstances, my father's call-up and conscientious objection and his absence both physically and mentally as he plunged into the never ending work of study and healing. Shortly after her delivery came the fear for his safety in Hull and the bombing of the Sanctuary there. Through all of this, she never faltered either as wife or mother, remaining a sure haven and support for my father every step of his way.

Cheltenham – Tudor Lodge

In October 1941, twelve months after the opening of the House of Divinity in Hull, Dr Letari cast his eyes further afield. The intensity of the air raids on Hull had eased and the work in the Hunslet factory was flourishing. He now wished to broaden the therapeutic base of the Sanctuary, always working towards greater use of homeopathic remedies in the healing of patients, both emotionally and physically. Over the years that lay ahead, he would steadily shift the emphasis in his mediator's healing work from a primarily psychic to a primarily homeopathic approach, while retaining his clairaudience and his extra-sensory capacity to diagnose by psychometry. For the further training of William's homeopathic skills, Dr Letari now required a facility that could offer after-care for those who needed it, accommodation for difficult cases that required close observation and an environment conducive to the treatment of cancer patients. Richards proposed Cheltenham as an ideal location.

Cheltenham is a large, rural spa town situated in Gloucestershire in the South-West of England on the edge of the beautiful Cotswold range of hills. It became a health and holiday resort after mineral springs were discovered there in 1716. The Sanctuary was kindly offered accommodation in a spacious house, Tudor Lodge, part of which was already being used as a Spiritualist church. The vacant section provided ample space for the proposed nursing home. With their usual attention to detail and excellence, Arthur Richards and William, under the guidance of the good Doctor, set about creating yet another house of healing, but this time with the possibility of having beds for a limited number of in-patients. Arthur Keith Desmond, the journalist who wrote *The Gift of Healing*, which chronicled my father's life up to 1942, was one of the first patients to stay a number of weeks at Tudor Lodge. He had been approached by *Psychic News* to provide the newspaper with an article about 'Lilley's ministry.' He was welcomed as both guest and patient. Apart from receiving physical and spiritual therapy for his ailments, the time he spent at Tudor Lodge afforded him the opportunity of interviewing Richards, my father and Dr Letari and observing the methods of treatment used in the clinic. He responded well and problems, which had resisted the attention of his conventional doctors, were resolved. The various forms of material therapy that were used to supplement spiritual healing intrigued him, especially the osteopathic, chiropractic and percussion therapy that were administered to him. Discussing these methods with William, Desmond posed a question that many have asked: 'Why should a spiritual healer need to use material methods?'

William replied:

> Let us assume that a patient comes to us with a displacement of the bones of the foot, or of the spine or shoulder. Possibly after one or two months under spiritual healing, the joint will be realigned. But why not manipulate it into position in two to three minutes and then apply spiritual healing to those tissues or organs where neither medicine nor physical healing can produce a cure?[11]

He went on to explain that homeopathy, biochemistry (Schüssler tissue salt therapy), chromotherapy (colour therapy) and osteopathy (manipulative therapy), were all necessary to alleviate and cure and did so because they applied definite laws of healing, which were universal. All such methods should be regarded as being essentially spiritual – as they had to be if capable of removing disease, suffering and despair. By comparison, much of the mental and physical suffering experienced by humanity stemmed from wrong and wilful use of powerful chemical drugs, which drove the effects of disease inwards.

Asked why he should expend so much time and trouble studying homeopathy when his spirit guides and helpers could transmit healing power in an instant and over great distances, William replied that it was the knowledge and power of homeopathy that needed to be passed on to his successors in healing. His mediumship had been developed to prove the truth of life-everlasting and the intimate interplay that exists between the spiritual and physical domains and to do so through acts of spiritual healing performed by spirit physicians. This had been planned by the Ramasôye and others for the specific purpose of not only bringing this vital knowledge and comfort at a time when the world was torn by strife and carnage, but also to promote for the future needs of humanity those forms of healing that were vehicles for spiritual healing; homeopathy being central to this endeavour. Whereas, his gifts, though natural and common to all, had, like a concert musician's, been honed to a degree of fineness possible to few, the gift of homeopathy and its kindred therapies could be passed on to many. There use would always be overshadowed by the healing power of spirit.

Colour therapy

At Tudor Lodge, Dr Letari had the opportunity to develop the application of chromotherapy, or healing the body by the use of colour, to a deeper level than had been possible in Leeds or Hull. It became and remained an important element in my father's analysis and treatment of patients. In his physical life, Lejan Tari Singh was a Brahmin, a member of the priestly or highest class in Hindu society. He spoke Sanskrit and was versed in the teachings of the Vedas, the oldest Hindu sacred texts, and the practice and philosophy of yoga. Allied to these teachings and disciplines was understanding of the chakras: the seven major energy centres of the subtle body (the soul, or intangible counterpart of the physical body), which vitalise, influence and control the functions and form of the physical body. As we shall consider in volume two, the energy frequency of each chakra is represented by a specific colour, with which it resonates and which it radiates.

These radiating colours are visible to the clairvoyant eye as the human aura: a nimbus or rainbow of colours, which surrounds and extends beyond the physical body like a halo. Emotional and physical dis-ease always has its origin in the energy system of the body (even when triggered by some impingement from without) and involves a change in the ordered function of the chakras, which is revealed by colour changes in the aura. Dependent on the profile of the disorder, one or other of the chakras will show a disturbance in energy frequency and this becomes visible in an alteration in the intensity and purity of its associated colour in the aura. From such changes in the radiation of the aura, the trained clairvoyant is able to make a chakra diagnosis of the patient's condition and monitor the effects of therapy. It has been found that the iris of the eye similarly provides a template for the diagnosis of emotional and physical disease.

Dr Letari regarded colour interpretation and colour therapy as of great importance. He considered colour as one of Nature's most powerful symbols through which she expresses unambiguously clues to her hidden power, nature and intention. Red, for example, pertains to the lowest and densest energy centre of the body, the root chakra and therefore represents the basic instincts of survival and propagation – animal aggression (flight or flight) and sexuality. At an organ level it represents the heart, the arterial system, the blood and all organs with a surfeit of blood, such as the spleen and thyroid. The red berries of the hawthorn (*Crataegus spp.*) indicate their value in the treatment of cardiac disease when the heart muscles are weakened; the red hourglass vividly displayed on the ventral abdomen of the black widow spider points to the value of its venom in the homeopathic treatment of angina (heart pain due to impaired blood flow). Red also stands for passion, anger and fever.

Likewise, our emotions are esoterically and idiomatically entwined with colour. Most of us are aware that colour elicits an emotional and often a physical response from us. We are drawn to certain colours and averse to others; some colours lighten our spirits, some have a depressing effect upon us; some of us prefer pastel shades, others need vibrant colours; some colours relax us, some cause agitation. When angry we see red; when depressed we have the blues; envy turns us green; indignation is purple; when cowardly we are yellow-bellied; and white or grey show our fear or anguish. Colour and our inner lives are entangled. When we are able to recognise a specific chakra predominance in a patient's symptomatic picture or by the organs primarily involved in their disease state, or see a strong relationship between the patient's emotional temperament and the emotional affinities of a colour, then specific colour therapy based upon this relationship often proves remarkably curative, or acts as a facilitator for the action of other therapies. Used in this manner, colour has a homeopathic effect. In volume two and subsequent books, I will have the opportunity to consider the interpretation of colour and its therapeutic uses in detail.

In Cheltenham, the windows of each patient's room had a section into which a pane of glass of the required colour called for in the patient's treatment could be inserted. Day patients would be exposed to colour rays appropriate to their emotional or physical condition for varying periods of time. Arthur Keith Desmond was treated with orange, which is the colour of the second or sacral chakra, for his chronic spinal problem. Sent to the nursing home as a reporter, Desmond left as a convert.

> For six weeks I lived in a rich, spiritual atmosphere. In a house of peace. A house where God's work was being performed. A house where the spirits came and healed. A house that left its mark on all who entered, and why not? For it was a different house . . .[13]

While the reporter's turn of phrase and rather florid journalese invariably made my father uncomfortable, and he never felt entirely at ease with the book Desmond wrote about him, despite its overall accuracy (I suspect it offended his modesty), one could never doubt Desmond's sincerity and commitment to the cause.

Today, through the insight, enthusiasm and enterprise of Ambika Wauters in Colorado, USA, a homeopath, psychotherapist and healer, originally from the north of England, we possess all the major colours in homeopathic potency. Focusing specifically on the colours of the chakra system, she captured the imponderable energy and essence of each colour by exposing an inert carrier medium (distilled water) to rays of light passed through a filter of the chosen colour. The colour-saturated water was then preserved by the addition of alcohol and run up into potency, or dynamic form, in the customary manner. Ambika has written a book on homeopathic colour therapy: *Homeopathic Color Remedies*, in which she details their relationship to the chakras, their individual qualities and case examples. It is a valuable book about an important subject.

From our earlier contemplation of the action of remedies in potency, it will be apparent that treatment by colour in potentised form must prove more deeply curative, when selected appropriately, than exposing patients to the prolonged effect of coloured light. But, in 1941, it was all they had, and it worked!

Bigotry

One cannot imagine a more relaxed and harmonious environment, ideal for convalescence and retirement, than Cheltenham, especially at a time when the Continent was seething with violence. Here, unlike Hull, there were no targets for *Luftwaffe* bombers; it was a haven of peace. However, bureaucracy is ubiquitous and when so far removed from the influence of a worldly metropolis is likely to be highly conservative, especially in the face of controversial, unorthodox activities. Such was the situation in

Cheltenham. When all was in place and functioning admirably, the Sanctuary's application to run a nursing home was peremptorily refused. City Councillors, the Clergy and the local medical fraternity had made common cause against Lilley and it was rumoured that the Cheltenham Woman's Knitting League, indignant at the 'goings-on' at Tudor Lodge, had thrown their not inconsiderable weight behind the decision. On inquiry into the possibility of the decision being reversed, the applicants were sternly informed that it was "unlikely to be varied."

Arthur Richards, never one to be daunted by authority, then engaged a matron and a nursing sister, both registered nurses, in addition to three assistants brought from the Leeds and Hull Sanctuaries and forthwith appealed to the local Council for a further hearing. The request was granted and William and Richards yet again faced interrogation by a committee, on this occasion made up of representatives of all three elements of their opposition – two Councillors, the local Bishop and two medical doctors. Their tone was hostile, suspicious and inquisitorial. Searching questions were asked. "How did Lilley heal? How long had he been healing? Why did he need a nursing home? Why pick on Cheltenham? What nationality was Lilley?"[13]

As we have previously recorded, the press had described William as a dark, short, stocky fellow. At that time, my father was 27 years-old, five-foot six-inches tall, muscularly built, particularly in the chest and arms, slightly overweight with a full face strengthened by a remarkably noble, Roman nose and a dimpled chin. His hair, which was pitch black, like his mother's, was rapidly receding, but this loss was compensated for by a virile amount of hair elsewhere and a fierce pair of the blackest eyebrows. His mouth was generous and his intelligent, hazel eyes were warm, and often twinkled with the mischievous humour, which so delighted and charmed his patients. He was often mistaken for a Greek, an Italian or a Jew.

Apparently, in Anglo-Saxon Cheltenham, in 1941, a foreign cast of countenance was already reason for suspicion of villainous intent. The information that he was a Yorkshire-man somewhat allayed their fears.

The doctors on the panel tried to trip William on his medical knowledge and failed to do so; Dr Letari's training of his pupil, William's avid reading and the past years of intense experience proved more than adequate for the occasion. Secular scrutiny having failed to unseat the presumptuous young man, the Bishop took over as interrogator, taxing him on spiritual grounds, querying his ability to cure by absent healing. William replied by carefully explaining to this man of God the dynamics of the spiritual realm, his psychometric and clairaudient gifts and the imminence of our companions of spirit. The pompous prelate then asked him why, if he could cure by absent healing, he needed a nursing home at all. When in response, William inquired of him, if he, the Bishop, when ill would believe he could be cured by absent healing, he retorted:

"Certainly not!"

"Very well" replied William, "it is for people like you that I require a convalescent home!" Deflated, the Bishop retired from the fray.

The Councillors were interested to know about the financial soundness of the House of Divinity. This was Richards' domain. He explained that it was a non profit-sharing organisation, any monies accrued being put back as capital. From this money and funds guaranteed by certain benefactors the cost of founding, equipping and maintaining the nursing home were funded.

Their next question was regarding how many patients Lilley had and how many were currently receiving treatment. They nearly had a fit over his answer, for he said that they had 20,000![12] The Bishop was outnumbered and Tudor Lodge received its licence.

Desmond summed it up:

> The three of them had walked in and upset the decision which was 'not likely to be varied!' Yes *the three of them*, for the good Dr Letari was there, too. 'I shall be with you,' he had said on the eve of the hearing. 'All will be quite well.' That is how a bit of history was made in Cheltenham on December 10, 1941.[12]

The call of the Capital

For all the energy and money put into this project it proved to be short-lived. Within a few months the accommodation at Tudor Lodge became inadequate to cope with the number of patients and the associated administrative work. The space occupied by the Spiritualist church was not available to them and the building on of annexes was too uncertain in wartime, due to lack of materials and labour. The option of finding larger premises locally was considered, but eventually discarded. Though reluctant to leave the restful surroundings of Cheltenham, which had proved so ideal for their mission, in March 1942, 'The Three' decided that since a move was unavoidable, it should be a decisive and long-term one, and one which would place the Sanctuary at the very heart and centre of British life. Undeterred by the bombing of the capital, which was intense, they headed for London.

References

1. Business man's Inspiration Over Spiritual Healing. *The Greater World* (646); October 12 1940. Frontpage.
2. Desmond AK. *The Gift of Healing – The Story of Lilley the Healer*. London: Spiritualist Press. 1943. p28.
3. *Ibid.*, p29.
4. "Spirit Doctor" Guides Cure Of Sick In Leeds Sanctuary Of Healing. *Yorkshire Evening News*; Friday, June 2 1939.
5. A Hunslet Spirit "Doctor." *Armley and Wortley News*; Friday, June 9 1939.
6. Leeds Objector Says He Is Healer, Not Killer; Tells Of Sanctuary In Factory. *Yorkshire Evening Post*; Tuesday, June 4 1940.
7. Desmond AK. *The Gift of Healing – The Story of Lilley the Healer*. London: Spiritualist Press. 1943. p33.
8. *Ibid.*, p34.
9. A Healer. *Manchester Guardian*; Friday, April 4 1941.
10. Desmond AK. *The Gift of Healing – The Story of Lilley the Healer*. London: Spiritualist Press. 1943. p35.
11. *Ibid.*, p42.
12. *Ibid.*, pp44–45.

14

THE MOVE TO LONDON

Consultations in London

The final decision to relocate to London was preceded by preliminary healing visits to the capital to test the waters and pave the way. The first of these was in the third week of January 1942. Arthur Keith Desmond kindly offered William the use of his flat. This afforded the journalist further opportunity to observe the healer at work. He reported this important extension of my father's work under the heading *Famous Healer Plans A London Sanctuary* in the January 31st edition of *Psychic News*:

> Lilley's personal healing mission in London has begun; 'personal' because he already had many absent healing patients in the metropolis and Greater London. Last week in a small flat in Central London, Lilley of Leeds sat and talked with men and women whom he had earlier diagnosed and prescribed for from a distance.... Let us follow Lilley-in-London and see what more we can learn of the methods of the medium and his spirit guide. What is the object in travelling 180 miles from his headquarters to talk to these grateful people? To check over the symptoms, and, in the light of his discoveries, to make any necessary changes in the medicines they are receiving – that is the main object.
>
> Symptomatology, he calls it, and there are no half measures about it, I can assure you. His thoroughness would be an object lesson to many doctors if only they would watch him. The patient is questioned and cross-questioned until every possible symptom is extracted from him. By the time Lilley has finished, he has filled the greater part of the specially printed case sheets that are part of every patient's file.[1]

Over the years, in addition to his intuitive and psychic perceptions, Dr Letari had developed William's abilities in homeopathic case taking, patient observation and analysis. The homeopathic consultation is the most searching of all medical interviews, structured to reveal the unique emotional and physical characteristics of each case, enabling the physician to find the closest possible match between remedy and patient. Dr Letari regarded homeopathy to be just as vital to the healing process as was spiritual healing. Under Dr Letari's tutelage, as well as through his own assiduous studies and his constant exposure to clinical situations, William had achieved a level of homeopathic expertise, which enabled him to analyse and assess a patient's emotional and clinical condition and devise an appropriate treatment regime independent of his spirit guides.

The diagnostic observations of the 'good Doctor' would be dictated clairaudiently to William and added to the homeopathic history of the patient.

> The better part of half an hour is spent thus with each patient; each without exception goes away immensely cheered and confident from their initial contact with the healer. He has brought fresh hope into their lives and been able to promise many of them a cure.[1]

After the consultation, for cases requiring direct 'laying-on-of-hands', Dr Letari would take over the treatment.

> When Lilley is entranced for treatment, always three, often four, spirit helpers accompany the 'dead' Doctor Letari. I asked Lilley where these stood in relation to the patient. At the head and foot, he replied, and on either, or both sides.
>
> When . . . Dr Letari turns his head to one side or the other in the course of treating a patient, he is actually turning to make some communication with these helpers from the Other Side whom neither you nor I can see.

This communication, which I often witnessed, was not audible, but telepathic and accompanied by an expression or gesture appropriate to a 'silent' instruction or comment he was imparting.

> But whether it is this simple action, or the replacement of a vertebra, or the breaking down of a lesion, or applying the incredibly fast percussion treatment to the patient's back, or picking his way about the room, not once while he is entranced do the medium's eyes open. Dr Letari can see better that way than you or I possessing normal earth vision![1]

He might have added – or when looking at an X-ray, or reading a medical report, or reaching for a stethoscope – because with eyes closed, Dr Letari was able, under any circumstances, to see and function unerringly like a sighted person. Only when he appeared on behalf of my father in court did he keep his mediator's eyes open.

Keith Desmond then went on to mention an essential component in psychic healing:

> Like the spirit helpers at these treatments, another invisible yet indispensable accessory is the psychic rod. This is a kind of ectoplasmic link between spirit guide and patient.[1]

William had told him that recently Dr Letari had been treating a man suffering from paresis (paralytic weakness) of the leg at Tudor Lodge.

Working with ectoplasmic stimulation of the semi-paralysed muscles he was able to temporarily restore movement, so much so that the limb which had been long inactive, kicked upwards with such involuntary force that it struck the entranced William a sharp blow on the arm and temporarily severed the ectoplasmic or psychic rod that was being used therapeutically; the abruptly withdrawn energy caused superficial burning of William's arm.

Ectoplasm

The term ectoplasm used here to describe undifferentiated, primal matter must not be confused with the biological definition of the word, which relates to the outer part of the cytoplasm: the jelly-like substance that fills the cell membrane and holds the sub-structures or organelles of a cell. Ectoplasm in the psychic or spiritual sense refers to the highly charged energy-substance that bridges the interface between energy and matter. It is a universal field of invisible, intangible, formless spirit-matter of the subtlest form, which can be used by spirit scientists as an instrument for influencing change on the physical plane. It can be manipulated with greater skill and precision than a laser beam or a surgeon's scalpel during psychic operations and can be materialised in varying degrees of density to give temporary physical form to a spirit entity that animates it. Being pluripotent (like the biological stem cells of the body) it can differentiate and diversify into any of the substances and forms of the material world and particularly any of the body tissues. Usually manifesting ephemerally at the will of spirit for a particular purpose and resorbing back into its undifferentiated, potential form when released from this control, ectoplasm can be congealed into a tangible, sustained form which is then subject to the forces of the relative dimension: death, decay and disintegration. Materialised ectoplasm is sensitive to bright light and if touched without warning, as William experienced, withdraws into the medium with such implosive energy that injury can be sustained.

Materialisation

Certain full-trance mediums have the power to be used by spirit guides as a channel for ectoplasm, which can be drawn from them to materialise and give transient form to a deceased soul. Such psychics are known as *physical* or *materialisation mediums*. The purpose of such a manifestation is to bring solace to the bereaved and to give irrefutable proof of life after death and continuity of existence. Whereas, ectoplasm is generally invisible other than to clairvoyant vision, depending on the development and sensitivity of the medium and the skill of the spirit scientists responsible for achieving the phenomenon, this energy-matter can be rendered more dense, becoming not only visible and recognisable as being the image of a loved one, but providing a temporary vehicle for the discarnate spirit to use for movement, expression and communication. Such advanced mediumship is extremely rare. Because this subtle matter is seen extruding from a medium's body, usually issuing from the mouth, the term ectoplasm (from the Greek *ektos*, meaning 'outside', and *plasma*, meaning something formed or moulded, which combined denote: exteriorised substance) was coined by Charles Richet (1850–1935), a French physiologist, who won the Nobel Prize in 1913 in recognition of his work on anaphylaxis, and who, in his later years, became devoted to the study of spiritualist phenomena. In 1905 he was elected president of the British Society for Psychical Research (SPR).

Helen Duncan

An exceptionally gifted materialisation medium was Helen Duncan (1897–1956), born Helen MacFarlane in Callander, Perthshire, Scotland. From an early age, she evidenced psychic awareness of future happenings, often dire and fearful, which distressed her Presbyterian mother, who urged her to keep her visions to herself, lest she be thought to be under the influence of evil spirits. Inevitably, rumours about her occult powers circulated, which together with her retiring nature and strangely contrasting capacity for aggressive hysterical behaviour, made her one apart in the community; an object of either fear, awe or scorn. At a time when everyone around her thought the 1914 war would be over in a few months, this sixteen-year old prophet of doom foretold that it would drag on for years and cost many lives. The slaughter that followed resulted in widespread increase of interest in Spiritualism through the hope it offered bereaved families of making contact with those they had lost.

In 1916, Helen, who already had a baby daughter, married Henry Duncan, a cabinet-maker from Dundee, who had been posted back from the front after developing rheumatic fever, which had left him with a damaged, heart valve. Due to Henry's weakened state of health and lack of work and Helen's repeated pregnancies, the Duncans were soon struggling financially. Encouraged by her husband, Helen started to augment her earnings at the local bleach factory by giving clairvoyant readings. Her success persuaded Henry that her mediumship could be developed much further and a home circle was established for this purpose. By 1926, her psychic gifts had so advanced that while under the control of her spirit guides, under séance conditions, she was able to manifest ectoplasm, which materialised from her mouth in an amorphous stream of luminous matter and would then build up into the recognisable form of deceased persons. Her controlling spirit guide was Albert Stewart, a tall, slim, well-spoken gentleman who had drowned in 1913, at the age of thirty-three. In stark contrast, Helen Duncan was five foot six inches (1.68m) tall, extremely obese and spoke with a very broad Scots accent.

A paradoxical psychic

To this day, Helen Duncan's remarkable mediumship remains a source of controversy and dispute. At its best, it was extraordinary and gave comfort and solace to many; at its worst, it had all the trappings of vaudeville and clumsy conjuring. Her gift was both her triumph and her tragedy – her pride and her shame. She and her spirit helpers achieved a degree of spirit materialisation, which was second to none and brought her fame, but it also brought high expectations and pressure to perform, which her deteriorating state of health could not support. In the early days of spiritualism, the late 1800s and early 1900s, much like operatic sopranos, it was thought that successful physical mediums, who were invariably women, should be of ample proportion, their bulk rendering them better able to provide the energy necessary for materialisations. Unfortunately, in the case of Helen Duncan, obesity and its complications contributed to her downfall. In all, she bore eight children, of whom only six survived childhood. She suffered from high blood pressure and chronic kidney disease, which caused pre-eclamptic fits during childbirth and eventually, in the early 1940s, she developed diabetes. She was a gross woman – coarse of speech, appearance and habit and notwithstanding her ailments remained undisciplined in her eating, she also smoked and was at times a very heavy drinker. The extreme demands of her exacting form of mediumship placed such toll upon her ailing and abused body that her gift was jeopardised and whenever it failed her, she apparently resorted to dissimulation. Spirit materialisation is a phenomenon particularly open to deception and conjuration; muslin, stockinette or cheesecloth concealed in or on the body providing an ectoplasm lookalike. Spiritualism had often been brought into disrepute by fake mediums, charlatans preying on the need and gullibility of the public, but unlike other mediums suspected of fraud, Helen Duncan was very high profile. In her case, the law reacted punitively.

A threat to national security

Helen's first brush with the law was in Edinburgh, in 1934, when she was found guilty of affray and fraudulent mediumship; he was fined £10 or one month in prison. In 1944, a more serious charge was laid against her, aggravated by the fact that she was seen as a threat to national security because at a séance in 1941, she had revealed that the warship HMS *Barham* had been sunk, months before this loss was officially announced. At a time when the invasion of Normandy was imminent, the authorities were alarmed that she might somehow have access to classified information and divulge it. On 19 January 1944, police raided the séance she was holding in Portsmouth. Allegedly, they found her compromised in faking a materialisation and arrested her under the Vagrancy Act of 1824. However, this was a minor offence and the authorities needed a more serious crime to restrain and silence her. Legal research revealed that by invoking the archaic Witchcraft Act of 1735, Helen could be tried before a jury for fraudulent 'spiritual' activity with the possibility of a prison sentence.

The trial, which took place at the Old Bailey, created a great stir in wartime London. In a tedious, drawn out affair, witness after witness appeared on behalf of Helen, testifying to her authenticity. Many of those called by the Defence were educated, articulate and prominent members of society, but it was all to no avail. It was as if the die had been cast even before the trial commenced. Counsel acting for Helen Duncan, requested that she be given the opportunity to demonstrate her powers of mediumship to the jury in a private séance as part of her defence against being found fraudulent. The judge refused her permission. Helen Duncan was found guilty of conspiracy to contravene the Witchcraft Act and sentenced to nine months imprisonment, which she spent in the notorious Holloway Prison. She was 46 years of age. By the time she was released in 1945, the allied forces were well on their way to winning the war and she was no longer deemed a risk to the war effort.

News of this outlandish trial came to Winston Churchill's notice and he felt obliged to give comment. On Monday, 3 April 1944, he sent the following caustic request to the Home Secretary, Herbert Morrison:

> Let me have a report on why the Witchcraft Act, 1735, was used in a modern Court of Justice. What was the cost of this trial to the State, observing that witnesses were brought from Portsmouth and maintained here in this crowded London for a fortnight, and the Recorder kept busy with all this obsolete tomfoolery, to the detriment of necessary work in the Courts?[2]

Helen Duncan was a paradox; a woman of unprepossessing habit and manner, loved by few and revered by many, yet gifted beyond the normal and sadly guilty of squandering and disgracing that gift; an unstable, immature soul filled with fear and uncertainty, yet one who brought consolation and comfort to so many. In mitigation, she was literally destroyed by the pressure placed upon her by Spiritualists who clamoured for more and more séances, more and more materialisations until she grew exhausted. Those who should have protected her were weak and probably like Helen, who had known poverty and hardship, became greedy for money and complicit in her simulations. I cannot comment on how much of her work was authentic and how much was fraudulent, but I can relate what transpired one night at a public séance in Doncaster, near Leeds, in the late 1930s.

Materialisation in Doncaster

My father, my uncle, Wilfred Overton, and Arthur Richards were invited to attend a Helen Duncan séance to be held at the nearby Doncaster Spiritualist church. Because of William's renown in the Yorkshire Spiritualist world and the respect with which he was regarded, he was asked with the help of Richards to ensure both before and during the séance that there could be no possibility of fraud. To this end, he examined Helen thoroughly and satisfied himself that she was not hiding anything on her person that could be used to fake materialisation. He escorted her to the cabinet which had been installed in one corner of the séance room and assisted in securing her wrists and ankles to the heavy chair in which she sat. Richards conducted an equally thorough search of the cabinet and its surrounds. Satisfied that all was above board, the three representatives of the Sanctuary sat close to Helen so that no one could approach the medium without them being aware of it. The red light that was used to illumine the room was sufficient for the sitters to witness phenomena, but dim enough to encourage trance, protect the medium and permit the visual manifestation of ectoplasm.

The first materialised figure to appear after Albert, the medium's guide, had opened proceedings was that of a clearly defined, short, elderly man who at first seemed disorientated and perplexed at finding himself in a dimly lit room and an object of interest to a group of silent, unfamiliar people. After Albert had courteously explained to him where he was and the purpose of the sitting, he relaxed and appeared to enjoy the attention he was receiving. He gave his name as James Wright, and with a marked Yorkshire accent told the sitters that he was a miner and that he had died the previous day and believed that he was to be buried on the morrow.

My father who was sitting close to him asked Albert if he might touch James. Albert graciously gave his permission. The consent of those controlling the materialisation was very important. William knew that if he touched the former miner without warning, the spirit helpers would not have time to stabilise the ectoplasm, which would flash back into Helen, causing her injury. He cautiously reached out and gently took hold of James' arm. It was warm and firm and replete with life. Whilst thus engaged, he studied the man's features closely and even in the dim, red light, to which his eyes had grown accustomed, noticed something highly characteristic, often seen in men who worked for years at the coal face and sustained injuries: a deeply etched scar across his forehead; a scar which in that light seemed highlighted with black, but which William knew would be the dark-blue of ingrained coal dust. William asked James where his body was lying prior to burial and the deceased miner gave the address of his home, which was not far from where the séance was being held.

No sooner was the séance brought to a close than William and his companions took leave of their hosts and hastened to the address that James had given and despite the lateness of the hour knocked upon the front door. The sad features of the lady who answered the door clearly told them that they had found the correct address. Though surprised and somewhat taken aback by the unexpected visit and their questions, she responded willingly: yes, she was Mrs Wright, her husband had died the day before and his body was still lying in the upstairs bedroom. William respectfully asked if she would mind their having a look at her husband, for if he proved to be the person they anticipated, they had wonderful news for her. They followed her up the narrow stairs to the bedroom above. William approached the bed and at his request Mrs Wright switched on the bedside light. There lay James Wright, cold and inert in death, though they had spoken with him but a few hours before. Across his forehead was the collier's scar that William had noted, with its tell tale blue highlighting exactly as it had appeared at the séance. William thanked the good widow and explained why they had taken the liberty of disturbing her. She looked at him, at first in disbelief, and then, recognising his sincerity and concern, in wide-eyed amazement as the realisation of her husband's complete continuity of existence dawned on her. Tears of joy mingled with her tears of grief and there was a visible lightening of her burden of bereavement. After sharing a cup of tea and a few more words about the small miracle that had taken place in Doncaster, her visitors departed, warmed by her grateful thanks for the blessing they had brought her.

Many years later, I recall my father, during the course of a lecture, recounting the cure of a young girl suffering from juvenile rheumatoid arthritis. It had been a difficult and aggressive condition, taxing his skills to their limits. The memory of the responsibility he had born in advising the parents to avoid the use of steroids (cortisone), in the face of medical opinion warning them that without such treatment their daughter would suffer permanent damage to her affected joints and be crippled, prompted him to say, with great emotion, that if he had been born to achieve only that single success in his practice of homeopathy, he would not have lived in vain. Similarly, in the case of Helen Duncan, that most inappropriate of mediums, whatever her history, one can say that if it were only for the materialisation of James Wright on a certain night in Doncaster, her gift was not in vain. His widow's grief was assuaged, and my uncle, Wilfred Overton, testified to me, all of forty years later, that the experience of that evening proved transformative for him. Although his previously narrow, world perspective had expanded vastly since meeting Dr Letari, the Helen Duncan séance added the priceless experience of tangible and incontrovertible proof of survival after death.

* * * * *

8/10 Bulstrode Street

The site chosen for the new nursing home was a large five-story house, one of a row of similar houses lining both sides of Bulstrode Street in Marylebone, Central London; the number on the door, 8/10. Today these houses have all been replaced by modern structures, which possess none of the distinction of the original buildings with their handsome doors, charming bay-windows, steeply pitched tile roofs, proud chimneys, many-paned attic windows, and, at street level, their metal railings and gates over which one could peer at the basement windows below. However, much to my delight when visiting London after many years absence, I found that despite the totally unfamiliar appearance of the street, No 8/10 still stands, undefiled, sandwiched between non-descript office blocks; the last evidence of how the street used to look. No visit to London is complete for me without a brief, nostalgic stroll along Bulstrode Street to view the façade that was so familiar and dear to me as a child.

The lion's den

Bulstrode Street is a quiet side-road leading off Wigmore St in the neighbourhood of Wimpole and Harley Streets, names synonymous with the

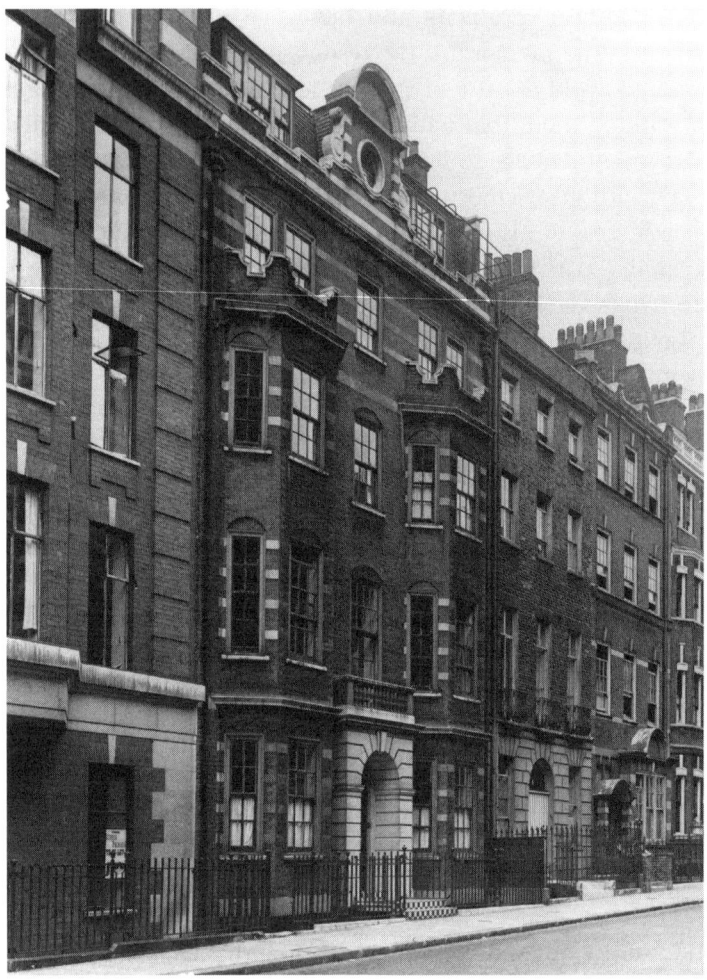

Figure 14.1 8/10 Bulstrode Street, Marylebone, London in 1942–48

higher echelons of conventional medicine. Daniel had entered the lion's den, the very heart of medical London, and the arrival of this interloper was certain to cause a stir. From the outset, it was clear that the transition from Cheltenham to London would not be without difficulties. Without delay, William and Richards applied to the London County Council (LCC) for a licence to open 'The Letari Nursing Home' as a massage and special therapy establishment. The application was at first rejected without reasons being given. Undeterred, William and Richards requested a hearing in order to present their case to the LCC in person. This was finally granted and they appeared as co-applicants before the Public Control Committee of the LCC. Though they stressed that in Leeds, Hull and Cheltenham, the

Sanctuary had been permitted to function as was now intended in London, the application proved unsuccessful.

Licence refused

All the leading London evening newspapers carried news of the story. The *London Evening Standard* Wednesday, December 9, 1942, reported details of the hearing thus:

> *Psychic Healer With 53,000 'Absent' Patients – LICENCE REFUSED.*
>
> William Henry Lilley, stated to practise as a psychic healer was refused licence to carry on a massage and special treatment establishment in the name of Letari Nursing Home, Bulstrode Street by the Public Control Committee of the LCC today.
>
> Mr RJB Dowell (for the chief officer of the Committee) said that Lilley claimed that the spirit of an Indian, Dr Letari, had trained and guided him in the art of healing.
>
> An LCC doctor said that Lilley had mentioned 'absent treatment' by a system of thought vibrations, and that he had about 53,000 absent patients in various parts of the world. The doctor said, "The main idea I got was that contact was established between Mr Lilley and any of these patients at certain times of the day, in the morning and in the evening. The nature of that contact I did not ascertain."[3]

The article also quoted Arthur Richards as saying that the work was not run for a profit and that his interest was to back Mr Lilley's great gifts.[3]

Looking back on these events, it is hardly surprising that the LCC viewed with some suspicion and doubt this medically unqualified, spiritual healer's application to open a nursing home in the West-end of London, his claim to eligibility based on the possession of unusual powers of healing.

The appeal

William and Richards had no alternative but to appeal against the LCC ruling. On the day of the hearing held at the Marylebone Police Court in January 1943, counsel acting on behalf of the Sanctuary brought forward five of the nine witnesses who were present, to testify how they had benefited from the spiritual and homeopathic healing received from Lilley and his spirit guide when conventional medicine had failed to clear their problems. There were two cases of multiple sclerosis, one of severe migraine, a twelve-year old boy suffering from hip disease, and finally a man with spinal arthritis and high blood pressure. All expressed their gratitude for the help they had received. The father of the young boy, giving evidence on his behalf, stated that under Lilley's treatment his son had been able to discard his crutches and calliper within a few months of treatment, whereas orthopaedic opinion had said he would be dependent on them for years. Thomas Powell of Sheffield, one of the multiple sclerosis cases, gave practical proof of his restored ability to walk unaided and avowed that since receiving treatment from Lilley, he felt better than he had done for twelve years. Edward Gunter, of Leeds, told the court that he had suffered from agonising headaches and nervous problems since his experiences in the trenches during the Great War and had received various treatments from the orthodoxy over the intervening years without relief. He now felt "wonderfully better." Asked whether he believed he had received more benefit from Mr Lilley than from other medical treatment, Gunter replied loudly and clearly, "Definitely."[4]

Unfortunately, despite these proofs of therapeutic success in the face of orthodox medical failure, the magistrate, Ivan E Snell, ruled against the granting of a licence. He was seemingly swayed by the LCC's Inspector of Massage Establishments opinion that even massage should not be given except under doctor's orders. In his summing up of what he described as a most important case, he accepted as indisputable evidence the testimony of Lilley's healing ability as expressed by the witnesses, but, in view of Lilley's lack of formal training, he was unable to accept the appeal. However, he did say that if Mr Lilley undertook only to do work upon the recommendation of a regular medical authority then he thought the LCC should grant a licence.[4]

While this comment sounded magnanimous, Snell overlooked the fact that collusion or co-operation between medical doctors and unregistered practitioners was seriously frowned upon and for the doctor carried the risk of being struck off the medical register, as had happened in 1911 to Dr FW Axham, who acted as anaesthetist to Sir Herbert Barker (1869–1950), the much respected osteopath, or bonesetter, as some called him. Barker's manipulative skills were such that they far surpassed anything known to the medical establishment and made him a household name. However, despite his clinical success, Barker's methods were never formally recognised or adopted by the orthodoxy, a fact that prompted Bernard Shaw, whose wife had benefited from Barker's treatment, to write in a letter to the *Daily Telegraph*, in 1920 stating that the General Medical Council . . . at that time exhibited every constitutional vice that a trade union or professional association could have.[5] The attitude of the GMC towards the unfortunate Dr Axham remained unbending and unforgiving until his death at 86, even after Barker was knighted in recognition of his work, and public sentiment called for Axham's reinstatement. Given this history, it was highly unlikely that the Letari Nursing Home would ever have achieved a licence through the mediation of a medical collaborator.

In his role as custodian of the public safety, restricted by bureaucratic protocol and limited to the materialistic perspective of the modern world, Snell, and those he represented, were devoid of latitude to consider even in the face of compelling evidence that an unseen team of accomplished spirit healers was the authority for the medical decisions made at the Sanctuary; an authority with far greater vision than their orthodox, physical counterparts, who, in general, possessed little insight into the origins and nature of disease. As a result, the medical trade union's monopoly was honoured rather than the needs of the public.

Psychic News reported on the aftermath to the failed court appeal on February 6, 1943:

> Neither WH Lilley, the famous psychic healer, nor his colleague, Arthur Richards, is daunted by the court verdict recorded last week. Indeed, Lilley and Richards feel that they have won a moral victory. Richards reminds me that ever since he has been associated with this psychic healing they have triumphed over all sorts of obstacles, and he is convinced that in the end they will win through in London. The court decision has made no difference to the number of patients requiring treatment from Lilley.[6]

Refurbishing

Indeed, as always, the publicity derived from these difficult challenges resulted in even greater public interest and many more applications for personal or absent healing. Before these demands could be met, however, there was work to be done at 8/10 Bulstrode Street. Dr Letari, unperturbed by these hindrances on the physical plane, advised William and Richards to press on regardless of the lack of a licence. To this end, it was necessary to move all the new equipment and furniture acquired for Tudor Lodge to London; but first the premises had to be prepared for their new role.

The building had suffered some bomb damage: the tiling of the roof had shifted, windows had shattered and rain damage had resulted; some of the ceilings had given way; the walls were badly stained; and there was a damp, musty odour pervading the building, which had stood empty for some time. Since the property was to be used as a Spiritualist nursing home and clinic, the Sanctuary applied to the Ministry of Health for help with labour and materials. Time passed and there was no response. On taxing the office of the Ministry with this tardiness, they were informed that there was no record of their application. A second application was refused.

Did they not know that there was a war going on?

A dilemma faced the Sanctuary even before it opened. Though not licenced to practise specific modalities, it was essential that the premises should meet all the criteria required of a medical clinic, but they were unable to meet these criteria due to official, wartime financial restrictions and due to lack of manpower and materials. Patients stepped into the breach and a small band of amateur decorators and handymen descended on 8/10. When word of this activity filtered through to the Ministry, its pride must have been piqued, because belatedly both paint and painters

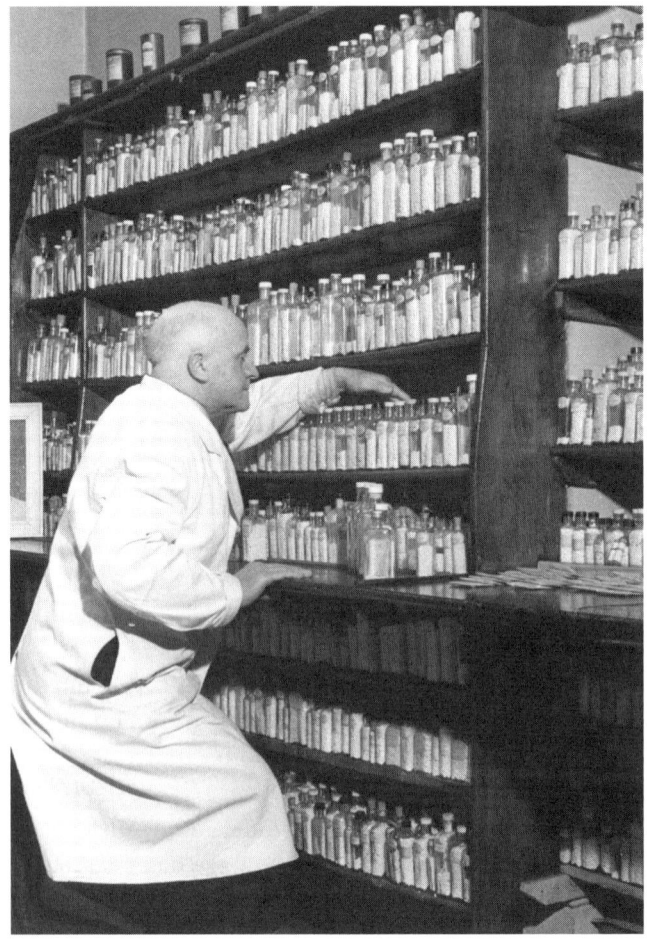

Figure 14.2 William Henry Lilley (senior) Dispensary, Letari Nursing Home, London. 1945

were made available. In no time at all, the house was looking resplendent and ready for the doors to be opened.

The five stories, including a basement and an attic, comprised some 30 rooms of which three became treatment rooms: two on the ground floor and one on the third floor. In addition there was a consulting room, a waiting room, a dispensary and a facility for in-patients. The rest provided offices for the secretarial staff that coped with the vast amount of correspondence that passed to and from the nursing home. On the third floor, was a lounge for the use of senior staff and visitors, in the centre of which stood a billiard table, providing a lunchtime recreation that replaced the table tennis of the Hunslet days. The attic became a home for my grandparents. Pop remained in charge of the dispensary and Sally, hearkening back to her years in service, became the housekeeper and cook, roles at which she excelled. The basement housed a general staff lounge, a dining room, and a large kitchen with a vast cooking range. As a youngster, the kitchen and dispensary were my favourite ports of call and there I would spend many hours watching my grandfather working magic with his bottles, pills and tinctures and my grandmother working equal magic with her cooking and baking. The entire building was made accessible by a wonderful 'electric cage-lift' that fascinated me and in which I rode at every opportunity.

Evacuation

My parents moved from Leeds into a ground floor flat in Cholmley Gardens, Fortune Green Road, West Hampstead, London and there we would live for the following seven years, apart from the time during which my mother and I were evacuated back to the family in Leeds during the bombing of London. Whilst there, much to my mother's consternation, I quickly developed a Yorkshire accent, which she was ever at pains to correct. Despite my youth, that time remains rich with images – images that made a particular impression upon me, such as the gargoyle-like gasmask I was issued with in case Hitler used poison gas in his attacks against Britain. I recall my Uncle Jesse returning from his shift at the mine, blackened from top to toe with soot; divesting himself of all his layered upper garments with one deft movement; sitting in a metal bath in front of the fireplace and by dint of the vigorous use of back brush and 'flannel' emerging as clean as a new pin; and then later, standing with his back to the fire, noisily sipping, with infinite pleasure, his tea from the saucer into which he had poured it from his cup – an exercise much frowned upon by my mother, but which I was highly desirous of emulating.

London and The Blitz

By 1944, we were back in London, as I remember well the blackout; the air raid sirens wailing their warning; my mother, or grandmother, May Overton, urgently getting me to crawl under my bed for safety; listening to the drone of the 'doodlebugs'[i] overhead and knowing that when that sound cut-out, I would hear the whistling of the flying bomb hurtling down upon us followed by a violent explosion that would often shake the flat and on occasion blew our windows in; the release of tension as the all-clear sounded; and the gaping void which had been the fishmonger's shop the week before when I stood on its saw-dusted floor waiting for my mother to make her purchases – memories never to be forgotten.

8/10 open for in-patients

During the first months of 1943, the alterations and refurbishing at 8/10 were pursued with such expediency and devoted enthusiasm that on 20 March *Psychic News* was able to report the following:

> **Milestone For Lilley**: Monday was a red-letter day in the psychic healing career of WH Lilley. On that day the first in-patients were admitted to his healing headquarters in the West-end of London. The necessary licences had been granted, and the matron was installed. It represented a triumph over great difficulties.
>
> Lilley has been inundated with requests for healing since he began his activities in London. Now Dr Letari, his spirit guide, has declared that no new patients are to be accepted. For the time being they must concentrate on the large number who are already receiving treatment.

Prominent Spiritualists of the day

Arthur Conan Doyle

Our move to London brought father into closer contact with the wider British Spiritualist world – a world which Sir Arthur Conan Doyle (1859–1930), the creator of Sherlock Holmes, had frequented and supported until his death. After losing numerous members of his close family, including his wife Louise in 1906 and his son Kingsley, who died from pneumonia in 1918, just before the end of World War 1, the Scottish physician and author

---

[i] Doodlebug (or buzz-bomb) was a popular name for the V-1 flying bombs developed by the German *Luftwaffe* and deployed against London and other British cities, They were designed to destroy 2–3 houses.

sought and found solace for his resultant depression in Spiritualism, which offered proof of life after death. He became a member of the *Ghost Club*, a research organisation, founded in 1862 to investigate psychic and paranormal phenomena. One of this club's earliest and most renowned members was Charles Dickens.

Oliver Lodge

Another eminent Spiritualist of this time was Sir Oliver Lodge (1851–1940), a distinguished British physicist and inventor, who, curiously, like Conan Doyle, was a member of the *Ghost Club* and also lost a son in World War 1. However, in contrast to Doyle, Lodge's interest in Spiritualism developed many years before his son died. His scientific work with the imponderable nature of electricity and magnetism fostered in him a deep interest in psychic phenomena and extra sensory perception, particularly telepathy, and he devoted much time to researching this faculty. He was a deep thinking man of charming disposition, highly respected and well thought of. An eloquent speaker, both in debate and in the lecture room, Lodge possessed an outstanding ability to elucidate the most complex subjects with ease and clarity. His broad, scholarly brow, equal to that of Hahnemann, testified to the brilliance of his scientific mind. He lived a year longer than the Master, passing on in his ninetieth year.

After his son Raymond was killed in action in 1915, Lodge consulted two independent psychics, Alfred Peters and Gladys Leonard, in the hope of contacting him. Despite the paternal emotions involved in this search, he maintained a scientifically critical attitude in evaluating the communications he and his wife received through their mediumship. Lodge was careful to discount any responses, which could possibly have been influenced by telepathy. After a number of sittings held over a period of several months, characterised by many searching questions and the cross checking of facts, the preponderance of evidence they accumulated convinced Oliver Lodge and his family that they had gained irrefutable proof of Raymond's spiritual presence. Through the mediums, especially Gladys Leonard, Raymond was able to provide them with information about events known only to himself and the family.

Lodge judged the evidence to be beyond the possibility of fraud, coincidence or telepathy and in 1916, in a book about his son's survival wrote, "I am as convinced of continued existence on the other side of death as I am of existence here."[7]

A telepathic experiment

This conviction would be strengthened many years later, towards the end of his life, when he devised an experiment between himself, William and Dr Letari, with my mother acting as go-between. Lodge came to hear of William and Dr Letari through the numerous articles about their activities that had appeared in *Two Worlds* and *Psychic News*. The phenomenon of 'absent healing' was of particular interest to him because of his lifelong interest in the power of telepathy and the transmission and reception of immeasurable influences by the human mind and nervous system. He conjectured that for healing to be extended between a medium and a patient through the agency of spirit doctors, regardless of the physical distance between them, the process must be paralleled by an ability of the guiding and entrancing spirit to define the thoughts and actions of a subject from afar. In order to test this, he determined to contact my father. At the time, William was still based in Leeds, but unlike most Yorkshire village households in the late 1930s, he had a domestic telephone service. This was ideal for the extra sensory perception test that Oliver Lodge planned with my father.

He set the time for the experiment at 8.00 p.m. At this time, William would sit at home in Leeds with my mother, Nancy, and go into trance. When this was achieved and Dr Letari was in full control of his medium, Nancy would telephone Sir Oliver in London and inform him that all was ready. Lodge would then perform some definite activity in his home and when he had completed this he would telephone back to Nancy and ask her to ascertain from Dr Letari exactly what he had done. On the chosen evening, after receiving Nancy's call that Dr Letari was present, Sir Oliver walked into his study, took down a copy of Gray's anatomy, opened it at a specific page and read a certain paragraph. He then replaced the book and telephoned my mother. Relaying to Lodge what Dr Letari said to her, Nancy told him precisely the sequence of his actions: the room he entered, the name of the book, the number of the page, and which paragraph he had read. She then proceeded to repeat after the Doctor, word for word, the text of the paragraph Lodge had chosen. When she had given no more than a few sentences from the paragraph, Sir Oliver stopped her and with audible emotion told her that there was no need to go any further, for she had given more than enough evidence of her husband's gift. She was asked to thank Mr Lilley and Dr Letari for making the experiment possible.

Had Sir Oliver Lodge lived longer, I am sure further tests would have been designed to give further proof to science of the immediacy of the spirit world and its vital interplay with the physical domain. However, by the time the Sanctuary moved to London in early 1943, Lodge had himself made the transition to spirit two years previously, and it was other leading lights in the Spiritualist world who now entered my father's life.

Maurice Barbanell

Amongst these, Maurice Barbanell (1902–1981) was the closest and most influential. A journalist and co-founder, with Hannen Swaffer and Arthur Findlay, of the Spiritualist newspaper, *Psychic News*, Barbanell served as editor of this periodical and its sister publication, *The Two Worlds*, for over thirty years. He was born in London, May 3, 1902, into a Jewish family, the son of an East End barber. His father was an atheist and his mother a *frum* (orthodox) Jewess. This religious difference lead to many arguments between the two, particularly because Barbanell's father refused to accompany his mother to any orthodox services. His father's influence prevailed and Maurice took on his father's atheism, but later, finding such a rigidly closed attitude contrary to his nature, changed to agnosticism, maintaining an open but critical outlook. This stance suited him well for his appointment as the unpaid secretary of the Ghetto Social and Literary Club in what he later called *"London's darkest East End,"* tasked with sourcing notable literary and artistic personages to address his society on their area of expertise. He was eighteen years old and already excelled at playing the devil's advocate at such meetings to ensure a lively exchange of ideas.

During his tenure as secretary, friends invited him to attend a séance; a new experience for him. It turned out to be a farcical affair conducted by persons unaware of the potentially serious nature of flirting with unseen realms and ignorant of the possible consequences of their levity. This flippant parody, although far removed from a serious introduction to the subject, left the teenage Barbanell with a "subconscious antagonism to Spiritualism." As is the way with such currents in our lives, which often first lick at our toes before sweeping us off our feet, shortly after this episode, in the absence of a celebrity speaker, the club hosted a young man, Henry Sanders, who spoke about his experiences in Spiritualism. Cast as he invariably was as speaker for the opposition and knowing his sentiments on the subject, at the close of the lecture, Maurice's colleagues eagerly anticipated him firing a sceptical and dismantling broadside with which to initiate a warm debate. His response surprised them. He said that this was a subject on which only those with experience could venture any worthwhile opinions.[8]

When the meeting was concluded, Sanders, recognising an astute and unbiased mind, approached Barbanell, and asked, in view of his comment about experience being essential, whether he would be prepared to personally investigate the subject. Barbanell willingly agreed, and, moreover, committed himself to spend six months pursuing this research before drawing any conclusions. Little did he realise that this investigation would occupy the rest of his life.

Entrancement
Sanders invited him to attend a home circle lead by a middle-aged woman, Mrs Blaustein, who was reputedly a trance medium, able to channel various entities of diverse nationality. On the date set, Maurice, accompanied by his fiancée, Sylvia Abrahams, attended the sitting, which was held in a very poor district in the East End of London.

The circle in the dingy block was composed of a mixture of young and old Jews who all seemed earnest though unprepossessing;[9] a far cry from the warm, hearty gathering in the room above a pub where my father received his initiation into the world of spirit. On that evening, Mrs Blaustein was as prolific as promised, but Barbanell was not impressed, and remained unconvinced that he had indeed heard 'dead' foreigners speaking through her lips. At one point during her trance state, her spirit guide picking up on his disbelief said pointedly: "You will be doing this soon."[10] Though still sceptical, he remained sensitive to his commitment and duly attended the next sitting during which a similar demonstration was given. At some point in the proceedings, which he found far from stimulating, he drifted off into sleep. On wakening, feeling rather embarrassed, he apologised for his lapse, only to find himself the centre of the group's attention. Much to his surprise and wonderment, he was told that he had been in a trance; his guide had given his name and said he had been training him for years and that, before long, he would be speaking on Spiritualist platforms.[10]

His lapse into sleep had actually been a mediumistic trance and as in all William's experiences, he had no recollection of what had transpired during his temporary absence from his body.

Sylvia, who in 1932 was to become Mrs Barbanell, wrote about the quality of the first communication of the spirit entity who later became known as Silver Birch; a beloved being who touched earth again for a short period in order to spread a spiritual message of wisdom from the beyond, important at any time, but particularly so when Europe and the rest of the world were about to confront a terrible ordeal.

The earth barriers that have to be overcome in initiating such a trance state are truly formidable, and the inspiring spirit had little familiarity with the use of English. On this first occasion, he spoke but few words, and these uttered in a husky, almost guttural tone.

But how different were those early manifestations from those of today! When the guide first announced himself at that sitting, he could barely string a few words of English together. Gradually, he learned to speak with greater fluency. It has taken him a long time to attain his present, rich vocabulary.[11]

Home circle

The presence of Sylvia at that first sitting, and her witnessing at first hand what happened to the young man she knew so well, must have been contributory to the quick transformation of this down-to-earth agnostic into a budding medium. Always a decisive man, disinclined to permit the grass to grow under his feet, Barbanell set about the formation of a home circle. This enabled Silver Birch to further his medium's development in the most favourable circumstances, gradually making the merging of his individuality with that of Maurice a progressively more simple transition. Although seeking to develop his mediumship as far as it would go, the young Barbanell disliked one aspect of his entrancement: the lack of awareness of all that was said and done while he was out of the body. He later conjectured that this reservation was probably due to vanity, but it was more likely due to his need to be always in control of his life. Honouring this, on the night after each sitting, when he lay in bed prior to sleep, the workers in spirit would give him a psychic replay of what had happened. This was both visual and auditory, unfolding before him as if he was watching a film at the cinema. As valuable as this was for Maurice, for his own spiritual development and to keep him familiar with the uplifting teachings that were being transmitted through him, as with my father's initial clairvoyance, this psychic process consumed energy which could be put to better use. This soon became no longer necessary, due to the intervention of the famous Fleet Street journalist, Hannen Swaffer.

Hannen Swaffer

Hannen Swaffer (1879–1962), a self-confessed agnostic and cynical newspaper editor, had Spiritualism brought to his attention when his close friend and secretary, Louise Owen, informed him that his former 'Chief,' Alfred Harmsworth, Lord Northcliffe, the powerful newspaper magnate, who had died two years before, in August 1922, had communicated through a medium at a séance she attended. Swaffer was certain that she had been deceived. "As an agnostic, I sneered at the idea," he wrote. However, sniffing a good story, he had his brother, one of his reporters, interview Louise to get all the details. This provided the basis for a newspaper story, which was circulated worldwide. Matters might have rested there, but

Swaffer had worked closely with Northcliffe for many years and knew him better than most. Larger than life, Lord Norcliffe was a man of immense ego and iron will, who founded the *Daily Mail* and *The Daily Mirror* and took ownership of both *The Times* and *The Sunday Times*. Through this wide readership, his editorials wielded great influence over both 'the classes and the masses.'[12] Such a man was not easily forgotten, and certainly not by Swaffer, who had great admiration for him. His curiosity was aroused and more so because he was acquainted with both Conan Doyle and Oliver Lodge, aware of their convictions and respected them both. Being a journalist and accustomed to probing things however apparently fantastic they might appear at first, he went out to enquire for himself.[13]

As was to be expected in a man of his pragmatic, no-nonsense nature, Swaffer set about his investigation with a critical and sceptical mind. He was helped in this task by the urgency of the departed Northcliffe to make known his continued existence. This he did through medium after medium, commencing on the very night of his passing through a circle led by a former Baptist minister in South Norwood, an urban district situated in South London. Whereas many have delved into the world of Spiritualism and after years of attending sittings have never had a personal experience that could be regarded as convincing, within four days, Swaffer had the evidence he needed – evidence, which converted him into a leading proponent of Spiritualism. He made note of the day it occurred; it was October 6, 1924.

Swaffer's conversion through direct-voice mediumship

Prior to Louise Owen's news of Northcliffe's return, Swaffer had been honoured by an invitation to attend a séance at the house of Dennis Bradley, a friend of some twelve years standing, who was a medium in his own right, but had never previously encroached on Swaffer with his belief. These Bradley-held séances provided a platform for various outstanding mediums and it was the custom of the circle to invite to each of the sittings some or other eminent person. Celebrities of every kind were numbered amongst the guests. When Swaffer attended, the professional psychic present was the remarkable American direct-voice medium, George Valiantine.

Although he received a communication, ostensibly from his grandfather, Swaffer remained sceptical and departed unconvinced. Bradley, having sensed his friend's uncertainty, and knowing what a prominent voice Spiritualism would have if Swaffer could be swayed, decided to telephone him some months later. It cannot be fortuitous that this call coincided with Swaffer's determination to uncover the truth. Bradley invited him to a private, direct-voice sitting without a professional medium and suggested that he bring with him Louise Owen and anyone else he liked. Swaffer accepted and took Louise and another close lady friend. That night there were six sitters – the three guests, Dennis Bradley, his wife and their son. Swaffer wrote that they all trusted and respected one another and would never have dreamed of trickery, particularly regarding such a sensitive and important matter.

In direct-voice mediumship, the spirit communication does not take place through the use of the medium's voice, as in the case of William and Barbanell, but through a temporary ectoplasmic voice box or larynx created by the skill of spirit technicians from power and ectoplasm drawn from the medium and sitters. A very light aluminium trumpet amplifies the sound vibration generated through this voice box. The quality of the communication depends on many factors: the presence, power and health of the direct-voice medium, the power, quality and compatibility of the sitters, the functionality of the ectoplasmic voice box that is created, and the variable skill of the spirit entities utilising this instrument to convert thought into speech. This skill must be likened to learning to skate – at first a very shaky, uncertain affair – because it must be understood that confidence and aptitude vary as much on the plane of spirit as they do here, and, although receiving assistance, few would-be communicators are spirit scientists or in any way versed in voice production between different spheres of frequency. In addition, the use of such a generic larynx robs the voice produced of its uniqueness, its characteristic pitch and inflection – it is never a perfect reproduction of the spirit's voice as it was when they were living on earth. However, despite these great difficulties, direct-voice communication can be very effective and impressive, especially when associated with high levels of mediumship, such as two outstanding mediums of the past, Estelle Roberts and Leslie Flint, were capable of. The authenticity of the communication and identity of the communicator must be judged not by similarity of sound, for even a physical telephone can render some voices difficult to recognise, but from personality, vocabulary, speech patterns, language and shared memories, all of which should reveal the individuality of the person.

The direct-voice séance needs to be conducted in total darkness because of the extreme sensitivity to light of the delicate ectoplasmic structure on which voice production depends. Whilst this is essential, it does unfortunately provide the charlatan every opportunity to produce fraudulent phenomena and deceive sitters, hence the importance of recognising the individuality of the communicator through their unique characteristics and not being impressed or swayed by the mundane, commonplace or non-specific or by mere physical sensations, such as the touch of a hand or a current of cool air.

The aluminium trumpet is an important prop. Being light it can be levitated with relative ease through psychokinesis (telekinesis). Because of the pitch dark of the séance room, it is customary to make the trumpet visible by placing a luminous band around the broad end of the instrument. The trumpet is usually placed on the floor in the centre of the ring of sitters. During a successful sitting it will be seen to lift up into the air and hover or move about, sometimes gently, sometimes vigorously, even making wide excursions from side to side, or up and down. Since the one seeking to communicate is usually manipulating it, the behaviour of the trumpet may provide an expression of their personality, much as the hand held microphone of a speaker or performer can do. Some being reserved, serious or focused will scarcely move or any movement proves slight, slow or deliberate, used for emphasis, others more expressive, emotional or urgent may display agitation or flamboyance. As vital as the trumpet is to direct voice mediumship, it is also an ideal tool with which to dupe the gullible sitter; an energetic trumpet is only a marvel when backed up by incontrovertible proof of a familiar entity's presence.

On the night in question, Swaffer and his friends sat in darkness listening to a gramophone recording of Galli-Curci, the great coloratura soprano. Soon they saw the trumpet lift into the air and for a moment hang there as though suspended, then begin to wave rhythmically to and fro as though conducting the music. This completed, it fell to the floor, only to rise again and move slowly across to Swaffer's friend and hover before her. A scarcely audible whisper emitted from the trumpet, which when repeated, after the entity had been asked to speak louder by Bradley, was heard to be *"Mother"*, followed by the friend's name and *"Darling,"* and then something about *"Kisses."* All of which would have provided no proof whatsoever of the mother's presence, if it had not been immediately followed by the utterance of unmistakable evidence shared only by Swaffer and the mother's daughter. That was the moment when Swaffer's eyes were fully opened to the truth of continued existence after death.

> Then I knew that Spiritualism was true ... that my friend's beloved mother, who had been dead for nine years, had really spoken to her and that we were in the presence of the living dead.... I knew that Conan Doyle was right and the sceptics were wrong.[14]

Again the trumpet fell to the floor. During the pause, Bradley turned on the gramophone to assist the gathering of energy, a tribute to the wonderful power and reach of the soprano voice. They did not have long to wait; the trumpet once more rose into the air. Bradley switched off the music. The voice issuing from the trumpet announced itself as Feda, well known in spiritualist circles as the young Hindu control and guide of Gladys Osborne Leonard, the gracious and irreproachable medium who had supplied Sir Oliver Lodge with evidence of his son Raymond's survival in the spirit world.

Bradley, a confident and experienced sitter, speaking on behalf of Swaffer, asked Feda if she could contact Lord Northcliffe and try and get him to speak to them. "I will try my best," whispered Feda through the trumpet.[15]

Another pause while the trumpet lay immobile on the floor. Another ascent into the higher reaches of coloratura virtuosity. When the trumpet sprang once more to life it showed no hesitation in selecting who it wished to communicate with; it made a determined bee-line for Swaffer and came to a halt within an inch or two of his right elbow and said: "The Chief! The Chief! I am glad to see you Swaff." The difference in the movement of the trumpet compared with how it had been controlled by his friend's mother was marked. It was immediately apparent that someone very confident and forceful was speaking. Swaffer was fully aware of his 'Chief's' presence clearly conveyed by style of speech and the assertiveness of both the voice and the gestures of the trumpet. After the initial greeting, the trumpet alternated its interest between the journalist and Louise. The voice urged them to continue direct-voice sittings and told them that there was a great work to be done for "God and the world." It finally bid them "Goodnight."

A few days later Swaffer lunched with Sir Arthur Conan Doyle at the Author's club and they exchanged notes. Northcliffe had spoken to Doyle at a sitting in New York some weeks previously, manifesting the same idiosyncrasies familiar to Swaffer, but new to Doyle who had never known him personally.

"Was Northcliffe an indiscreet man?" asked Doyle.

"The soul of indiscretion," replied Swaffer.

"I was surprised by him," said Conan Doyle. "He told me a lot of family things that almost made me blush."[16]

Northcliffe persisted in his desire to be heard, and, by his presence at sittings, to spread and increase confidence in communication with the spirit. But, he was particularly focused on Swaffer and appeared at every mediumistic circle that Swaffer attended. As anticipated, therefore, he announced himself at a sitting, with Evan Powell as the medium, to which Swaffer had invited Maxwell Aitken, Lord Beaverbrook. Beaverbrook had been a press colleague of Northcliffe, was the owner of the *Daily Express* and the London *Evening Standard*. In 1942, he became Winston Churchill's

Minister of War Production and later Lord Privy Seal. Yet again, Northcliffe gave voice to his concern for society and the world, and stressed how, if humanity could be enlightened to a complete and unshakable certainty of life after death, it would change the future. He shouted "My God, Beaverbrook, if only you knew how difficult it is. This is the new revelation. Don't you understand? This is the great reality."[17]

Northcliffe's personal purgatory was to observe from afar "the vast newspaper machine of his own creation being used for purposes out of harmony with his new found convictions,"[17] and not having the power to change its policy. Most striking to Swaffer, who had known him very well, was the shift in his drive from gratifying a much-inflated ego to being a propagandist for Spiritualism, world peace and universal improvement, while still manifesting the same dictatorial eccentricity. It is to be hoped that in some measure he was able that evening to sway the sentiments of Beaverbrook, if only on a personal level.

Birth of the *Psychic News*

Swaffer had already met and worked professionally with the young journalist, Maurice Barbanell. They became very close friends, a friendship made all the more intimate because of their shared interest in Spiritualism. It naturally followed that Swaffer was invited to attend the Barbanell's home circle and was introduced to Silver Birch. Barbanell wrote: "He was intrigued by my mediumship and came to love Silver Birch."[18] Up to that time, Silver Birch's teachings had been limited to the immediate circle. Swaffer, the newspaper editor, seasoned journalist and propagandist, deeply impressed by the wisdom he heard from the lips of the spirit guide, realised that these teachings would be wasted if not brought to the ears of a larger public. This concern burgeoned into the vision of a Spiritualist periodical newspaper, which would serve the many people interested in understanding spirit contact and life after death and also provide a platform to disseminate the words of Silver Birch. One can well imagine the unseen Northcliffe egging him on with glee, because his pursuit of Swaffer had certainly been part of some greater plan. With his usual enthusiasm and decisiveness, Swaffer proposed that Maurice should himself edit such a paper and that it should be called *Psychic News*.

At first, Barbanell was uncertain about this role because he feared that he would be criticised for publicising his own mediumship in the newspaper that he edited. Swaffer suggested that to avoid this anxiety, he should publish the articles reporting Silver Birch's words, but withhold the identity of the medium. On this condition, Barbanell agreed to the plan. Thus, in

1932, the *Psychic News* was born, just a few months before a detestable megalomaniac would be appointed Chancellor of Germany. The timing for a periodical whose prime theme would be eternal life could not have been better. *Psychic News* abruptly ceased publication in July 2010.

The Hannen Swaffer home circle

Until then Barbanell's guide was affectionately known only by a nickname which seemed inappropriate to the serious work which would appear beneath his name. The intermediary he used to gain proximity to the gross vibrations of earth was a Native American Indian, therefore when asked to choose a formal name, he selected Silver Birch out of respect for his mediator. The sittings continued to be held at Barbanell's home every Friday evening and each week the words of Silver Birch appeared in *Psychic News* as the teachings of the Hannen Swaffer home circle. At first the anonymity was successfully maintained and speculation, about who the medium of this wise, spirit seer was, abounded. Swaffer, however, true to his nature and his desire to spread the word, was always inviting his celebrity friends to these sittings. Although guests were always sworn to secrecy, a point was reached when Barbanell realised that it was no longer possible to keep the secret, and, in a special article, he finally announced that he was in fact Silver Birch's medium.

With the advent of Hannen Swaffer, and the launching of the *Psychic News*, recording every word that Silver Birch uttered became imperative. This task, in the days before tape recorders, became the responsibility of two shorthand writers, first Billy Austin, who was Barbanell's assistant editor, and then Frances Moore who served in this capacity for many years and was called "The Scribe" by Silver Birch. This material, apart from appearing in the weekly periodical, became the contents of a number of books, which are still in publication and have illuminated the minds of a multitude of readers. Once recording was initiated, the bedtime playbacks of the sittings for Barbanell's benefit were no longer necessary and the psychic energy needed for this process could be preserved and used in other ways.

A deeper awareness

The modern mind tends to regard what has been related so far about William, Dr Letari, Barbanell and Silver Birch, about guides, mediums, trance states, ectoplasm, materialisations and talking trumpets, as being supernatural, delusional or just fantasy, material for films and novels but of little relevance to life in the modern world. For some it even smacks of Satanism. As Swaffer remarked:

to the average, conventional Christian such phenomena are accepted as fact only when they occur two thousand years ago and in Jerusalem.

Yet in all of us, there is a childlike level of consciousness that responds instinctively and intuitively, in defiance of our intellect, to the mysterious and magical, silently acknowledging the existence of other dimensions of reality. Caught unawares, exposed to a thought, an emotion, an image, a phrase, a melody, an evocative ambience, a thrill courses through us as we touch something precious, something exquisite, something extraordinary that stirs us to our depths and arouses a surge of emotion that washes over us, catching our breath, stirring our heart, bringing tears to our eyes and causing our hair to stand on end. We are multidimensional beings and promptings from our eternal source ever seek expression, but can only do so when the externally directed mind is arrested and diverted to a deeper level of experience and the aesthetics of the esoteric. The clutter of materialism chokes our innate sensitivity and awareness; to apprehend and assimilate the science of the spirit, we must recapture the open curiosity and supple adaptability of our infancy; then we can find nourishment for the unfulfilled yearnings of our inner being at the banquet table of the most high.

References

1. Famous Healer Plans A London Sanctuary. *Psychic News*; 31 January 1942.
2. Gaskill M. *Hellish Nell: Last of Britain's Witches*. London: Fourth Estate; 2002. p297.
3. Psychic Healer With 53,000 'Absent' Patients – LICENCE REFUSED. *London Evening Standard*; December 9 1942.
4. Lilley Loses His Appeal. *Psychic News*; January 30 1943.
5. Psychic News . . . Should doctors be the judges of medical orthodoxy? The Barker case of 1920. *Journal Of The Royal Society Of Medicine* 2002; 95(1): 41.

15

SILVER BIRCH – WISDOM FROM BEYOND THE GRAVE

I grew up with the example of my parents, the wisdom of Dr Letari, the teachings of Silver Birch and the security of being raised in a homeopathic household; a combination of influences, unique, as all our life experiences are, but also rare. To have, from the cradle, parents who were lovers to the very grave; a spirit father, a Brahmin versed in the Vedas and homeopathy, who taught me the philosophy of a higher form of medicine; words of a master seer from far beyond to guide me; and the gentle power of Hahnemann's legacy to heal my ills, was a blessing beyond evaluation. Even now, more than three score years and ten later, I wonder at such good fortune and need to pinch myself mentally to know it is real. My grandmother Overton rightly told me that I was born with a silver spoon in my mouth, and that being a Friday's child, I should always be loving and giving. In over forty years of practising and teaching homeopathy, I have discharged this responsibility to the best of my ability, whereas, given the frailties of human disposition, I often failed to do so in my private life. Yet even when I faltered, the teachings of my spirit mentors ensured that I did not stray too far and soon found my bearings.

In times of doubt, fear, self-pity, resentment, impatience or intolerance, the light and wisdom of spirit, as inimitably expressed through the simple eloquence of Silver Birch, can bring back the balance and higher perspective required to change the trials of life into rich opportunity. Always central to his message are the qualities of love and service, qualities that can make us all Friday's children.

Who was (and is) Silver Birch, the spirit guide of the Hannen Swaffer home circle? This is a question best answered by the spirit guide himself and those closest to him, for the answer sheds light on the science of the spirit world.

Hannen Swaffer tells us:

> Silver Birch, as we call him, is not a Red Indian. Who he is, we do not know. We assume that he uses the name of the spirit through whose astral body he expresses himself, it being impossible for the high vibration of the spiritual realm to which he belongs to manifest except through some other instrument.[1]

Sylvia Barbanell expresses, with a simplicity and directness equal to that of the guide, a few words about his identity and mission:

> The personality of a dead North American Indian cloaks the anonymity of his true spiritual status, for he has returned from the Beyond to serve and not to be revered.
>
> The mission that Silver Birch has undertaken is to teach the eternal truths to those who will listen. The wisdom he expounds is always simple and direct. He is not interested in what we call ourselves. He has no use for religious labels, creeds or dogmas. Silver Birch tells us that if we would serve the Great Spirit we must serve our fellow-men, for within each one of us is the spark of divinity, which is part of the Great Spirit, the Perfect Law, or whatever conception of God we may serve.[2]

The Great Spirit is the supreme deity of the native-American Indian nation, a people who live far closer to the essence of life, nature and the creation than the white man who ravaged their civilisation. Their philosophy, which transcends religion, is universal, cosmic and both pantheistic and monotheistic, recognising divinity in all things and the presence of an all-presiding beneficent power or law: The Great White Spirit, a feminine and masculine omnipotence that governs life with love and wisdom. They are intensely conscious of the deep connection and intimate interplay that exists between the spiritual realm of departed ancestors and our physical world. The spirits of the wise and the beloved move among them, inspiring, tending and sustaining. Life is an act of worship, suffused with spirituality at every level. Part of the tragedy of their nation is the loss to so many of the precious, innate consciousness of divine immediacy that was always their birth-right, due to the erosive and corrupting influence of the materialistic world of the white man. The philosophy of Spiritualism at its purest level, is not religious but spiritual, and is one with that of the Amerindian. It is not surprising, therefore, that a number of enlightened and caring spirits of that race returned with the selfless mission of bringing to the Western world their consciousness of the sacred significance and inherent beauty and perfection of every moment, at a time when that world was torn asunder by two disastrous wars.

Outstanding exemplars of the work that was achieved during those harrowing years, incorporating not only wartime and its aftermath, but also the dire period of the great depression, were Red Cloud, the guide of the direct-voice medium Estelle Roberts, whom Barbanell described as one of the most versatile of mediums, and White Eagle, the guide of Grace Cook, who focused on spiritual teaching and healing through colour therapy. On a less conspicuous level was the dedicated protective role of my father's 'gatekeeper,' White Hawk.

Silver Birch has fortunately left us with details of this mission, how he came to be involved and from whence he came.

> Silver Birch is not my name. It is the name of the Indian spirit I use as a transformer that enables me to lower my vibrations and reach your world. The name does not matter.[3]

Not only did he consider his name and identity unimportant, he also did not wish to be thanked personally for the wisdom he imparted, firstly, because it derived from a source higher than himself, he being only the messenger of the enlightened beings who inspired him, and, secondly, because he wished to obviate the tendency of disciples down the ages to put more devotion into worshipping the teacher than into the observance of what is taught, as has happened in Christianity and in the glorification of Eastern gurus. Ardent disciples are inclined to set aside their reason and self-determination in favour of adoration and obedience to meaningless rituals that will by some inexplicable process pave their way to redemption. This tendency towards hero worship is not absent from homeopathy, and in science pumps up the arrogant hubris of the pre-eminent proponents of scientific atheism.

> I insist on this (not being thanked as the source) because I deprecate very strongly an aspect I have seen too often. It is known as guide worship, and we do not desire worship. The only power that is to be worshipped is the Great Spirit, the infinite spirit, the supreme creator, the acme of all light, love, wisdom, truth and inspiration.[4]

> Your world has for too long concerned itself with teachers whom it has aggrandised into exaggerated positions and has forgotten what they came to teach. What does it matter whether I am a teacher of great distinction or a lowly beggar, so long as the seal of truth stamps what I say?[5]

The spirit world, or heavenly sphere, represents an ascending hierarchy of dimensions of spiritual attainment ranging from the lowest and grossest vibratory level of planetary life, with which we are familiar, to the incomprehensibly sublime and exquisitely refined realm of the illustrious, radiant souls who stand spiritually in closest proximity to the perfection of the Great Spirit. In contrast to the resplendence of these celestial spheres, our world, despite its physical beauty, appears cold, grey and unattractive.

When the spirit, now named Silver Birch, had attained the necessary level of spiritual enlightenment, he was approached by his teachers and requested to fulfil an important mission on Earth. His initial response was reluctance to forsake the harmonious tranquillity of the higher spheres of existence in order to descend into the murkiness of the lower reaches of the creation.

> I did not want to come back to your world. It has very little to attract once you have passed beyond its vibrations. The realm or sphere, which is my natural habitat has a radiance and translucence that you cannot understand, clogged as you are by matter.[6]

His desire to be of service to struggling humanity was more powerful than his initial reluctance and he agreed to take on the task. For this to be fulfilled, careful preparation was necessary. Due to the fineness of the plane he dwelt on, it was necessary for him to find a compatible intermediary on a lower level of vibration through whom he could gain access to the vastly denser and more ponderous physical dimension. This was the Native American spirit whose name he adopted. Through his spiritual standing and his dwelling on a lower spiritual level, this spirit was able to act as a transformer for the higher source. Once this bridge was achieved, Silver Birch was in a position to find an instrument through whom he could express the message he was charged to deliver. There was nothing random in this choice, it was determined by the special spiritual destiny of a particular incarnating soul, and in keeping with ancient wisdom that tells us: "many are called, but few are chosen." Both William and Maurice Barbanell were chosen because of who they were spiritually before their training commenced. The connection between guide and medium was initiated at conception and strengthened as the spirit began to express itself. From that early immature period, Silver Birch played an inspiring and moulding role in his medium's development through infancy, childhood and adolescence.

> I accustomed myself throughout the days of boyhood to all the mental processes, to all the physical habits. I studied my instrument from every aspect – mind, spirit and physical body.[6]

He instilled in the youth an interest in religion – an interest and critical standpoint that produced contempt for formal religion with its dogmas, creeds and superstitions, and made him an atheist. Once this was achieved, the slate was clean, uncontaminated by prejudice, programming or preconceived ideas. He was ready for the introduction of other perspectives. Silver Birch guided and persuaded him through the events, which led up to his first trance state – so crude and awkward in comparison with what would be achieved – yet so vital. His progress was swift and Silver Birch soon perfected his control to the point of being able to express his ideas fully without the intrusion of the medium's unconscious mind.

Soon a nucleus of sympathetic souls was formed, which became the Hannen Swaffer home-circle from which the message of spirit could be disseminated, first via its mouthpiece, *Psychic News*, and later through a number of books, which are still in print.

The Message

Much of the emotional distress – anxiety, fear, anger, resentment, depression and other negative and often destructive feelings – that besets millions of people throughout the world stems from ignorance of spiritual truths, which if known with complete and utter certitude, would provide understanding of life's purpose, give adversity spiritual meaning, impart a sense of personal significance and value, and dispel doubt and uncertainty. The failure of the various religions, particularly those of the Middle East, with which the religious mind of the Western world has been indoctrinated, to present a spiritual science supported by precepts based on true knowledge of the occult and free of superstition, fable and futile ritual, has left society rudderless and prey to the growing influence of a godless, empirical science devoid of a sacred dimension. Humanity needs to have an unassailable conviction of the immediacy of a loving, universal intelligence; of a hierarchy of spirit beings who guide and care for the incarnated soul at all times; of personal and collective divinity; of kinship and connection with all life; of survival after death; and of the spiritual nature of a creation governed by laws that are perfect and express truth, wisdom and love.

Life after death must be understood to mean the survival and continuity of the individuality, in its entirety, in circumstances harmonious and beneficial to the further progress of the soul, based on who it is and not what it believes. Survival must not be perceived as a ghostlike, nebulous, intangible, bodiless state, fraught with either the vacuous ennui of purgatory or the perils of hell, but as a substantial and vital life experienced in an environment more real than that which we inhabit on earth. There are no halls of judgement, no hell-fire or brimstone or eternal damnation and no trumpets to herald the resurrection of believers. Death constitutes a natural and blessed passage from a transient, limited physical state, filled with perplexing polarities and paradoxes, and release into our true, untrammelled state of spirit, bearing the fruits or famine of our life on earth. We are answerable only to ourselves: through service and love we prosper, through selfishness and prejudice we stagnate. Such knowledge, which is more substantial and durable than belief, faith or hope, provides the basic trust to face and triumph over the challenges of life without faltering. It is what humanity urgently needs, hence Silver Birch's descent to our world. It is worthwhile that we should consider the message he brought.

It is not new, but fresh, simple and rational, devoid of religious mythology, free of ritual and guru worship or any teachings that bring about difference, distinction and division, which are the cause of most of humanity's strife and suffering. Judaism falls away, Christianity falls away, Islam falls away, mere belief and faith fall away, and in their place stands the Truth that is enshrined in the heart of all religions: the pristine, purity and perfection of a loving, serving philosophy based on absolute trust in the spiritual nature of all things, the indivisible oneness of all, the immortality of life and the wisdom, perfection and truth of an all-seeing, all-loving Creator – the Great Spirit.

He emphasised, time and time again, the omnipotence, omniscience and omnipresence of the 'supreme creator,' the perfect Law that lovingly and wisely permeates, vitalises and governs the creation, and affirmed the eternal, indissoluble, sentient bond that exists between the creator and the created. Just as we are bonded and linked to our divine parent so are we all, as children of the divine, bonded and linked to one another in a vast spiritual family, differences of colour and race being an illusion.

> The summit of all attainment is the Great White Spirit, the infinite power of love and wisdom that has devised the boundless universe in which we live and has brought natural laws which ensure that everything and everybody come within their framework.
>
> Nothing exists apart from the Great Spirit, therefore the Great Spirit is all. . . . You cannot separate yourself from the Great Spirit because the Great Spirit is imminent in all creation . . . the infinite creator, the supreme arbiter whose love and wisdom are responsible for the majestic universe and whose perfect intelligence devised all the natural laws which encompass every manifestation of being, majestically mighty or microscopically minute, and has made provision for all and everything that exists. So perfect is the operation of these natural laws that nothing and nobody can be outside their scope.[7]

Spirit, and the qualities and values of spirit, are central to life. Spirit is the core reality, the mainspring of existence. Spirit is the dynamic essence out of which every manifestation of life is formed, whether it be a plant, a tree, an insect, a bird, an animal or a human. Spirit is the spark of divinity embedded within every being and within everything that expresses life, no matter what form it takes. The human being is a spirit with a soul, mind and body, not a body, mind and soul with a spirit.

The purpose of the soul's descent and birth onto the earth plane is to quicken the spirit, or inner divinity. This can best be achieved through exposure to the polarities of earthly existence and to a variety of circumstances, which demand the exercise of personal choice and free will and the expression of latent qualities that can only be called forth when confronted with difficulty and adversity. The circumstances of life are designed to enable the soul to exercise its divine potential and emerge stronger as a result. In the attainment of its goal, spiritual enlightenment, the soul must perfect all its gifts and to achieve this must go through light and dark, sunshine and rain, fire and flood, in order to be tried and tested. Earth is the training ground, the school where the soul learns the lessons of life essential for the journey beyond death and for its development to a higher state. The purity of spirit is like gold hidden within the dross of the lower self and it is necessary that the life process should grind this away to reveal the gold of spirit. Like fine steel, the soul must be tempered by fire and hammer in the forge of life.

> For that reason I say to you again and again that what you regard as the bad experiences can be the best ones for you. It is not in the sunshine that the soul finds itself, but in the storm. It is when the thunder rages and the lightening flashes.
>
> You must be sharpened, purged, refined. You must experience the heights and the depths. You must have the variety of experiences that earth provides for you. In this way the spirit emerges stronger, fortified, ready for what awaits it when death comes.[8]

Law governs everything, and the Deity is the Law. Although the Deity is ultimately benevolent, indeed, infinitely so, it is also the Law, which is inexorable, yet just, remorseless, yet perfect, resolute, yet loving, and it is the Law, which in its wisdom and love brings the rain, the storm, the lightening and the fire, which cleanse and purify.

Although we grow through overcoming adversity, the traumatic extremes of life that we see all about us, are not essential to the growth of the soul and are not imposed by the Great Spirit, but are the consequence of human behaviour. In answer to a question regarding this paradox, Silver Birch answered:

> Wars are not made by the Great Spirit; disease is not given by the Great Spirit. These are the things that the children of matter have brought upon themselves by the misuse of their free will. There are lessons to be learned, but they can be learned without the brutalities and the hideous cruelties that the children of the Great Spirit perpetrate against each other. Do not mistake the doings of man for the acts of the Great Spirit.[9]

The natural law of cause and effect is intrinsic to the universal Law. As we sow, so shall we reap. This sequence is inescapable, both in this life and in the next. The law applies to all of us, no one has the power to thwart it. It may often seem that the reprobate and delinquent profit and thrive at the expense of the good and innocent, but there is always a spiritual debt incurred by the offender. There will be perfect retribution for the villain and perfect compensation for the victim; the account will be settled; balance is always maintained. The operation of this law is to be seen in the events, circumstances and situations that we experience. Although we are always inspired, supported and assisted by our spirit guides and are never alone, we are responsible for our own spiritual progress; only by our own actions and thoughts can we further our progress; we have to write our own spiritual examination, no one else can do it for us. No one can die on a cross for us. A life of selfishness brings about certain unavoidable consequences and stunts the expansion of the soul. Through a life of kindness, tolerance and altruism, the soul steadily grows in stature. The soul reaps its own reward and makes its own punishment. After passing to the next life, the soul will find itself on a spiritual plane in keeping with the progress it has made, shared with kindred spirits entertaining like values, interests and aspirations. The law of spiritual gravitation is infallible, we will always find ourselves with our spiritual equals. Birds of a feather will flock together, be they vultures or eagles. We create our own heaven or our own hell, but either will be as we wish it to be, at a vibratory level that is compatible with our inherent nature and level of spiritual progress.

> You are what you make yourself to be by your own conduct, by your own actions, by your own thoughts, by the whole of your life. And although that reality may not be visible in your world, the moment you pass the threshold of death, severing yourself from your physical body, you manifest as you spiritually are – no higher, no lower. You take with you just that character which you have moulded by your life. . . . Now see what happens (after death to the earth plane). You go to that sphere for which you are spiritually fitted. You have no desire to go lower, unless it be temporarily, on some mission to help those less fortunate than yourself. You cannot go to higher spheres because it is impossible for you to express yourself in any higher vibration than that which you can register. And your associates are those of like spiritual growth and like mental spirituality.[9]

The beauty of the spirit realm

Silver Birch extols the beauty of the spiritual domain; a beauty, which becomes evermore exquisite, glorious and sublime the higher one ascends through the spheres. Many who fear or resist death do so because of their fear of annihilation, fear of the unknown that looms before them, fear for the loss of their individuality, reluctance to leave their loved ones or to give up things that give them joy or which they are dependent upon in this world. But as the guide tells us there are more reasons for tears at the birth of a baby into this uncertain, potentially perilous life than there is reason for tears at the death of the body and the release of the soul into the beauty and security of the Life Beyond.

> To die is not tragic. To live in your world is tragic. To see the garden of the Great Spirit choked with the weeds of selfishness and greed and avarice, that is tragedy.[10]

For the spirit descending into the lower vibratory levels closer to the earth plane, the experience is extremely uncomfortable and unpleasant, the milieu through which they must move becomes progressively more dull, dense, oppressive, heavy and gross.

> And the nearer you get to the belt of matter, the more clumsy and difficult it is for the spirit to express itself. I never like to come back. The only things that make me do so are the promise that I have given to serve and the love of all of you, which gives me some compensation.[10]

We would require full consciousness of the contrast between the higher levels of the spirit world and this world to be able to truly appreciate the immense sacrifice made by great spirits when they return to work amongst us. Only love could motivate such a gesture.

> You have not tasted the joys of the world of spirit. There is nothing in your world of matter with which you can compare the life of the spirit, freed from the trammels of the flesh, escaped from the prisons of the body of matter, with liberty to go where you will, to see your thoughts take shape, to follow out the desires of your heart, to be freed from the trouble of money. No, you have not tasted the joys of the world of spirit.
>
> You, who are encased in matter, do not yet comprehend beauty as it can be. You have never seen our light, colour, scenery, trees, birds, rivers, streams, mountains, flowers – and yet your world fears death.
>
> This is the world where the artist finds all his dreams come true, where the painter and the poet realise their ambition, where genius has full power of expression, where the repressions of earth are swept away and all the gifts and talents are used in the service of one another.[10]

To have a clear-cut vision of the world that awaits us, to be able to anticipate its grandeur and magnificence, and to possess this foresight from birth is a huge asset and when coupled to the absolute, unshakable conviction of immortality, knowing that death is impossible, enables one to endure the tribulations and tragedies of the physical life with greater equanimity and fortitude, even in the face of what seems to be the greatest loss we can experience in life: the loss of a child, sibling, partner or parent.

The beloved spirit speaks on:

> To die is to enjoy the freedom of the spirit, which has been imprisoned behind the bars of the material body. Is it tragic to be released from suffering, for the soul to come into its own? Is it tragic to see colours, to hear music that does not belong to material expression?[10]

He tells us that there is no earthly painter, musician or writer who could through their art capture, record or describe, the sublime glories of the colour, music and landscape of the spiritual world. Our world is but a pale reflection of these beauties. However, the lower the spiritual sphere, the more its appearance resembles conditions on earth because its vibratory level is more dense. The vibration of the higher spheres is far finer and as one ascends their beauty becomes more and more transcendent.

Every night when we pass into the sleep state, we 'die' to the physical world and every morning we are 'born' again as we emerge from sleep. While the body sleeps, the soul is out of the body in a state of astral projection, connected to the body by an ectoplasmic, umbilical astral cord. The un-evolved soul remains close to the body and is relatively inactive while the body sleeps, but the more evolved the soul becomes, the more it participates in the activities of the spirit world and gains experience according to its stage of spiritual consciousness. On waking, the average soul will be unable to consciously recall what has happened during astral projection, because the lesser cannot contain the greater, or some images and memories will be retained, but often in a fragmented or distorted form. On an unconscious level nothing is lost, and the experience and knowledge gained always prove of value. The evolved soul that has reached a more advanced stage of consciousness has the ability to recall astral experiences, initially coming as spontaneous flashbacks, later in more continuous and extended form. This faculty can be developed through training. The more the soul progresses, the more prepared it becomes for the transition to spirit at the death of the body. To the soul well acquainted with spirit, death is like walking from one room into another without the least distress, confusion or lapse in consciousness.

The reality of spirit

When asked if the body we use in the spirit world is as real and solid as the one we leave behind, Silver Birch replied:

> Far more real and far more solid than the one you leave behind in the world of matter, for your world is not the real world at all. It is only the shadow cast by

the world of spirit. Ours is the reality and you will not understand reality until you pass into the world of spirit.[11]

Spirit to spirit is more real and authentic than physical to physical. This is understandable, because in the physical state, matter of a dense, low vibratory form stands between those who wish to communicate. Through facial expression and body language, a mask (the persona) can be donned to conceal feelings and emotions. In speech, thoughts have to be transformed into the symbols of language by the speaker and then interpreted and changed back into thought by the listener before they can be appreciated, which does not necessarily result in full understanding of what the speaker is trying to convey, and, besides, the subtle meaning of the symbols will often differ between the two. To further confuse matters, even without wish to mislead, words chosen do not always accurately voice what has been thought. As adept as we may become in the art of conversation and expressing ourselves, the process remains cumbersome, witnessed in the number of 'umms, errs, I mean-s, you know-s,' etc., that we frequently utter. Even the verbal mastery of a Shakespeare is inadequate to spontaneously express the totality of our thoughts, which are immaterial, while our language is material. Furthermore, speech, being an excellent vehicle for dissimulation, is not a reliable source of truth.

In contrast, in the world of spirit, there are no such barriers or possibilities of deceit, the spirit etheric body is radiant and far more sensitive and responsive than its physical counterpart; its boundaries are less defined and permeable. Through clairsentience, feelings and emotions pass freely between souls at the same level without importuning or impinging inappropriately. Communication is by means of thought without language, a skill that the newly born soul has to learn. Feelings and thoughts emanate openly, therefore the soul is never masked – it cannot escape scrutiny, there can be no deception or hidden agendas; its degree of radiance indicates its spiritual standing and the colours of the aura faithfully portray the emotions. In the spirit world you are known for who and what you are.

The imminence of spirit

It must be realised that although throughout our lives we are physically confined during our waking hours to the earth plane and a physical body, nevertheless, we are as much spiritual beings now as we ever will be, and, since everything created is in essence spirit, although we manifest on the lowest plane, we exist in the spirit world now as much as we ever shall. Under normal circumstances, however, we remain totally insensitive to this. Our lack of awareness of our spiritual identity and the spiritual milieu in which we dwell was not always so. Over centuries, our world has become coarsened through its materialism. In times past, human beings knew that spiritual gifts were the natural expression of faculties that belonged to their inner, eternal reality. Consideration of ancient texts and scriptures, lends proof to the conclusion that the exercise of the psychic faculties was far more common in those distant times than it is now. Our ancestors were conscious of the existence of other dimensions interpenetrating our own and these were accessible to them. The Native Americans, and other peoples regarded by Western society as unsophisticated, have, to a varying degree, retained this consciousness, and live in a world peopled by the spirits of the departed, who interact with them and can intercede for them. Young children, newly arrived on the earth plane, often display sensitivity to the presence of unseen persons or friends, indicating the presence of still-functioning psychic faculties, which later lose their acuity and finally, due to the impinging world and parental imprinting, cease to operate. We witness the same psychic perceptiveness in our dogs, cats and horses, a faculty that remains well developed throughout their lives. Unhappily, in the majority of people today these faculties have atrophied or closed down through disuse, and the number of psychics who can register the vibrations of spirit are very few.

Silver Birch tells us that we are all living in prisons with five tiny windows: the tiny apertures of our physical senses. Unless they are seen, smelt, touched, tasted or felt, we are oblivious to the happenings about us, and to the busy, teeming, unseen world with which we are surrounded, because we cannot register its vibrations. Our five faculties are the physical counterpart of our largely dormant, five etheric or psychic faculties, which, when developed, can give us sensory access to finer vibratory levels.

Speaking of the intermingling of dimensions, the guide says:

> It is all one universe, with many worlds in it. All life is one life, but it has many gradations. Life is one; the universe is one; there is no boundary; there is no frontier. Those who have passed from your ken are in the same universe as you are, but they are registering different vibrations, they are functioning on a different plane or aspect of consciousness. But they are here, even though you cannot see them, just as you are in our world, even though you cannot know it.[11]

Healing the sick

In addition to delivering the urgent message of eternal life, love, service and spiritual unfolding, a vital aspect of the plan initiated on the highest sphere of the spirit realm is the healing of the sick. In this aspect of the mission, the work of Silver Birch and Dr Letari, and other mediums and healers of the time, came together. Sickness of the body always indicates an associated sickness of the mind and soul, and healing is required on all three levels. Orthodox medicine lacks the method, understanding and reach to bring about such a cure. Limited by its material nature and oppositional strategy, it can at best only relieve, control and suppress the external manifestations of disease. The causative level of the mind and soul are beyond its influence even when it modifies perception, mood and behaviour through the action of psychotropic (psychoactive) drugs. Behind the pharmaceutical mask of normalcy, the soul still carries its burden of anxiety, fear, grief, paranoia, anger, resentment, hatred and depression; nothing is learnt, nothing is resolved. The healing process must touch and cleanse the soul so that the perfect, spiritual nature within can unfold and become the leading force in the patient's life.

The focus of Silver Birch's ministry was on touching the soul through spiritual instruction; the focus of Dr Letari's ministry, even though he commenced it by providing evidence of divine healing through direct laying-on-of-hands and absent healing, was on touching the soul through homeopathy.

Silver Birch always gave support, encouragement and advice to spiritual healers, advice which is just as pertinent to the homeopathic physician.

> What is important is to touch souls. Then the power of the spirit can quicken the flicker of divinity into a beauteous, lambent flame, so that the majesty of latent divinity shines through . . .[11]

> The healing power, which is divine in origin and in essence, is among the most important forces streaming into your world today. It is a very sick world. There are increasing numbers of diseases caused by the stresses and strains of the inharmonious conditions in which too many people live. Your so-called civilisation has divorced man from nature which provides some of the sources of his energy.[13]

He explained that disease is due to the natural balanced unity of body, mind and soul being out of harmony and that healing was the restoration of that harmony.

Emphasising, as he always did, the essential and beneficial role of suffering in the growth of the soul and the awakening of the spirit, Silver Birch asserted that the very essence of healing was that the healer should have personal familiarity with the pains of life and in consequence have suffered, because such experiences provide the compassion and empathy needed to successfully tend the afflicted. This is how the laws of life work, hence the old adage of 'the wounded healer.'

Suffering and spiritual growth

The following words uttered by Silver Birch are extremely profound and far-reaching; he was addressing healers at the time:

> So you suffer, and in your suffering, your spirit begins to come into its own. As a result you are able to unfold your healing gift and know what others feel when they come to you to be healed. Pain and suffering are regarded as miseries; they are not. They have divine parts to play in the evolution of the individual.[12]

Suffering is a word that chills the heart, but it must be understood that the suffering alluded to is far less the anguish and agony experienced in Germany as these words were uttered, and far more the suffering we all experience on our journey through life: the suffering imposed by our own, personal inner demons; our sense of isolation, loneliness and separateness; our delusions of being unlovable, inferior and unworthy; our anxieties, doubts and fears; our dependencies and needs; our losses and bereavements; our moral deficiencies; our emotional and physical illnesses; and particularly all the problems and trials we heap upon ourselves through wrong thinking and wrong acting. The paradoxes and polarities of physical life are essential to its purpose and possibilities. There must be light and dark; sun and shade; heat and cold; storm and calm; flood and drought; feast and famine; so too, pain and pleasure, sickness and health, just as there must be birth and physical death. Every emotion has its equal and opposite: love can transform to hate and hate can transform to love; only the coward can be courageous. The polarities sustain one another – one cannot exist without the other – this is the law of relativity – and the law is good! Life needs to be variegated and textured, it must intrigue, perplex, appal and enthral and offer opportunity to love or hate, to create or destroy, to be the hero or the villain. The most blessed gift we are given after that of our divinity is our freedom of choice and it is through exercising this gift judiciously, with care and love, that we express divinity. How could we do so if this life unfolded without the need for choice and decision over opposites, with no peaks or valleys, all level, monotonous and devoid of challenge or triumph? The soul must confront the choice between vice and virtue.

Think of the satisfaction and pleasure we derive from reading an exceptional book, or seeing an outstanding film, in which the wide range of human emotions is authentically depicted, touching us to the very quick, enabling us to identify with the characters and their fiction, sharing their pains and pleasures, their despair and joy. Would we have the book of our life written otherwise? Would we truly wish it to be insipid, indifferent and trivial, a book to be ignored or put aside? In moments of despondency and gloom, we may, indeed, evaluate the content of our lives in this way, viewing it as colourless, futile and worthless, but therein lies the delusion, the drama and the dilemma. The challenge to morality and grace does not have to be heroic to be significant, as the soul becomes finer and more translucent to the brilliance of the spirit, the enigma of life's events becomes more subtle and sophisticated in testing virtue.

Life is a symphony exquisite in counterpoint, a canvas rich in chiaroscura, a tapestry elaborate in design, yet simple in theme. The theme is always the unfolding and spiritual realisation of the individual soul. No matter what this entails, the events that take place in that soul's life are in every aspect perfect, fashioned with this sole objective and evidencing the divine law, which is wise, just and loving. Often in its misery and fear, or when surveying the tragedies of life, which can escalate to monstrous proportions, as during the Holocaust, the soul cries out in anguish to the silent heavens, "How can there be a loving God, when such terrible things are permitted?" Yet, there is a loving, wise and all-powerful, beneficent, universal consciousness or Great Spirit, which permeates all life and which created both the perpetrator and the victim, and loves them both. That paradox must be understood and explained.

The enormity of such a horrifying episode in humanity's history, magnifies the paradox to such vast proportions that one loses sight of God, immortality and the destiny of the individual soul caught up in such a catastrophe. The observer abandons objectivity, becomes entangled in group passions and identification, and caught up in subjective, emotional responses about injustice, barbarism, inhumanity, Jews, gypsies, homosexuals, Nazi's and Germans. For where in this vastness of hatred, cruelty, vicious sadism and unbounded evil can one detect the thread of truth, perfection, wisdom and love that constitutes God?

It is only when we consider the spiritual path of the individual soul caught up in the destructive seizure of a world event that we can cease 'to see through a glass darkly,' and identify the eternal thread that indicates the loving presence of the Great Spirit. From an early age, I was fortunate to be the recipient, through discourse with Dr Letari and familiarity with the teachings of Silver Birch, of many insights into the immaculate Reality, which stands behind the perplexing contradictions and hideous distortions which relativity presents to our human senses, emotions and understanding.

Divine beneficence

Firstly, as Silver Birch has told us, **the Great Spirit does not will wars and the horrors associated with human conflict, or the suffering of disease**, these are the consequences of our misuse of our freedom of choice; we must not "mistake the doings of man for the acts of the Great Spirit".

Immortality

Secondly, all the actors on the stage of life are immortal; no matter what ghastly tragedy is being enacted, no one can die; all the participants are, without exception, spirit beings cloaked with the attributes of soul developed in the course of their odyssey towards perfection.

Mystic truths, driven from our perception through our focus on what seems to be reality, or consigned to fable by the barren imagination of science, are captured and embodied in our myths. In this realm, unrestrained by the narrow paradigms of the intellect, we can glory in our divine heritage. Like the demigods of Greek legend, we are born of the gods and of mortals. In the act of conception, the god and mortal in us unite and the demigod is born, the imperishable, indestructible hero, or heroine, whose quest is the holy grail of spiritual excellence. The mythical demigod, an immortal hybrid, typified by the Greek heroes Herakles, Perseus and Theseus, although not yet a god, possessed unusual powers that approached those of a deity. These are akin to the latent, awesome spiritual powers within us all. In legend, these heroes fought and overcame all manner of evil in the form of vile humans or vicious beasts. We, in turn, cast in the same mould, must fight and overcome similar adversaries that dwell within our lower selves, the base characteristics of temperament and habit that hinder the progress of the soul. These encounters can only be enacted on the world's stage, which provides the extreme polarities against which the soul can test its moral fibre.

The spiritual teachings of all religions admonish us in one form or another to turn our cheeks to aggression, to love our enemy and to do unto others as we would be done by. These are the exercises that progressively transmute us from soul to spirit. Such precepts are meaningless if there is no aggressor, no enemy and no one we can hate or harm. All the players acting out these roles are present on our stage; there stands a Hitler, but there also stands a Mother Theresa; there stands a Himmler, but there also stands a Schindler; a motley multitude of saints and sinners make up the divine cast, all equally immortal and all possessing the freedom of choice with which to put our, and their, virtues and vices to the test. This is the school of life and there are sweet and bitter lessons to be learnt. For as Dr Letari told me time and again – *we are angels in training*! We must be familiar with every note on the keyboard of life.

Shakespeare inimitably paints this theatrical setting of life in the well-known, melancholic monologue delivered by Jaques in his play *As You Like It* (Act 2, scene 7, 139–143):

> All the world's a stage,
> And all the men and women merely players:
> They have their exits and their entrances;
> And one man in his time plays many parts,
> His acts being seven ages.

The seven ages of man which Jaques then catalogues pertain to a single life and its sequence of stages from infancy to old age, but, standing alone, these five lines have a far more profound meaning and pertain to the evolution of the soul, necessitating many different roles and many exits and entrances as the soul ascends to ever-higher levels of attainment, a gradation often referred to as 'seven spheres within seven spheres.'

Reincarnation

This brings us to the **third point** in understanding suffering and its catalytic role in the soul's progress: **reincarnation**. The eternity of existence of the spirit that extends limitlessly both into the past and into the future is punctuated at times by the soul once again descending to the earth plane for the purpose of exercising what it has learnt, reaping what it has sown in the past, facing unresolved issues, repeating trials as yet un-surmounted, gaining further experience, or returning in order to fulfil some service in the world. This cyclic return of the soul is known as reincarnation, also referred to as the transmigration of souls, or, given the name of the Greek equivalent, *Metempsychosis*. In ancient Greece, the precepts of Orphism, a religion structured round the mythical poet and musician Orpheus, who descended into Hades or the Underworld and returned, and the mythology of the risen hero-god, Dionysos, proposed the immortality of the soul and a cycle of successive physical lives, which the soul would eventually transcend through secret initiation rites and ascetic observance. Plato, in his Socratic dialogue, Phaedo, has his master, shortly before his death, state: "I am confident that there truly is such a thing as living again, and that the living spring from the dead".

Although a central tenet of the majority of Indian religious traditions, and intrinsic to Buddhism, most sects of the Middle-Eastern religions,

Christianity, Islam and Judaism, do not accept that the soul reincarnates. Notable exceptions are the contemporary followers of Kabbalah and the Rosicrucians. Christianity cannot accept reincarnation because it would overturn the elaborate system of political theology built around the concept of Christ as the saviour and redeemer of sins, a promise offered believers as reward for their loyalty to the creed. Such vicarious suffering on their behalf has seductive allure for those who wish to live their lives as they will, to 'sin,' and be exonerated through averred belief and through observance, tithes, penance, ritual and confession. All of which are alleged to provide painless passage to some poorly conceived, nebulous heaven of which their religious leaders can explain little. Press button salvation for many is the order of the day, and is particularly in keeping with the instant demands of the technological age. By contrast, reincarnation indicates spiritual self-determination and accountability and holds the soul responsible for its own redemption through expiation and loving service. Fortunately, many followers of the Middle-Eastern religions, while accepting, often without question, absurd interpretations of sacred texts, live an exemplary life based not on superstition and observance, but in harmony with the eternal philosophy inherent to all religions.

Though reincarnation is generally referred to as a belief, tenet or doctrine, both Silver Birch and Dr Letari present the principle of multiple lives as a scientific fact and not a religious concept. Even without the sort of proof that would satisfy modern scientific research and without personal memory of past lives, the principle of reincarnation should, nevertheless, make complete sense to anyone seriously contemplating life's critical role in the evolution of the soul. Life has immense purpose; it is a rite of passage, a baptism of fire, through which the purity of spirit becomes the light of the soul. It is immediately clear from our own life experience, that one lifetime, no matter how long, complex or colourful, cannot achieve such an extreme metamorphosis. As with any performing artist in this world, there must be many entrances and many exits, many diverse and demanding roles played before the soul becomes consummate in living the life spiritual, and receives the accolades of its peers. We must sip from many cups in our pursuit of universality. These varied roles must, therefore, require the soul, which retains its unique individuality from one life time to the next, to be variably male or female, heterosexual or homosexual, of any race, black, white or brown, of any nationality, and to be born into any religion. This fact immediately exposes the error of seeking identity or exclusiveness in any gender, race, nationality or religion or of harbouring any gender prejudice or any racial, nationalistic or religious pride or intolerance. Such discrimination and arrogance is based on childish ignorance and must prove futile, divisive and destructive. The world of today bears witness to this. No one can be spiritually Christian, Jewish, Muslim, American, British or Chinese, or any other religion or race. We are all immortal children of the divine, universal intelligence, one family, one people, all on the same spiritual path and we need to embrace and uplift, not hinder, hurt or distance one another.

Everything, from the electrons around the protons and neutrons of the atomic nucleus, from the vast orbits of planets about their suns, to the planetary and lunar phases of Earth, moves in cycles; so also the transmigration of the soul. After every spring, follows summer, after every summer follows autumn and after every autumn follows winter; then miraculously out of the transient death of winter spring bursts forth anew, blessing the world with resurgent life and creative vigour, preparing the way for the fullness and splendour of summer. This is the way of nature and we are part of nature and so it is our way too. A complete life has a sequence of spring, summer, autumn and winter and each season is precious and sacred, each brings its own treasure of soul experience; but just as no single cycle can produce the mighty oak, so too the soul requires many life cycles to attain its full majesty and display the 'annular lines' of its experience and maturity.

Each incarnation is like attending a grade at school. In the earlier stages of soul growth, the periods between each incarnation will be relatively short and as the soul matures through experience, and manifests more spiritual qualities, so the intervals grow longer until eventually incarnation to the earth plane is no longer necessary, or, as in the example of Silver Birch, and other great souls, a descent is made through intermediaries for a particular purpose. The lessons to be learned are inherent in the situations, circumstances and events of life, which are perfectly tailored to the needs of the soul. Nothing is by chance, coincidence or fortuity, everything happens when and as it should and is designed for the soul's progress, there are no mistakes and no accidents, everything happens according to law and the Law operates and governs through truth, wisdom, perfection and love. Certain lessons will be learned by the soul, others will be missed, resisted or ignored. Such lessons have to be repeated, often in the course of a single incarnation and sometimes through many cycles. The soul's failure to resolve or meet a challenge positively causes it to stumble into events, which repeat themselves, especially when relationships and unwise habits are involved. Thus the soul is given many opportunities to master a particular lesson. Within the tapestry of each soul's destiny, the pattern of compensation and blessing or reparation and suffering will be woven, not as reward or punishment, but as the inevitable consequence of good or bad action.

The reincarnation cycle is always human, and although some souls may make little if any progress during a specific incarnation, and others may even slide backwards, the accumulated experiences of life incrementally bring about the evolution of the soul; an upward spiral of sublimation leading on to transcendence. Animals belong to a parallel, spiritual hierarchy always ascending and refining, but always distinct from that of humans.

Given the spiritual nature of the cosmos, and its immensity, it is inconceivable and implausible that Earth should be the only planet in the infinite vastness of the universe to have produced life forms. There are millions upon millions of planets throughout the universe, which support life. Like Earth, these living planets provide soul experience for the legions of spirit beings populating all dimensions of the creation. The entire cosmos is our home; consequently, we are not restricted to planet Earth when we incarnate. This applies to our past as well as our future descents into the realm of matter.

The spiritual purpose of a productive life is to be of service to the creation and to be a source of love and light to others. Service comes in many forms ranging from the simple smile given to a stranger, to imparting knowledge, and to selfless acts of benevolence and altruism. It can also entail the bringing of pleasure and joy to others through all the arts and crafts: painting, sculpture, architecture, music, dance, literature, poetry, fashion, cuisine, photography, stage and cinema, and all things aesthetic, wholesome and uplifting. It is clearly not only for the spreading of spiritual knowledge and healing the sick that gifted souls descend into the physical sphere, it is also to give expression to their creative flare. These gifts may be called upon anywhere in the universe. Since the Renaissance, the Western arts reveal distinct periods in which exceptionally gifted artists, sculptors, composers, writers and poets, etc. have incarnated, enriching the world with great works of genius; indicating a huge determination of creative energy and talent to planet Earth during a relatively short time span. This happens on all planets when the civilisation and culture it sustains reaches a certain level of sophistication. In this we see a conjunction of planetary preparedness and the inherent and imperative need of the soul not only to love and give service, but also to create. This urge may bring about incarnation, as in the case of Bach, Mozart and Beethoven, during which the gifted musician serves as a highly accomplished channel or medium for music composed by groups of musicians working together in the spirit world. However, the composer is not merely a channel, but a full participant in composing the music that he or she is inspired to transmit. This can be well understood since during sleep the composer is able to commune on the astral level with musical colleagues in spirit. Collaboration of the two worlds is evidenced in the remarkable work of Shakespeare, Dickens and Tolstoy. The same planetary need, attraction and response that drew such creative minds to Earth, accounts for the concentration of high quality mediums incarnating between the late 1800s and the middle 1900s, a time of great activity in the astral world due to the large number of traumatised souls transiting to the afterlife, and the widespread grief experienced on the earth plane.

Our role and activities during our incarnation may be different and more modest than those of a Michelangelo, Rembrandt or Keats, nonetheless, each one of us has a significant and critical part to play in the universal plan and we too have beloved souls who accompany us through life, lightening our burden, protecting, prompting and inspiring us. Those closest and dearest to us often dwell in spirit, working assiduously for our benefit, sharing our trials and our joys, laughing with us and weeping with us, unrecognised and unacknowledged, but dedicated in their service to us. Others stand beside us physically, often shoulder to shoulder, pacing the earth with us, sharing in our destiny, possibly not for the first time, but as old and tried friends. Those united by love, interest, past association and common purpose are often drawn into the cycle of re-birth during the same period of Earth time.

Along the road we traverse in life, there will always be individuals we meet, who have significant influence on the unfolding events of our lives; these contacts, whether brief or prolonged, are never by chance, they are always predestined. Some come to stay, other encounters are short-lived, even fleeting, but nonetheless full of import. They appear in order to teach, prompt, support or point out the way, drawn to us by our conscious or unconscious aspirations; or they come to light attracted by less wholesome traits that we nurture, consorting in our decline and downfall should we yield to their negative influence. Despite all the blessings and love that surround us at all times, through our own inclinations and freedom of choice we can still court the disasters inherent in the dark side of life. Many of us only seem to grow through repeatedly falling and hurting ourselves, until through torment and travail we recover our senses, take stock of our lives and respond to the inner prompting of common sense and conscience.

Intrinsic to the peerless beauty of the divine scheme is the narrative of the hero's quest, which down the ages has been central to the myths and legends of all societies and cultures. In this timeless adventure, the soul, male or female, sets out on a seemingly impossible mission, which only he or she has the purity of spirit to achieve. This unique, inborn quality is known only to the Great Ones who secretly protect and foster the child, ensuring that through circumstances and the intercession of others the developing soul is aided in the preparation essential for the attainment of the divinely appointed goal, which when fulfilled will benefit humanity. Certain astrological, or other occult signs, reveal the child's birth or presence to those whose evil designs will be dashed if the child succeeds. They do everything in their power to ensnare or destroy the elected one. Sometimes flight from the motherland becomes imperative. Many hazards and temptations test the virtue of the young initiate, who, though vulnerable, repels the demons of fear, doubt, greed, pride, power and lust and remains inviolable. Finally, shed of moral impediments, the soul embarks upon its quest, sometimes astride a trusted steed, the fleetest of its kind, gifted with psychic perception and able to communicate with its charge telepathically. Often the mission entails a return to the land of the hero's birth and direct confrontation with the enemy. After surmounting many obstacles and facing many perils, which cause even this indomitable being to sometimes flinch and falter, yet always sustained by the divine powers of its animal companion and help from unexpected sources, the soul prevails, the enemy is vanquished and the quest fulfilled. In some versions, the attainment of the goal and final triumph demand the sacrifice of the soul's physical life.

From childhood, the hero's story, in all its variants, is dear to the human mind and heart, which intuits the reality of the adventure within the metaphor and identifies with it. It reflects in allegorical form the drama of all our lives. It is our story; it was William and Maurice's story. As told by Tolkien, we are all ring bearers with a divine mission in life, which only we can fulfil, to cast the ring of corruption and power, the false-self, into the cauldron of purification so that the true-self may rise like the mythical Phoenix from the ashes. The story is reflected in the myths not only of knights and maidens, but those that surround great souls such as Zoroaster, Moses, Jesus and Mohammad.

Cause and effect

In our search for God in the worst that life can offer there is a **fourth aspect** of the relative plane that we must analyse and that is a law intrinsic to life, to perfect justice and to spiritual progress: **the law of cause and effect, also known as karma**; the inevitable sequence of sowing and reaping that which we have sown. Through the action of this law, there is always perfect compensation for suffering and perfect reparation for the perpetration of wrong. The retribution should not be misconstrued as vengeful, malicious punishment, or the coldly dispassionate exacting of payment for moral debts accrued in this life, or past lives. Although the consequences of past action lead to the events which bring 'suffering', these events are always perfectly designed to prove spiritually catalytic and salutary to the soul experiencing the ordeal, and the soul is never abandoned, but helped in every possible way to achieve rehabilitation and insight. Even if only a glimmer of compassion or remorse can be evoked, progress results.

Therefore, when we try to make sense of the horrors of persecution and genocide, we must bring together our knowledge that both perpetrators and victims are immortal souls, no participant can die; that the intrinsic evil witnessed is man's inhumanity to man, exercised through his free-will, and is not willed, sanctioned or condoned by the universal consciousness; that the souls implicated in the events are both sowing and reaping their own deserts; and that what appears to be divine indifference or injustice is the playing out of individual destinies. The reasons for each soul facing a particular ordeal or challenge are complex and unique to that soul, and are always governed by perfect compensation and reparation brought about by the law of cause and effect.

Before the Holocaust, there was a seething, collective energy in the German people, which created a force field that drew incarnating souls within the ambit of developing events. The irresistible pull upon the soul to enter the vortex of violence depended on resonance between the soul's spiritual need to atone or attain and the template for fulfilling this need provided by the impending circumstances. The same laws that attracted highly gifted souls to Europe during and after the Renaissance, producing the eruption of artistic genius that enriched our civilisation, in the late 1800s and early 1900s, acted with ominous portent. Those souls drawn to the European stage, where they would play the roles for which they had been prepared and rehearsed through their past life experiences, came from many different levels of the spirit world, souls in transit, many new to Earth, not Jews, not Germans, not Poles, not Russians or any other nation or race, but souls intent on giving expression, through their free-will, to the light and dark within them. On that stage, primed with high drama, appeared many heroes, many villains and many victims, all archetypes of the human state. Lost to our sight are the unseen army of angelic beings, who, trained through their own familiarity with suffering, assisted and inspired the afflicted.

To contemplate the enormity of the Holocaust from an impersonal perspective and without losing trust in the imminence of a just and loving God, it is imperative to remember the cosmopolitan nature of the souls in contention, the spiritual dynamics presiding over all events and circumstances and the hidden morality running through the catastrophe and through the experience of each individual who was involved. It was a cosmic catharsis and should not be seen simply in terms of evil perpetrated by Nazis against Jews. To do so is to mislead ourselves with conclusions distorted by the residual passions and pains of identification with religion, nation or race, a delusion which supplies the ingredients that ensure the perpetuation of hate, prejudice and victim consciousness.

To make sense of the paradox of a loving and wise, omnipotent, omniscient and omnipresent divinity and the co-existence of extreme suffering, it is essential to grasp the interplay between divine benevolence and love on the one hand, and the action of the immutable laws of the creation on the other hand, of which free-will is an essential element, indispensable to the evolution of the soul. The ancient Greeks were conscious of this pivotal paradox and depicted it mythologically in the tension existing between the godhead, Zeus, and the three fates, the trio of goddesses, collectively known as the Moira, who, although vaguely conceived, represented destiny, 'man's lot,' or fate, in that our birth and death and the critical events which evolve between these extremes are predetermined. In the structure of the myths, it appears at times as if the Moira are independent of Zeus's will, or even above it. In a sense, they represent the fundamental laws of the universe, which even Zeus may not transgress.

The relativity of evil

Silver Birch explained that through its relationship to humanity, evil extends beyond the grave. The transition between this life and the next entails the setting aside of the physical raiment worn through life, but not the character, inclinations and individuality; these are preserved intact and unaltered and determine the spiritual level that the soul will dwell upon. The more carnal, selfish, acquisitive and egotistical the soul is, the lower the plane it will inhabit, and there, as in life, it will consort and conspire with souls of similar disposition. These lower planes are close to the vibratory level of earth with which they intimately interface, permitting such low souls to revisit the environs they previously frequented, and there vicariously satisfy the unresolved desires and urges which still prompt them. Bent on mischief, indulgence and subversion, they gravitate to places and people emanating disharmony and dissipation. Where revellers gather together and degeneracy and debauchery reign, particularly when alcohol and recreational drugs have removed inhibition, these dissolute souls feast and sate themselves on the emotional turmoil and wantonness that ensue. In this decadent scenario, we witness the indulgence of free will and the potential for dire consequences, despite the presence of an omnipotent loving God and the protective influence of the individual's spirit helpers. The same dynamics are played out in many homes when, despite loving parents, and against all advice and good example, the children pursue a hazardous path of self-indulgence and experimentation.

> The world of spirit is entirely composed of human beings who once lived on earth. It is not a world full of angelic cherubim. It is a world filled with a variety of human beings ranging from the very poor in spirit to the highest in saintliness. It is composed of the people in your world, and until all people in your world live lives that are clean, unselfish, filled with service and kindliness, there will always be a proportion in our world who include the undesirables and those who will still have to be helped and watched.
>
> A lot of them are not amenable to our influence. We cannot reach them. They become amenable to our influence only when they are touched in some way so that they are ready to be helped.[13]

Christian thought entertains the concept of a devil, or fallen angel, Satan, a demonic and evil being who wields an insidious and destructive power which can impinge upon human lives and seduce its victims to pursue a path of wickedness. His power is such that he can challenge God and undermine his works. This belief perceives evil as an autonomous, intelligent, dark energy that is pervasive, capable of preying on the pure and innocent and seeks the spiritual downfall of man. Evil in this sense is given an absolute value, the equal and opposite of virtue. In the light of Silver Birch's message, evil, unlike love, has no absolute or eternal quality, it is relative and utterly dependent on the thoughts and actions of humanity on this plane and the next, and though its intangible influence exists as a field of negative energy which is pervasive, the band on which it vibrates is narrow and pools around places, persons and circumstances where it finds resonance. Evil has no predatory power; like a virus, it is opportunistic and seduces the vulnerable; the seed is in the individual and germinates through imprinting, conditioning and example and grows through habituation. Sensitives who are not vulnerable to a specific evil influence may, nevertheless, be clairsentiently aware of its vibratory presence, which is very disquieting, but, unless there is some affinity with its influence, it has no power to do harm. Virtue is the armour of the soul.

However, the presence of many unpleasant, 'undesirable' souls in the lower spheres of the spirit world can be disruptive to the work of mediums and those seeking to spread spiritual truth.

> There are unfortunately, forces which are not charitably disposed towards the spread of truth, wisdom and knowledge and whenever they can they seek to use their influence . . . that it is why it is unwise for individuals to attempt the unfoldment of psychic faculties when they are alone. There is no power there to enable a control or guide to build up sufficient strength to ward away interlopers and the undesirables.[13]

It is not surprising, given the current intense antipathy of scientific atheists on the earth plane to religious belief and all forms of complementary and alternative medicine, and their belittling of any perspective differing from scientific reductionism, that similarly arrogant and prejudiced souls residing in the spirit world, and still ignorant of spiritual truth, desire to disrupt and sabotage the work of those intent on bringing this knowledge to humanity. Leopards do not easily change their spots; the passage to spirit does not filter out egotism and bigotry.

Religious indoctrination

However, their activities remain only an annoyance and cannot be compared with the difficulties caused by the indoctrination of so many in this life with spurious religious teachings that ensure that the soul is ill-prepared for the transition to spirit, which renders them confused, disorientated and unable to adapt to their new circumstances. Their belief becomes their reality. While this is true in life, it becomes even more so in the spirit world where thought is pivotal and creates the world in which they live. If they are convinced that they have been consigned to purgatory, then so it will be, and the soul stagnates in a state of spiritual inertia unable to move forward and embrace the incomparable opportunities of its new world. It might seem that it should be fairly easy to persuade the misled soul of the truth. With some it is, but with the majority of religiously afflicted souls, the belief system with which they were brainwashed, often from birth, serves as compensation and security for a dysfunctional soul troubled by fear, shame and guilt. Their survival and redemption depends on the belief being true, it is imbedded in the psyche and an immense amount of energy has been invested in self-indoctrination. They cling to this protective shield, and, as in this world, join communities of souls with similar convictions, which further confirms and intensifies their fanaticism.

Silver Birch is a gentle, loving spirit who preaches profound truths, which if followed lead to the unfolding of the higher nature and a deeper understanding of life and the afterlife. When considering the history and present role of the orthodox religions, he is severe in his judgement and condemnation. They constitute a serious hindrance to spiritual progress, which requires freedom of the mind and soul, devoid of bigotry, division and the restricting, retarding influence of doctrine and dogma based on superstition and ignorance. In this critical stance, he, like Richard Dawkins, sees religion as a major cause of ignorance, conflict and strife, but he goes much further in analysing its destructive influence.

> The bondage of creeds is one of your world's worst afflictions. It is worse than pestilence and disease, far worse than the physical sufferings of the body through illness, for it is an affection of the soul. It puts the spirit in blinkers.

He speaks with respect of Jesus (whom he calls the Nazarene) as a fellow messenger and teacher, but reproaches the Churches.

> They have surrounded the Nazarene with fable. They have magnified him into the Great Spirit of life. . . . I am impatient with Churches because they betray the Nazarene whom they seek to serve. I am impatient because they remove him so far from humanity that he ceases to be an example and becomes a god, dwelling in the high heavens beyond the reach of the children of matter.

> Over the doors of the churches is not written: 'We are loyal to truth and truth alone.' Rather does it say: 'We preach by creed, we espouse doctrine, we practise ritual, we are tied to ceremony.' The Churches are the means of opposing truth.

> That is why we have come back to your world – to ask you to give no obedience to any one man, to any one book, to any one church, to any leader, to any being whether in the world of matter or the world of spirit, but only to learn obedience to the laws of the Great Spirit, for they alone are infallible and unerringly right.[14]

The teachings that Silver Birch left to the world are precious gems best appreciated by reading the books that have been compiled from notes taken during the séances of the Hannen Swaffer home circle. His message always affirmed that the purpose of life is the spiritual enlightenment of the soul, which can only be achieved through loving service to the creation; that the path will entail obstacles, opposition and suffering; that the soul has the inner power to prevail, no matter the challenge; and that we are never alone, but always accompanied and sustained by those in the spirit world. His simple eloquence always provides balm and inspiration to the beleaguered soul.

> We are concerned with the reality of life, trying to teach your world that it cannot find peace and real happiness in shadows. Shadows exist because they are cast by the light, and the light is spiritual reality. We desire always to draw attention to the vast potentialities of an infinite spirit, not only ruling through the universe, but in fragment, resident in every individual.

> It is within that you will find that vast treasury where true riches are stored. It is within that you will find the strength to help you in times when you need it and

when all the resources of matter fail; when all earthly friends have fled; when you seem to be alone, uncared for and neglected. Even then, you can know that the warmth, the companionship and the love of beings from another world are still with you.[14]

References

1. Swaffer H. Foreword. In: Austin AW (ed). *Teachings Of Silver Birch*. London: Spiritualist Press; 1962.
2. Barbanell S. (ed). *More Wisdom Of Silver Birch*. London: Psychic Press Limited; 1945. pvii.
3. Riva P (comp). *Light From Silver Birch*. London: Psychic Press Limited; 1988. p201.
4. *Ibid.*, p205.
5. Storm S (ed). *Philosophy of Silver Birch*. London: Psychic Press; 1972. p25.
6. *Ibid.*, p23.
7. Riva P (comp). *Light From Silver Birch*. London: Psychic Press Limited; 1988. p15.
8. *Ibid.*, p25.
9. Barbanell S (ed). *More Wisdom of Silver Birch*. London: Psychic Press Limited; 1945. p81.
10. Austin AW (ed). *Teachings of Silver Birch*. London: Spiritualist Press; 1962. pp120–121.
11. Riva P (comp). *Light From Silver Birch*. London: Psychic Press Limited; 1988. p111.
12. *Ibid.*, p113.
13. Barbanell S (ed). *More Wisdom of Silver Birch*. London: Psychic Press Limited; 1945. pp188–189.
14. *Ibid.*, p198.

16

HEALING AND TEACHING

The opening of the Letari Nursing Home

When the new Sanctuary opened its doors at 8/10 Bulstrode Street, William received a telegram from Sylvia and Maurice Barbanell, which read: "May this be the beginning of even greater work and greater success."

This telegram must have meant a great deal to him because he kept it amongst his important papers. As I write, it lies on the desk before me. It is dated Monday, 2 November 1942 – posted all of seventy years ago.

Barbanell officiated at the formal opening and reported this event in the *Psychic News*:

> I opened on Monday the Letari Nursing Home in the West-end of London, where WH Lilley will now treat his patients.
>
> Its opening is a triumph for the dogged endurance of Lilley and his colleague, Arthur Richards. Men of lesser mettle might have given up in despair because of the difficulties, which often seemed insuperable. They had to obtain all sorts of permits from the Ministries of Health and Supply. They had to satisfy many inspectors.
>
> At first out-patients only are being treated. Later, arrangements will be made to receive in-patients.[1]

From the outset, the Letari Nursing Home was a hive of activity. The day began early and went on into the early evening. It was the usual mix of consultations, spiritual healing while in trance, the acute and chronic prescribing of homeopathic remedies, chiropractic manipulations and then the immense task of dealing with the mountain of correspondence from the British Isles and the rest of the world. This was made up of reports from patients on treatment, each of which had to be analysed for the follow-up homeopathic prescription and personally answered, and appeals for diagnosis and absent healing, which were also answered individually, each reply being accompanied by a homeopathic prescription decided on by William and Dr Letari. When I was old enough to remember, the oak desks at which the typists laboured, the smell of ink and stationary, the overflowing waste paper bins, the relentless rapping of the typewriter keys and the staccato pings of the carriage returns, impressed my young mind.

Diagnosing for the orthodoxy

Being in the heart of medical London and having a reputation for making accurate psychic diagnoses at a time when medical science lacked many of the sophisticated diagnostic methods it possesses today, my father was often approached by medical doctors, both general practitioners and specialists, to help with difficult cases. This collaboration began in the early years before the Sanctuary opened in Hunslet and at that time involved my mother, who through working at the clothing factory was available on the telephone. She told me that frequently Dr Letari would anticipate these calls and give her the names of those who would telephone, what time she could expect the call, what would be asked and what she should tell the doctor. It was this evidence of medical interest that made my mother realise the great importance of the work William was doing.

While still in Hunslet, he was requested by a group of specialists to attend the Leeds General Infirmary in order to have his diagnostic skills tested. The results so impressed his audience that he was made a considerable financial offer to make his gift professionally available. As attractive as the incentive was, especially to a young married man on a modest salary, Dr Letari advised his mediator to decline. The gifts of spirit were not for sale. Reflecting on that time, my father told me that he was only too glad to extricate himself from their clutches because they also wanted to do physiological experiments on him while in the trance state. On the only occasion that Dr Letari permitted this, the specialists stuck pins into various zones of his body to test his reaction to pain. They failed to elicit any response. When pressed to submit to further tests, Dr Letari refused knowing full well that one thing would lead to another, they would never be satisfied and his mediator would be used as a guinea pig to satisfy their curiosity. Similar overtures and promises of reward were received in London, but William kept the doctors at arm's length and only consented to aid with diagnoses. At the time, he found it curious that although his reputation resulted as much from the results he achieved with the remedies he prescribed as from his gift of diagnosis and absent healing, the specialists he dealt with expressed no interest whatever in the homeopathic treatment that played such an important part in his success. They were only interested in the diagnosis and not the cure. He came to realise that more often than not the medical mind is stubbornly closed to alternative forms of therapy.

Scotland Yard

Throughout his career, my father's healing work was so conspicuous that whereas many lesser known spiritual healers and professional homeopaths passed unnoticed or were ignored by opponents, he was soon seen as a danger either to orthodoxy, to religious creed or even to public morality, and therefore targeted. The Letari Nursing Home had been in operation somewhat over a year when, as my father put it, ". . . there came the knock upon the door." Inspector Chesney of Scotland Yard, under instruction from the Home Office, had come to investigate the nursing home in response to a number of complaints and suspicions that had been lodged by certain parties, obviously intent on doing harm to the venture. These complaints ranged from exploitation of the public for exorbitant financial gain, to suggestions that the work being done in the establishment was potentially immoral, since the Absent Healing pamphlets issued by the nursing home were calculated to excite the sensibilities of women. The inference that there was a potential brothel on the boil and possible tax evasion left the authorities with no alternative but to investigate. For good measure, the nursing home was also charged with the illegal use of labour and paint during a time of war restraints.

The investigation lasted two months, a time of great stress to all involved in the healing work, which went forward without faltering. The forensic audit revealed that the nursing home was being run at a loss and would not have been able to meet its financial commitments if it had not been for the sponsorship received from its patrons. All the other charges were found to be equally unfounded and the nursing home was free to continue operating. During this time, Inspector Chesney was in frequent contact with my father and became intrigued by the work he was doing. I have no doubt they spent some time together in the third floor room in which the billiard table stood. They became friends, and when the investigation was brought to a close, the Inspector, who was experiencing health problems became a patient and met Dr Letari. Through Chesney's enthusiasm for the cause, William gained many patients from Scotland Yard.

William meets Silver Birch

It was during this time, when problems and hindrances beset them from every direction that William and Arthur Richards received an invitation from Silver Birch to attend Hannen Swaffer's home circle. The details of this meeting were published in *Psychic News*, October 31, 1942. When given the opportunity to question the spirit sage, William spoke of the problems attending the opening of his healing clinic in London's West End, the opposition, prejudice and barriers to be surmounted.[2]

Silver Birch reassured him:

> My son, you have been raised up because the Great Spirit has endowed you with gifts that must be used, and there is no power on earth that will prevent those gifts from being exercised if you will co-operate to the fullest extent with those associated with you from my world. You speak of difficulties and obstacles; they were made to be overcome. But remember you have invited some of them. You have asked some of these troubles to be visited upon you. You have not chosen to work in silence. You have behind you those who are capable of guiding you through all your difficulties and who have given evidence of their ability for many long years. They have guided you over many difficulties and through many perplexities and at any time when you look back and contemplate the road you have travelled, you will see quite clearly the guiding finger of the spirit.
>
> You are a healer. You will heal. No one can stop you, unless you stop yourself. You have a power which must be expressed. It is a power which does not belong to your world; it comes from the higher spheres of life. That power will be a boon and a blessing to thousands of sufferers. There is no authority in your world that will stop that power from being expressed if you choose to express it. You must not allow any fear to take even temporary residence within your being. You must have complete confidence that those who have led you so far will not fail you now, for there is still a broad path to be traversed, there is still a wide sphere of service to be accomplished. Have no fear. Just as the power of spirit has triumphed over what in days gone by seemed insuperable difficulty, so once again it will be victorious, and in the years to come you will be able to pause and smile at problems that then will be regarded merely as shadows.
>
> There is work to be done. There are so many who require the healing touch. There are so many troubled souls. There are so many fearful minds. There are so many racked with disease and illness. And you can help them with the gift that has been given to very few. I wonder if you know how richly you are blessed and endowed.[2]

These words were of great importance to my father for they came from a great soul whom he held in high esteem. Although never without the inner voice and supporting presence of Dr Letari, encouragement and confirmation coming from such an additional source at a critical crossroad were wonderfully empowering. The guide's words proved prophetic because no matter the difficulties which lay ahead, and these were considerable, the work of healing, upon which he had embarked, though on more than one occasion threatened by officialdom, remained unhindered until many years later when his health began to give way.

When asked by my father about the difficulties which often arise in the treatment of disease, Silver Birch replied that disease results from humanity stepping outside the laws of the creation and that there is no panacea for any particular disease manifestation:

> If there were correct living there would be no disease. Disease, in essence, is caused by disharmony, discord, by the failure to live life according to the laws of the Great Spirit. Always the healing power has to be adjusted to the type of illness. There is no such thing as one vibration that is capable of healing all manner of disease. Success in psychic or spiritual healing consists in finding that vibration of power, which is exactly needed for the disease.

This statement is in perfect keeping with the principles of homeopathy; asserting that disease results from a negative change in the ordered vibration of the healthy body and that healing requires a precise, corrective adjustment of that vibratory change.

Silver Birch then referred to the failures in healing that occur and stressed the necessity for the healer to develop spiritually and thus be in harmony with the laws of healing. As in homeopathic therapy, it is never just the song – it is always the singer and the song in unison that create the harmony of healing.

> Where there is failure, it is not necessarily a criticism of the world of spirit, or of the particular healing guide, or even of the instrument. So many factors are in operation all the time. The most important thing for you to consider is this. How can I live my life so that I am completely and perfectly in harmony with the power that uses me? For the more you abolish all the differences between you and your guides, for you know there are more than one, the easier it is for them to transmit through you just the right vibration which is necessary every time.

> There is a whole range of healing power in our world, for there are doctors and scientists constantly engaged in research, but they are dependent on the instruments at their disposal as to the amount that can be transmitted, as to the type of rays and vibrations that can be used. That is the part you must play, in the growth of your soul, the unfoldment of your mind and the equipping of your own body.

No healer could possibly receive better advice than that which Silver Birch imparted to my father that evening. Whereas it is possible to be a villain and remain a brilliant surgeon, a healer and any physician using energy medicine, such as homeopathy, must possess the essential moral integrity to be an unresisting channel for the healing process. Spirituality and the healing vocation must walk hand in hand.

Frank Leah, the psychic artist

One evening, not long after we had settled into our flat in West Hampstead, Arthur Keith Desmond, the special correspondent for the *Psychic News* and author of the book about my father, *The Gift Of Healing*, visited us. As usual, the conversation between Desmond and my father turned to Spiritualist matters and to the various mediums that were prominent in the movement at the time. During the discussion, Keith Desmond brought up the name of Frank Leah (1886–1972), a remarkable psychic artist renowned for his exceptionally accurate portrait drawings of deceased persons, who worked from his studio in Kensington, London.

Leah, the eldest child of a large working class family, was born in Stockport, England. He showed artistic skill from an early age, producing great likenesses of people in caricature. When just twelve years old, he sold his first cartoon to a local newspaper. Confident of his ability and determined to develop it further, he left home at fifteen for Ireland and settled in Dublin where he trained as a draughtsman and developed his skill as a portrait and landscape artist. His work won him great respect and after working as an illustrator for a number of newspapers, he became at various times, the art editor for five Dublin journals. A collection of his portraits of Irish theatrical personalities was donated to the national Library of Ireland. Possibly keened by the otherworldly milieu of the Irish consciousness, Leah's own inherent psychic awareness began to unfold with the development of exceptional clairvoyant, clairaudient and clairsentient powers, which permitted him to identify and draw the portrait of spirit sitters. Not only was he able to see and converse with the spirit entity posing for him, but as part of the psychic process of creating a lifelike portrait, he would often vicariously experience the events and sensations associated with their passing. He once commented about this saying: "I have died over one thousand deaths."

Eventually, the insistent prompting of his psychic gift moved him to return to England, and once there, to devote himself to giving the bereaved the most convincing proof possible of the continued existence of their loved ones, portraits of such accuracy and detail that they might well have been photographs. In addition to these portraits he was able to relay messages from the deceased to their families, which contained vital details, leaving them with no doubt about the immediacy of those they mourned. In 1943, the year after the evening we are considering, a book on the work of Leah by Paul Miller was published titled: *Faces Of The Living Dead: The Amazing Psychic Art Of Leah*. This book has recently been republished and bears witness to his truly extraordinary ability, both as a medium and as an artist. Leah died at the age of 86, after over forty years exclusively devoted to painting the portraits of 'The Living Dead.'

Talking of Frank Leah put a thought into Desmond's mind and he told William that he would like him to meet Leah. Caught up by the enthusiasm of the moment and suiting the action to the word, Desmond immediately phoned Leah from our flat and introduced the two mediums, each so renowned in his own field.

Lilley chuckled and asked of Leah, "Do you ever see a Hindu gentleman walking around your studio?" Leah replied, "Oh, yes. I feel sure he is here now. The vibration is so strong!" The artist's mediumship is frequently demonstrated in this manner in the course of telephone conversations. To this many can testify.[3]

Leah's clairvoyance and clairaudient sensitivity was so acutely developed that he was known to have described and given details about a deceased spirit before the prospective sitter on the other end of the telephone had time to give a name and ask for an appointment. The intent to establish contact on the part of the sitter would be sufficient to give the departed spirit the cue to appear before Leah's inner eye. On one occasion, when very tired from all night Air Raid Precaution (ARI) duty, he unintentionally fell asleep in his chair before his morning bath, and during this very short nap, a man appeared vividly before him, who after relating his story told him that his daughter would be telephoning shortly for an appointment. Half an hour after he awoke, the telephone rang, and as he anticipated, the caller was the man's daughter, hoping that her father would appear to the artist for his portrait. This anticipatory knowledge was similar to Dr Letari's giving case details of a patient and their diagnosis to my mother before any doctor had telephoned for help.

With my father on the telephone, the contact between Leah and Dr Letari was particularly strong and Leah, without hesitation, commenced describing him to William and gave him important details from Dr Letari's life on earth, all of which confirmed that the Doctor was beside him as he spoke.

He told William that Dr Lejan Tari Singh was born in Peshawar, India, in 1889 (in 1942, Peshawar was not yet situated in Pakistan). He was a Hindu of the Brahmin caste and 'died' near his birthplace, at the mouth of the Khyber Pass, on April 18, 1914, just two months after my father's birth on 25 February, when he was only twenty-five years of age. Leah went on to supply details about Dr Letari's medical education in Calcutta, giving the exact address of the college he attended. On qualification, he left India and studied surgery for two years in England before returning to Peshawar to commence practice. Two years after his return, during riots against the British, a man was shot in the street outside the building in which Dr Letari was working. Without thought for his own safety, he dashed into the street to assist the injured man, and while he was tending him, a stray bullet wounded him severely in the abdomen. For a week he lay in a coma. His colleagues tried desperately to save him, but he died without regaining consciousness. Leah continued by describing Dr Letari's features, his figure and his mannerisms. In particular he stressed the intensity of his eyes – one of his outstanding features – and his short stature. This last point was very conclusive, because Dr Letari was only five-foot-one in height.

Very impressed, William turned to Keith Desmond and told him that no one had ever given him such an accurate description of his guide.

In an article written for *Psychic News*, Keith Desmond supplied more details about that special evening when two very gifted mediums met.

> Almost every fact tallied with what Lilley already knew of the 'dead' doctor – with one exception. Leah said the doctor wore a moustache. At the time Lilley could not agree.
>
> But when, in response to the artist's pressing invitation, I took Lilley down to his studio the same evening, Dr Letari himself, through his entranced medium told us that from 1910–12 – two years before his passing – he wore a moustache during his visit to this country (England) to study surgery.[3]

While William remained entranced and Dr Letari and Keith Desmond continued to talk, Leah, intent on capturing the portrait of the spirit guide, approached his drawing board and "executed a lightening, but detailed portrait of the Hindu who is beloved by thousands."[3] Leah was noted for the speed with which he could accurately sketch the features of his subject. Some could be completed in a few minutes, but he was known to have produced good likenesses within half a minute and one fully recognisable drawing took no more than nine seconds. The eyes were critical to him, and once he had captured these, the remaining contours of the face followed rapidly. His initial sketch would often follow a telephone call and the further filling in of detail would take place later when the person wishing for a spirit portrait visited his studio. Some would take considerably longer because spirit sitters can be as difficult and idiosyncratic as their 'living' counterparts.

When William returned from his short visit to the astral plane, an excited Keith Desmond showed him the picture. His reaction was immediate and spontaneous. He exclaimed, "That's the doctor!"

However, Leah was not yet satisfied. He told them that he needed time to add more detail, which would render the drawing an even more faithful likeness of his clairvoyant image of the doctor.

This did not take long. The following day, he informed them that the finished sketch was waiting. William was delighted with it and told Leah that Dr Letari wished to personally thank him, therefore, as on the previous evening, William went into trance.

Healing and teaching 411

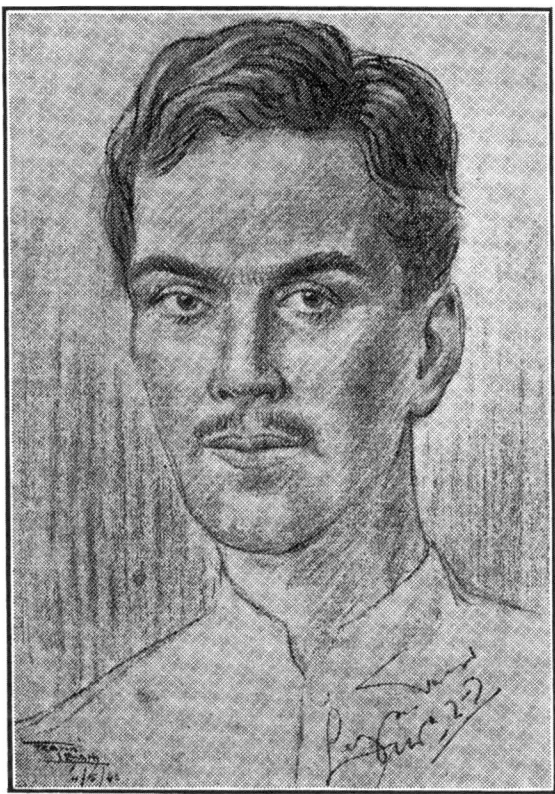

Figure 16.1 Frank Leah's Portrait of Dr Letari

Whereupon, in his own characteristically courtly manner, addressing the artist, the guide said: 'If you will give permission, I would consider it a great privilege to sign it.'[3]

Which he did, and added, beneath his signature, symbols which indicated his calling, his status and his religion.

Contemplating the image of himself, he then declared that if he had seen the portrait as his own reflection in a mirror, he would have been well pleased at the spectacle. It is this reflection of Dr Letari that contemplates me from the wall of my study as I sit before my computer.

This portrait became as well known to the public as the photographs of my father that appeared with newspaper articles written about the work of the Sanctuary. A small print was always included with the homeopathic questionnaire that every applicant for psychic healing received.

My spirit father

Dr Letari was involved in my life from conception, advising and helping my mother through her pregnancy and later with all the anxieties and uncertainties of tending a first baby. It was he who prescribed homeopathic remedies for me when I suffered from severe whooping cough at three years of age.

I had just turned four when I was present at a trance address that my father gave. I was apparently well behaved and fascinated by his transformation. Maurice Barbanell was present, and after the address took me aside and questioned me about what I had seen. He was so charmed by what I had to say that he included our exchange as a tailpiece to his editorial in the next edition of *Psychic News*, dated October 21, 1944.

> Asked what he thought of a trance address given through his father, four-year-old David Lilley, son of the famous healer, said, 'Daddy is talking funny.' While the boy accepts Dr Letari, the healer's guide, David believes, in some childish way, that the 'dead' doctor is in Daddy's head.[4]

However, I was five before I retained a memory of his presence. I can remember exactly where I was at the time – sitting on his lap in the treatment room on the third floor of 8/10. My mother must have been present, but only the doctor is in the image. Most clear to me is the complete acceptance and understanding I had regarding the fact that the person holding me was not my father but a loving, protective, wise being from the spirit world, who, though unseen, was always present and one of the family. This never seemed strange or unusual to me. His voice, accent, vocabulary, facial expressions and mannerisms were markedly different to those of my father and remained consistently so throughout our long relationship, which commenced in 1945 and ended in 1972, some four weeks before my father's death, when his mediator was no longer strong enough to go into trance. On the occasion of this first recollection, I remember him saying that as I grew up he would tell me many wonderful stories about many wonderful things. It was a promise I would never forget and one that he kept – and in great measure. In a sense that first meeting with him was also my baptism for he gave me my spirit name, a name I had carried with me through past incarnations and which I will take forward with me into the lives of the future. He never called me by any other. To my father, I was always David.

From that moment, Dr Letari instilled in me the precious knowledge of my deathlessness. Would that all children could be given that consciousness: the unshakable conviction of their immortality, an unassailable fact, unadulterated by fantasy and religious superstition. With that eternal awareness deeply inculcated, the events of life become far more significant and meaningful and can be appreciated as part of the essential schooling of the soul. Life, with all its ups and downs, retains a sacred aspect, which fortifies the stoicism of the soul through adversity.

An avalanche of correspondence

The war on the continent was raging, but life in Britain went on as usual and the demand for absent healing from the Sanctuary increased steadily. This multiplied significantly after *The Gift Of Healing* was published. The Leeds healing centre remained open for applicants, but with the headquarters now established in London, all the post received in Hunslet had to be forwarded to Bulstrode Street. Most of the letters were bulky, containing either handkerchiefs or other personal articles sent in for psychometric analysis. Eventually the entire process became too cumbersome to continue. An article in the *Psychic News* referred to the problem and the solution, which was made possible by the further development of William's diagnostic mediumship.

> His post bag became so swollen that it was found impracticable to post him hundreds of letters and articles. On the instructions of his spirit guide a new method was devised. Lilley merely receives a list of the names and addresses of applying patients. Then looking at the list, he gives the diagnosis right away. So widespread were the number of applications, as a result of the recent series in *Psychic News*, that at one time there was a danger of the whole elaborate Leeds organisation breaking down.

The press of patients did threaten to overwhelm the Sanctuary. How my father managed to cope with the extreme demands made upon him during those years is hard to imagine, let alone explain, and I suspect the continuous pressure to perform must have insidiously initiated the changes, which eventually contributed to his early death. In addition to his intense work at the nursing home during the week, William was invited by numerous Spiritualist churches scattered around England to give addresses to their congregations at their Sunday services. Although it was Dr Letari who took the platform, nonetheless, the extensive travelling and prolonged trance states all took their toll on his mediator.

During a conversation with Maurice Barbanell, he confessed to feeling the effects of his continuous labours. This prompted Barbanell to add an editorial tailpiece in the June 9, 1945, edition of *Psychic News* to the effect that a famous psychic healer, after a hard day's work, had said to him in the last week, "I feel so tired that I am going to put myself on my absent healing list."[5]

This comment was typical of the delightful sense of humour he always retained even in the most exacting circumstances.

Lecturing

Like Silver Birch, Dr Letari was an excellent and inspiring orator and although he spoke primarily about the origins of disease and its management, his message was always threaded-through with the same uplifting spiritual truths that his fellow guide was spreading.

Over the years, the demand for these appearances increased and they developed from short discourses into substantial lectures delivered to larger and more informed audiences, but still under the auspices of various Spiritualist churches or societies. The subject matter of the lectures became more complex and profound as Dr Letari expounded on the spiritual science of divine healing and on the philosophy of disease causation, teaching the hereditary and miasmatic nature of chronic disease as elucidated by Hahnemann and his followers. As their content deepened, his lectures also became more controversial, not only in the eyes of orthodox medicine, but also to many Spiritualists and other spiritual healers.

Ectoplasm dispute

During such a lecture, Dr Letari explained how he utilised ectoplasm generated from his medium and assistants to isolate benign and malignant tumours, while the healing process he initiated, assisted by carefully selected homeopathic remedies, brought about their absorption and elimination. This method could prevent metastatic spread and in cases where this had already occurred, could isolate the metastases (secondaries). Dependent on the degree of destruction, restoration of damaged tissues was also brought about. The energy required in the production of the primal matter, which acted as a barrier and as a pluripotent substrate for tissue regeneration, was rapidly restored to the medium and the assistant donors without untoward effect. Restoration of damaged structure was more easily achieved when the lower organs or tissues were compromised, e.g. the skin, fibrous tissues and bones, and with greater difficulty when the higher organs were involved, e.g. the nervous system, pancreas, etc.

It is remarkable how human nature so easily adopts an archetypal rigidity and entrenched stance once a concept has taken root and then resists and derides any model that presents a contrasting view. This can be anticipated among the orthodoxy, but is less expected among the eclectic.

Dr Letari's explanation of his use of ectoplasm, excited a controversy amongst Spiritualists who had never heard of ectoplasm being used in this way, and resulted in a flurry of correspondence in *Psychic News*. At the forefront of the opposition was Harry Edwards (1893–1976), the well-known non-trance contact healer, who expressed his scepticism in articles he placed in the periodical.

> To assert that ectoplasm can be dissociated from the producing medium and that it can be intelligently maintained within the body of a second party is outside all known experience . . . it is incomprehensible according to known facts.[6]

His criticism was based on the common knowledge that when ectoplasm was extruded from a materialisation medium, such as Helen Duncan, it temporarily adopted the features and form of a spirit entity, but did not take on an independent existence. It remained an extension of the medium and when the phenomenon was concluded it immediately withdrew into the medium's body.

In response to the questions the controversy raised, Dr Letari expanded on this subject to his helpers at the Sanctuary and to a *Psychic News* correspondent. He told them that ectoplasm could be used in many ways and for different purposes. Although all ectoplasm takes form from the slowing down of energy frequencies, the vibratory level used for materialisation differs from that used in healing. In the case of materialisation the ectoplasmic structure employed is a temporary, or 'artificial,' creation for the express purpose of allowing the deceased to reveal themselves; it is usually tenuous, but even when in its most dense form remains ephemeral and does not require the qualities essential to ectoplasm being used for healing. He emphasised that although ectoplasm provided the primal material for the restoration of tissue it was the animating, healing energy of the body itself, stimulated spiritually and homeopathically at soul level, that vitalised and patterned the tissue and restored function.

The resistance to concepts that range beyond pre-conceived boundaries is not restricted to the world of reductionist science. The same blinkered prejudice exists even in metaphysics. Harry Edwards remained un-swayed in his disbelief.

> All previous knowledge has shown that any kind of ectoplasmic structure emanating from the medium's body is part of his total organism, that any interference with it adversely affects the medium, that it has never been possible to

dissociate even a portion of the structure from the whole, that all structures that emanate from the medium return to him immediately the need for the externalisation has ceased. All these definite laws are violated by this new healing theory.[7]

Today with the advent of tissue transplants and stem cell therapy it is easier for us to understand the concept of an ectoplasmic graft of pluripotent capacity linking with the capillary and nervous systems of the recipient and restoring tissue structure and function, but, in 1944, such advanced medical technology still lay in the future. Dr Letari stated that a miracle is a scientific phenomenon beyond our present knowledge, but governed by natural law.

The Witchcraft Act of 1735

This was only the beginning of the friction that developed between Dr Letari and the established fraternity of spiritual healers. However, before the rift deepened, my father's prominence led to an unavoidable clash with the law and even greater publicity for his work. He was engaged by the Ravenswood Spiritualist Society to give a trance address entitled: *The Science of Spiritual Healing*, at the Stamford Hall, Altrincham, in Greater Manchester, on Sunday, 8 August, 1944. This was to be a follow-up to an address, which he had given at the same venue on 4 June, entitled: *The Gift Of Spiritual Healing*, which had created considerable interest. Eight days before the meeting, the President of the Church received a letter from the town clerk returning the rental paid for the hall and intimating that the magistrates of Altrincham City Council had refused permission for the meeting to be held. The secretary of the Society, RS Corbett, telephoned the police for clarity in the matter and was informed that the meeting savoured of conjuration aggravated by the fact that money was being taken. Police Superintendent FJ Morris informed the secretary that if the meeting were held it would be illegal and there could be police action. He added that the police were not suggesting that Lilley was a fraud. The genuineness of his mediumship was not at issue. Nevertheless, voicing the rather convoluted thinking of the authorities, the Superintendent said that Lilley would be breaking the Witchcraft Act 1735, simply because of giving a trance address. A 'dead' man was advertised as going to speak through him. That made him guilty of pretending to conjure up spirits. Ironically, the posters advertising the meeting clearly indicated that the proceeds of the silver collection would be in aid of the Altrincham General Hospital and the building fund of the Society. Reserved seats were 2/6 (12.5p); otherwise admission was free. At a meeting of the Altrincham Borough Council, held in response to public protest, the mayor revealed that Altrincham General Hospital had written to the promoters of the meeting asking that the hospital should not be associated with it.

The ban was obviously a consequence of the conviction of Helen Duncan earlier in the year on the charge of fraudulent witchcraft. At the time, the precedent set by this strange case had alarmed Spiritualists in Britain. Quite realistically, they feared the possibility of a witch-hunt, and just the sort of action that was now being taken against my father. The repercussions were potentially manifold: the organisers of such meetings could be found guilty of complicity and the audience regarded as accessories. If the Altrincham meeting was illegal then so too was every Spiritualist séance!

The Society decided that defiance of the law, which in this case was archaic and discriminated against religious rights, was the correct policy. My father, who ran the greatest risk of being arrested, agreed to deliver the address, come what may. The attendance at the previous lecture, and the interest it had generated, indicated that a large auditorium would be required.

Since the spacious Stamford Hall was now out of bounds, an alternative venue had to be found. The Society decided to approach two of the largest chapels in Altrincham and request that the protest meeting be held on their premises. The Rev WG Barnes of the Hale Road Baptist Church, after placing the matter before his deacons, informed the Society that they could not sanction the use of their premises for a meeting connected with Spiritualism, and the Rev Harry Fletcher of the Oxford Road Methodist Chapel said that he would not lend his Church for purposes which were against its beliefs. Such doctrinal prejudice and lack of Christian goodwill explains much of Silver Birch's distaste for the Churches and their canons.

Thwarted on every side, it was finally decided that the meeting should be held at the Society's own modest venue. Loudspeakers were installed to cope with the anticipated overflow. JB McIndoe, President of the Freedom Fund, involved his organisation by occupying the Chair, ensuring that if arrests were made he would also be implicated. Fortunately, despite the fact that Corbett informed the police that the meeting was going to be held on the Society premises, there was no police interference.

This ban on freedom of worship and free speech, especially since it invoked the archaic Witchcraft Act, created a furore at the centre of which Hannen Swaffer wielded his acerbic pen. He sent letters to the *Times* and the *Manchester Guardian* expressing his indignation and warning of how such a law threatened public liberty. In the *Psychic News* he wrote:

> Spiritualism is now at the mercy of any cowardly and anonymous bigot who calls up the police, as one did in Altrincham.⁸

On 14 October 1944, the matter was brought up in the House of Commons by Mr Brown, MP for Rugby. Protesting against the police's use of the Act, he informed the House:

> ... trance addresses were a normal feature of Spiritualist services, and if Spiritualists were not to hold services on the ground that there might be an offence against an act 200 years old their work must come to a end.

Herbert Morrison, Home Secretary, explained that the Altrincham Town Council had cancelled the letting of the hall because of a complaint from a member of the public, who felt that in view of the grief and mourning caused by war casualties, a meeting at which a 'dead' doctor would supposedly give an address was most inadvisable in the public interest. He then limply responded to Brown's challenge:

> Local feelings and local circumstances arise. I should be taking a great responsibility if I took personal responsibility as to whether each particular meeting is to be held or whether the owners of halls are to let them or not.⁹

However, the widespread public outcry against the banning of the meeting in Altrincham did have the desired effect. From that time on, no local authority ever ventured to repeat such a banning, and, in 1951, the Witchcraft Act was finally repealed with the enactment of the Fraudulent Mediums Act, which protected the public against exploitation by bogus psychics.

The need for responsible healers

In the meantime, Dr Letari and William pressed on regardless, ranging as far afield as Glasgow, Manchester, Leeds, Sheffield and Southampton, amongst many other destinations. In his addresses, Dr Letari became ever more outspoken about his views on the role of healers, their need for training and the necessity for homeopathic support for all spiritual healing. This push for the educated healer was first reported in the *Psychic News* of September 2, 1944:

> Dr Letari, the Hindu guide of WH Lilley, the healer, was in a provocative mood when he spoke through his medium to a large congregation in Salem Church, Leeds, last Saturday.¹⁰

The justification for this statement sprang from the direct attack Dr Letari made on the limitations of laying-on-of-hands as practised by the healing mediums in the Spiritualist movement. He first explained that a healing medium was not just a channel or robot under the control of a spirit guide. The healer played a personal and essential role in the act of healing, and must be medically informed. It was essential that the medium should have knowledge of the basic medical sciences, be conversant with disease patterns and diagnosis and be able to identify cases that required orthodox medical intervention. He called for responsible healing, based on knowledge and not just faith or superstition.

He urged the healer to consider that apart from hereditary disease, which is the result of the incorrect thinking and acting of ancestors handed down through the generations to the present time – broken precepts, which have to be made good or they will continue to pollute descendants for an eternity – it is the soul that produces disease and it is only through acting upon the soul that disease can be eradicated.

> Doctors do not sufficiently realise this. They try to cure the physical body without getting to the spiritual cause. Doctors fail in their work because they are trying to cure the effect instead of the cause. Often they merely treat a Latin name. Is it possible for the soul to be diseased? I say yes! It is diseased in its thought![10]

He then made what was regarded as a most contentious statement. He said:

> The mere laying-on-of-hands will not heal. Do you really think it is possible to take stones out of kidneys by the laying-on-of-hands? No, we must come down to science. Down to fact and away with belief.[10]

He noted that there was, indeed, a great law that operated through the laying-on-of-hands, but it had to work through the soul of the patient to be able to bring about curative change. He also said that it was the law acting through the soul and not the laying-on-of-hands that brought about the cure.[10]

The soul of the patient is as much a factor in the process of cure as the medium.

In this he was intimating that the laying-on-of-hands simply directed to the physical effects of disease could prove superficial and palliatory because it did not address the deeper reasons for the peripheral signs and symptoms.

Questioned about how absent healing works, he explained:

> There are three factors, just as there are in ordinary healing. There is the soul of the patient, which, through faith, works on his own physical body. Then there is the soul of the medium directing its force from a distance. Thirdly, there is the spirit guide.
>
> In my own case, I contact the patient wherever he is and direct the triple thought-force throughout his body by working on his own soul and mind. Thus you have

the combined mental power of three spirits manifesting in the one physical body.[10]

At the tea break, the audience were invited to submit their written questions. There were so many it was only possible to answer a few. One important question, which is highly pertinent in our times, was about assisted euthanasia and whether incurables be assisted to make an easy entry into the spirit world.

According to the *Psychic News* report, Dr Letari's answer was emphatic.

> *No!* Often, these are the people richest in spirit. I meet many of these who are tender in years, but how strong in spirit are they! Only the physical body is suffering. That is part of their evolution. All the time, the spirit is progressing. When the time comes for them to leave the physical body, they will reap the reward in the hereafter.

The *Psychic News* correspondent rounded off his report with the following words:

> It was a great meeting and an important address. The echo of Dr Letari's words will be reverberating for a long time. He has given Spiritualists and investigators plenty to discuss.[10]

Reverberate was a good word to describe the reaction amongst many Spiritualist groups and the response of certain individuals, but it was some time before it gained a voice.

The *Psychic News* report on the Letari Nursing Home

At this time, *Psychic News* sent one of its reporters to interview my father at 8/10 Bulstrode Street to obtain first hand information on the combined spiritual and homeopathic work being done at the nursing home. His was a fresh face, and he had an intelligent, investigative enthusiasm that appealed to William. He showed the reporter round the premises and familiarised him with the organisation and administration that was essential for the efficient running of a busy healing centre. The reporter was interested not only in the spiritual aspects of the healing work, but also in specific case histories and the remedies that were successfully prescribed and why they were selected. He wrote a definitive article on the work being done at the Sanctuary entitled, *The Case Book Of A Psychic Healer*, which appeared in the *Psychic News*, September 9, 1944.

> In his healing centre in the West-end of London, WH Lilley is treating people by the score who have been to doctors and found no relief for their pains. I have been going through some of the case histories in his files – there are thousands now – and have picked out examples to show what the spirit world is doing to demonstrate that, in co-operation, healers here and healers in the life beyond are extending the boundaries of our knowledge, and at the same time are effecting cures.[12]

It soon became apparent to him that many of the cures took a long time to effect. They did not evidence the much-vaunted miraculous and even instantaneous transformations in health that are often recorded as being characteristic of spiritual healing. The files revealed a different story. They documented a carefully conceived strategy of therapy, which while incorporating a spiritual element when required, was particularly founded on the considered application of homeopathic remedies, covering the full range of potencies from mother tinctures to the CM ($10^{-100,000}$) and even MM ($10^{-1000,000}$) level. Such treatment was often augmented by colour therapy and spinal manipulation with percussion and massage. The latter administered not only for the chiropractic reduction of vertebral subluxations and restoring mobility, but also for its laying-on-of-hands effect, and its modulating action upon the chakra energy centres of the body.

The reporter gave details of a woman suffering from rheumatoid arthritis who had been under orthodox therapy for four years before consulting the Sanctuary. She had received a great amount of analgesics (pain killers) and in addition gold therapy and thyroid extract, which had caused an unwanted loss of weight. Orthopaedic surgery to the lower spine, instead of bringing relief had resulted in increased pain and weakness and what she termed, 'spinal debility.' She had previously been severely affected by a smallpox vaccination, which caused a widespread outbreak of septic skin lesions.

As harsh, toxic and suppressive as gold therapy is, it did not prove as obstructive to the healing programme instituted by Dr Letari and William, as modern day steroid therapy would have.

Unfamiliar with the inquiring exactness of the homeopathic consultation, the reporter wrote:

> In this healing centre, attention is paid to every detail of pain experienced and the mental condition of the patient. There is nothing haphazard, for the intimate details of this one patient's condition show what improvement was experienced in the first year of treatment. Weight after 18 months of treatment had increased, and instead of long paragraphs giving particulars of pains, there are a few words after each visit to indicate the reaction. Towards the end of the treatment given by Lilley and his spirit guide, Dr Letari, this comment appears: 'All conditions show good progress.'[12]

Those with homeopathic knowledge will be interested to know that in the sequence of remedies used to effect these changes, Thuja, Malandrinum, Sycotic co and Causticum played a significant role.

The reporter continued:

> Proof consists of curing a patient. In all the work done by Lilley and his staff, the greatest attention is paid to symptoms, for to them and their spirit instructors they are the language of disease.[12]

In the waiting room, he met an old man in his seventies accompanied by his wife and daughter and questioned them about the reason for his visit, the treatment he was receiving and how he was responding. The ladies were only too eager to give him their story; this was to be his last appointment and they had come with him to express their gratitude for his recovery. They told him that the father of the family had for some months been suffering from severe urinary symptoms with frequent urging to urinate even when his bladder contained very little urine. He had complained of a burning pain in his bladder, pain extending up into the kidney region on both sides, and, the man added on his own behalf, a constant ache in his testicles. His daughter remarked that since the problem began her father had become very withdrawn and depressed, which alarmed them considerably, making them fear the worst. His family doctor referred him to an urologist who, though he did not suspect cancer, advised the immediate removal of the prostate, which he said was probably harbouring chronic infection. However, when the family questioned him, he admitted that he could not guarantee that the operation would prove successful. The family, practising Spiritualists, declined and arranged for him to attend the nursing home.

After speaking with them, the reporter asked William to give him the details of the treatment the patient had received on his road to recovery. My father showed him the case history.

> The treatment consisted of Mountain-grape because in the form in which it was prepared (30CH), it had just the right vibration to produce the desired effect. In less than a fortnight an improvement was reported. In just over five weeks the cure was complete. The intense pain and discomfort had disappeared.[12]

The mountain grape, Oregon grape or *Mahonia aquifolium*, as it is known to herbalists, who use it in quite substantial, material doses, is a remedy which has been successfully employed in treating conditions of the urinary tract, liver and spleen. It possesses a particular affinity for elderly men suffering from genito-urinary problems and has gained a reputation for making '*a new man of an old one.*' A North American plant, growing along the west coast from British Columbia to northern California, it was introduced into the homeopathic materia medica by Edwin Hale (1829–1899), who pioneered the use of many Native American herbs. Its scientific name is *Berberis aquifolium* and it belongs to the Barberry family, or Berberidaceae.

The reporter noted in his article that this case was in direct contrast with that of the woman with rheumatoid arthritis,

> . . . whose long treatment was a record of the progress of pain from one part of the body to another (from the centre to the periphery in accordance with Hering's law of cure) until she showed by unmistakable signs that she was well on the road to recovery.[12]

He asked William why the 30th potency had been prescribed and not a more materially potent (lower potency) or more energetically potent (higher potency) one.

Speaking particularly of a potency higher than the 30th, William answered that it would be like putting a Spitfire engine into an old motor car chassis. The moment the engine started up, the chassis would fall to pieces.

> In this instance, as in many others, the medicine had to be suited to the age and condition of the patient, so that the natural healing forces in the human constitution could be brought to bear.[12]

The higher potency though possibly the most effective when the symptom match between remedy and patient is most congruent can be so energetic in its effect that it overtaxes the strength of a constitution already weakened by prolonged disease or age. In these cases a lower potency such as the 30th is to be preferred.

William spoke frankly about his failures. He said that no healer, or physician, who understands the nature and difficulty of his work, would claim that he, or his method, could cure everyone who seeks relief. Sometimes, as Paracelsus tells us, the time for healing for the specific patient has not yet come. He or she will only be cured by the physician "only when the hour of recovery strikes for the patient; all who go to him before, go to him in vain".

Though they spoke at greater length on this topic, the reporter did not include my father's further comments in his article. Remarks William made when similarly questioned in February of the same year give more detail:

> I never think it is because the patients are not in tune with me. It is perhaps because we do not know enough. It is hard to explain. For instance, there are cases simple to diagnose, where the symptoms are easy to obtain and analyse and yet the patient takes months to be cured – or fails to be cured. At other times there are cases with chronic medical histories and structural change, which, nevertheless, respond quickly to treatment.

> If patients are not cured, then I believe that I have not yet the means to achieve it. I will go so far as to say this, that I believe that patients I have failed to cure, could have been cured. The reason for the failures is that I am not yet sufficiently developed to express the great power which Letari and others have at their command.

The healer is always developing.

> There are cases now, which are simple to handle, which even five years ago would have baffled me. I would have failed with them then.

He stressed the need for the personal development of the healer *at soul level* in order to become better perfected as an instrument of healing.

> I am trying to become all that I ought to be by following the very simple rule laid down by Dr Letari: Test all things; hold fast to that which is true.[11]

Another precept he held dear was that given by Polonius to his son Laertes in Shakespeare's Hamlet (*Act 1, scene 3, 78*):

> This above all: to thine own self be true.

William explained to his interviewer that spiritual instruction and counselling were always important elements in the healing of the sick; patients need to be lead into a new system of living based upon spiritual truths and with cognisance of their spiritual status and powers.

Another case investigated by this very thorough man from the press was of a London barrister who had become increasingly hypersensitive over many years until even with eyes closed he would react with discomfort to the movement of someone's hands some distance from his body.

> To the Spiritualist that will be easily understood, for the human aura is to them a fact and its extension beyond the body is seen commonly by clairvoyants.

> This lawyer's condition became so acute that he could not listen to his clients. He was in pain if he tried to sleep in a certain position, and he had to be careful not to make any sudden movement. Shaving, washing his face, the pressure of the bedclothes, all caused the pain to start.

> He had suffered from quinine poisoning due to an overdose during the last war.[12]

After only three days of taking the medicine prescribed by William, the lawyer whose condition had been progressively deteriorating for years, causing him great distress and pain, reported that all his pains had diminished and he could bear pressure on his face.

This rapid response deeply impressed the reporter, as well it might, because the many doctors and specialists that the barrister had consulted had been unable to explain or treat his symptoms. The suggestion that the high doses of quinine he had received almost thirty years before might in some way be implicated was either dismissed or ignored.

The reporter wrote that the medicine given by Lilley after psychic diagnosis was 'simple.'[12] He was correct in saying the remedy was simple, but wrong when he ascribed its choice to psychic diagnosis. William, like any trained homeopath, required no input from Dr Letari to enable him to prescribe for the suffering lawyer. The symptoms of hyperaesthesia, oversensitivity of the nervous system, and opening up of natural boundaries, which usually protect us from excessive sensitivity to external impingements and the emotions of others, is typical of the symptom picture induced by quinine. The homeopathic law of similarity informs us that what a poison can cause when given to a healthy person it can cure when administered in potentised (dynamic) form to a person suffering with the same symptomatic picture. The answer to the problem was therefore extremely simple. What quinine could cause, quinine could cure. William gave the lawyer China 200 (homeopathic potency of quinine) once per day for three days, and in a very short time he was completely cured.

The last entry in the case sheet read: "Patient to report any aggravation, otherwise no further medicine required."[12]

The clinical significance of this little case is enormous, yet if it were submitted as proof of the efficacy of the homeopathic method, the orthodoxy would discount it as anecdotal and therefore invalid.

Dr Letari on spiritual healing

At a packed meeting at Blackley, in Greater Manchester, held on Sunday, 19 November 1944, Dr Letari expanded on his previous advice to spiritual healers. He opened the meeting with a heartening comment on the change that the war in Europe was taking.

> My friends, I rejoice at having this opportunity of speaking to you because we of the spirit realise that you are on the eve of peace, which will open out a new world, a new life, and we hope, light in darkened places.[13]

He was anxious as always to dispel superstition, misconception and wishful thinking on the part of those who embraced Spiritualism and spiritual healing and at the other extreme to dispel dependence on mechanistic medicine. He often stated that the orthodox religions repressed the soul as much as orthodox medicine repressed disease.

Although divine healing had been practised since ancient times, it was during the past fifty years that it had emerged as a movement and Dr Letari was concerned that those who practised as healers should be responsible and knowledgeable.

> I have during the past twenty-one years of experience with my medium been able to realise the faults of Spiritualism. I am aware of all things that seek to break down that great service that Spiritualism can give to humanity, and it is with that purpose in mind I come here to you, to give you some idea ... of the conditions, which are detrimental to its progress.
>
> Spiritual healing is not just the Laying-on-of-Hands – it is a science based on facts.
>
> From both the healer and the patient's perspective: It is a phase of one soul's progress. The forces of destiny are at work, which operate synchronistically through the application of natural law. The healing that I am privileged to extend to my patients is not based simply on religion, or upon belief, but upon scientific facts which can be examined; facts upon which we can build.
>
> I know that my words at my various lectures have caused concern. They have caused argument – in fact, in the Psychic papers they say I am provocative. I feel in one of these moods today because we of the spirit are fighting.
>
> I have told you I do not bring religion to you. It must be fact. Because we realise that laying-on-of-hands is insufficient, we realise that prayer is insufficient.[13]

He said that Spiritualists and the followers of other religions, due to ignorance, superstition and misguided teachings had a distorted concept of what transpires when spiritual healing takes place.

> When I come through my medium, I do not bring a great power. I do not give all that is necessary to make a cure. Because of my clearer vision I am able to give to my medium knowledge and wisdom that enables him to cure rationally and in tune with the infinite. Therefore, the spiritual healing that I represent is healing based on rational methods, rational facts, and not just the idea that some power flows down from the heavens and is curative.[13]

Healing the sick must be likened to any creative act. There is inspiration received from a higher plane which works in consort with the innate gift of the creator – the healer, the artist, the sculptor, or the musician – who must have the required training, skill and knowledge to bring into being the artistic work visualised – the cure, the painting, the statue or the composition. When Michelangelo confronted a block of marble, though prompted, aided and inspired by unseen influences, no great power descended from on high to miraculously release the sublime image he had conceived from the formless slab before him. He needed, beside his spiritual gift, the carefully selected tools of his art and the deftness to use them. So it must be with healing the sick; even to the point that the healer may on occasion require the assistance of a surgeon to resolve elements of the case that require physical intervention. However, for work at the soul or causative level, the finest tools of all for the healing artist are the potencies of homeopathy.

Dr Letari's address, as edited in the article, led to much misunderstanding, and, in some quarters, consternation, therefore, using the framework left us by the editor, I have restored details essential for fuller understanding of his discourse.

> The spirit world from which I have come is a world of consciousness in an environment of the finest matter. Consciousness acts upon this milieu, creating the reality of the soul. It is not a world such as your earth plane. It is simply consciousness. Consciousness expresses memory built by experience. When we have finished with our physical body, our soul, mind and consciousness persist. Without consciousness there would be no buildings, no churches, no palaces, no flowers, no trees in the spirit world, but with consciousness there are all these things and in an abundance and variety inconceivable to those on the earth plane.
>
> The consciousness, which is a quality of the soul, first manifests in life when the physical vehicle, which has developed from the union of two cells, followed by multiplication and differentiation, reaches a certain critical point of development and quickening. The physical body, which temporarily houses the soul consciousness, is the product of years, centuries and ages of evolution. It is the repository of all the errors of our ancestors and taints the indwelling soul with the imperfection of inherited disease characteristics, thus distorting the soul's perspective and its consciousness.
>
> Reincarnation permits the karmic assets and debts of the soul to be carried forward from life to life. On the debit side of the scale are unresolved propensities, unrequited desires and the need for reparation. To process these, the soul requires the tempering effect of life experience, which is predestined accordingly. Inescapably entangled in this cause and effect state is the miasmatic inheritance of chronic disease, which is deeply implicated in the health and behaviour of the soul.
>
> You who are here are gaining experience through the world of matter that will enable you to find your position when you take up the greater life. This physical life is not only determined by your soul qualities, but also by your constitutional state of health, by the functions of the body systems, especially the endocrine glands, which can prove intrusive. If these glands are out of harmony, you think and feel differently, you think and feel wrongly. Suppose we have a man, who is a good man, who loves his family and home. He receives an injury to his head. What may happen? That man from being good may become evil. He becomes a drunkard, a sexual maniac. He forgets his home, his wife, his children. Can you realise now how we must include the physical with the spiritual.
>
> Everything must be used for spiritual healing that has been given to us by our Creator – osteopathy, chiropractic, light, colour, herbs, homeopathy, etc. – to restore to man his healthy body and mind. I appeal to the medical profession to try and understand that those in the spirit world are endeavouring to give them

> a wider understanding of the spiritual essence of man. I deplore the fact that most regard their patients as little more than an assemblage of tubes and matter.
>
> I diagnose by the interpretation of a patient's vibration or aura. I can read quite clearly whether the patient is suffering from rheumatoid arthritis, cancer, glaucoma, stomach ulcer, TB, etc; all due to underlying causes handed on to patients by their ancestors. The simple laying-on-of-hands would only be getting rid of the effects and not the cause.
>
> I am aware how members of past audiences have noted in my lectures my insistence on the importance of the underlying (miasmatic) causes of disease, even the common cold. When I know the cause, no matter the diagnosis, I can cure it, though certain destructive results of the disease may be irreversible.
>
> Spiritualists should cleanse their minds of all the peculiar theories of the spirit world obtained from the séance room. Facts are wanted, not theories.
>
> After 25 years on the earth plane and 30 in the spirit world, seeking to bring laws to the world for its healing, I am not interested in rapping a table or throwing a trumpet around. I am only interested in my patients. There are few leaders (among Spiritualists), but many among the masses, that want the truth. Come forward and help those of the spirit who are fighting for the light of the future.[13]

He then invited questions. There were many, and a few are worth considering. In response to a question about a foetus dying before it has a chance of quickening Dr Letari said.

> If anything should happen to the foetus before the quickening period, before the physical brain is perfected, then there is no consciousness in spirit. If anything happens after that time there is consciousness, which passes into spirit unfiltered by experience and will require education in the spirit spheres.[13]

Another member of the audience wanted to know if it was possible for Dr Letari to cure a patient through absent healing during a patient's sleep to which he replied,

> Yes, but it will take much longer than if the patient also attends my mediator and receives the additional healing of homeopathy.[13]

Asked about life in spirit, Dr Letari dealt with it briefly:

> Each individual life is made up of experience and reactions to experiences. Then, comes the time when the individual passes to the spirit world. Consciousness is released, and past experiences, joys, sorrows, griefs, etc. are taken forward into spirit.
>
> If one has always loved art and beauty and music etc. then one will sense and experience these things and respond to them because they existed in the mind as consciousness. Goodness or evil are in our consciousness, which then gives either reality. The world of spirit is a world of consciousness, because we are the sons and daughters of the universal consciousness.[13]

References

1. Barbanell M. Lilley's Nursing Home. *Psychic News*; November 7 1942.
2. *Wisdom Of Silver Birch*. London: Psychic Press Ltd; 1944. pp76–77.
3. Desmond AK. Guide Praises Psychic Sketch. *Psychic News*; May 30 1942.
4. Barbanell M. Editorial tailpiece. *Psychic News*; October 21 1944.
5. Barbanell M. Editorial tailpiece. *Psychic News*; June 9 1945.
6. Edwards H. How Is Ectoplasm Used In Spirit Healing? *Psychic News*; March 4 1944.
7. Edwards H. How Is This Spirit Healing Done? *Psychic News*; May 13 1944.
8. Swaffer H. Our Fight For Religious Freedom. *Psychic News*; October 14 1944.
9. Banned Spiritualist Talk: Morrison Explains. *Yorkshire Evening Post*; October 14 1944.
10. Spirit Doctor Explains How He heals The Sick. *Psychic News*; September 2 1944.
11. Healer Has Treated 16,000 Patients. *Psychic News*; February 26 1944.
12. The Case Book Of A Psychic Healer. *Psychic News*; September 9 1944.
13. The Application Of Spiritual Healing. *The Two Worlds*; December 1 1944.

17

CONTROVERSY AND INITIATION

Misconceptions

1945, a memorable year that commenced with Maurice Barbanell making his editorial in the January 5 edition of *Psychic News* a response to the large number of letters he received from his readers expressing their concern or confusion regarding the statements made by Dr Letari at the meeting in Blackley, which *Psychic News* had reported in its December 1 issue. The letters were not sent with a view to having them published, but to gain Barbanell's opinion. Questions ranged from: were there truly no trees, buildings, etc. in the spirit world, did the incarnating soul only link with the developing foetus when quickening took place, was laying-on of hands completely valueless? All of which exemplified Dr Letari's words: that we, one and all, create our own reality through our consciousness, which interprets what we see, hear and experience according to our own perspective, often creating misconceptions and misunderstanding even when there should be clarity.

Being at the centre of controversy only served to keen public interest in the remarkable healing team of spirit guide and homeopathic medium. The public in Britain and abroad wanted to know more about them.

In a letter to Arthur Richards, dated 21 March, 1944, Barbanell wrote:

> Dear Arthur
>
> I thought you would be interested to know that we had a cable from South Africa for 100 copies of *The Gift Of Healing* to be sent to Durban. It is good to know that our knowledge is spreading.
>
> sincerely,
> Barbie.

By the end of 1945, 6,000 copies of *The Gift Of Healing* had been sold.

On March 17, of the same year, in a short paragraph, *Psychic News* announced the author's death the week before, and revealed that Arthur Keith Desmond was the pseudonym of Victor Hyde MC. No further information about the author was given.

An indignant medical bigot

Interestingly, particularly in the light of all the hostility and contumely that homeopathy and other forms of alternative medicine are currently being subjected to, an article entitled, *I Accuse These Doctors*, appeared in the *Sunday Pictorial*, July 8, 1945, which specifically derided homeopathy and rebuked the medical doctors who were using it in the treatment of their patients. Little has changed in the intervening years. The writer of the article, Dr Thomas Arkwright, a medical doctor, showed all the personal affront and indignation that modern day critics of this gentle and effective therapeutic method display. He writes with the emotional intensity of one whose deepest religious belief has been outraged.

> It is time in my view that the menace of homœopathy was exposed, for as it is there are thousands of simple people who believe in it and several hundred doctors who practise it. They are in my view letting down the medical profession, whether they realise it or not.
>
> Homœopathy is balderdash and poppycock. It is dangerous poppycock, propagated by men who have had a scientific training, and who therefore ought to know better. Unfortunately there are a lot of patients as well as doctors who believe in it. I know I am washing my profession's dirty linen in public in exposing this nonsense, but if it cannot be washed in private there is no alternative. For washed it must be if medicine is to retain public respect and to do its job in the relief of pain and suffering.[1]

This diatribe was precipitated by a short explanatory treatise on the science of homeopathy, which was first published in 1940; it was written by Sir John Weir, a consulting physician to the Royal London Homœopathic Hospital, who became the King's physician. Arkwright demonstrates all the animosity, prejudice, arrogance, and ignorance of the subject he disparages, evidenced by the empiricists of today.

Peace in Europe

However, the public mind in 1945 had other priorities to occupy it than trees and palaces in the afterlife, and accusations of quackery in this life.

The war in Europe had come to an end. On 8 May, the Allies received the unconditional surrender of Nazi Germany and Adolf Hitler's Third Reich collapsed. I was not yet 5, but the immense energy generated by the people of London on V-E Day, etched the sounds and sights of that day into my consciousness, never to be forgotten. I remember everywhere the profusion of Union Jacks, at least one hanging from every window, the constant, exultant peal of the church bells, the intense excitement and joy to be seen on every face and the mass of milling people on the pavements and in the streets. Accompanied by my parents and my cousin, Ronnie, I ventured forth from 8/10, clinging to my small flag, and we joined the jostling throng that was heading for Buckingham Palace. Fortunately, we had set off in good time and managed to avoid getting caught in Trafalgar Square, or The Mall, and found a place amongst the press of people in front of the Palace. I can still recall exactly where we stood on the right hand side with our backs to Green Park and with a good view of the balcony where we knew King George VI and Queen Elizabeth would appear. As the promised moment approached, a vast murmuring arose amongst the multitude, moving wave after wave through their ranks until reaching crescendo pitch it broke forth in the universal cry: "We want the King! – We want the King! – We want the King!" I was hoisted up upon the shoulders of my cousin and so had a grandstand view. I added my tiny voice to the insistent chant and felt as if my chest, small as it was, would burst with pride. At last the doors to the balcony opened and shortly afterwards the King and Queen emerged to be greeted by a vociferous cry from the thronging populace. The beloved figures were the very symbol of the nation and its victory; archetypal parents with whom their jubilant children wished to share their triumph. And then, a great roar erupted as the warrior of words joined them, he who had rallied his people and fought the Nazis with his heroic rhetoric, Winston Churchill, another archetype: the tenacious and obdurate bulldog, giving his characteristic, two-fingered victory gesture.

Experiences like this, at so young an age, prove formative at a deep level, and I carried forward from that day, apart from an awareness of being British, which later was at odds with my greater awareness of being nothing of the sort, impressions which fortified my interest in symbolism and archetypes. It also gave me consciousness of the immensity of the stage upon which our lives are enacted, even when apparently parochial, and the importance of every role we play, no matter how ordinary or mundane it may seem.

A Spiritualist platform for homeopathy

After the war, it was rations, coupons and queues, but at 8/10 business as usual and on-going weekend lectures throughout the country, at which William was usually supported by Richards, who would chair the events. From a Spiritualist platform, Dr Letari and William were bent on spreading understanding of life eternal, a cosmos governed by law, life's spiritual path, the role of disease as both catalyst and impediment to spiritual unfoldment, the chronic, miasmatic nature of disease, which touched body, mind and soul and the curative power and elegance of homeopathy. They sought above all to stimulate an ever-widening public interest in Hahnemann's legacy – in effect to create a homeopathic public.

On Sunday, December 9, 1945, Dr Letari addressed a packed Co-operative Hall in Nottingham. He told his audience that he had come to give them an understanding of spiritual healing as something tangible, something factual and not dependent on belief.

> What is spiritual healing; is it a science or just a religion? I can assure you it is a science of religion, but as all branches of science, it has within it laws which must be upheld and understood; laws which cannot be disregarded, for if goodness is to be received, these laws must be understood to their fullest extent, for without law there can only be chaos and healing becomes haphazard. Healing is not just a matter of laying-on-of-hands with a prayer, but the application of the laws of creation; those laws of life that create health from disease and which must be understood and put in motion. Without understanding, the healer cannot hope to reach those pinnacles of healing, which with wisdom, he is destined to attain.[2]

His message to healers (and this was intended to include all who sought to heal the sick, including the orthodoxy) and to the public was becoming more insistent and more specific. Always, he was speaking to a wider audience than those sitting in the auditorium, knowing that his words were being recorded and would be published. He stressed yet again how necessary it is for the spiritual healer (and all healers) to understand the body both in health and disease, to understand the laws that govern healing and to know that the body is the gateway to the soul, and that in any sickness it is the soul that is diseased and needs to be cured. He insisted that the medium, who was content to be a "robot for the spirit," would never attain success. *All healing involves mediumship*, which requires a complete co-ordination between the spirit world and the physical healer. Awareness of this collaboration, and commitment to it, together with an understanding and application of the laws of disease causation and cure, opens up a greater power of healing than has yet been known and which will be at the command of the healer. He went on to explain that he could not heal disease, that no one can heal disease – only Nature can achieve this. He and all others were only Nature's assistants, but by the wise use of law, method and art, Nature's capacity for healing was enhanced. It is not possible to cure everyone, for there are always those who are incurable, but with trust, knowledge and the skill to use it, the 'sphere of incurability' becomes less and less.

Dr Letari repeated yet again that laying-on-of-hands needed to be administered with the same vibratory precision with regard to the disease state of the patient as was the case with homeopathy. When this resonance was not achieved the healing would fail to cure. The combination of spiritual and homeopathic healing, both of which work through energy frequencies, must prove more efficient and bring greater success.

> He also pointed out that another error of the spiritual healer is if his patient suffers from headaches the healing will be given to the head, and yet the headache may be produced by an imbalance of the liver, or a toxic condition of the bowel. Therefore such treatment is but palliative, as if one had taken an aspirin.[2]

This type of healing, although not posing any risk to the patient, could otherwise be equated with orthodox medical practice, which was "too apt to try and treat a Latin label rather than to understand the true processes of disease."[2]

He then entered into a far deeper consideration of the origin and nature of disease manifestation than he had done before. The theme of the chronic inherited nature of disease would become characteristic of all his future lectures.

> He went on to the subject of diagnosis and of the three principle disease forces, which he termed psora (susceptibility), sycosis (gonorrhoea) and syphilis, and their combined consequences tuberculosis and cancer. He spoke of how these disease forces were the root cause of every disease known to mankind. For example gonorrhoea or syphilis may have been contracted three or four generations ago, passed down through the generations, until now the great, great grandson has rheumatoid arthritis or some other disease. The medical profession would treat the patient for rheumatoid arthritis, whereas in truth he is suffering from inherited sycosis (the result of uncured or suppressed gonorrhoea).[2]

Dr Letari also asserted that these chronic inherited states were implicated in diseases affecting not only the mind and body, but also the soul, and he stated that the recent war, and indeed all wars, stemmed from such disease, which created diseased thinking and feeling. This knowledge was critical for the healer. An article reporting the message he delivered at a later address in Hastings stated:

Knowledge of spiritual truths – which he directed towards healing – and overcoming the greater root cause of disease, ignorance – represented the crux of his work.[3]

Silver Birch's message to William

In the heat of this unremitting commitment to the cause of healing and homeopathy, William and Arthur Richards were once again invited to attend the Hannen Swaffer home circle. The details of the meeting with Silver Birch were published at length in the *Psychic News*, December 15, 1945.

> *Silver Birch Gives Guidance To A Psychic Healer – "Thousands Will Rejoice Because Of Your Ministry."*
>
> Praise, encouragement, guidance and a warning were expressed by Silver Birch, guide of Hannen Swaffer's home circle, to WH Lilley, one of our outstanding healers. It was two years since this guide had spoken both to Lilley and Arthur Richards, his associate in his healing mission.
>
> "I love to meet my old friends," said Silver Birch, "those who work with and for the spirit, and my heart is filled with rejoicing at the tremendous progress that has been made. I told you before – and I only speak for those who have sent me, I am nothing of myself – that the power of the spirit would sustain and would triumph, and that as fast as difficulties arose, so they would evaporate. I think that has happened. The work that Lilley does today is greater than the work he did yesterday and the work he will do tomorrow is greater than that which is done today. Only those whose lives are given in full service know the unspeakable joy that comes from the constant feeling of the nearness of those appointed to guide, to guard and to uphold you. You are very fortunate. You are richly blessed and still you are only at the beginning. The years that are yet to unroll will make the field of service larger and larger and thousands will rejoice because of your ministrations. Lift up your heart in thankfulness and know that there are not many who can contemplate a life dedicated to the service, which you will be able to accomplish."
>
> *Then came a warning to the healer that he should be careful not to overtax himself. The guide told Lilley:*
>
> "Give your inspirers – who are counted as men of great worth in my world – complete confidence and know that they will not strive to take you any further than they know you can go. Bear in mind though, that it is a physical body that has to be used and it is very easy to succumb to the temptation of doing too much. It is hard to resist the cry of the afflicted, the agony of those who suffer when you know that you can help them. But always remember that you

> have a paramount duty to your own body, which is the temple of the spirit. If that body becomes tired, then that condition restricts the amount of spirit power that can be transmitted through it. It is very necessary to be careful. The power of the spirit flows, not in one continuous, unceasing stream, but in well-regulated measure, and you must close the tap again and again. Otherwise nothing will come. The body must be fit, for upon that body depends the power of the spirit, the rays, the forces which can come through it."

Since we are all on a spiritual path, this advice is pertinent to us all. While exercise is essential for the maintenance of health and optimum performance, excess, to which many are inclined, depletes the energy pool, which has to serve not only physical and mental needs, but also the spiritual sphere. Excess expenditure of physical energy devoted to exercise must impoverish other more subtle and urgent areas of endeavour. Indulgence in extreme forms of exercise can prove a very selfish activity, serving only the athlete. I can speak from personal experience since I became addicted to marathon running during my forties. In the case of my father, Silver Birch's words were particularly relevant and would contribute to him initiating great changes in his life, but constitutional damage had already been sustained and would inevitably shorten his life.

Silver Birch told the sitters that plans were being unfolded in the higher spheres of spirit for the advancement and spread of spiritual truths on the earth plane. He said that humanity in general had lost its way and was stumbling and falling in the darkness of spiritual ignorance.

> "It has been given to a few people, a comparative handful, to guide mankind to those paths which will bring certitude and peace, understanding and all the lavish bounty that the Great Spirit freely provides ... in all ages the greatest tasks have been performed by the smallest numbers."
>
> *Knowing what was destined, Silver Birch spoke further:*
>
> "No body of men, however mighty they may be considered in your world have the means or the ability to thwart the power of the spirit which has now come through you and other instruments."
>
> *Speaking in more general terms he then added:*
>
> "I wish that you, and all of those who work with us, could tear away the film that prevents your eyes from seeing so much of the radiance of the greater life which is there. If you could see what goes on behind your world's activity you would understand more of the purpose of life itself. Ours is a highly organised

> state of being. Each one of us is responsible to higher beings and all are subject to supervision. At any time we have problems – for we have problems – we can consult those with greater knowledge and obtain from them the answers we seek. Your world does not stand still; neither does ours. We have in it minds who have given years of service to the investigation of all these forces of the Great Spirit and they bring their knowledge to be used through instruments like yourself."
>
> *Silver Birch closed the sitting with words for my father alone.*
>
> "Have no fear, and know that the power which works through you is part of that vast power which fashioned the whole universe, which regulates the ebb and flow of the oceans, which holds the stars in their appointed places and causes the sun to shine. Know that this power is part of that same power which breathed into man and woman and made them living souls. The universe is ruled by inexorable law, law unceasing, unfailing, as every part of the universal whole works in accordance with the divine scheme. There has never been a failure in the divine scheme because the power that devised it, the power that organised it, the power that sustains it, is infinite. That part of it which works through you will wrap you around like a cloak of love, shield you in adversity and keep you always, so that you will know protection is yours."[4]
>
> *Finally Silver Birch gave a personal message to William for Nancy:*
>
> "I am very sorry that the Lilley lady is not here because I have much love for her and she should have been here by your side. Will you please give her my love and tell her that her unswerving loyalty and devotion is not unknown or unrecognised. That in return a wealth of affection comes to her from all who are associated with you in your work and they never forget that it is she who has made it possible for it to go on."

At the end of the sitting, the scribe, Frances Moore, who always noted in shorthand every word that Silver Birch uttered, handed William the last page of her shorthand notes on which the guide's message to Nancy was written. On the reverse side, she had kindly reproduced the message in longhand. Mother treasured these words for the rest of her life, and, thirty years later, I found the original note amongst her papers.

This was fated to be the last sitting of Hannen Swaffer's home circle that William would attend. Huge decisions, encompassing a vast change in his life, were looming on the horizon.

South Africa calls

The Gift of Healing had generated a great deal of interest in South Africa, even more than in the other British colonies, and as a result the Sanctuary had acquired a large number of absent healing patients, distributed throughout the country. This interest spread to Northern and Southern Rhodesia (later Zambia and Zimbabwe) and South West Africa (later Namibia). Due to the wish of its members to hear the message of Dr Letari and to witness the healing work he was doing, the South African Society for Psychic Advancement approached my father with the request that they might host him on a lecture tour of all the major cities in British southern Africa. Although not setting a specific date for the tour, William, after consulting with Dr Letari, accepted the invitation and proposed that it should take place in the second half of 1947. With so many patients in the region, and the tour likely to increase this base, they saw the possibility of opening a healing branch in South Africa, much as they had done in Hull. After the sitting with Silver Birch, William mentioned the likelihood of this tour to Barbanell, who responded enthusiastically. My father later confirmed his decision to go, and Barbanell included a short report in the *Psychic News*, February 2, 1946.

> Another medium who is going to demonstrate his powers overseas is WH Lilley, who is planning to visit South Africa and establish a branch of his healing mission. But more of this anon.[5]

Margaret Tara's baptism

However, the séance, in which father received the words of warning from the guide, was not the last time that he and Silver Birch would meet on the earth plane, and when they next came together, I would be present. My mother had fallen pregnant, and fully six years after my birth, on 26 July, 1946, with a midwife and my father in attendance, she added a baby girl to our family in the front room of our flat in West Hampstead. She was named Margaret Tara Lilley, her middle name being given her by Dr Letari. This became her spiritual name when she was baptised by Silver Birch in the lounge of our flat six weeks later. To Dr Letari, however, she would always be, the "Little Mem" (Little *Memsahib*).

On that Saturday afternoon, it was like a whose-who of Spiritualism in Cholmley Gardens. I still have an image of the large number of people who were present at the ceremony and of Silver Birch holding my baby sister, who was as good as gold, and looked like a tiny angel in her baptism robe. I know that I was well aware of it being Maurice Barbanell, and not Silver Birch, who approached me afterwards while everyone was chatting and enjoying tea and cakes. Although I cannot remember what he said to me, I can remember his delighted reaction to my response and his drawing the attention of others who were standing-by. Apparently, he engaged me in conversation about transport facilities in the afterlife and the likelihood of there being cars, buses and bicycles there. I told him, with all the certainty of my six years, that there was no need for these because spirits moved about by 'thought.' I do not know whether I achieved mention in the next *Psychic News* editorial, but if so, that issue is missing from our press cutting's book. Certainly, my observation was stored in the family myth and often repeated with amusement and pride.

The healing controversy

In May, 1946, William gave trance addresses in both Portsmouth and Southampton, entitled *My Healing Mission*, in which he expanded on the themes already expounded in Nottingham earlier in the year. As previously related, Dr Letari's insistence on the need for healers to be trained in the basic medical sciences, and to use homeopathy in conjunction with the laying-on-of-hands, had not gone down well with many healers and some of the Spiritualist rank and file. The various reports in the psychic press about the meetings in Portsmouth and Southampton, which detailed Dr Letari's uncompromising stance regarding these principles, caused a great deal of debate and both opposition and support. Although he had attended neither of the lectures, Dr Sidney John Peters, an ex-MP, doctor of law and himself a spiritual healer, felt moved to defend the cause of the untrained lay-healers. Ironically it was Peters, who, while still an MP, had written a glowing review on *The Gift of Healing* in the October 2, 1943, edition of the *Psychic News*. On that occasion, he wrote that he always carried the Frank Leah portrait of Dr Letari in his pocket; the book's publishers, Psychic Press Ltd, had distributed the portrait in postcard size. He was unreserved in his commendation of the book and of the healing work upon which it was based.

> *The Gift of Healing* . . . portrays the life and work of one of our greatest spiritual healers, WH Lilley, whose fame is world-wide.
>
> One of the most arresting points so well established in this book is the fact that spiritual healing as such *can and should** be linked up with what might be called material methods of healing. Rarely is it found in my own experience of healing that healers do exemplify this in their work
>
> Lilley has devoted his life to acquiring medical knowledge in spheres which often the spiritual healer may have felt himself incompetent to launch out upon, and he is thus a shining example of what devotion and concentration of mind and purpose can accomplish.

> I must say that I was astounded when I first met Mr Lilley, and mentioned three cases I was personally in contact with. Within a few moments of giving the names and addresses and ages of these three people, I was confronted with a clear exposition of their maladies, etc. which I could vouch for myself. In one case, I was able to have confirmation of a deep-seated cause of the trouble, which I had not suspected.
>
> Only one thing troubles me after reading this book, and that is the longing that this marvellous development of spiritual gifts should be acquired by others, who can enlarge upon this gracious work of healing the sick, when Lilley and his helpers pass on.
>
> We cannot look to the orthodox churches for this power, which they lost so long ago.[6]
>
> (* my italics)

In contrast, three years later, Dr Peters, acting on hearsay, wrote a critical letter to the *Psychic Truth*, which was published in December 1946. In this letter he was at pains to dissociate Dr Letari from Mr Lilley and ascribed all statements with which he was in disagreement to the medium and not his guide, i.e. that it was useless for mediums to try to diagnose or heal without having medical knowledge or to think that by thought or prayer alone they could heal sick people at a distance.

> I have spoken with many healing mediums up and down the country during the months I have been able to devote more of my time to propagating our cause since I gave up my seat in Parliament. I can assure readers I am convinced that where a person has the urge, motive and desire to heal and render service to suffering humanity there will be given the power to heal through the healing guides, whom from all accounts Mr Lilley has sought to decry.[7]

Dr Peters focused on what Dr Letari said about disease suppression through the administration of general, non-specific, spiritual healing and the deleterious effect such blindly directed healing could have.

> He (Mr Lilley) says that possibly a medium may have healed a skin or other complaint, but sent back into the patient's body the actual *cause* which they cannot diagnose properly without medical knowledge, and thus cause further trouble to the patient.
>
> I would venture to remind not only Mr Lilley, but those who heard him that the whole of the available evidence, which is enormous, proved that what Mr Lilley has said is devoid of foundation.[7]

How similar his response was to the similar reaction of medical doctors today when they are told that the suppression of eczema by tar preparations or steroids has grave consequences for the general health of their patients. Their ignorance of the law of healing is akin to that of Dr Peters and the healers who rallied behind him. The medical knowledge that Dr Letari always alluded to was not just knowledge of anatomy, physiology, biochemistry, pathology and orthodox, clinical diagnosis, but the deeper knowledge of the laws of disease causation, diagnosis and healing and the laws of cure as laid down by Hahnemann and his followers.

On the evidence of an informant, Dr Peter then incorrectly reported that one of the meetings had almost resulted in pandemonium through questions put not being answered and that many people had left the meeting.

Once again, reality is in the eye of the beholder, and in this case proved to be a prejudiced distortion. Mrs E Homer, the organiser of the Portsmouth meeting wrote a letter of appreciation to the Sanctuary:

> Thanks for a glorious evening, the Portsmouth people are delighted, you left them full of love in their hearts and with an urge to seek deeper and obtain greater knowledge of healing.

The organiser of the Southampton event wrote:

> We do thank you all so much for coming here and being such a help as you all were in every way.

In his letter, Dr Peters went on to reassure the 'dear souls' who were despondent after attending the meetings that spiritual healing could be theirs, notwithstanding anything they may have heard from Mr Lilley.

He continued:

> I wholeheartedly regret having to write this letter, but the sooner Mr Lilley, whether under control or not, stops making these statements the better for all concerned. In my humble view he has done our cause an infinite amount of harm.[7]

He closed with these words:

> Knowledge is of course very useful, but it is by no means essential, and I have known cases where my own medical knowledge has been a hindrance, for it has predisposed me to do something which the healing guides stopped me from doing.[7]

Letters flew back and forth for some time after this, but most importantly and publicly between Dr Letari and my father on one side and Dr Peters on the other. These were published in the Spiritualist periodical, *The Two Worlds*. The difference of opinion between the two became known as 'The Healing Controversy'.

E Smith, Stonestile Lane, The Ridge, Hastings wrote the following to *Psychic Truth* (published January 1947):

It is necessary for me to protest against the ill-advised criticism conceived by your correspondent Dr SJ Peters concerning the well-known spiritual healer, Mr WH Lilley. The criticism should have been directed against the guide, Dr Letari, and not against his instrument. It is also surprising that Dr Peters refers to second-hand information.

It has been my privilege to attend a lecture given by Dr Letari at Sleaford, Lincs, and to have a copy of a lecture given at Coventry. Neither of these lend any support for the criticisms from Dr Peters; on the contrary they show that our lecturer, Dr Letari, emphasised the need for knowledge of the laws governing such healers and the powers at their disposal. What is wrong with this?[8]

It was Dr Letari who responded to Dr Peters, and did so at some length for the benefit of the wider public (I have inserted editorial points for greater clarity; the headings were added by the editor of *The Two Worlds*):

> Because it was I, and not my medium who made such statements, 'that caused the greatest confusion and distress both to healing mediums and those coming on in the work', I feel that I must meet the welcome criticism of Dr Peters.

He then paraphrased points from the third aphorism of Hahnemann's *Organon*:

> May I first give four laws of healing that apply to mankind and to spirit alike, be it by healing-power vibrations (frequencies), homeopathic medicine or any other kindred branch (of healing). The healer must be able to:
>
> 1. Perceive what is to be cured in every individual case – *this requires the correct diagnosis.*
> 2. Perceive what is curative within the healing agencies at his disposal – *this requires knowledge of spiritual and medicinal laws.*
> 3. Know how the healing should be administered and with what frequency repeated.
> 4. Perceive the obstacles to cure that must be removed and how to accomplish this, *so as to ensure that the cure shall be permanent.*
>
> *The Law of Vibrations*
> Keeping these precepts ever before us, we are able to pass from the visible to the invisible; from the known to the unknown, from the physical to the spirit. There is no law which is not in its turn governed by law; law is the very existence of all things; all normal life is governed by law with which it is in harmony; but disease is paradoxically a perversion of the law (in relative terms) although within the law (in absolute terms). The vibration (frequency) of the life force (of all individuals) has a constant, which is ordered and fixed, and is capable of measurement, as is the frequency of a perfect note; the vibrations of a sick person, however, are changed and discordant. The symptoms and signs of their sickness depend upon this perverted vibratory change. Hence it is essential to use healing frequencies (spiritual and/or medicinal) to perfect a cure. Each healing frequency (e.g. homeopathic remedy) has its own particular mode of motion and action.

No two vibrations of healing are alike. When given as a specific, i.e. matched in rhythm and character to the diseased state, then the cure takes place, for harmony is restored. This is healing administered according to law and requires knowledge of the law. Is the selection of the specific vibration (essential for cure) to be random? This is indicated by Dr Peters, on the basis of an approach in ignorance, for he states quite definitely that medical knowledge is a hindrance to him. I agree, but only when the knowledge is too little. Then it becomes dangerous.

A Lawless State:
In most cases the healer has been told by a medium or spirit guide that he has a gift of healing. Believing this, the person begins to heal. His spiritual gifts are undeveloped, therefore, he has no direct communion with his spirit guide. His first patient may suffer from head pains. Healing to the head will be given, but the head pains may be the effect of some liver condition. Such treatment will be simply to apply an 'aspirin' in the form of healing power, but with what result? The head pains will recur until the root cause is specifically treated. In this approach, there is neither knowledge of the physical, nor of the spirit. This is the lawless state that Dr Peters advocates. Many spirit guides when questioned, prove equally, and in some instances more ignorant of the vital laws of healing, than the healer. Let spiritual healing speak for itself in its progressively vivifying, recreating, uplifting and healing processes . . . that it is of law and order.

Spirit 'Cure-All'.
Too much stress is placed on spirit guides. It would seem that whosoever we are, we have a universal or spiritual 'cure-all'; a vibration that can cure everything from the common cold to cancer; that can be applied by any healer to any patient for any disease. How foolish this is. We of spirit are subservient to law, just as you are on the material plane. We may not transgress the law.

Our friend infers that disease cannot be suppressed by spiritual healing. This shows a lack of observation and inexperience. All life works from within outwards and from above downwards, while disease processes work from without inwards and from below upwards (Hering's law of cure and of disease progression). Both life and disease are permeating and are within – and not upon the surface or localised. One can never see disease any more than one can see life itself. It is but an expression that one sees. Therefore he, or she, who applies healing to that expression without having considered the true internal cause, is as guilty of suppression as is the medical doctor who uses chemical or surgical means. An expression or effect is removed, but the root cause remains within only to express itself outwardly again at a later date; or it will establish 'new' disease processes, which are more threatening and more difficult to eradicate.

Again I say, the healer and the spirit guide must have this knowledge, and be able to direct the power of healing according to the law of cure; otherwise . . . nothing but a suppressive action will be accomplished. Healing power cannot be administered at random. In my mediator's dispensary are hundreds of homeopathic remedies, each with its own specific vibratory force. These cannot be given at random; they have to be chosen carefully according to the law of similar frequency. This law of similarity applies equally to the healing given by spirit guide and healer, who have at their disposal a spectrum of healing rays. Random therapy, homeopathic or spiritual will occasionally bring about a cure, but the majority will not benefit.[9]

Dr Letari remarked on the extensive study and training that was required of scientists working with atomic energy and likened this to the spiritual healer who "deals with and must control ethereal forces, which by comparison make atomic energy most crude." Surely knowledge and training for such work was essential?

> Too long has spiritual healing been ridiculed and rightly so. Now the time has come for it to take its rightful position, *as the basis of all science* (spiritual laws are fundamental to physical laws and are scientific, not based on faith or religion).

If his critics had sought to fully comprehend and appreciate the positive nature of his admonishment, urging them to acquire and use knowledge and method to improve their competence, rather than experiencing it as a challenge to their integrity and the validity of their work, they would have noted that he did not refute spiritual healing or absent healing, indeed, especially during the early years of his association with William his mission had primarily taken this form, and that his addresses throughout the country were always followed by demonstrations of spiritual healing.

> My lectures throughout this country have been to give knowledge of law to potential healers, and only to those who have not this knowledge; so to warn them of the pitfalls, but above all to teach them truth.[9]

Silver Birch speaks with two famous healers: Parish and Lilley

In his letter of protest, Dr Peters had referred to the wonderful work of WT Parish as an example of what spiritual healing was capable of achieving. Parish, a pioneer in British spiritual healing, commenced his healing mission after his wife was diagnosed with inoperable cancer in 1929. A Spiritualist friend suggested the possibility of psychic healing and Parish, desperate for help, attended a séance during which the presiding spirit guide informed him that he had natural healing power and would be the one to cure his own wife. This he did through laying-on-of-hands over a period of nine months. With this proof of his psychic ability, he commenced his work as a spiritual healer, a career that was rewarded by many remarkable cures and lasted until his passing in January 1946. He and my father met at the Hannen Swaffer home circle, in 1943. At the time Parish was practising in East Sheen, near Richmond, Greater London. Like all meetings this was not by chance, but it was also at the request of Silver Birch, who wished to convey his thoughts and encouragement to them. The two wives, Peggy Parish and Nancy Lilley were present.

Though addressed to two healers, his words are for us all:

> Remember the power of the spirit is supreme. Even you, who are old workers, do not fully realise what the power of spirit can accomplish provided you give it the right conditions. It is not merely an empty phrase, for the power of spirit is the power of life itself. It is the vital, energising, dynamic mainspring of all being, and it is the power, which in many diverse forms is at the disposal of those evolved beings, who co-operate with you in your tasks.
>
> Where you provide the right atmosphere, the right conditions, where your hearts and minds are filled with the single, inflexible purpose, where you are resolute, unyielding, unmoved by the storms and stresses, the tempests of your world, and stand like a rock knowing that none of these will be able to deflect you, there you provide us with the perfect instruments.
>
> When people rush hither and thither and never stand still, they do not give us the opportunity of pouring this power through them. All growth of the life forces is accomplished in the stillness, where there is receptivity. And when you stand still and allow the power of the spirit to suffuse and flood your being, then you are indeed instruments, for through you that power can stretch and reach and touch others, and bring the healing, the comforting, the teaching, the tenderness, the sympathy and all the love and life that yearns to reveal itself in your world.[10]

My father, a great orator in his own right, told me many years later of this meeting and even then marvelled at the magnificent eloquence of the great soul who addressed them, his words flowing like liquid, caressing, uplifting and inspiring, bringing such confidence and trust in the power of spirit that suffering and obstacles were seen in a different light and could be transcended, knowing that behind all events the hand of the Creator moved with wisdom and love.

Silver Birch told them that their work was vital and that they were pioneers and shining exemplars, and though they might at times wonder what they had achieved and whether it was worth while, they could not judge, because unknown to them others were fired by their example.

He explained how the spirit influenced their work:

> Here you have Parish and there you have Lilley – two great healers, both responsible and receptive to the power of the spirit, two instruments inspired by the same source, but working on different lines – each according to his nature.
>
> Wherever there are instruments ready to serve, there comes to help them those in my world skilled in just those capabilities best suited for the individual

> purpose. Each instrument is a study in himself. Each has a different make-up. All the phases, physiological, psychological and etheric characteristics, the constitution of the individual, the faculties, the capabilities of the mind, the emanations of the aura; all these in turn have to be studied so that the right kind of spirit helper can be called upon to assist in the great task.
>
> I wish you could all see with the eyes of spirit. I wish you could see what is happening all the time that you are at work and we are at work with you – it is a wonderful sight.[10]

In his reply to Peters' argument that the healing work of Parish proved him wrong, Dr Letari pointed out that Parish was an exceptional healer and an exceptional man, not without knowledge, an adept in Yoga, and one who had gained mastery over himself. His gift was an expression of his spiritual attainment. Parish could not be compared with the majority to whom he was addressing his concerns.

In concluding his letter, Dr Letari reiterated how essential the need for medical knowledge of the body in health and disease was to both guide and healer. Without this knowledge the healer is entirely dependent upon his guide. When this obtains even greater laws have to be brought into operation to make diagnosis and cure possible: the healer must develop trance and clairaudient mediumship. In most cases the healer lacked these psychic gifts and was working blind.

> My comments are based upon the concept 'cure' in its true interpretation and not in the loose sense such as the patient feeling better because of religious, emotional or psychological uplift (placebo effect).
>
> This subject of spiritual healing is so vast; it is not possible to deal with even the elementary principles in the confines of a letter. I am however, prepared to meet Dr Peter and his guides, or any group of healers with him, in a full discussion, either publicly or privately.[11]

Dr Peters response in *The Two Worlds* a week later was to express his disbelief that Dr Letari was the author of the letter under his name, or, if so, that it was "coloured by Mr Lilley's mind" and further he objected "that there was no need to develop an essay on Mr Lilley's particular views on healing."

He then reiterated his previous statements and again refuted those of Dr Letari. He asserted that Mr Lilley had not considered *magnetic healing* and *'radiatory'* healing when expounding on healing methodology. He affirmed that in magnetic healing the healing medium first attracts the type of energy necessary to counteract the particular disease and then applies it to specific centres, and secondly he attracts to himself and absorbs those forces which are producing the disease, drawing it forth from the patient. In 'radiatory' healing, a process simpler and safer for the healer, the outflowing stream of radiant energy is directed to the centre nearest to the location of the disease.

Obviously stung by a comment made by Dr Letari that his opinions stemmed from inexperience, he wrote rather pretentiously:

> I am really not interested in Mr Lilley's attempts to show that I am 'inexperienced' when there is no known method of healing, ancient or modern, of which I have not made a complete study. Surely Dr Letari should know this, and of questions I put in the House of Commons on advanced methods of healing by members of the medical profession and which the Minister of Health could not answer correctly.[12]

It would seem, however, that he had failed to incorporate the *Organon* or other works on homeopathic principles in his exhaustive studies.

He declined participating in an open debate as he felt it might lead to contentiousness, create animosities and prove detrimental to the cause of Spiritualism; he proposed that tolerance for different methods of spiritual healing was the best way forward for all.

William enters the debate

It was evident that with this letter Peters wished to stand down from the controversy, but his inference that the letter he was replying to was the brainchild of Mr Lilley and not Dr Letari, his assertion that debate would create division rather than resolution, and his explanation of *magnetic* and *'radiatory' healing*, prompted my father to take up the gauntlet. It was also his urgent wish to bring healers together as a united and informed body, and to protect both healers and patients from their own ingenuousness.

He replied to Dr Peters in *The Two Worlds*, January 24, 1947, in a letter entitled *Throw off the Shackles of Ignorance*. He urged that discussion and evaluation were of prime importance for the furtherance of spiritual healing, which was not a question of opinion and conjecture, but a matter of science, and that debate should be encouraged with one thought in mind; "the advancement of spiritual healing through the revelation of truth."

He opened with this comment:

> Doubt is inferred by Dr Peters whether Dr Letari or I had replied to his first 'open' letter; the assurance has been given. To satisfy our friend, I now take over, since Dr Letari's offer to meet in a debate publicly or privately, has not been accepted.[13]

After a preamble, in which he reiterated Dr Peter's objections, he wrote:

> When we first begin to study any science, we should first ascertain the laws that govern, and not the reverse, i.e. strive to apply a science independent of its laws.

He emphasised that the medical knowledge referred to by Dr Letari in his lectures extended well beyond the basic medical sciences; these were but the nuts and bolts of the knowledge required by the responsible healer.

He continued:

> Life is a vital power, and when acting in harmony with the body preserves it as a harmonious whole; disturbances of the life force mean disease; absence of the life force means death. Bodily death means an absence of spirit and soul, which give the body this vital principle; therefore changes or perversions of the life force, which constitute disease, must indicate that there are primary changes, firstly in the soul (the spirit is our innate divinity and is therefore eternally perfect).[13]

He insisted that we must know how the soul gives its life-force to the body and regulates its physiological processes and be able to interpret the emotional and physical changes which indicate a perturbation in the frequency of the life force.

> Dr Peter's infers that soul emanation, or the psychic aura, does not come within the category of medical knowledge, but I do not agree because the only difference is that one manifestation (soul) is finer than the other (physical). One must understand these finer forces just as surely as the physical.[13]

This principle accorded with Dr Letari's use of colour therapy for the colour changes in the aura which soul-based disease causes. For therapists who lack the clairvoyant gift necessary to visualise the human aura and diagnose from it, knowledge of the specific therapeutic power of each colour and the indications for its use are an invaluable substitute.

William then questioned Dr Peters assertions about *magnetic* and "*radiatory*" healing. In the instance of *magnetic* healing, he asked how the healer could possibly determine the type of energy necessary to counteract a disease when he had no knowledge either of the ray forces or of the disease to be cured.

> Also if he does not know the disease, how can he 'attract to himself and absorb those forces which are producing the disease?' In *radiatory* healing we are told the 'radiant energy' is directed to the centre nearest the location of the disease. Again I ask Dr Peters, how does the healer without the requisite knowledge, ascertain and specifically determine the location of the disease? Let me remind our friend, that disease is never located, but only the effect, or symptoms. Treatment so applied must be to the effect only, therefore, suppressive or palliative in action.[13]

My father pointed out how Dr Peters' criticism of Dr Letari's lectures was at variance with his own statements made in his review of *The Gift of Healing* only three years before; his opinion had so changed that he now blamed Dr Letari's advocacy to healers, of the very methods he had previously so warmly extolled, of doing an infinite amount of harm to the cause of healing. William repudiated this and asserted that any harm done to spiritual healing rather lay in the contradictory opinions and lawless theories expressed by Dr Peters. Furthermore, until spiritual healing became ordered and based on a solid foundation of knowledge, the evaluation of its healings, which too often amounted to exaggerated claims, would remain "mythical, haphazard and unexplainable." He attacked the exemption from knowledge claimed on the supposition that the spirit guide possessed the necessary knowledge. Such a state indicated that the medium was then a mere automaton, totally dependent, and, when not in communication with the spirit guide, either impotent or a 'fake.' Moreover, it presupposed a collaborative union of ignorance and wisdom, which was absurd.

We are all, in varying degrees, mediums. Years later, when father and I were discussing mediumship, he explained that for inspiration to flow from the spirit realm to the world of matter, a channel is required that is highly attuned and sensitive to what is being transmitted, just as silver and copper wire are able with minimal resistance to transmit electricity, and yet lead cannot. Music could stream through Mozart because he was a gifted musician – he was like pure silver. Healing, a vocation that blends knowledge, art and spirituality, similarly demands freedom of flow, facilitated by sincerity, compassion, trust and love.

In his letter, William wrote that he realised that it could be said that Jesus and other great spiritual masters healed the sick without the knowledge that he advocated. In answer, he asserted that by virtue of their spiritual standing such masters possessed both the wisdom and power to use natural law to the highest degree, and that any comparison between such personages and the spiritual healers for whom Dr Peters was the voice would be incongruous.

> Is there a person living who dare claim the powers of the Master?[13]

In conclusion, he called upon all spiritual healers to "throw off the shackles of ignorance" and make themselves worthy of the trust placed in them.

> Collective effort with knowledge and wisdom will surely place spiritual healing on a pinnacle which will command the respect and admiration of future generations.[13]

Publically, this brought the controversy to a close, but unfortunately did not bring about a united front, nor did it induce my father's fellow healing mediums to consider homeopathy as an adjunct to their work. Nevertheless, as previously, the increased exposure that the heated correspondence had brought him resulted in even greater public interest.

Controversy and initiation   451

On Sunday, April 27, 1947, William was in Northern Ireland and gave two lectures in Belfast each attended by over a thousand people. On July 10, 1947, a similar number attended his address in the Victoria Hall in Hanley, Stoke-on-Trent. The occasion was the centenary meeting of the Potteries and District Council of Spiritualist Churches. After the address, Dr Letari gave healing to a number of patients from the audience.

War is symptomatic of disease

In those years, the team was indefatigable. Time-off was minimal. In the practice at 8/10, and from the platform, the mission was threefold: to teach the truth of life everlasting and the soul's spiritual destiny, to heal the sick and to spread awareness of homeopathy as the means of treating body, mind and soul. The recent war, from which Britain was still struggling to recover, with its overtone of perverted minds capable of initiating and perpetrating the most heinous atrocities, provided Dr Letari with material proof of the desperate need for healing at soul level. Lest with time, the monstrous distortion of the soul, which made such happenings possible, should mistakenly be thought resident in the few, he pointed to the participatory congruence and compliance that the hideous doctrine of hatred had found amongst cohorts of minions. There were certainly those who were appalled by the acts they were ordered to carry out, but there were also those who relished it. These energies were present amongst the children of every generation of every nation and every race. Only spiritual knowledge and homeopathy could expunge the taint that warped the soul.

> He stated that the last war – and all wars – were the result of disease; disease of the soul. A diseased soul led to a diseased mind and body. The wars and troubles that beset humanity today were the direct result of spiritual ignorance and disease. Knowledge of spiritual truths – which he directed towards healing and the greater root-cause, *ignorance* – represented the crux of his work.[14]

This report of a lecture delivered by Dr Letari, under the heading, *Lecture by Famous Spirit Doctor at Hastings*, appeared in the *Psychic Journal* in June 1947, and gives us a glimpse of the message he was spreading.

Homesickness

The lecture was timed to coincide with my parent's visit to the boarding school near Hastings where I had been sent, as was the custom of the time, at the tender age of six. I am still acutely aware of the intense pangs of homesickness, which made a misery of my life there. Each night, I sobbed myself to sleep, overwhelmed by feelings of utter desolation and abandonment. This was intensified by the austere formality and rigid discipline of the school tradition, captured by the school uniform, which consisted of a pin-striped, long-trousered suit, white shirt and tie. The shirts were cursed with detachable stiff-collars, cuffs and studs, which were the bane of my life each morning. My memory of the place is one of dismal darkness and oppressive wood panelled halls and passages. The only relief from the heartless tedium of life there was the Sunday morning ramble over neighbouring farmlands, exciting minefields of fresh and ancient cowpats, on our way to the village church. I recall, one weekend, my grandma Overton, accompanied by a lady friend, taking me out for the day. That day arrived like a long awaited oasis. It turned out to be grey, dismal and drizzly, very like my inner world. We sat under a shelter on the promenade, protected from the rain, but not the cold, looking out to sea. Despite the ice-cream cone that should have claimed my attention and lightened my heart, all I was conscious of was the hollow, aching in my stomach, which heralded my return to prison. Unbeknown to me, life was preparing me for what lay ahead, introducing me to painful experiences of human emotion, which would stand me in good stead, when, in the years of the future, the truly forsaken related their sufferings to me. A chord of compassion would be struck, quickened by familiarity, granting me entry into many dark and secret places.

My parent's visit was most timely. The excellent reputation, which had persuaded them to select this school, must have been achieved prior to the war. Although the standard of education had been maintained, all other aspects of the institution, from the kitchen up, had gone into sad decline, especially the upkeep of the premises and the monitoring of pupils' cleanliness and clothes, of paramount importance at a boy's school. Immaculately white stiff-collars and cuffs were more important than whiteness of teeth or holes in socks or underpants. My mother was horrified by my unkempt appearance and I was summarily removed from the school, just before the summer holidays. On arriving home, I was immediately put into a hot bath and scrubbed from top to toe with uncomfortable attention being given to a very grimy neck and ears.

Meningitis

Whether it was the conditions at the school, or, more likely, the deep unhappiness I had experienced, no sooner was I home than I developed a painful sore on the left side of my neck. Knowing how things can be in a doctor's home when children are sick, I think, like the cobbler's son being without shoes, the sore was neglected. It soon led to a general infection, which put me into a high fever and very soon a critical state. I lay in a semi-coma for three days with raging temperature, jerking limbs, violent head pain and wild delirium, with horrid, glaring gargoyle-like faces leering at me. Amidst the mental confusion and severe pain that seemed to paralyse my brain, I still remember those nightmarish apparitions, which seemed bent on my perdition. For years my mother kept a diarised account of those terrible days in which she had meticulously recorded the temperature readings, my symptoms and the remarks of Dr Letari, who tended me throughout. Looking at those notes after I had qualified as a doctor I could only marvel at my mother's utter confidence in the good Doctor and my father. No hospitalisation; no antibiotics; only homeopathic remedies, the love and care of my parents and the spiritual treatment of Dr Letari. Our neighbours, refugees from Nazi Germany, with whose children I often played, were aghast at my almost moribund state and remonstrated with my parents about the necessity of calling in a 'real' doctor to save my life. When this did not happen and my condition remained serious, the mother of the family, a large, big-bosomed, controlling woman with a heavy German accent, who loved feeding me on liver-sausage and sauerkraut, out of fear for my life, threatened to call the authorities. Fortunately, this proved unnecessary because that very night the crisis was reached.

The infection had concentrated on the left side of my head causing my left eye to bulge forward conspicuously (proptosis) due to pressure behind the eyeball. With this localisation, I became more conscious of my circumstances and for the first time of Dr Letari ministering to me, which he had been doing daily. Considering the extreme nature of the signs, I was remarkably free from pain. That evening, Dr Letari told my mother that he needed to perform a spiritual operation to relieve the pressure and bring the infection to a close.

I lay on the bed to which I had been confined for so many days and the Doctor made passes over my head and face, sometimes making the lightest contact, so light it seemed like a breath of air or the touch of a feather. After a while, his hands focused on the region of my left forehead, eye and nose. Although I was not in sufficient possession of my faculties at the time to be able to remember exactly what he did, I have observed him performing spiritual operations on so many occasions that I can accurately describe how he must have worked. His hands moved with extreme dexterity, suppleness and speed, while manipulating some invisible material through rapid pianist-like movements executed between the first two fingers and thumbs. The left hand would be held close to the area of the body being operated upon, concentrating the energy at the desired point while the right hand, with the fingers in constant motion as described, moved more slowly up and down a trajectory focused on the same point. This would continue for some time depending on how critical or complicated the procedure might be. This highly concentrated action would be interspersed with more generalised passes over the area of treatment, characterised by the final short, sharp, casting-off gesture of the hands, as if ridding them of drops of water. At times, he would briefly look either to left or right of him or to the head or foot of the bed and like a conductor with a slight nod of the head or raising of the eyebrows cue unseen helpers. The treatment would be completed by a number of full body passes moving and dispersing energy always from above downwards. Finally, the good Doctor would resume his seat and discuss what had been achieved and then close with a short prayer either in Hindustani or Sanskrit, always followed by the words: "Now I will bring my mediator back."

When my treatment was completed, Dr Letari told my mother that I would shortly experience a severe nosebleed and that she should prepare for this, but not be alarmed. A large bowl and a towel were brought and the Doctor and my mother sat quietly beside me while I lay peacefully on the bed. It was not long before I felt something trickling down my throat and experienced the unmistakable taste of blood. Then the haemorrhage came! My mother had to act swiftly or I would have choked. She got me into the seated position and supported me, since I was as weak as a lamb. I remember hanging my head over the bowl for what seemed an age as strings and strings of black clotted blood continually issued from my left nostril. This went on for some time, gradually easing off until it finally ceased. This considerable haemorrhage proved to be the turning point. I was convalescent for many days, but my recovery was complete. The proptosis rapidly subsided, leaving me with nothing more than the slightest heaviness (ptosis) of the left upper eyelid, often only noticeable when I am tired, but in latter years more constantly apparent; a small price to pay for a bout of bacterial meningitis, which so often proves fatal or leaves severe neurological damage.

My mother's diary shows that I received Belladonna 10M (deadly nightshade) during the period of initial intense fever and hallucinatory delirium, followed by Apis 200 (honey bee) when I ceased to urinate; in the final phase, as symptoms became concentrated on the left side, I was given Lachesis 200 (bushmaster snake). With typical British stiff-upper-lip stoicism, shown even at six years of age, I had never told my parents about the depth of my unhappiness at boarding school. If I had, my father would have probably given me Capsicum (Cayenne pepper), a remedy frequently of value in the treatment of intense homesickness. The plant is a member of the Solanaceae family and hence closely related to Belladonna, which so clearly matched the early symptoms of my illness. It is possible that Capsicum, given for my emotional state, could have prevented the development of meningitis. However, that would have robbed me of an essential experience. In the event, the therapy I received was a fine example of the successful combination of spiritual and homeopathic healing – the very method my father wished to propagate amongst healers.

My illness proved of incalculable value to me; a profound experience, which at an early age gave me complete confidence in the power of spirit and the magic of homeopathy. Nothing can take the place of personal experience. It was an initiation rite, essential for the vocation I was to follow. It also addressed constitutional, hereditary tendencies. My recovery, unmarred by any suppression of disease, would ensure that much negative patterning from the past was resolved. In that regard there was still work to be done, but the illness was an important healing step towards future health.

I was still bed bound when I told my parents that I was determined to become a doctor like my father. This decision never changed and provided me with all the motivation I needed to further my education.

After the summer holidays, I was sent to Claremont Boarding School in the countryside near Beaconsfield, which proved to be like a breath of fresh air in comparison with the grim misery of Hastings. I was still beset with twinges of homesickness, but managed to cope much better and enjoyed an environment which was truly idyllic.

It was here I commenced piano lessons, developed an interest in nature and acquired a life-long love of mythology. My teacher introduced us to both Greek and Norse legends, to the magic worlds of Heracles and Achilles, and of Sigurd and Loki, imparting a fascination for these timeless stories that I never lost. On reflection, I regret that I was unable to finish my schooling there, but that was not to be, and there are always reasons and compensations for the way things are.

The events that would dictate why I would only be at Claremont for just over a year were already falling into place. As related earlier, interest and enthusiasm for his work had resulted in my father being invited to tour southern Africa. Although this had seemed still remote late in 1945, when the invitation was received, time had flown, and in the middle of August 1947, shortly before I started at my new school, my father departed for South Africa.

The *Psychic News*, as always, was first with the news. On August 23, 1947 it reported:

> **Off to South Africa**: Mr WH Lilley, the well-known healer, started for South Africa last Monday on a healing tour among his 2000 patients in the Union. He will be back in this country before Christmas.

References

1. Arkwright T. *I Accuse These Doctors. Sunday Pictorial*; July 9 1945.
2. Précis of Dr Letari's Address at Nottingham. *The Searchlight of Spiritual Truth*; February 1946.
3. Lecture by Famous Spirit Doctor: WH Lilley at Hastings. *Psychic Journal*; June 1947.
4. Silver Birch Gives Guidance To A Psychic Healer. *Psychic News*; December 15 1945. p5.
5. Barbanell M. *Psychic News*; February 2, 1946.
6. Peters SJ. Behind The Scenes With A Great Healer: Healer MP Praises New Book On Healing. *Psychic News*; October 2 1943.
7. Peters SJ. Ex-MP Healer Takes Up The Cudgels. *Psychic Truth*. December 1946.
8. He Makes A Protest. *Psychic Truth*; January 1947.
9. Letari Dr. Medical Knowledge Is Essential To Both Guide And Medium. *The Two Worlds*; January 10 1947.
10. Silver Birch Speaks With Two Famous Healers. *Psychic News*; December 25 1943.
11. Letari Dr. Medical Knowledge Is Essential To Both Guide And Medium. *The Two Worlds*; January 10 1947.
12. Peters SJ. Toleration In Healing Methods. *The Two Worlds*; January 10 1947.
13. Lilley WH. Throw Off The Shackles Of Ignorance. *The Two Worlds*; January 24 1947.
14. Lecture by Famous Spirit Doctor at Hastings. *Psychic Journal*; June 1947.

18

A PLACE IN THE SUN

Vision of a different future

William's four-month trip to Southern Africa was a great success. Dr Letari gave trance addresses and healing demonstrations to packed audiences in Johannesburg, Pretoria, Durban, Cape Town, Windhoek, Bulawayo and Salisbury. Everywhere he went he was warmly received and shown great hospitality. Coming from bomb-damaged London, food rationing and a serious economic downturn in post-war England, colonial South Africa appeared to William not only a land of milk and honey, but also a land of opportunity for a different kind of life with his young family. For twenty years he had devoted every waking moment to the cause of healing and lived under immense pressure; a life driven by numbers – letters, patients, diagnoses, treatments, trances, addresses and cures, but never by money. In South Africa, he saw the possibility of extricating himself from a life that was profiting him little financially and slowly wearing him down, and of building a future for his family. He could not have wished for a better opportunity for bringing him to the attention of the South African public and building on the considerable patient base that already existed.

Significantly, Arthur Richards was not involved in this trip; William had made all arrangements personally with various Spiritualist associations and the President of the Society for Psychic Advancement, David Lepato. The experience of being free of his arduous schedule for four consecutive months, and at the same time feted and favoured by all the representatives of the many organisations that hosted him, broke the pattern of interminable labour and made him long for a more tranquil life. To work, most certainly, but with reasonable hours interspersed with time at leisure, something he and my mother had never enjoyed.

A star performer

Richards was an A-type personality; a man of considerable means who had transferred his achievement driven focus from engineering to philanthropy, and found in William the means to fulfil this ambition to the highest degree. As much as Dr Letari, working from spirit, created the healer and the homeopath, so Richards working from the material plane created the gentleman with business expertise, who could move in any society with ease and confidence. Richards had the shrewdness, assertiveness, influence, contacts and the money to make things happen and through his generous sponsorship gave my father's career a flying start. He had provided welcome and persuasive support for William during his conscientious objection and through the confrontations with the Cheltenham authorities and the London County Council, but inevitably, through his combined role of mentor, promoter, organiser, administrator and sponsor, he had control of almost every aspect of the younger man's life. Although Richards was mindful and respectful of Dr Letari's wishes, William was the star of his philanthropic show, which while serving altruism also served his egotistic and entrepreneurial drives. In consequence, there was the ever-increasing push for William to perform both in the nursing home and on the platform with insufficient concern for the dangers of fatigue and burnout. The warning of Silver Birch was not without reason.

The spiritual and charitable nature of the mission meant that at first no fee was asked for direct or absent healing. All that was required of distant patients was a stamped, self-addressed envelope. Only later was a charge made for the homeopathic remedies that were prescribed and this was always nominal. The addresses that Dr Letari gave throughout the land to many thousands of people were all by invitation of Spiritualist Churches, and created no revenue; being far-flung, they cost the Sanctuary heavily in transport and accommodation. As a result, William, his gift and his knowledge were the financial prisoners of Richards' philanthropy. Despite his success and celebrity, my father remained a salaried man of very modest means. I know that my schooling in England was only made possible through considerable sacrifice on the part of my parents. While Richards could well afford the generosity of his altruistic aspirations it was at the expense of the one he promoted and sponsored.

Decision

One may justifiably ask why Dr Letari and others connected to my father did not advise or insist upon more financial independence on the one hand and moderation of the workload on the other, but that would be to discount the control, for better or worse, that we must exercise over our own destiny. We always remain central to the path we follow; we are not pawns to be moved passively and acquiescently over the chessboard of life by our guides and inspirers, or for that matter, by those who would subvert us; our self-determination is an essential element in our development, which is never overruled by those who overshadow us. However, advice and gentle persuasion are always given, often unconsciously during our waking hours, or more directly, but still for us unconsciously, during our nightly sojourns in the astral world. In addition to these influences, my father had the conscious immediacy of his clairaudient faculty. Advice there was, but freedom of choice is always entangled with disposition and all its foibles and frailties and seldom results in prompt response to words of wisdom. It was the trip to South Africa that proved the essential catalyst. By the end of the tour, William had made his decision and it was a momentous one: to emigrate to South Africa and commence a new life.

He returned to London with a sense of elation. My mother was not surprised by his sudden determination to leave England. She was relieved. They shared everything, and she was well aware of the stresses and frustrations he was exposed to despite the continuous accolades and success that rewarded his efforts. She was witness to the spiralling intensity of his work and its tiring effect. She knew it could not continue. His letters from South Africa were filled with wonder and excitement about the open, vastness of the land, its multi-facetted beauty, the richness of its wild life, its profusion of unfamiliar fruits, the glorious weather and the magnificent thunderstorms of the Highveld. And then there were the many special people that he met, who surrounded him with their enthusiasm, support, gratitude and friendship. On that trip, he forged bonds that would last the rest of his life. Of particular importance was the friendship of HP (Lassie) Smit, who lived in Pretoria, the administrative capital. He was a typical Afrikaner both in feature and form, a rugged, powerful man; his broken nose testifying to his earlier prowess on the rugby field; his sheer physicality masking a very astute intellect. His deep pride in his birthright and passionate love of the land and its fauna and flora were only matched by his deep commitment to the cause of Spiritualism in which he played an influential role. His interest in nature and his culture extended to the use of '*boereraad*,' the folk medicine of the Dutch pioneers. From this it was an easy step for him to adopt a broader herbalism and the concepts of homeopathy, which he appreciated as spiritual medicine. My father could not have had a better host or companion on his introductory tour than Lassie Smit. It was he, who sensing my father's thoughts and deliberations, encouraged him to seriously contemplate the move to South Africa and promised him every possible support and assistance if he should make such a decision.

Nancy backed William fully. Any anxieties she may have felt were eased after she spoke with Dr Letari and he told her that although the decision was "Bill's," it was in perfect keeping with the intentions of spirit. The work in Britain was complete; my father's future lay in South Africa and would move forward under different conditions and with a different goal.

This was not palatable news for Arthur Richards. For some time he had been aware of William's determination to become increasingly more involved in the administration of the nursing home and his affairs. This independence had been made very clear in William's decision to go to South Africa and his handling of all the arrangements beforehand, but he was unprepared for the marked change that the trip had wrought on William. Richards' vision for the future was more fame and success for his charge, and more honour and respect for himself as the selfless benefactor. Although Dr Letari's quiet insistence, that this radical change was essential for the future work of his mediator, carried considerable weight with Richards, who held him in the highest esteem, the relationship between ACR and WHL, as they often spoke of one another, became strained and would never be the same again. The decision was a huge disappointment to Richards, and I am sure that in some measure he felt betrayed, taken advantage of and possibly rejected. However, he played his role through to the very end at 8/10, and the preparations for the transition, which proceeded throughout 1948, unfolded without hindrance on his part. It was decided that on my father's departure, the Letari Nursing Home in Bulstrode Street would be closed, as also the subsidiaries in Hunslet and Hull. Eventually new premises were purchased in Luttrell Ave, Putney, where Richards had a home on the banks of the river Thames. From there, Richards would continue to co-ordinate absent healing and homeopathic medication for patients in the United Kingdom.

I was first apprised of my parent's intentions when they picked me up from Claremont at the close of term before the summer vacation. Usually, I was put on the train in Beaconsfield and my parents would be at the station in London to receive me, but on this occasion they drove out to the school from London in our black Austin 10 motor car. I remember well its small double rear windows, large prominent headlights and the silver winged Austin insignia above the grill. I thought the car rather handsome, and still do. I recall on the journey back to London, my father stopping on a grassy verge, and father and son taking a slow stroll down the quiet country byroad, while my mother remained in the car tending to my baby sister. I was not quite eight years old, but father addressed me as an adult, telling me his plans and asking me what I thought of them. I was both excited and anxious. I knew I was going to miss Claremont, where I had at last settled in and was enjoying my schooling. He reassured me, explaining what a wonderful outdoor life awaited me in South Africa, that he was sure there would be a good school for me to attend and that in our new country we would be able to have far more family time together. We then went on to spend our last English summer holiday in Bournemouth.

Vaccinosis

Shortly before I returned to Claremont, we all had our obligatory smallpox vaccination in preparation for our emigration, which was to take place at the end of January 1949. Hardly had I returned to school when I developed an intermittent fever and within a day began to break out in cowpox lesions, firstly in the genital area and then severely to my face, especially about my lips and nostrils, which became swollen, crusted and very unsightly. This affliction was further evidence that cobbler's children have no shoes. In the rush of events, father had omitted to give us all protective doses of Thuja (northern white cedar) or Arsenicum album (white arsenic), two remedies of great value in preventing the adverse effects of vaccination or immunisation. I was the only one to develop this state of acute *vaccinosis*, and I did so in a most conspicuous manner.

The school doctor and matron realised from the typical lesion on my arm that I was suffering from vaccination reaction and notified my parents. My father asked that if possible no treatment should be given. During the fever, which was mild and lasted only a few days, I was confined to the school sick bay. Because of my frightful appearance it was debated whether I should be sent home to avoid causing alarm amongst my peers. It was finally decided that I could stay on, but I remember that for many days I was not permitted to sit at table with other pupils during meals. I was placed at a small table of my own, some distance from the rest, as if I had a dreaded contagion. My food had to be liquefied as I could only feed through a straw. I felt very much like a pariah – a loathsome creature to be avoided, or kept at a distance. Soon medicine arrived from my father: Malandrinum 200 (the nosode of 'grease', a skin infection of horses) to be taken once per day for three days and Thuja 30 to be taken at first twice daily and then less frequently as I improved. The medication speeded my recovery and soon I was accepted back into the ranks. Although they had been so severe, and so repulsive, the lesions dried up and scaled off without the slightest scar.

This brief, but significant, illness proved more traumatic to me emotionally than physically because of the repulsive lesions I developed and the isolation they caused. This was made worse by my sensitive age and the exposure of being at boarding school. It served an important purpose, almost as important to my development as the meningitis of the previous year. It was the second stage in the clearing of inherited miasmatic debris from the family past. Such a florid response to smallpox vaccination is indicative of a sycotic constitution; a constitution harbouring the long-term effects of suppressed or inherited gonorrhoea (sycosis), often handed down through many generations. My body's ability to vigorously externalise and reject the grafting onto my constitution of the disease pattern of cowpox indicated a similar pattern or template resident in my system, which in voiding the effect of the vaccine weakened or erased itself; a very crude form of homeopathy and far from free of risk. The Malandrinum and Thuja were given to ensure that this process was complete. Both these remedies, apart from their ability to eliminate the untoward effects of vaccination, are major anti-sycotic remedies.

One of the most characteristic indications that a patient has a predominantly sycotic (gonorrhoea related) inheritance is the presence of a yellow-green catarrhal discharge from any of the mucous membranes of the body (similar to the characteristic discharge of acute gonorrhoeal infection). Babies will often give early evidence of the sycotic *miasmatic taint* when they develop a purulent conjunctivitis (eye infection with pus) with a yellow-green discharge that accumulates in the eye corners or gums-up the eyes during sleep[i] and likewise when, after every nose cold, they develop a yellow-green nasal catarrh. Another typical sign of underlying sycosis is the development of herpetiform (herpes-like) eruptions, i.e. vesicles upon the skin, such as recurrent fever blisters (*Herpes simplex*), genital herpes (*Herpes genitalis*), severe chicken pox, shingles (*Herpes zoster*), smallpox, and the cowpox vaccination blisters that I developed. To the homeopathic physician these clues are of great importance, pointing to a group of remedies that is most likely to be helpful for the patient.

In my case, the sequence of meningitis followed by vaccinosis was further confirmation of underlying sycosis. One of the most important organisms capable of causing meningitis is *Neisseria meningitidis*, (meningococcus)

---

[i] Here I am not referring to acute gonorrhoea *Ophthalmia neonatorum*.

which is a diplococcus (double coccus), very closely related to *Neisseria gonorrhoea*, the organism that causes gonorrhoea and is implicated in sycosis. Therefore, weakness in the blood-brain barrier, which normally prevents invasion by organisms from the blood into the central nervous system, is intrinsic to the sycotic miasm. This holds good regardless of the infecting organism, be it viral or bacterial. I did not have a lumbar puncture performed on me, so the organism implicated in my infection remained unknown, but this proved no hindrance to treatment or cure, since the symptoms and signs were explicit and provided sufficient guidance for prescribing purposes. In the long term, the diagnosis of sycosis proves of greater importance in the on-going treatment of a patient than the short-term diagnosis of meningitis, since it reveals why the meningitis was possible in the first place and assists in the future selection of remedies to address this vulnerability. By assisting the body to cure itself, Dr Letari and my father removed the most aggressive and dangerous layer of my sycotic inheritance; the *vaccinosis* took this process of cure a step further. There was still work to be done because in South Africa I became susceptible to sinus catarrh, of the tell-tale greenish-yellow type, after winter colds, and developed a large, ugly looking wart on the inside of my left elbow. The typical viral warts of children are also a sure-sign of a sycotic taint. For both these problems, Thuja once again came to my help.

The meningitis could have cost me my life, but it did not, and with this outcome, we witness the healing power of illness. The falling away of a layer of sycosis removes simultaneously a veil of the soul that shrouds the perfection of the indwelling spirit. The healing is at the level of the soul. If the illness had taken my life, it could only do so physically, I am immortal and my time for passing from the earth plane would have come, neither too early nor too late. In touching the physical plane, even for a short time, the soul is quickened, and the loss to those who grieve, though painful, is seasoning for the soul; and remember always, that in the scale of eternity the parting is but for the blink of an eyelid. Suffering is as much in the eye of the beholder as is beauty. Immersion in the abiding Reality of spirit, permits the eye of the soul to focus above events.

If antibiotics had been used to save my life, the healing power of my illness would have been blocked. The antibiotic removes the external challenge, and the energy of the constitutional miasmatic state, which seeks expression through the illness, moves to a deeper level of activity, more chronic and more inveterate. Sooner, or later, the inner condition will demand release either emotionally or physically, or through both outlets. The veils of the soul become more opaque and the occlusion of spirit becomes evident in unwelcome behaviour, e.g. irritability and impatience may dethrone tolerance. There is continuity in life and in disease

This does not mean that antibiotics should never be used.

Faced by meningitis, or other life-threatening and aggressive infections, especially in the young, the weak and the elderly, an antibiotic may be the only way in which life can be saved, or severe damage avoided. One does not throw away life; it is precious; much better to live and fight another day. *However, we must fully understand the process in which we are involved*, and know that the resolving of an infection by chemical means is not a cure, it is a truce through compromise, and the combatants still face one another across a divide. The prescribing of antibiotics is an act that carries great responsibility and should be carefully considered and only resorted to when a more natural conclusion cannot be expected in the light of the patient's condition and the experience of the physician. With growing experience in the use of homeopathic remedies in emergency situations, the seasoned physician is able to prescribe with greater confidence for an ever-wider range of conditions. It is remarkable to witness the rapidity with which the correctly selected homeopathic remedy can act in the face of an acute challenge. In the instance of my illness, which was extremely threatening, I was fortunate to have the assistance of hands-on spiritual healing in combination with homeopathy. Few patients have the benefit of such a defence, and, therefore, their treatment must suit the circumstances!

In evaluating my illnesses, it is essential to see nothing random or arbitrary, to know that they were instructive and essential for my progress on various fronts. There is a blessing in even the most appalling events, and, though it is often difficult to comprehend, there are no exceptions to this fact. Life plays out as it must and its goal is always ascendant. As we shall consider in more detail later, there are archetypal forces at play in all our lives and these become apparent when looked for with insight. The aggression of my first illness pooled on the left side of my head and behind my left eye, and the seemingly trivial wart that developed later was on the inside of my left elbow. Nothing is coincidental; everything is according to law. The left is our intuitive and creative side, related to the archetypal feminine principle within all of us, regardless of gender. It is the stage upon which my life has predominantly been played out and therefore, as is invariably the case, the side that was most vulnerable in my youth. In contrast, the scientific reductionist lives out his pragmatic life on a predominantly right-sided stage, which is archetypally masculine and governed by the intellect and logic.

The left side is also the side upon which the sycotic miasm principally works out its energy and this is always in conjunction with disturbance of the second chakra, one of the seven important energy centres of the body.

The world of the homeopathic remedy archetype has still to be considered, but in the light of my *vaccinosis* experience we may take a peep into this magical realm. Thuja, from the northern white cedar, the very tree that gave Hahnemann's clergyman his gonorrhoea-like urethral discharge after he chewed its leaves, is a profoundly sycotic remedy, i.e. in its proving symptoms it displays the characteristics of the sycotic miasm most markedly. It is strongly left-sided in its effects. One of the most distinguishing emotional feelings that its provers experience is a sense of being soiled, dirty or blemished, a very common observation of those who have contracted gonorrhoea. They also feel disliked, an object for contempt, if not loathing; alone, rejected, separate and isolated. This may be associated with the sense that their blood is dirty or has been poisoned, or that there is something wrong with them; something that no one must know; something they must hide from others. In my boarding school seclusion, an archetypal pattern was played out, which found me leper-like, an object of rejection, ostracised, isolated from my peers, feeling defiled and even in my own eyes repulsive. I remember particularly how ashamed I was of the genital lesions when the school sister applied dressings. The archetypal role of pariah is perfectly matched by the archetypal nature of Thuja and when the two meet in a healing process a cure will be achieved; a cure that transpires at an archetypal, soul level.

An enigma is presented in the fact that neither my parents nor my sister, no more than a year old at the time, showed any signs of reaction to the vaccination other than a mild local blistering, slight malaise on the part of my parents and a short-lived fractiousness in Margaret. Why? Medical foolishness would inform us that nothing untoward transpired; that the family were successfully fortified against the likelihood of contracting small pox and nothing more. Is that so? It is well known and acknowledged that smallpox vaccination can have dire consequences, including demyelinating encephalomyelitis; so much so that when, through successful vaccination programmes, the disease reached such a low incidence that the risk of vaccination outweighed the risk of contracting smallpox, routine vaccination was wisely discontinued. But this knowledge has not translated into a suspicion that even in those who show little or no reaction to vaccination, something insidious and potentially destructive has been imparted, which at some time must manifest itself through physiological imbalance or pathology, if not in this generation then in generations to come, because life is a continuum. Nor has the definite evidence of negative reactions to vaccination been a warning to the orthodoxy that possibly all immunisations expose recipients to deleterious effects. The policy of medical scientists to disavow anecdotal evidence, on the one hand robs them of proof of the power of homeopathy to heal, and on the other hand robs them of the indications that immunisation can harm. As a result, heavy immunisation programmes with an alarming number of components are being vigorously promoted and legislated, even in the face of widespread concern. In practice, the experience of having a child develop grand-mal epilepsy one week after DPT immunisation (diphtheria; whooping cough; tetanus) or seeing a child emotionally and intellectually regress after MMR immunisation (measles; mumps; German measles) leaves one uneasy, even when statistics fail to support one's disquiet and medical authorities 'poopoo' any suspicions.

The severity of my experience, which I repeat was not by chance and proved salutary to my health and my thinking, left me with the conviction that whereas my body, harbouring a sufficiently similar sycotic patterning, was able to eliminate the miasmatic power of the vaccine; my parents and sister failed to do so and thus absorbed its considerable energy with inevitable negative effects. In consequence, and due also to further observations made in my practice, none of my four children have received any form of immunisation and this abstinence is being extended to the next generation of Lilleys.

The proven demyelinating effect seen in certain cases of *vaccinosis*, should by comparison draw one's attention to the demyelinating nature of multiple sclerosis (MS), one of the many autoimmune diseases in which the body produces antibodies which mistakenly attack the body's own tissues; in MS this attack falls on the myelin sheaths of the nerves. When confronted by similarities, we should look for relationships. The similarity between the extreme pathological process of *vaccinosis* (demyelinating encephalomyelitis) and that of MS, should make the responsible observer at least query the possibility that immune programmes, designed to elicit immune response through the introduction of disease products (vaccines), could, through their intensity and the diverse and inherently morbid nature of the substances used, provoke various aberrant responses of the autoimmune type; the type being dependent on the pre-existing constitutional profile of the recipient.

Autoimmune disease constitutes the rejection of one's own body, be it the myelin sheath, as in MS, the pancreatic islets of Langerhans in diabetes, or the synovial membranes in rheumatoid arthritis. Slipping into archetypal mode, the rejection of self can be perceived as the playing out of the pariah consciousness, the self-loathing and self-condemnation which belong to the sycotic miasm: "there is something wrong with me – I must hide it – I must reject it." This presents us with certain links: sycosis + immunisation = more sycosis = pariah archetype = autoimmune disease. Knowledge such as this was at the heart of Dr Letari's mission. It was not new to homeopathy; it was new to the public whom he wished to inform.

Immunisation remains a controversial subject even amongst doctors, but the controversy should not be so much whether to vaccinate or not; this must be determined by the circumstances: the threat to an individual or to society posed by an invading organism and the conditions existing within specific communities, weighed in the balance against the risks inherent in immunisation. The controversy is therefore rather about the risk factor. Medical orthodoxy largely disregards this or does not accept it. In this ostrich-like attitude lies the danger. As in the case of antibiotics, if we opt to use immunisation, *we must be aware of the process we are involved in*. However warranted, we must understand that immunisation grafts a disease pattern onto the constitution of the recipient and there must be negative consequences, which need to be addressed. Homeopathy can protect against these dangers and neutralise after effects.

* * * * *

Farewells

Once the decision to emigrate was finalised, William paid a special visit to Dudley Everett at Nelson's homeopathic pharmacy (see Chapter 9). Everett had given him invaluable advice during the setting-up of the Sanctuary's comprehensive homeopathic dispensary at Letari Nursing Home. While thanking him for all the help he had given in the past and bidding him goodbye, William placed a large order for remedies in all potencies. These were to form the foundation for the new dispensary he would attach to his practice in South Africa.

The rest of the year proceeded smoothly, and in December I closed the Claremont and Beaconsfield chapter of my life, of which I retained many happy memories. The time spent there had benefitted me in many ways. By the time I returned from school, my parents had already left West Hampstead and moved in with my grandparents at 8/10 Bulstrode Street.

There, I attended a farewell party given for my father's students. It was held after the final lecture of the year. During the late 1940s, Dr Letari had encouraged William to commence homeopathic lectures for interested members of the public, to spread a deeper knowledge of homeopathy, and

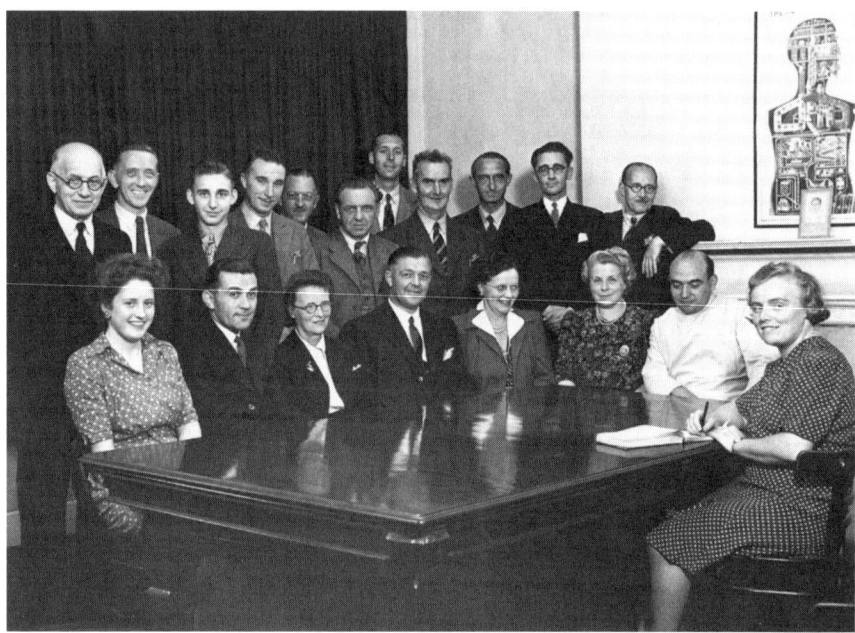

Figure 18.1 Letari Nursing Home: Student group. 1948

also to provide tuition for those wishing to pursue homeopathy as a profession. It must have been a great blow to the members of this small, but select group when they heard of father's intention to leave England. I remember the great respect and affection that was shown my father and how Arthur Richards held the stage. The students presented me with a silver serviette ring inscribed with an ornate $\mathcal{DJL}$, which I still possess. A picture of the group sat around the covered billiard table captures my father's diffidence and the central position that Richards so enjoyed (see Figure 18.1).

Christmas and New Year 1949 were spent with my grandparents in the upstairs apartment at 8/10. Images of the time are patchy, but I remember well the heavy snow that fell that year, tobogganing on Hampstead Heath, and being given a Hornby electric train set for Christmas and on the day, despite my eagerness, hardly managing to get my hands on my present as my father and grandfather commandeered it. Early in January as a parting get-together, we spent a Sunday with the Richards family at their house in Putney, and they took us up the Thames in their motorboat. It was a very exciting day for a young boy, hence the impressions remain vivid, and especially of our passing through the many locks we negotiated on our voyage. Though the weather was cold and overcast, it remained dry. I had no concept of the sun, blue skies and heat that awaited me a few weeks later, six thousand miles to the south.

January fled by and on the 19th the Lilley family boarded a Sabena DC 6 for South Africa via Brussels, with, in those days, many stops on the way. At the height of his fame, William, with never a backward glance, turned his back on his celebrity and headed into a new future.

* * * * *

> It is not my intention to give a detailed account of our life in South Africa, but only to touch those aspects that relate to the story I have so far unfolded.

A new beginning

Lassie Smit met us at Palmietfontein, which in 1949 was the South African international airport situated close to Johannesburg. He lived in Pretoria, so this became our immediate destination. Here, my father set up temporary practice in the house of Mrs Ross; I always knew her as 'Aunty Ross.' She lived at the very end of Jacob Marais Street, close to the Pretoria railway station, which at that time was a residential area; today it is in the very heart of the city. Mrs Ross was both a well-known medium and a leading Spiritualist in Pretoria and a close friend of Lassie Smit. William soon decided not to move to Johannesburg, but rather to live in the quieter and more relaxed atmosphere of the capital. In February, with the guidance of the ever helpful and attentive Lassie, my parents bought a house in Waterkloof, a suburb of Pretoria, and there I lived, with breaks for study and marriage until December 2007, when my wife Paddy and I moved to our present apartment in Cape Town, fully sixty-four years later.

Severance from England

With my father's absence from England, Arthur Richards lost his focus and drive and the administration of the Putney Sanctuary fell into neglect, so much so that early in 1952 my father insisted that it be closed and the property sold. From their correspondence it is apparent that their roles had reversed, William was at the helm, giving instructions and Richards though resisting had to comply. My grandparents, Pop and Sally Lilley, who had continued in their previous roles at Putney, left the foundering ship and retired to Woodlesford, a small village outside Leeds. They came out to South Africa to spend a three month holiday with us in 1956, my last year at school, and shortly after there return, Pop died of a heart attack at 65 years-of-age. Grandma lived on until her ninety-second year, outliving the passing of her youngest son by eight years.

Once Putney closed, all continuing ties with England were broken and to the Spiritualist world it was as if William had simply ridden off into the sunset. He had dominated the stage and featured in most editions of the various Spiritualist periodicals for over ten years, and then suddenly there was utter silence. He would only be briefly heard of again in England in 1953, but to thousands of patients he literally vanished in 1949. The disagreements about the running of the Putney Sanctuary caused an irreparable rift between William and Arthur Richards, and long before Richards' death in 1958, they had ceased corresponding.

The Pretoria practice

Father's new practice in South Africa was a repeat of his experience in England. No sooner had he opened his doors than he was under pressure to find time for all the people who wished to see him. In 1950, he moved from Jacob Marais Street to new rooms in Proes Street. The building had been constructed by a grateful patient and was named Letari House. He stayed there for three years and then, in 1954, finally moved his practice to the centre of the city, establishing himself in more spacious premises in a wing of the fifth floor of a building aptly called City Centre. In the shopping arcade below he opened a health shop for the general public. He practised at City Centre until his death in 1972.

He was soon in demand by various Spiritualist and esoteric organisations to give trance addresses. The Johannesburg societies and Spiritualist churches had a disproportionate number of Jewish members and this predominance was soon reflected in my father's practice. He often said that his most loyal and supportive patients came from the Jewish community and from Afrikaners from the '*platteland*', the rural farming areas, even though he never managed to get his Yorkshire tongue round their language.

The first South African naturopathic and homeopathic college

When he opened the first formal college for the training of professional homeopaths in South Africa in 1951, half of his students were Jewish. Dr Letari and my father shared the task of teaching. From the outset, Dr Letari moved my father more and more to the forefront and changed the emphasis of his practice from psychic healing to homeopathy and chiropractic. Within a few years, he was no longer referred to as the famous medium, but rather as the well-known homeopath. This was not due to any diminution in his psychic gifts, which remained acute until his death; it was in line with Dr Letari's major objective: increased public consciousness of homeopathy. Parallel with this, it was essential to establish a register of qualified homeopathic practitioners, hence the training he and his mediator made possible. At the time, medical doctors practising homeopathy in South Africa were virtually non-existent.

The course extended over a period of three years and was held in Pretoria every Thursday evening. Alongside their study of the materia medica and the clinical application of homeopathic remedies, the students were instructed in the basic medical sciences, colour therapy and chakra science. In addition, Dr Letari gave spiritual discourses imparting to the students knowledge of our divine nature, our spiritual quest, the miasmatic nature of disease and its influence upon the unfolding of the soul. After the first group of students had qualified, William discontinued the Pretoria course and together with Tom Watson, a South African naturopath and homeopath, established the Lindlahr College of homeopathy, naturopathy and osteopathy in Johannesburg. The College was named after Henry Lindlahr, one of the foremost pioneers of natural therapeutics. William became a guest lecturer. The first group of students graduated in 1956 and a number became leading figures in professional homeopathy in South Africa. During this time, William also became co-founder of the South African Naturopathic and Homœopathic Association, the first organisation to represent the naturopathic and homeopathic professions. This organisation was to prove pivotal in the political struggle for recognition that lay ahead.

Through the difficult times that South African homeopathy experienced in the 1950's and 1960's, during which he was always an inspiring and central figure around whom the homeopaths rallied, his war-cry was always for unity, something that was foreign to homeopathy's history; a fact which frequently blighted progress. Often I heard him, when discord threatened to disrupt the common cause, exhort his colleagues with the words: "Either we stand together or we will most surely hang together!"

Spiritual universality

With dissociation from his Christian roots and the strong Masonic influence of Richards, the overtly religious tone of the Hunslet 'House of

Divinity' and the Letari Nursing Home in London fell away. In these Sanctuaries, the main treatment rooms were dominated by an altar draped with a deep-blue material embossed with a large central silver cross flanked by two smaller crosses, indicative of the triune God, a logo which was echoed on the breast pocket of the white coats of the healing staff and on the letter head used for all clinic correspondence. In City Centre there were no altars, the stationary carried no religious insignia and the practice was no longer called the Sanctuary. William, consistent with his deepest conviction, was now able to present his spiritual universality, devoid of religious sectarianism, which, while embracing all religions, shed difference, and in so doing rose above them. He felt that to be a Christian, Jewish or Muslim homeopath, or indeed a homeopath of any religious conviction, was incongruous, an anachronism and a hindrance to the full flow of healing power, which, to be optimal, needs to be untrammelled by doctrine or dogma, enabling the physician to be receptive and sympathetic to the divergent philosophies of patients. He pursued a spiritual path, not a religious one and so obviated belief, bias and prejudice. He regarded the great spiritual teachers of the past, whose adoration and sanctification have degraded into the religions of the world, in the same way as Silver Birch. During one of William's visits to the Hannen Swaffer home circle, the beloved guide of Maurice Barbanell expressed through a parable of light and darkness, the role these masters have played in the spiritual evolution of humanity:

> Once upon a time, the world was very dark, and along came a man with a little torch and he held it aloft, and it cast gleams of light around him.
>
> And those who dwelt in the darkness were attracted to the light, and they drew near until the rays were shed upon them.
>
> Time went by, and the torch began to flicker. And then one who lived in the darkness of fear and foreboding, which he now knew was part of the darkness, and was killed by the light, grasped the torch and rekindled it with such vigour that the illumination was cast even wider.
>
> And so through all ages, someone has arisen to hold aloft the torch of life, each adding his own lustre to its luminosity, until gradually the light has been spreading in ever-widening circles. At no stage has the torch been allowed to be extinguished.
>
> That is all. Hold aloft the torch of the spirit, feed it with the lustre of your own souls so that each one of you helps to dissipate and dispel the gloom in which so many needlessly live.
>
> That is important. The rest of the things that many people worry about do not matter. When all is said and done, the physical body gets an excessive attention, the spiritual body and its requirements are very much neglected.[1]

Initiation into the power of spirit

In 1952, scarcely three years after our arrival in South Africa, my initiation into the power of spirit took a further step. My father became dangerously ill. One afternoon, while visiting a patient, he was attacked by two Rhodesian ridgebacks. The male sank his fangs into my father's left calf causing a very ugly wound. Characteristically, my father neglected himself. The wound turned septic, but drained well as it had not been sutured. Although oozing continued for some time, the wound began to show signs of improvement and father seemed well enough when he left for his consulting rooms on a Thursday morning some six weeks later.

We had been joined in Pretoria by a good friend of my mother's, Mary Brown, a spinster, whom Nancy had worked with in the textile factory in Leeds. She worked closely with my father, acting as his practice manager and personal secretary. She jealously protected him from the demands of patients, and as previously related, became affectionately known in the practice as the 'battle-axe.' After his morning list on that particular Thursday, she became concerned about William when she noticed how pale and absent he seemed to be. There was a light sweat on his forehead, although the day was cool. He had no appetite for the usual light snack she placed before him, and more ominously no interest in his customary cigarette. She noticed that his hands were not steady, his body seemed stiff and his movements were slow.

Determined as always not to yield to the weaknesses of the body, my father rallied sufficiently to be able to see a number of patients in the afternoon, before a patient, who knew him well, burst out of the consulting room after a few moments in great alarm calling on Mary and the nurse for help because she was certain the doctor was seriously ill. He was as pallid as the walls, sweating profusely, seemed distracted and had difficulty articulating. Every now and again he would shudder as if chilled to the marrow. He resisted the nurse's insistence that a doctor or ambulance be called and told Mary that he would drive home. The journey back to Waterkloof was a nightmare for Mary. She, who had never learnt to drive, had to steady the wheel to keep them on the road, because he kept involuntarily jerking it to one side or the other. As she put it later, "I nearly had a heart attack when he drove through a red traffic light." Fortunately, they were ahead of the rush hour traffic and no police officer witnessed their uncertain progress, otherwise William would have been arrested for drunken driving. When, by some miracle they arrived home safely, he remained slumped at the wheel unable to get out of the car. Afraid to leave him for a moment, Mary had to use all her strength to assist him. Finally she got him to the gate, opened it and with him hanging onto her managed to shuffle him halfway along the garden path to the front door, where he seized up completely, locked in the intensity of the rigors, which shook him from head to foot.

That terrifying frame is frozen in my memory, for it is what I saw as I looked out of the study window. My mother, who was waiting their arrival, ran out to help, and between them, she and Mary, managed to lift and drag my helpless father into the bedroom, onto the bed and into his pyjamas. Speech was difficult for him because his jaw muscles were tightly contracted, but he managed to tell mother not to call a doctor, because although he was very ill, he was going to be all right. He asked her to give him a dose of Nux vomica and then lapsed into unconsciousness. One cannot even imagine the agony of anxiety and uncertainty my mother felt at that moment. Her instinct was to get medical help as quickly as possible, but my father's last words rang in her ears. As she had proved with my illness, she had profound trust in William and Dr Letari. They had walked a long and difficult road together and she had witnessed many wonders, but now she could communicate with neither, and William lay before her critically ill, unconscious, bathed in cold sweat, and jerking spasmodically. Any delay could cost him his life. What should she do?

Keeping her presence of mind, despite the desperate fear that clutched her, she sent me off to find the Nux vomica and phoned the person closest to my father, someone she could rely on to give her good advice: Lassie Smit. He had just returned from work and lived only a few kilometres away. He was with us in less than fifteen minutes. While waiting for him to arrive she managed, with Mary's assistance, to get a few drops of Nux vomica between my father's clamped lips. Nux vomica is derived from a strychnine containing plant and hence homeopathically suitable for treating spastic and convulsive conditions.

I was caught up in my mother's fear and greatly relieved when I saw the burly figure of Uncle Lassie coming down the passage towards my parent's room. The door remained slightly ajar and standing in the passage, hardly breathing, I was able to hear their hushed voices. Lassie Smit was of pioneer stock, a practical man, familiar with afflictions that can befall one in the wilderness when injuries and wounds are sustained. He knew of father's recent bite and on seeing his condition realised that William was showing signs of tetanus and regardless of what "Bill" requested, they would have to get him to hospital immediately. No sooner had he said this to my mother than William went into his first convulsion. It was extremely violent and he uttered a terrible cry as the breath was driven from his lungs. Hearing this ghastly sound and the bed responding to the tetanic spasm that convulsed him, I felt as if the world I knew was disintegrating around me. The door was closed on me, and I hung suspended in the dreadful moment, straining with all my might to hear what was happening. I was not yet twelve, but even as I type these words, I can recall the intense fear I experienced that night. I was terrified that my father was dying. Our African housekeeper, helped at intervals by Mary, was caring for my five-year-old sister at the other end of the house, thus sparing her from the extreme stress of the situation.

After the attack, which had racked him severely, William lay comatose and inert. Both Mother and Lassie were shocked to the core by what they had seen and mother realised the urgency of her friend's advice. They were about to suit their actions to his words, and call for an ambulance, when mother saw William's lips move and then heard him speak. His voice was scarcely audible, and bending over him with her ear close to his face, she thought at first that it was William speaking, but then realised that it was Dr Letari's voice she could hear. He had entranced William. Scarcely above a whisper, the good Doctor confirmed that his mediator was gravely ill and that in the course of the following hours he would experience many convulsions, but that he, Dr Letari, would remain in the body taking the fits while the spirit doctors in attendance would give healing. He told her to have faith and not to fear for all would be well. He warned her that later he would be unable to speak to her, but to reassure her, in response to her questions, he would be able to squeeze her hand: twice for 'yes', and thrice for 'no'.

Mother told me years later that she prayed that evening as she had never prayed before. From 6.00 p.m. until 10.00 p.m. my father passed from one violent convulsion into another, eventually with scarcely a pause between them. Throughout, he was bathed in sweat and the seizures arched him violently from his head to his heels (opisthotonus, a characteristic of tetanus). She and Lassie Smit sat by him and prayed throughout this time, and always between the attacks there came the reassuring double squeeze from his hand in reply to my mother's anxious question as to whether all was still well. After enduring almost four hours of this terrible experience, Dr Letari once more spoke and told my mother that his mediator would suffer one more convulsion, which would be more severe than any of those previously experienced, and then the attacks would cease. And so it was! The storm had passed!

Dr Letari then instructed them to keep my father awake for at least the next two hours and only then to permit him to sleep. With that he withdrew from William's body and my father slowly regained consciousness. He was exhausted, as weak as a kitten, and unlike Dr Letari, only a few moments before, scarcely coherent. Throughout that dreadful time, I had kept my vigil at the door of my parent's room, often with my ear pressed to the woodwork. I had heard the convulsions and had suffered the added torment of filling in what I could not see or understand with my imagination. Now, I was at last called in. Father was sitting at the end of the bed, his eyes glazed and unresponsive to my presence. I was shocked by his appearance; he seemed so reduced and fragile. I watched as Lassie Smit placed a cigarette between his lips, and there it dangled with a life of its own, wavering with his every breath, threatening to fall. Finally, Lassie managed to light it and instinctively my father drew on it. He was an adept smoker and I anticipated that the smoke would come curling out of his nostrils in the lazy way it always did, but he was unable to inhale and simply blew it weakly back out of his mouth. Lassie then, holding both his hands, drew him to his feet and very slowly walked him up and down the length of the room; all the while the cigarette hung precariously from his slack lips. He was severely unbalanced, only able to shuffle, and if Lassie had not held tightly on to him, he would have fallen. So, by degrees, they coaxed him into slow, gentle movement, which proved the best way to keep him awake. Finally, after midnight, they permitted him to fall into a deep sleep from which he only awoke at daybreak.

The following day he could scarcely move. He felt as if he had been in a fight and run a marathon at the same time. His entire body ached. Every muscle felt bruised, beaten and strained. Thanks to Lassie's intervention during the convulsions, he had bitten his tongue only slightly. My mother plied him with many doses of Arnica during his recovery and the remedy proved invaluable. Three days later, this indomitable man was back at work.

Nothing ever happens without good reason. In this drastic event, we witness the playing out of a major event in the fortunes of our family; an event in perfect keeping with the entangled destinies of Dr Letari, his spirit helpers, my father, my mother, Mary, Lassie Smit, my sister and myself. For each of us, the happening had a particular reason and purpose for taking place. Although, in our eyes, a miracle transpired that Thursday evening, there is no such thing as a miracle, all was according to plan and according to natural law.

Having from birth both a biological and a spiritual father, I was comfortably familiar with the intimate interplay that exists between the realms of matter and spirit. I never doubted my spiritual, immortal state. I knew that whatever befalls me, and however difficult circumstances might be, every experience is an opportunity for growth and that life, with all its valleys and peaks, is a spiritual adventure and not the dire reality it often seems.

My severe illness gave me proof of the power of spirit and in particular of the wisdom and skill of Dr Letari as both spiritual physician and mentor.

My father's close encounter with death reinforced my trust and confidence in the spirit, revealed to me the extent to which our spirit guides and helpers play a role in our lives and the healing power that is at their disposal. While this event was not designed for me alone, it played a vital part in my future, equipping me for the work I would do, underpinning my trust, and giving me the right to express spiritual truths, not just from a stance of belief or faith, but from a vantage point of experience and knowledge. I also knew that life happens as it should; that regardless of our wishes certain experiences are unavoidable; that no matter what happens it has to happen; and that we are always surrounded by loving support and assistance. These become all the more potent when we participate creatively in what is unfolding, are willing to ask for spiritual and physical help, have complete trust and know, without the least doubt, that no matter the outcome it will be correct. We come seemingly naked and alone into this world, and at the end of our life on the physical plane, we leave, seemingly naked and alone, taking nothing from this mortal existence with us, other than the experience. All the comings and goings in life, even of those whom we come to love, all the calamities and the triumphs that mark our path, are the ineffable expression of a loving, cosmic intelligence that longs for our immersion in its inexpressible bliss. Let the experience of life be a spiritual one, filled with love and service to others.

Above all, these events enable me to write these words and tell this story, which can inform and uplift others, because the same laws are operative in all our lives. While the scientist would tell us that what I have written is only anecdotal and therefore cannot be accepted as proof of anything, that we have no laboratory evidence of meningitis or tetanus, no results of lumbar punctures or cultures; we do have two very clear clinical pictures of a severe order, that were cured by means other than those which would have had to be used by orthodox medicine. Neither can be dismissed as a spontaneous remission or placebo effect. While my experiences cannot be yours, I must share them with you, because they happened and I was witness to them.

Too strange to tell

In 1975, I was approached by a Johannesburg physician specialist, Dr S Levin, FRCP, who, being interested in spiritual and faith healing and unorthodox medicine, requested me to furnish him with details of my father's life and work. His intention was to present a lecture on psychic healing and to have an article on the subject published in the *South African*

Medical Journal. He had read *The Gift of Healing*, but needed more facts, especially about my father's life in South Africa. I was pleased to provide him with a synopsis. His request had come on cue, as do all cues. My father had been gone three years, but my mother, Nancy, was still with us, and only sixty-one. On receiving Dr Levin's letter, I was in a position to ask my mother to fill me in on details I did not know. This was something I would have omitted to do, because of my own circumstances, a youthful complacency that procrastination is affordable and my mother's apparent good health. In making my notes for Dr Levin, I captured facts that would have been irretrievably lost to the family.

His response to me on May 18, 1975 was:

> Your last missive was a splendid summary; just what I wanted, and presented in interesting manner and felicitous language.

> My thoughts on the matter are as follows: irrespective of orthodox medical training, the fact is that unorthodox healing, including faith and spiritual healing, fulfils a public need and there are sincere folk who provide this requirement. Among many in South Africa, your late father was pre-eminent. It seems to me, therefore, that a summary of his life and work should at least exist in the annals of our medical literature; perchance a future investigator may value its presence. For my part, the history of medicine, especially of unorthodox medicine, interests me, and in publishing, I will utilise much of your description verbatim. I shall do nothing definitive however, without showing you a final draft when the time comes. I may present a paper at the coming Congress in July, but will more likely submit one to our Journal (*SAMJ*) or to the *Bulletin of the Adler Museum of the History of Medicine*.[2]

As I expected, his submissions were rejected, providing further evidence of the closed state of the orthodox scientific mind, but his words sat in my unconscious and almost 40 years later added to my determination to write this summary of my father's life and work. Interestingly, I had a parallel experience in 2004 when I gave a weekend seminar in London on three important universal archetypes and their homeopathic counterparts: Zeus and Stannum; Ares and Ferrum; Aphrodite and Cuprum. During the course of the weekend, I was interviewed by a representative of the Society of Homeopaths, whose members made up the majority of my audience. The intention was to publish a background article on me in their journal. In the course of the interview, I was asked how, being a medical doctor, I had come to adopt homeopathy as my prime mode of therapy. The question could have received a simple answer: my conviction of homeopathy's superiority stemmed from witnessing my father's many successes achieved at a causative level and by natural means, compared with the hazardous chemical approach and the preoccupation with disease effects of orthodox medicine. However, by some twist, our conversation took a different turn, which surprised me as much as it must have surprised my interviewer. The story of my father spilled out and I do believe we both became equally engrossed in the remarkable events. Months later, I was back in England, giving an address at the University of Keele in Staffordshire on matching the profiles of certain serial killers to homeopathic archetypes, when the person, with whom I had shared so much, approached me apologetically and told me that my father's story had not been deemed appropriate for publication in the Society of Homeopaths' journal, *The Homeopath*. I was neither surprised nor disappointed: the story was even too unorthodox for the unorthodox. In retrospect, I was rather pleased because in such an article I would have pre-empted myself. To do the story justice, it was essential to first research certain aspects of my father's history, as I have now been able to do, and to tell it fully and accurately.

Ectoplasmic surgery

A year prior to the tetanus experience, Dr Letari gave me a remarkable demonstration of psychic healing with the use of an ectoplasmic, psychic rod. Rebecca, our Zulu housekeeper had returned from a holiday presenting with a huge abscess on her thigh. The skin was taut and shiny and looked to me as if it would burst at any moment. It was exquisitely tender and she shied away from any contact. Despite the ripeness of the abscess, the pus it contained was not superficial, but situated deep within the muscle due to a severe blow she had received. Rebecca had come to our home from a missionary school in Natal as a young girl of seventeen. She spoke excellent English and came to us under the recommendation of her headmistress, Miss Louie Farmer, who was an ardent disciple of Dr Letari and William. During my father's tour of South Africa in 1947, Miss Farmer had invited William to come to her school to give a spiritual address and healing demonstration to the senior girls. Rebecca had met both my father and Dr Letari on that occasion and had complete trust that they would help her abscess. My father told me that Dr Letari wished me to be present when he gave her treatment.

For the demonstration, we kept a side light on so that I would clearly see what took place. After making a number of passes over the inflamed area without touching the skin, Dr Letari started to concentrate the energy bringing it to a focal point over the apex of the swelling. The fingers of his left hand while moving rapidly against one another remained poised in this position while the fingers of his right hand, also in constant motion, moved up and down an invisible path as if creating a spiralling, vibrating rod of power which was directed through his left hand to the desired point. Not for even the briefest moment did he touch Rebecca. Within a few moments, I saw a burr hole begin to appear, steadily deepen and then slightly widen as the energy penetrated more deeply. It was as if he had concentrated the rays of the sun through a magnifying glass onto her skin. Rebecca showed no sign of pain or even discomfort. As the vent deepened, liquid pus began to spontaneously well up from the depths. Dr Letari applied pressure, as after a surgical incision, and persuaded the pus to escape more freely, which it did in copious amounts. Even then the young woman did not flinch or show any sign that he was hurting her. Mother acted as nurse, swabbing away the purulent matter, which eventually gave way to more wholesome blood and serum. Before leaving us, Dr Letari recommended Pyrogen twice daily and the use of Arnica and Calc-sulph in alternation until the condition was completely resolved. Rebecca made a perfect recovery.

As will be realised, what I have related could have been achieved with a surgeon's scalpel and an antibiotic, but in comparison, how elegant, painless and non-invasive was the spiritual technique, and when it was all over there was the certainty that the body had achieved the final result and in consequence had been strengthened, not weakened as when chemistry is resorted to.

However, this was not an exercise for the sake of comparison, but rather a demonstration of what can be achieved through the application of spiritual law. It formed part of my education.

References

1   Silver Birch. Parable of Light and Darkness. *Psychic News*; December 25, 1943.
2   Levin S. Letter to David Lilley; May 18, 1975.

19

MIRACLES AND MAGISTRATES

Tubercular osteomyelitis

In 1944, an eight year old boy, Desmond Jackson, living in Krugersdorp, a high veld town west of Johannesburg, developed a constant pain in his left upper arm, associated with tenderness and swelling. Treatment from the family doctor proved of no avail. The parents were referred to physicians and orthopaedic specialists. His condition was finally diagnosed as tubercular osteomyelitis; in which the TB organism, *Mycobacterium tuberculosis*, causes a destructive infection of the bone that attacks all components, including the bone marrow, and can spread to neighbouring joints. X-rays revealed that Desmond's left humerus was diseased from the elbow to the shoulder and his lungs were clear. He was admitted to hospital, and remained there for fourteen months while he received intensive anti-tubercular therapy. Finally, he was discharged, but suffered continuous bone pains. In spite of all the treatments he had received, the deep-seated inflammation was still active. He would sing hymns at night to try and forget his pain. The condition worsened, the symptoms increased and his general health deteriorated with loss of appetite and weight, night sweats and recurrent low-grade fevers.

When all medication failed to halt the tubercular process, the Jackson's were informed that the only way to save Desmond's life was to amputate his arm at the shoulder joint. The matter was urgent because the infection was threatening to involve the shoulder and elbow joints and was endangering his life. The desperate parents were unwilling to submit their son to such an extreme measure and looked round for other alternatives. It was at this time that Dr Letari and William made their tour of South Africa. When news of my father's ability as a healing medium and homeopath came to their ears and they heard of the difficult cases that he had successfully treated, the Jacksons contacted him and asked for Desmond to be placed on the absent healing list.

It was a huge responsibility to take on such a case and even more so at a distance; what hope could there be of success? Dr Letari was not dismayed. He knew that the spiritual co-ordinates governing the destinies of the prime players were favourable and would be played out to a successful conclusion.

Once contact was made and absent healing commenced, Desmond's condition improved, the pain was less. Within twelve months, the upper end of the humerus, which had been eaten through, began to protrude through the skin at the top of the arm. What looked to be deterioration of his condition proved in effect beneficial. A vent had been created through which purulent matter could escape, thus relieving the pressure within. Nonetheless, the arm was in a shocking state, constantly discharging pus through the vent; the surrounding skin and soft tissues were indurated, immobile, adherent to the deeper structures and an unhealthy bluish-purple colour. The appearance was that of some malignant process.

From the outset, absent healing was augmented by a series of homeopathic remedies, given strategically according to need. Among these were Tuberculinum, a nosode prepared from the tubercular organism *Mycobacterium tuberculosis*; Calc-phos (calcium phosphate), which is a specific tissue salt for the bones, and capable of playing an anti-inflammatory, anti-tubercular and reconstructive role; Phosphorus, which in its toxic action attacks and destroys osseous (bony) tissue and is particularly suited to the treatment of constitutions vulnerable to tuberculosis that disseminates to the bones; Silicea, a powerful anti-tubercular remedy acting upon the periosteum (sheath of the bones) and the connective tissue, while promoting immune response, resolving suppurative processes, absorbing scar tissue and rebuilding damaged tissues; and Symphytum officinale (comfrey or knitbone), the pre-eminent bone vulnerary (healing remedy). The open vents exuding pus were cleansed and irrigated with a diluted mixture of healing tinctures, containing Echinacea angustifolia (purple cone flower) a member of the daisy family, which is a potent antiseptic when used either topically (superficially) or systemically (internally); Calendula officianalis (marigold), another daisy, suited to the treatment of open wounds, such as lacerations and abrasions, but also burns and suppurating lesions; and Symphytum, which in addition to its specific effect on damaged bones has an anti-tubercular effect and the ability to assist in the healing of indolent, suppurative processes with ulceration.

After our arrival in South Africa, early in 1949, direct contact healing became possible. The boy's condition had been stabilised and his general health had improved, but much work was still required. The disease was still present, but at a lower grade. The continued confidence the parents placed in Dr Letari's advice and treatment at this point was surely the greatest miracle of all.

The upper end of the bone was protruding even further, at the other end the infection had encroached on the elbow joint, which had become swollen, inflamed and tender. With treatment, this was first contained and then improved, but damage to the joint had already been sustained and movement of the joint was limited.

Spiritual surgery would be of prime importance in achieving the result that Dr Letari and his team of helpers envisaged. This could only be achieved by degrees and had to run parallel with continued psychic and homeopathic treatment to promote Desmond's ability to fight the tubercular infection. His natural defence against TB was constitutionally impaired, but this innate susceptibility was exacerbated by the toxic inroads of the disease itself and also by the anti-tubercular drugs he had received, which having failed to overcome the infection, now contributed to the overall poisoning of the young boy's system. Sulphur, a remedy prepared from potentised flowers-of-sulphur, was one of the first remedies given. It has the power to eliminate the deleterious effects of previous drug therapy, and being the major substance related to planetary volcanism, it archetypally matched the entire nature of the destructive process, which significantly mirrored volcanic activity as it vented thick pus, like molten magma, onto a swollen, scarified surface.

As, over a period of years, the tubercular activity slowed and finally came to a halt, Dr Letari was able to proceed with the necessary surgical and reconstructive work. Early in treatment, it had been essential to ectoplasmically seal-off the ends of the diseased humerus to prevent further spread upwards or downwards and thus preserve the integrity of the shoulder joint and limit the damage to the elbow. Fortunately, in Desmond's case, the synovium (lining) of the shoulder joint, which is extremely vulnerable because of its rich blood supply, had not been attacked. The necrosis of the bone, which had created the pathological fracture through the upper part of the humerus, permitting it to protrude through the tissues of Desmond's arm had also involved the rim of bone remaining beneath the head of the humerus. This posed the greatest threat and had to be sealed-off with ectoplasm.

Although the shaft of the humerus, tunnelled and honeycombed by marrow destruction and necrosis, was still tethered at the base, the body, aided by the laying-on-of-hands and the action of remedies, started to abort the diseased bone further onto the surface. The open sinus that had formed at the top of the upper arm made this process easier. It looked as if a long, narrow ship, which had sunk prow-first, was now reversing its passage, thrusting its stern into the air. The freeing of the bone to permit this extrusion necessitated the ectoplasmic severance of the muscle fibres still attached. As it raised up through the parted, damaged tissues, this large sequestrum, made up of almost the entire shaft of the humerus, swung outward, away from the line of the arm at an acute angle. Only the distal (lower) part still remained submerged in the surrounding tissues, attached by muscle tendons, fibrous tissue and ligaments at its base. As the infection subsided, the discharge from the open areas had become less purulent and more serous (like-serum), and the parted tissues beneath the externalised bone showed granulation and were slowly closing.

A far more remarkable process accompanied the freeing of the diseased bone: the recreation of the humerus out of ectoplasm. This new bone was continuous with the preserved and healed proximal (upper) and distal

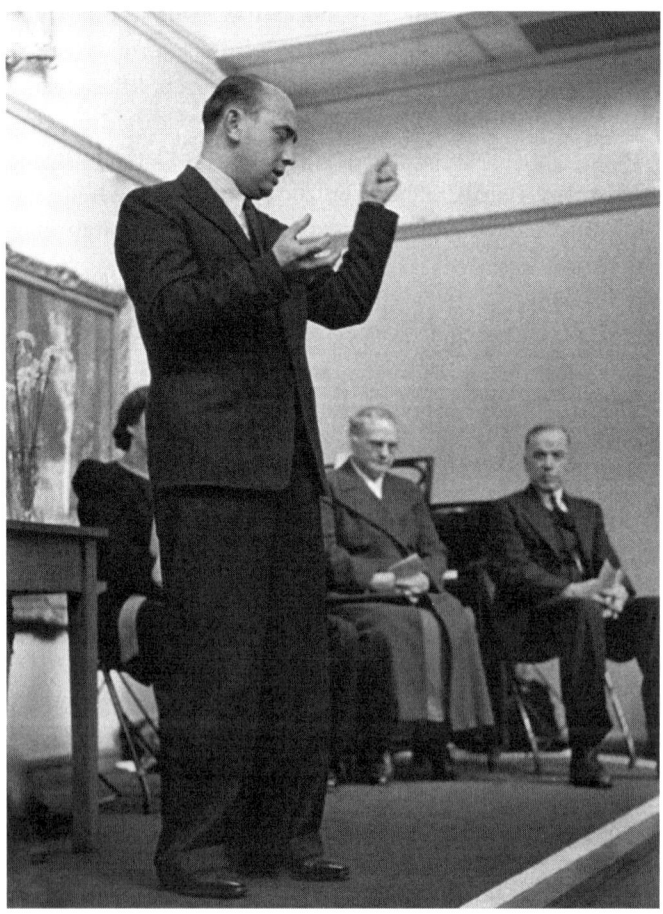

Figure 19.1 Dr Letari lecturing before a healing demonstration. Johannesburg 1953

sections of the original bone. All the muscular attachments necessary for normal mobility had to be restored. When the healing had reached this advanced stage and only a few further treatments were needed, Dr Letari and William were given the opportunity of concluding the procedure during a public demonstration.

After our arrival in South Africa, Dr Letari had continued giving trance addresses to various Spiritualist churches and groups, as he had in the UK. His message was definite: he insisted that psychic gifts should serve altruistic goals, not self-pride, and those mediums, who entered into the field of spiritual healing, should acquire knowledge of the body in health and disease in order to practise in a responsible manner. He also encouraged his audiences to follow the homeopathic mode of healing. He discouraged the pursuit of psychic gifts and psychic phenomenology and urged rather the quest for spiritual development, which in turn would open the doors to psychic attainment, appropriately, at the right time and in the right manner.

Public demonstration, Johannesburg, 1953

In early August 1953, William was invited by David Lepato to give a trance address and demonstration of spiritual healing in Johannesburg. It was expected that there would be a great response from the public, and it was decided to hold the event in the Selbourne Hall of the Johannesburg City Hall, which could hold almost 2000 people. On the night, the hall was packed beyond capacity with people standing at the back of the hall and in the aisles. I had just turned 13, and sat next to my mother in the front row, filled with pride at being my father's son. My father sat alone on one side of the stage and on the other, at a table, sat David Lepato, Lassie Smit and my father's nursing sister, Mrs Hopkins. In the middle of the stage on three chairs, well spaced out, sat the three patients who would receive healing. Desmond Jackson was one of the patients, his arm concealed beneath a swathe of dressing.

David Lepato acted as chairman and after welcoming the audience, gave them a brief history of Dr Letari's and William's relationship and of their healing mission in the UK and South Africa. This was followed by an eloquent prayer and invocation delivered by Lassie Smit. During this time, Dr Letari entranced my father. While directing only half an ear to what was being said, my attention was concentrated on him, and I knew the moment Dr Letari was in control by the changed expression on my father's features; a change I had become so familiar with. When Lassie Smit brought his invocation to a close, Dr Letari rose to his feet, and, after a short prayer in Sanskrit, addressed the audience in his gently accented English.

I will leave Lassie Smit to give his account of that eventful evening, an evening that created a great stir. He wrote an article for *Two Worlds*, which was given front page prominence in the August 29, 1953 edition. The article included a photo of the arm taken two days prior to the operation. This clearly depicted how the disease had ravaged the boy's arm.

> ***Spirit Doctor Removes Diseased Bone – 2000 See It Replaced With One 'Made From Ectoplasm.'***
>
> At a memorable meeting held in the Selbourne Hall, Johannesburg, Dr Letari and his instrument, Mr WH Lilley, demonstrated amongst other cases of remarkable healing, a psychic operation which is unparalleled in the annals of medical science.
>
> Having been interested in Spiritualism for many years, I am aware of the powers of the spirit and the wonders that can be performed by those loved ones who return to us from the other side of life.
>
> On this memorable occasion I witnessed a 'miracle' of healing. It involved the painless and bloodless removal of a diseased humerus from the arm of Desmond Jackson, a 12-year-old boy who was suffering from tubercular osteomyelitis and who could not have been expected by medical science to live long.
>
> I was privileged to assist Mr David Lepato, president of the Society for Psychic Advancement, who sponsored the meeting and was its chairman. I was, therefore, never more than a few feet away from Dr Letari during the entire 'operation.'
>
> An address of spiritual healing was followed by some practical demonstrations. Dr Letari gave a brief history of each case before giving psychic healing.
>
> When he came to Desmond Jackson, he furnished a complete case history as well as details of the treatment he was about to give. He told the audience that he would remove the diseased humerus from the arm and replace it with a new bone fashioned out of ectoplasm.
>
> Dr Letari explained that he would first give treatment in order to produce a state of anaesthesia of the arm, so that the boy would feel no pain. To stop the bleeding, he would ligature the arteries with ectoplasm and divide the muscles of the arm in order to permit the bone to be removed.
>
> The doctor then requested all present to be still and to project their thoughts and goodwill and love toward the patient.

Following this detailed description, the bandages were removed from the boy's arm, revealing an arm that seemed little more than putrid matter. I could clearly see the bone protruding through the skin.[i]

According to Dr Letari it had been brought into this position by previous treatment and to prepare the patient for this particular operation. From my vantage point on the platform, I was able to watch the reaction of the audience, which was one of amazement. Many turned away from the distressing sight.

After the removal of the bandages, the arm was held by the attendant nurse, Mrs Hopkins. The doctor began the healing process required to release and remove the bone, using only his hands, with deft movements carried out so quickly that it was impossible for the onlooker to follow them all.

When this was completed to the doctor's satisfaction, he took the bone and slowly and carefully withdrew it from the arm – a sight never to be forgotten. It was impossible to express one's feelings during those moments. I did not know whether to laugh, to cry or to pray, such was my amazement.

I could see in the audience that some had fainted, others were overcome and had to leave the hall, while most wept. To give vent to their feelings of gratitude, mixed with wonder, they joined in singing, *'Praise God from whom all blessings flow.'*

Dr Letari held up the bone for the audience to see. Taking the boy's arm, which could be seen by all in the audience, he revealed an incision approximately eight inches long (the upper four inches had already closed from earlier healing) and about two inches deep, through which the bone had been removed – in other words I as well as others, could clearly see 'inside' the boy's arm!

There was no bleeding and no pain had been experienced by the patient who, during the entire procedure, calmly watched as an interested onlooker.

We had witnessed a 'miracle,' but an even greater one was to follow when Dr Letari told us that he would now continue with the healing needed for the rebuilding of the new bone. The hands of the beloved doctor moved over the incision, again with remarkable speed, the fingers working so quickly that at times they were a blur. After a few minutes his work was complete.

He asked the boy to stand up, and to lift his arm above his head, a movement impossible unless a bone had been replaced in that arm. From my position,

---

[i] This picture is somewhat misleading, because the arm was in fact no longer putrid. However, the severe purple discolouration of the arm, the irregular swellings and hollows in the chronically inflamed and scarred flesh, together with the serous fluid that oozed from the open area around the protruding bone, was shocking to see and gave an impression of putridity.

> only a few feet away, I could see that the wound had been neatly closed. There was no bleeding and no pain.
>
> On the table before me lay the bone as proof to myself and nearly 2000 people that what we had seen was not a dream, but a reality.[1]

The images of that evening remain with me. The emotions in the hall were electric. I was caught up in the intensity of it all, and when the audience spontaneously broke into a song of praise, my throat was choked and the tears flowed down my cheeks. When David Lepato brought the proceedings to an end, there was a hubbub. Groups of people gathered together unable to contain their excitement. Everyone seemed to be talking at once. It took an age for us to extricate ourselves from the numerous people who wished to give their thanks to my father and to tell him how the evening had affected them.

William supplied some further details to the *Two Worlds*, in a short, supplementary article, which was included on the front page of the same issue alongside Lassie Smit's narrative. In it he informed readers that four treatments, given over a period of three months, had prepared Desmond's arm for the operation that had been performed at the Selbourne Hall.

> Naturally this 'operation' became the talk of Johannesburg attracting representatives of the press who communicated with me for permission to interview the boy and his parents and to obtain the opinions of orthopaedic specialists in Johannesburg.
>
> Their immediate opinion was that such an operation was impossible, and that a bone could not be removed in such a manner from the arm. The press accompanied by medical specialists took the boy to hospital where he was X-rayed extensively. The radiologists report was that a perfectly normal, regular, healthy humerus was evident. This is certainly the answer to our critics who often say that the cures by way of spiritual healing are never permanent.[2]

The cure of Desmond Jackson remained permanent. His health was fully restored and although he would always bear the scars of the disease that had nearly proved fatal, and would never be able to fully straighten his arm, he went on to enjoy a normal, active life, swimming and even boxing. When my father died twenty years later, Desmond wrote to my mother to reaffirm his gratitude for all that William had done for him, and to let her know that he was still in good health. The bone became a relic of that momentous occasion, an occasion that would never be repeated. I still have it in my possession, but having given this account possibly the time has come to dispose of it.

Desmond Jackson's psychic operation was a turning point in my father's career. His name was established throughout South Africa and Dr Letari retired into the background. The guide's long-term objective had always been that his mediator should be the healer, the teacher and the homeopath, and that time had now come. The psychic aspects of diagnosis and healing would always be intrinsic to William's work, but apart from a few exceptions, public demonstrations and trance addresses fell away. William himself mounted the platform and lectured on the causes of disease and their cure through homeopathy and naturopathy (correct living). Treatments under trance, except for members of the family, became very much the exception, and then only in the practice setting. To the public he became first and foremost a homeopath and chiropractor.

The 'knock upon the door'

In 1953, the year of the Selbourne Hall demonstration, father had his first clash with the monopolistic power of the medical orthodoxy. As in England, his practice in South Africa had become well known. Many of his successes were achieved with patients who had previously attended practitioners and specialists either in Johannesburg or Pretoria. Inevitably, his popularity and success finally stirred the ire of his medical peers and he was reported to the Medical and Dental Council. The wheels of the bureaucracy turned, and one day there came 'the knock upon the door.'

William was summoned to appear in the Pretoria Magistrates' Court on five charges of 'performing acts specially pertaining to the calling of a medical doctor, in that he did examine, diagnose and treat for gain.' He was singled out, from all the professional and lay homeopaths practising in South Africa.

In the hope of providing evidence for the prosecution, prior to the trial a police stooge, Mr HA Truter was sent to consult William, posing as a new patient. My father soon 'smelled a fish' and anticipated that there would be some sort of official follow-up to the deception.

The proceedings of this court case had quite the reverse effect to that which the complainants and medical authorities had wished to achieve. The proceedings were avidly covered by all the Pretoria and Johannesburg papers and in consequence provided a platform for giving anecdotal evidence of homeopathy's efficacy. The courtroom was packed with supportive patients, and those brought forward by the prosecution as witnesses to prove the charges against the defendant were eager to testify how they had been helped.

The *Pretoria News* gave the case front-page status:

> **Accused Man Cured Her Daughter, Mother Tells Court.**
>
> A Pretoria woman described in the Pretoria Magistrates' Court yesterday how her young daughter had been cured of a form of epilepsy after receiving powders from a man on trial in the Court. She was giving evidence in the case of WH Lilley, of Letari House, 276 Proes Street, who was charged with illegally practicing as a medical practitioner. Mrs M Bands told the Court that her daughter had suffered from 'Petit Mal,' a minor form of epilepsy. Doctors could do nothing more for her.
>
> She wrote to Lilley and received a questionnaire. She completed it and posted it to him. She paid 16 shillings for the powders, which helped her daughter 'tremendously,' the witness said. She used the powders for little over a year. When each lot of 28 powders was finished, she reported progress to Lilley.
>
> She had been at her 'wits end' about her daughter as the child was affected mentally by the illness. She was now completely cured.
>
> Another witness, Mr EN Welch said that he had suffered an illness while he was in the army for which he was pensioned off. Lilley treated him. To say that Lilley had done him a 'great deal of good' would be a gross understatement. He was now completely cured.[3]

The next day the *Pretoria News* carried the following news story:

> **Court Told Of Cure Of 'Dying' Daughter.**
>
> A French lady, Mrs Monique Perkins related to the Court how her daughter had developed epilepsy in 1949. She was then three-years-old. She attended several doctors, but her condition remained unchanged. Although the drugs prescribed had reduced the fits, they also dulled her emotional and intellectual state. In 1952, she had become very ill and despite medication developed multiple grand-mal attacks, one attack leading into another.
>
> "She was in a dying condition, completely paralysed on one side and could not talk."[4]
>
> Medical opinion did not give her long to live.
>
> Questioned by Counsel for the defence, the witness said she had previously taken her daughter to the best specialists in Pretoria and Johannesburg.
>
> "Lilley came to our house. He sat on the bed and watched the child. He said that he had hope that he would be able to help us. He did nothing, but just sat on the bed and looked."

She went on to relate that homeopathic powders had been prescribed and her daughter's condition had progressively improved, the paralysis and inability to speak had cleared and she was now free of fits.

I knew this girl and watched her mature into a young woman. In her twenties, she still remained free of epilepsy and of any after effects from her illness. It would be difficult for the scientific atheists to pass off her cure as either placebo effect or as a spontaneous remission.

On February 18, the Magistrate, Mr PJ van den Berg, who had been deeply moved by these heartfelt testimonies, passed verdict saying,

> I have reliable people before me who testified that through your skill you were able to cure children classed as hopeless by the medical profession. It hurts me to find you guilty. Although the defendant has contravened the law, it is clear that Lilley's first aim was to alleviate suffering.

A crowded court heard the magistrate caution and discharge Lilley after taking as one all five counts against him.[5]

Needless to say, the unprecedented publicity achieved through this trial, underlined by the sympathetic attitude of the magistrate, caused the practice to bulge at the seams. There must have been gnashing of teeth among those who had sought to close him down. Undeterred, William continued to practise and those who wished him ill bided their time.

William defends himself

Two years passed without incident, and then, in 1956, my final year at school, he was again summoned to appear in court, charged once again on five counts of contravening the Medical, Dental and Pharmacy Act. During the first court case, defence Counsel had represented him without success, now William resolved to defend himself.

The full Court proceedings lie on the desk before me. The front cover reads: Pretoria Magistrates' Court, September 24, 1956. *Regina versus Lilley*. Magistrate: Colonel GA Watermeyer, on the Bench. Public Prosecutor: Mr HJH Theunissen.

Studying the proceedings, it is touching to read how patient after patient, both those produced as witnesses for the Crown and those representing my father, attempted through their evidence to shield and protect William. Since it was evident that the treatment he extended to his patients did not fall within the definition of an act pertaining to the special calling of a medical doctor, the case for the prosecution hinged on two points: did he make a diagnosis and did he treat patients for gain? During the hearing, all the patients adamantly asserted that medical doctors had made their diagnoses and that apart from the medicines they had been prescribed, all payments made to my father were donations, given out of gratitude.

My father had designed a questionnaire, which new patients to his practice had to complete on making application for their first appointment. It prompted the patient to give extensive details regarding their personal and medical history, their circumstances, their emotional life, their dreams, their symptoms and bodily functions, and their preferences and aversions regarding food, temperature, weather, etc. It drew forth all the characteristics and nuances, which are important to a homeopath and need to be teased out of every case to reveal the uniqueness of the patient, regardless of their medical diagnosis. All the patients brought forward as witnesses at the trial had come to my father armed with their diagnoses, X-rays, laboratory tests, etc. It had not been necessary for him to give an orthodox medical diagnosis. Therefore, the question whether the use of the questionnaire could be construed as making a diagnosis in terms of the law would prove critical to the outcome of the case.

On the day of the trial, as in 1953, the Pretoria Magistrates' Court was crammed to capacity with members of the press, interested public and a large number of patients. I accompanied my mother. Considering what faced him, I was impressed to see how relaxed and composed my father was before the trial. I can still see him now calmly checking through his prepared notes before the proceedings. How far he had come, this son of a Yorkshire miner. This time it was all up to him; his career was at stake, Dr Letari was not going to entrance him, he had no legal training and no lawyer to consult; yet he showed no signs of apprehension. The same could not be said for either my mother or myself.

Amongst the Crown witnesses there was a young boy who had been treated by my father for eczema and the effects of polio, a patient with rheumatoid arthritis, a case of haemorrhoids and another of epilepsy consequent to head injury. All gave testimony that they had consulted the defendant because they were dissatisfied with the results of the conventional treatment they had received.

The mother spoke on behalf of the young boy. He had responded well to treatment. His eczema, which had proved resistant to drugs and ointments, cleared after a couple of months, and there had been a remarkable improvement in the strength and muscular girth of his leg.

> The prosecutor asked: "Since the treatment has your boy progressed?"
> The mother answered: "Well, he can walk now and he can run, and where his leg was three quarters of an inch thinner than the other leg it has caught up and is only a quarter of an inch thinner."[6]

The mother also testified that she had consulted the accused on her own behalf for contact dermatitis of the hands and face. She had received homeopathic powders and her skin cleared up completely.[7] Under questioning, she averred that she had provided Lilley with the diagnoses as given to her by the specialists she had seen, and that although she had paid for her powder prescriptions, all other payments had been in the form of donations to express her appreciation.

The second Crown witness suffered from rheumatoid arthritis and had been given an appointment with my father after she had completed the questionnaire. Before seeing him personally, she had been sent homeopathic powders through the post.

> She was asked, "Why did you approach Lilley?"
> She answered, "Because the doctors could not help me."

She told the magistrate that she had seen several doctors, all of whom had confirmed her diagnosis. She was asked what her condition was like when she first saw the accused.

> "I could not walk; my husband had to carry me."
> The Magistrate asked, "Did you obtain relief from his treatment?"
> She replied: "Well, I have no pain. It is only that I cannot walk properly; and that is coming right. The stiffness is now leaving my limbs."[8]

While under medical treatment her weight had been ninety pounds (41Kg); it was now 150 pounds (68Kg).

Her husband was also called to the stand. He told the court that his haemorrhoids had cleared up wonderfully after being treated by the accused; he had filled in a questionnaire prior to treatment being given; he had received numbered powders for which he had paid; and he had given a monthly donation of £5 to the Sanctuary, as the practice was still called before it moved to City Centre.

The fourth case for the Crown was that of a six-year-old boy who had developed epilepsy after a head injury. The mother had not been happy with the treatment that was given by a paediatric neurologist who had prescribed drugs and warned her that he thought the child would require special schooling. Despite treatment, the young boy had continued to experience frequent epileptic seizures and his memory and concentration were clearly impaired. Twelve months before the trial, the mother wrote to my father. The letter, which was produced in court, stated "I am writing to you in desperation."[9]

During cross-examination, William asked her:
"Twelve months ago you wrote in desperation. Are you in desperation now?"
"No, my child is almost cured."
The Magistrate then asked:
"When you say your child is almost cured, what do you mean? Does he still get these attacks of epilepsy?"
"Very, very seldom, Your Worship."

This was a marked improvement. The child was completely off all anti-epileptic drugs. The reduction in fits had been attended by an improvement in the boy's cognitive ability and his emotional state. During the year following the trial, continued improvement resulted in no further attacks.

This case closed the evidence for the prosecution because the last Crown witness had been withdrawn. If homeopathy itself had been on trial, the anecdotal evidence produced by the prosecution would have persuaded any jury of its superior efficacy in curing the incurable; but it was William who was on trial, not homeopathy, and healing the sick was no mitigation for the offence he was charged with: breaching the monopoly of the orthodoxy.

William then opened his case for the defence. Reading through the proceedings it is remarkable to note how a man unschooled in legal procedure and protocol, under personal attack and without a lawyer to consult, managed to marshal his forces, question his witnesses and present his argument with such composure, determination and clarity.

First to appear was Eileen Jackson, the mother of Desmond. She was followed by Desmond himself, now 20 years old, and he in turn by three other witnesses, each eager to speak in defence of the man who had helped them.

It was all to no avail; that is as far as the judgement was concerned, but in terms of gaining the sympathy of the court, enthralling the audience and giving the press a story, the day was far from lost.

In passing judgement, the magistrate, Colonel BA Watermeyer, after mentioning that the case had excited a fair amount of interest,[10] carefully explained the perspective of the Court. Drawing on legal precedents, he said the Court had to consider the charge of 16 shillings for the powders and the voluntary donations of grateful patients as evidence of practising for gain. This left the Court with the more difficult issue of deciding whether the accused did in fact make a diagnosis. Every patient questioned had filled in a questionnaire for the accused before receiving treatment – a very exhaustive enquiry into the patient's mental condition, eyes, ears, throat, chest, heart, stomach and so on, covering the whole body . . . in other words the patient was required to disclose the whole of his case history to the accused. Did this amount to a diagnosis? The magistrate felt that it did – and elucidated on his conclusion further:

> Although (the accused) accepted the doctor's diagnoses . . . he wanted the information in the questionnaire because it was personal to the individual, and he required the information to individualise the case. In other words, he said to the Court, he required this information in order to determine what treatment to give the patient. He argues that a dozen people can be suffering from the same disease and each require a different treatment, and in order to apply that treatment he has to elicit this information. What does this amount to? It amounts to this: he accepts the doctor's diagnosis, and from the questionnaire he does in fact make a supplementary diagnosis.[11]

This judgement beggared the fact that the supplementary diagnosis went far beyond the conventional and stood well outside the definition of an act pertaining to the special calling of a medical doctor.

In conclusion, Colonel Watermeyer said:

> I accept that patients consulted the accused as a last resort, after the ordinary medical measures had failed, and according to the evidence they benefited from his treatment . . . but unfortunately that is not the test here. The only point I have to decide is whether there was a diagnosis. I am quite prepared to accept that he is a man of honour and good standing.
>
> It is with some reluctance that I find the accused guilty. Speaking as a man, I will say the accused has the Court's sympathy in this matter. . . . I don't want to say any more now, and I do not desire to impose a penalty of any magnitude.
>
> The accused is fined a very nominal penalty of £1 on each of these counts.

Hardly had he concluded with these words, when William's patients quickly made a collection and placed the required amount before the surprised magistrate – an expression of their loyalty and support. Despite the verdict, there was a lot of jubilance in the courtroom at the final outcome. For those who had brought about the trial and sought to harm William's work, it was another Pyrrhic victory since the publicity it achieved benefited both his practice and homeopathy in general.

Needless to say, William pressed on intrepidly, without so much as a pause, daring the authorities to do their worst. Those implicated in the attacks must have taken stock of the situation and realised that their efforts had resulted in the public becoming more aware of the therapeutic power of homeopathy and of its ability to help when orthodox medicine fails. They must have concluded that it would serve them better to let the matter rest.

The case that set a precedent

Seven years elapsed before the next knock upon the door.' In all probability there would have been no further move against William if it had not been for an act of betrayal by a member of his staff. After a number of years in his employ, this person gave him good reason to dismiss her and she in retaliation, knowing of the past court cases, reported him to Medical and Dental Council. The Act had not been changed since 1956, therefore in terms of the law, he was still practising medicine illegally. Council had no alternative but to press charges.

This event, fraught with stress, particularly when vocation is at stake, is an example of how important free will is and of how no matter the immediacy of communication between guide and medium, the exercise of option, choice and decision-making must lie with the incarnated soul. My father's smoking habit, which was so detrimental to his health, is a simple instance of this self-determination in operation. It would be valid from the observer's viewpoint to ask why Dr Letari did not warn his mediator of the vindictive nature of this woman and advise him against employing her, but that would have been contrary to cosmic design. There are occasions when such a warning falls within the design; then it will certainly be given, either directly or intuitively. In this instance the decision lay squarely with my father, the result was part of his destiny and intrinsic to the universal plan. It was to prove pivotal to the future of homeopathy in South Africa.

On the 27 of March, 1963, William once again appeared in the Pretoria Magistrates' Court charged with contravening section 34(a)(1) of Act No 13 of 1928, as amended, in that he did wrongfully and unlawfully practise as a medical practitioner or perform acts specifically pertaining to the calling of a medical practitioner, for gain. An alternative charge served against him was that he did unlawfully hold himself out to be a medical practitioner. Advocate Melamet represented him.

The prosecution called upon the employee and her husband to give evidence and in addition three patients from my father's practice, two middle-aged spinsters and a police officer who had genuinely approached William for treatment of his spine. Two more ardently committed homeopathic patients than the two spinsters could not have been chosen. Years later, I inherited them from my father, and they both remained patients in my practice until I retired from full-time practice in 2007.

Once again I attended the proceedings. I was twenty-two and had qualified in medicine the previous year. At the time, I was serving my internship at the Pretoria Academic Hospital.

Miracles and magistrates 497

The trial clearly exposed the malicious intent of the wife and husband team, and in addition once again confirmed the benefit experienced by patients attending William's practice. In passing judgement, the Magistrate SR Nagel stated that he agreed with the defence that no evidence whatsoever had been led to substantiate the qualifying charge of practising for gain, since all monies received by the accused were in payment for medication given; that the acts performed by the accused did not specifically pertain to the calling of a medical practitioner; and that the accused had at no time represented himself as such. William was found not guilty on all charges.[12]

This was a huge step forward, not only for my father, but also for South African homeopathy. A precedent had been set, which protected him and his fellow professional homeopaths from further prosecution and provided a platform for future, successful lobbying for the recognition and rights of the profession. By association, this extended to other non-medical healing professions: chiropractic, osteopathy, acupuncture, Chinese traditional medicine, Ayurvedic medicine and others. William's court case set the stage for what has become a unique situation in South Africa: the establishment of a statutory body, the Allied Health Professions Council of South Africa (AHPCSA), which governs matters relating to all the registered non-medical

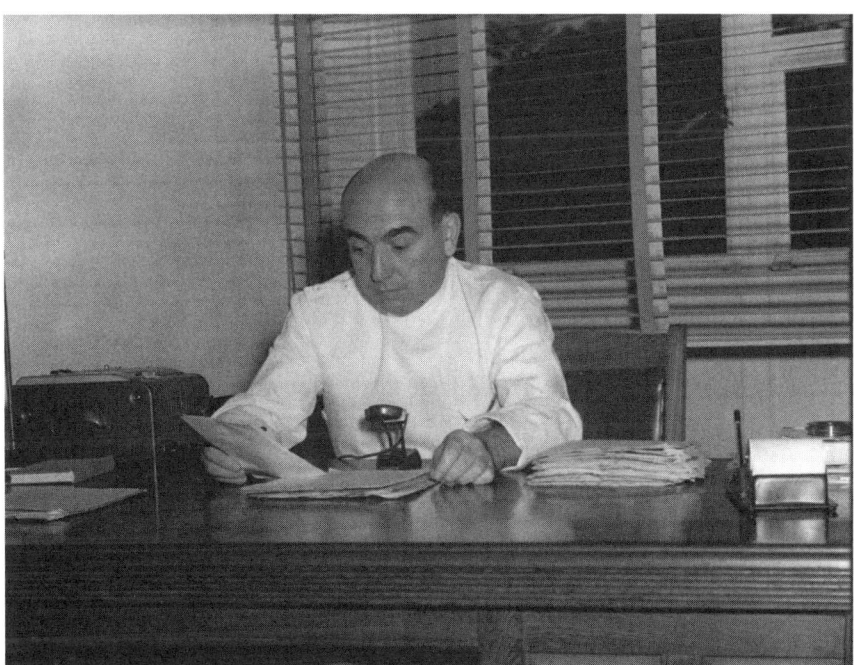

Figure 19.2 William dictating letters to patients on a wire recorder. 1954

health professions. Professional boards have been created which represent the various professions and interact on their behalf with the AHPCSA. Most importantly, standards of education have been established for all the professions under the Council's jurisdiction. In the case of homeopathy and chiropractic, two universities provide five-year courses of instruction for students wishing to enter the two professions.

For the rest of his lifetime, my father remained the leading figure in the fight for homeopathy's recognition in South Africa. He was not only involved as a homeopathic practitioner, but also as the director of a homeopathic manufacturing and distributing company, Homœopathic Biochemic Laboratories (HBL). In this capacity, he became the South African agent for Madaus homeopathic pharmaceuticals, Cologne, Germany and for New Era biochemic preparations, London, and he also imported remedies from Jso-Regensburg, Germany. His eclectic interest in homeopathy extended to homeopharmaceutics, and as chronicled earlier, following the example of Jenichen, he developed a 'super-succussion' method of potentisation, permitting him to achieve the very high potencies, which he used in his practice. In the 1960s, he was central to representations made to the Medicines Control Council for the registration of homeopathic remedies in South Africa. As in Britain, through his lecturing, clinical successes and political prominence, he was largely responsible for establishing a widespread homeopathic public in South Africa. This influence remains in evidence today and is his most enduring legacy.

A blessed upbringing

I have often been asked what it was like growing up in such an unusual family. Looking back over the years, I can answer that I always had a sense of being blessed. Blessed in having two loving fathers, one on the spirit plane, who introduced me to the wonders and mysteries of the creation and my own spiritual nature, and blessed in having a father on the material plane who through his manner of living exemplified the pursuit of excellence and devotion to healing. To my sister and I, the truth of survival after death and the spiritual purpose of life was part of our daily consciousness. During my early years, I felt our family was different and very special and finding others of my age either indifferent to the existence of higher dimensions or entertaining what appeared to me as strange and implausible beliefs magnified this. With maturity, I understood that our blessings were only different from those of others in being tangible and constantly manifest. Dr Letari was ever present in our lives and always involved, as guide and confidant in all major happenings in the Lilley household. It was he, not my father, who would advise us on homeopathic medication. When necessary, he would also administer direct spiritual healing. His regular visits to us through the mediation of my father were always special occasions and left us comforted and uplifted. He was, and still remains, a deeply loved member of our family.

Another question often asked is whether I inherited my father's psychic gifts of clairaudience and psychometry. The answer is negative. It was never intended that I should develop in that direction. My father's transition from healing medium to homeopath explains why this was so. The ultimate focus and goal of the Ramesôye and Dr Letari's mission was the furtherance of homeopathy as the perfect method to bring about the healing of the soul, mind and body. To this end, my father's own gift of healing, distinct from that which he channelled, was increasingly expressed over the years through the practice of homeopathy and through manipulative techniques that enabled him to influence the energy centres of the body (chakras) by spinal adjustment and articulation. Whereas before our emigration from England, Dr Letari had delivered all the public addresses, after 1956, the reverse was true. William had become the lecturer and the healer. While through William's mediumship, Dr Letari had been able to give tangible evidence of spiritual healing, this was only a springboard for a far more important message: *the spiritual healing power of homeopathy* – a power that is available to all physicians, regardless of overt psychic gifts, and which can be harnessed through education and experience.

After my recovery from meningitis, I was determined to become a doctor and a homeopath. There was never doubt that I would first study conventional medicine. Dr Letari was adamant that I must receive a medical education, be able to speak with the authority of a qualified medical doctor and never be vulnerable to the attacks my father had been subjected to. He had imparted the same education to his mediator, and he had unsettled psychic healers by urging them to at least acquire knowledge of the basic medical sciences. He told me that he would not commence my homeopathic education until I had achieved my medical degree.

I was fortunate that in moving to South Africa, I was able to benefit from the excellent education I had received at Claremont. After only a term at my first school, I was promoted from standard one to standard three, which resulted in my being two years younger than my peers, entering matric at fifteen, and final year medicine at twenty-one. This got me off to an early start in my postgraduate studies in homeopathy and osteopathy, so that by the time I was twenty-six I had acquired the basic skills I would require. My schooling was received as a day pupil at the Pretoria Christian Brothers

College (CBC), which proved an excellent introduction to the idiosyncrasies of the Catholic faith. The Irish Brothers were a curious mix of harsh disciplinarians, who ruled the classroom with leather strap and fear, and noble souls who were examples of devotion and kindness. On completing my schooling, I was faced with the decision of whether to attend medical school at the Witwatersrand University ('Wits') in Johannesburg, where instruction was through the medium of English, or to apply for entrance to Pretoria University ('Tuks'), which was an Afrikaans institution. I had been introduced to Afrikaans at a relatively late age and progressed so poorly in the language that I failed the final school examination. Intending to join my father in practice in Pretoria where Afrikaans was the dominant language, I decided that an Afrikaans based medical education would serve me well in my future practice. Though I struggled at first, I never regretted my decision. The homeopathic consultation is very searching and for those of my patients who lacked fluency in English, it was a boon to able to express their deepest feelings in the comfort and confidence of their home language.

On finishing my hospital internship at the end of 1963, I spent six months sitting-in on my father's consultations; a wonderful introduction to the art of homeopathic case taking, case analysis and case management. As a newly qualified medical doctor still plump with crammed knowledge and fresh, hospital experience, I was deeply impressed by my father's medical acumen and clinical skills. I sat by his side and avidly absorbed as much as I could of his manner and method. This period of observation and osmosis was of incalculable value and stood me in good stead for when I would no longer have him to turn to.

It was my father's wish that I should attend the Royal London Homœopathic Hospital (RLHH) and attain Membership of the British Faculty of Homeopathy (MFHom), before entering practice and studying further with him. Since my sister Margaret had just completed her schooling, my parents decided that it would be ideal for her to accompany me to London in order to spend a year at finishing school in Kensington. Both the long course in homeopathy and the Cygnet's House year commenced in September therefore the timing was perfect. In addition, my father, possibly aware that his years were few, decided that the four of us should first enjoy an extended trip through Europe, something we would never have the opportunity of doing again as a family. The holiday would end in England in time for us to start our further education. It was my father's special gift to us, one that Margaret and I have cherished ever since and over which we often reflect.

On 13 May 1964, we flew from Johannesburg to Athens to commence an adventure that is still vivid in my memory. It commenced with a cruise to the Greek Islands, including Rhodes and Crete, then to Ephesus and up the Bosporus to Istanbul. This was followed by an archaeological tour of the Peloponnesus where I stood on the soil familiar to the heroes of my youth: Mycenae, Argos, Olympia, Delphi and Sparta. From there we travelled to Italy, Switzerland, and on to Cologne in Germany, where we visited the Madaus homeopathic laboratories and plantations, and then to Amsterdam and Paris, arriving in London on 6 July. This idyllic experience was followed by a seven-week holiday together in England. In London, my father took ownership of a white S-type Jaguar with red leather upholstery and gleaming spoke wheels, a car that gave him great joy and which he treasured during his remaining years. In this new acquisition, we proudly and comfortably journeyed to Leeds to stay with my grandmother in Woodlesford. This was our first return to my origins since our departure in 1949; then I was eight, now I was nearly twenty-four and Margaret eighteen. William and Nancy were fifty. It was warming to see how my parents set aside their sophistication and blended so comfortably and naturally into parochial, Yorkshire village life. The years apart melted away and family ties were renewed.

On returning to London, my father accompanied me to the RLHH where I enrolled for the long course, which included lectures, ward rounds and outpatient clinics in the basement of the hospital, an area I would come to know well. From there he took me to Nelson's Pharmacy and introduced me to Dudley Everett, who was glad to see him again after so many years. They had remained in communication through the regular orders that my father placed. I found lodgings in Muswell Hill in North London, and would spend a happy three years there while I lay the foundation for my future work.

Eventually, the time for parting arrived; the Jaguar was freighted to Southampton and a few days later, on 27 August, the four of us travelled down by train. My parents were sailing back to South Africa on the Transvaal Castle, a mail ship of the Union Castle Line; they would disembark at Cape Town on 10 September. It was a poignant moment for all four of us as the vessel started to pull away from its berth, keened by the closeness we had experienced during the wonderful four months together. Suddenly, I was aware that father's waving figure had disappeared from where he had stood beside my mother. He did not return during the time that Margaret and I stood like heavy-hearted orphans on the quayside watching the ship drawing further and further away. My mother's first letter to me, written from the ship, described how he had been overcome by emotion and had retired to their cabin greatly distressed. He had not looked well and she had insisted that he see the ship's doctor who had found his blood pressure to be markedly raised. This was at first attributed to the intensity of his emotions, but became a more settled problem. It was the first intimation of what was to become a remarkable and irreversible decline in his health.

Visits to Grandma

So began an invaluably chapter in my life, which I owe completely to the foresight and generosity of my father. During my stay in London, from September 1964 to December 1966, he supported me financially while I devoted myself first to the study of homeopathy and then during my final year to the study of osteopathy at the London College of Osteopathy, Dorset Square. I fulfilled my responsibility by intense study. I lived the life of a recluse with my nose buried in my books, when I was not attending lectures or outpatient clinics at the hospital. On the occasional holiday, I did not travel or do anything adventurous. I headed with my books up the A1 to Leeds and spent my time-off in Woodlesford with Grandma Lilley. I knew that when I arrived a huge Yorkshire pudding, with sliced roast beef, onion gravy and 'mushy' peas would be waiting for me; a dish I find irresistible to this very day. It was during these visits that I taxed 'Gran' with tales of my father's youth. Even forty years later she still pondered why she had decided to walk to Kippax on that icy afternoon and how she had managed to get there on time.

Near death experience

Uncle Jesse, my father's second brother, often came round for a chat. He was still a miner, very much a man of the Yorkshire countryside and a true, rough diamond. His hands were strong, gnarled and like his face seamed with coal dust ingrained in every cut or abrasion he had suffered in his many years below ground. The only resemblance to his younger brother lay in his short stature, his stockiness, his good-heartedness and his mischievous sense of humour. In 1964, Leeds United, under the management of Don Revie, had just been promoted to the English Football First Division and I often accompanied my uncle to their stadium at Elland Road and became a staunch supporter of the team that would achieve so much, even when their more than robust style of play brought them into disrepute. He also introduced me to the 'dogs'.[ii]

[ii] Greyhound racing.

When he was younger, he had kept and raced whippets (dogs similar to greyhounds) and it was not very long before I was coaxed into going to the races with him. The first occasion was in the middle of winter, and I cannot recall ever feeling as cold as I did that night, but never was a mug of hot tea more welcome and enjoyable as we jumped up and down to keep warm on the icy terraces. He told me of the times between the wars when he would go ferreting for rabbits on the nearby estate and how the occasional gift of a brace of his poached gains to the local police constable kept him out of trouble. The times I spent in Woodlesford were happy and carefree, and being with him and meeting his friends in the local pub, gave me a sense of my Yorkshire roots, which has never left me.

One day, as we sat over a cup of tea before the fire in Grandma's kitchen-dining room, he addressed me in more serious vein. This was presaged by the fact that he had put in his teeth, a refinement usually reserved for football matches and special occasions. More often than not he would do without them, which resulted in his features so falling-in that I imagined the tip of his nose would touch his chin, and this, together with his twinkling eyes and glimpses of bare gums as he nattered away, gave him an impish look that belonged in a book of fairy tales. On this occasion, his demeanour changed and though our relationship had become that of buddies, he spoke to me as an uncle. He gave me a pointed look and said earnestly, "David, never be afraid of death!" Surprised, I waited for what was to follow. He spoke to me of life in the mines; the harsh, claustrophobic conditions, the extreme effort and difficulty of working with pick and shovel at the coalface and the constant danger. One day, while on shift, a tunnel collapsed and he was pinned beneath the fall. Fortunately, his mates managed with great difficulty to free him and get him above ground. He had been severely crushed and suffered broken ribs and severe lacerations to his back. He was transported by ambulance to Leeds Infirmary where he developed secondary infection that led to septicaemia and threatened his life. He passed into a prolonged coma.

During this period of absence from the earth plane, he had an uplifting spiritual experience. He found himself in a most beautiful landscape, utterly different from anything he had ever experienced. Like many village people in the mining community, he had never been further afield than the popular seaside towns of Blackpool on the Lancashire coast or Scarborough and Bridlington on the Yorkshire coast; his television was a small, black and white model. In this out-of-the-body experience, he saw magnificent vistas complete with mountains, lakes and grasslands. He knew as he was experiencing this vision that it was not a dream, but a reality more intense than life. It was accompanied by a sense of great peace and deep happiness that washed over him and even seemed to penetrate him. The next sensation he could remember was the feeling of being drawn inexorably downwards from a state of light, air and exquisite beauty towards a dark, grey, dismal abyss that took the form of a murky tunnel into which he was pulled with the deepest reluctance. It was as if he was sinking from warmth, bliss and tranquillity into something cold, indifferent and ugly. The process of descent quickened and he became conscious of his body lying inert at the end of the tunnel. A feeling of unwelcome coercion swept over him as it sucked him in. A moment later, he opened his eyes to find himself in the unfamiliar setting of the hospital. At first, he was confused and uncertain of himself and his whereabouts, but conscious of an overwhelming sense of sadness and loss. When he finally regained his wits and heard of the fears that had been entertained for his life, he realised that during his life-threatening illness, he had been through a 'near-death' experience; that for a time he had been in 'Heaven.' Apart from his family, the few people he told explained his vision away as being the result of toxic delirium.

Both he and I knew differently.

In this traumatic experience and its aftermath, archetypal energy is seen at work, playing out a universal theme, recorded in myth and legend, manifest in our lives, and reflected and matched by a similar motif in a homeopathic remedy. The mythological divinity associated with mining, be it of coal, gold or any other mineral, is *Hephaistos* (Roman: Vulcan) the divine blacksmith who toils in his underground smithy fabricating wondrous objects for god and man alike. He is the God of Fire and Volcanoes and the divine patron of blacksmiths, craftsmen, artisans, inventors, industry and technology. His symbols are the smith's hammer, anvil and tongs, and by extension the pick and shovel of the miner who produces the coal essential for the blacksmith and for industry. As we shall consider later, the homeopathic archetype most closely associated with the nature and attributes of Hephaistos is Sulphur and this relationship extends in varying degrees to all the sulphates and sulphides. Given this association, it is not surprising to find that Sulphur is one of the most frequently indicated remedies for the ailments of coalminers, but also on a more subtle level for their inherent nature: their values, sentiments, eccentricities and habits. In this sense, Sulphur is aligned with the Hephaistos archetype present not only in many miners, but also in members of the extended mining community – even if they happen to emigrate to South Africa!

Within the coalmine, the element sulphur is in close association with the element carbon, the main constituent of coal. When the two come together, they form carbon bisulphide, from which the homeopathic remedy Carboneum sulphuratum (Carb-sulph) is prepared. It is a very toxic substance, noted for the violence and suddenness with which its symptoms emerge and its tendency to attack the nervous system. It is a remedy that has proved effective in combating the toxic effects of coal-gas inhalation and is therefore closely associated with Hephaistos, Sulphur and the nature and ailments of coalminers. Considering this relationship, the proving of the remedy furnished significant symptoms relevant to Uncle Jesse's near-death experience: "Visions of magnificent grandeur" and the sensation of "Falling into an abyss" or "Falling into a hole." In addition, a 44 year-old bipolar patient, whose father was a mining engineer and took the patient to see a mine when he was six, responded positively to treatment with Carb-sulph. He recorded having had two very relevant dreams: "*Falling through space*" and "Of being crushed in a mine." Interestingly, as a youth he had been struck on the head by a golf club, which had resulted in reading difficulties.[13] Once more, we see the connection between the archetype and conditions commencing suddenly and associated with physical trauma and violence. My uncle's experience indicates that Carb-sulph should prove suitable for certain cases of blood poisoning (septicaemia).

> In these anecdotes we are given hints of the universal entanglement of soul, myth, destiny, situation, happenings, temperament, miasm, constitution and substance; all subject to universal law; all ordained and blessed. The study of homeopathy takes the student into a world of magic and 'miracles'.

References

1. Smit HP. Spirit Doctor Removes Diseased Bone. *Two Worlds*; 65 (3431): August 29 1953.
2. Lilley WH. X-ray Confirms "Miracle." *Two Worlds*; 65 (3431): August 29 1953.
3. Accused Man Cured Her Daughter, Mother Tells Court. *Pretoria News*; January 1953.
4. Court Told Of Cure Of Dying Daughter. *Pretoria News*; January 1953.
5. "It Hurts Me To Find You Guilty." *Pretoria News*; February 18 1953.
6. *R v Lilley* [1956]. Notes of Court Proceedings. Pretoria Magistrates' Court. September 24. p3.
7. *Ibid.*, p2.
8. *Ibid.*, pp7–8.
9. *Ibid.*, p8.
10. *Ibid.*, p33.
11. *Ibid.*, p34.

12 *Ibid.*, p47.
13 Morrison R. Carbon: *Organic and Hydrocarbon Remedies in Homeopathy*. California: Hahnemann Clinic Publishing; 2006. pp375 + 378.

20

MASTER AND PUPIL

My Faculty tutors

I was fortunate to attend the Royal London Homeopathic Hospital at a particularly favourable period; some very experienced and outstanding physicians were involved in the training programme. This clinical and academic strength was enhanced by the wide diversity of focus and approach presented by the tutors. I was enriched on a number of levels. I was also favoured by the relatively small classes, which permitted a good deal of personal interaction with teachers. Whereas other students only attended the lecture modules, I was present at out-patient clinics each day, and derived immense benefit from sitting-in with a number of physicians, all of whom had their particular and personal way of taking a case history, evaluating symptoms and managing patients. It was an added advantage that due to the many months I attended the clinics, I was present at follow-ups and able to monitor the progress patients made. Although I benefited from the instruction I received from each of my tutors, there were four who proved particularly important to me.

Although they never met my father, I think it is appropriate to write a few words about these exceptional physicians, who in one way or another laid the foundation of the homeopathic knowledge upon which Dr Letari and my father would build. They were contemporaries of William and represent the medical side of the homeopathic coin for which he had great respect. Each in their own way was influential in shaping homeopathy at the time and hence also the physicians who followed them.

Margery Grace Blackie

In 1964, Margery Blackie (1898–1981) had just been elected Dean of the Faculty. She had an assured, direct manner, and brought a clarity, vigour and passion to her lectures, which imprinted the remedy pictures indelibly in my memory. Her enthusiasm for the 10M potency was particularly contagious. I soon knew without doubt that once the correct remedy was chosen, there was nothing that a dose of the 10M could not achieve. Her respect for the work of Douglas Borland led me to thoroughly study his incomparable booklets on *Influenza, Pneumonia, Digestive Drugs, Children's Types*, etc., which to this day remain the mainstay of my clinical work. I had just turned twenty-four when I first met Margery Blackie and knowing I was not only unschooled in homeopathy, but also to a large degree in medicine and life itself, she was especially encouraging and supportive. Advice was given, as would a maiden aunt to an untried nephew. There was no discussion; she knew better than I how I should conduct myself. Visits to her London home and practice at 18 Thurloe Street, Kensington, for tea, sandwiches and cakes were mandatory, and did much to incorporate me into the homeopathic family over which she presided with matriarchal authority. She and John Raeside were my examiners in the final clinical examination held in May 1965. When it was all over and she congratulated me on achieving the MFHom, I received a little sermon about my future followed by the reassurance that all I now needed was experience. How right she was. It seemed a very correct choice when I heard in 1969 that Dr Blackie had been appointed the Queen's homeopathic physician; a queen for a queen!

Donald McDonald Foubister

Between 1964 and 1966, I was privileged to spend considerable time with Donald Foubister (1902–1988) in the paediatric out-patient clinic. He was one of the kindest, most gentle, caring and compassionate people I have met. His love for the children under his care was palpable and it was particularly touching to see him interacting with Down syndrome children and their parents. His treatment helped these children's progress and widened their parameters of expression and independence. It was from him that I learnt of the use and value of the Down's nosode. He regarded the syndrome as an extreme expression of the sycotic miasm, the miasm of excess, hence the extra chromosome and the increased mucus secretions. Like Margery Blackie, he was a bridge to Douglas Borland and Margaret Tyler, who in turn were a bridge to James Tyler Kent and John Henry Clarke; a notable homeopathic pedigree. During the time I spent with him, he was consumed with his study of the nosode Carcinosin, prepared from cancerous breast tissue. It dominated his thinking and became his passion. I was too new to homeopathy to fully appreciate the importance of his intense preoccupation with this relatively new, and rather poorly understood remedy. Indeed, I got the impression that many Faculty members at the time felt that he had got a bee in his bonnet; but what a bee it turned out to be! I was intrigued by the frequency with which he found it indicated, either as the central constitutional remedy or as a supportive nosode. The broader picture of the remedy was still taking shape in his mind and he shared his thoughts with me as he mulled over its scope and symptoms. He had already perceived its relationship to Folliculinum, a sarcode prepared from the ovarian follicle, which has a specific effect on the female hormonal cascade from progesterone to oestrogen. It required the combination of passion and focus which he brought to bear on Carcinosin and the insights of his compassionate nature, to recognise its inner mystery: its relationship to the injured and dominated feminine, and hence to Bellis perennis, the common daisy, Sepia, the cuttlefish, and Lac caninum, milk of the dog. It was only years later that I came to understand his love for this remedy. In my practice, it is one of the most frequently prescribed remedies and has proved a boon to so many patients. I surmise that Carcinosin would have been the constitutional remedy for this wonderfully gentle, loving man.

Liewelyn Ralph Twentyman

Ralph Twentyman (1914–2010) was born in the same year as my father, but came from a background of affluence, which could not have been more different from William's origins. I can remember clearly, as if it were yesterday, the impression he made on me when I first met him in 1964, talking to colleagues after a lecture he had just given. He had a cup of tea in his hand and was holding forth to his rapt audience. He seemed larger than life to me, someone who stood out from his peers by virtue of his sheer presence, his sense of humour, his confidence and forthrightness, all amplified by the breadth of his formidable intellect, his mastery of words and not least of all, his booming laugh. His influence upon me was not so much homeopathic, through insights into the remedies of the materia medica, or methodology, but rather through understanding of the deeper aspects of the creation and human nature and kindling in me an interest in anthroposophy, Freud and Jung. I spent as much time with Twentyman in the out-patient clinic as I did with Foubister, but conversations with him were less about remedies and patients than about broader issues which concerned him, the reductionism of conventional medicine, the morbid psychology of miasmatic disease, psychosomatic phenomena and the metaphorical mystery of life. It was a rich world of images beautifully captured by his eloquence, which could verge upon the verbose, but never ceased to enthral. We found common ground in our love of mythology, and I was inspired by the connections he perceived between the gods of the Greek pantheon and the metals of the materia medica, the relationship imparting to them archetypal significance. In this regard, he suggested I read *The Secrets of Metals* by Wilhelm Pelikan and *Living Metals* by LFC Mees, which proved invaluable to me. His own book, *The Science and Art of Healing*, provides insight into the scope of the fertile, enquiring mind that I was exposed to. His influence continued long after I returned to South Africa through the *British Homœopathic Journal* of which he was the editor from 1958 until 1979 when he retired. The wide range of articles written by like-minds were eagerly awaited, read and preserved. Of particular importance to me was the work of William Gutman, Edward Whitmont and Karl Koenig.

John Robertson Raeside

John Raeside (1926–1972) assisted Margery Blackie in the running of the long course at RLHH during the time I was studying there. He was a close friend of Ralph Twentyman and, like him, also deeply interested in an anthroposophical approach to homeopathy. He was very active in the proving of new remedies. I remember him particularly for his kindness, gentle manner and his willingness to spend time after lectures explaining and elaborating on aspects of the materia medica. His deep love for his subject was evident. One particular late afternoon chat we had was very important to me. The other students had departed and we were alone enjoying a quiet moment when he gave me an impromptu talk on the cuttlefish from which Sepia is obtained. He had touched on this remedy earlier. He had recently carried out a proving of the edible clam (*Venus mercenaria*), and was well versed in the natural history of the mollusc family. He possessed a wide knowledge of cuttlefish biology, morphology and behaviour. He drew comparisons between the appearance, structure and habits of this advanced mollusc and the mental and physical attributes of those who needed it as a constitutional remedy for their ailments. It was the first time I had heard metaphorical relationships and parallels taken to such lengths; it was a revelation to me.

John saw in the shape of the animal and its tentacles a similarity to the uterus with its fallopian tubes and fimbriae (finger-like extensions of the tubes which reach out and gather an ovum released from the ovary), revealing Sepia's remedial affinity for conditions of the female pelvic organs. This beautiful creature is a master (or mistress) of camouflage, capable of a spectrum of colour changes to match its environment and to display its moods. Raeside likened this characteristic to emotional changeability and capriciousness, the ability to don various personas in keeping with the demands of society and the tendency for emotions to play freely over the countenance. The beak-like mouthparts used for shredding its prey indicated a capacity for spite and the ability to reduce others through cutting remarks directed with shrewish intent and insight into their vulnerabilities. The large, eloquent eyes, like the owl, spoke of high intelligence and wisdom. The cuttlefish possesses an ink sac from which a black pigmented secretion can be ejected into the surrounding water when the animal is threatened, indicating a gloomy response to life's challenges; a tendency to melancholy and black moods. He mesmerised me with a magical world of archetypal analogies, links and correlations. I was filled to the brim. Today, such detailed investigation of resemblance and comparison is common to modern homeopathic remedy analysis, but in 1964 this approach was still in its infancy. I hastened back to Muswell Hill and wrote down all he had told me and this formed the basis for my very first lecture on Sepia delivered to a captive and very dutiful audience, my sister Margaret.

On another occasion, John and I took a leisurely stroll around Queen Square, adjacent to the hospital and there ended up sitting on a bench close to the statue of Queen Charlotte, the wife of King George III, discussing the universality of the ancient Hindu texts, the Vedas, and the spiritual teachings of the Bhagavad Gita. It was always a pleasure to be in his company and to experience the way he thought. At the time he was in his late thirties, but already possessed wisdom beyond his years. It was a great sadness for me when, in 1972, I heard of his death in the Staines air disaster in which a BEA Trident airliner crashed shortly after take off for Brussels. There were no survivors, and an entire generation of British homeopaths travelling to a homeopathic congress in Belgium were lost. Dudley Everett of Nelson's homeopathic pharmacy was on that fatal flight. It is a sobering thought that if my father had not decided to emigrate, I could have been with them.

Elizabeth Wright Hubbard

During 1966, I trained as an osteopath at the London College of Osteopathy. It was a full time course, but still afforded me time to visit the RLHH for further experience. I was fortunate to attend a lecture held in the hospital Faculty boardroom given by Elizabeth Wright Hubbard (1896–1967), the doyen of American homeopathy. She gave a masterly exposition of Nitric acid and Thuja. The following year she died at the age of 71, but left a number of books, which are of inestimable value for any student of homeopathy. I remember at the time wondering if I would ever have the honour of giving a lecture to my colleagues in that room. This came to pass when I delivered a three-day seminar to Faculty members in February 1999.

Starting practice

Once I had achieved my qualification in Osteopathy, my preparation for future practice was complete and I returned to South Africa. My father had already reserved rooms for me on the fifth floor of City Centre, just down the passage from his suite. He had fully equipped them and in the consulting room stood a brand new Zenith chiropractic couch, specially shipped out from America; his gift to me for having completed my studies. Never was a son better groomed and provided for. Nor did I have the anxiety of establishing myself and slowly building up a practice. On my very first day, I found myself facing twelve patients – a combination of old stalwarts from my father's practice, among them the two spinsters who had defended him so loyally, and new patients who had applied to join the practice and been referred to me. This was the least number of patients a day that I would see in the following forty-one years of practice. Within a short time, I was seeing twenty a day and this built up to an average of thirty. Each day was a homeopathic and osteopathic marathon.

My spirit tutor

In January 1967, Dr Letari and my father took over my homeopathic education. Having my rooms so close to my father's was a great advantage. We were not permitted to share rooms because South African law at the time did not permit medical doctors to be in any way associated with non-medical practitioners. However, I had only a short passage to negotiate to be with him, and each lunch break we would review the cases I had seen in the morning and he would give me his observations. The same scrutiny of my case taking and methodology was continued in the evening. Until my first marriage in October 1967, I continued to live with my parents and this provided an ideal period for instruction. Thursday evenings were reserved for my sittings with Dr Letari. At first, these were weekly, and later at least once per month continuing until shortly before my father's death in 1972. Sometimes, my mother would join us, but usually we were alone. In addition to these sittings, there were many occasions when, as a family, we would come together to share time with our spirit father.

Unless I needed to read from case notes, we would dim the room or simply rely on the light shining in from the street. Dr Letari always sat in the wing-backed rocking chair that stood in my parent's lounge. This chair is now a much-treasured possession in the apartment Paddy and I have in

Cape Town; it has become the favourite of my three-year-old granddaughter, Vega Belle, whenever she is watching television.

My father and I would sit in silence; he with his eyes closed, his ankles crossed and his hands resting on his knees. A minute or two would pass during which I would see his face relax and his breathing slow and deepen. An observer might have thought that he had lapsed into sleep. My first indication of the good Doctor's presence would be the subtle animation of my father's features, which while still in repose, changed expression. His countenance mysteriously became that of another. Time seemed to stand still, and no matter the tribulations I might be experiencing, I would find myself immersed in a sense of tranquillity and timelessness. A brief period might elapse before he spoke, as if he was adjusting to the earth vibration or silently communing with other unseen personages. If I was sitting somewhat to one side, he would turn his head to look directly at me with closed eyes. When he finally spoke, his first words were always, "Greetings..." addressing me by my spiritual name. His voice, while speaking through the same voice box as my father, was always deeper in tone and his accent, rendered less Indian with the passage of years, was completely devoid of any trace of the slightly Yorkshire vowel sounds retained by my father. He never mastered the English 'r', replacing it with a 'w.' This resulted in 'spirit,' a word he often used, becoming "spiwit." He never ever used the terms Mr or Mrs, always referring to others as either *sahib* or *memsahib*; hence, he always referred to Lassie Smit as "*Sahib* Smit" and Mary Brown as the "*Memsahib* Brown."

Another distinguishing characteristic, differing markedly from my father's everyday vocabulary, was Dr Letari's elevated language. Like Silver Birch, he used beautiful metaphors and images and his teachings were couched in lofty words that inspired courage and trust, no matter the circumstances. He was always calm, always sure and always spoke from the objective vantage point of spirit. In the worst situations, even during my father's final illness, when he had difficulty in speaking to mother and myself because of William's failing heart, his message of trust remained the same, his words lost nothing of their majesty and his vision was fixed upon distant horizons that defied death. Even on the last occasion that we spoke together, a few weeks before my father's passing, when William was devoid of the energy that had thus far sustained him and was withdrawing more and more into himself, Dr Letari came through with words of comfort and reassurance and directives regarding the running of the laboratory and my future. He shared our lives with all the ups and downs that are inevitable on the physical plane, but stood back from our emotions and the vast majority of our decisions, generally restricting himself to delivering wise advice and encouraging us always to look at the broader picture from a spiritual rather than a materialistic viewpoint. Directives were always long term and encompassed important goals that should be achieved to fulfil the path of destiny. This extended to giving us guidance regarding our future in South Africa during times when the political situation was uncertain and even threatening.

Spirit optimism

We emigrated to South Africa in January 1949. In the previous year, on 4 July 1948, the National Party, the political party representing the aspirations and beliefs of the white Afrikaner nation, came to power, defeating the United Party led by the veteran, international politician, soldier and philosopher, Jan Smuts. Because of their fierce antipathy towards the British, residual from the time of the Boer War, many of the leaders of the National Party had been sympathetic towards Nazi Germany during the war. The policies of this party, which was essentially fascist and tribal, included legislated racial segregation (*apartheid*), the enforcement of white supremacy, the promotion of the Afrikaner culture and the establishment of a republic, preferably outside the British Commonwealth. The latter was achieved on 31 May 1961.

We found that we had come to a land where the white man was privileged and all other races were legally discriminated against. In City Centre, a seven story building, there was a sign over the lifts that read '*Europeans Only*' and the Afrikaans equivalent '*Blankes Alleen.*' This was an example of 'petty apartheid', but other laws were far more harsh and restrictive. Over the years, growing unrest, incidents of violence, including the Sharpeville massacre, international condemnation, economic sanctions, increasing political, cultural and sporting isolation, the interminable border war and the defiant hard-line response of the Afrikaner driven government, created great reason for concern in all who realised that white domination was not only unjust, but also untenable. There was a diaspora of the white, intellectual elite, the 'brain drain,' as ever increasing numbers of the wealthy and talented sought a safer future for their families in other countries, especially Australia and New Zealand. Friends, acquaintances and colleagues were amongst those who left. Dr Letari, however, remained confident and repeatedly reassured us, not only regarding our personal safety, but also about the long-term outcome for South Africa. He was unswervingly positive about the country's future and assured us that it was where the Lilley family should remain. Likewise, although he foresaw problems lying ahead for homeopathy because its very existence challenged the science of conventional medicine and the vested interests of the pharmaceutical industry, he predicted that these obstacles and setbacks would prove temporary. In representing scientific truth and the medicine of spirit, homeopathy was irrepressible and would not only survive, but gain in strength through acceptance by the public and the support of enlightened scientists.

Spirit reticence

Dr Letari, like Silver Birch, attached no importance to his own identity, spiritual status or previous life on earth. When Keith Desmond was looking for a story from the deceased doctor, the only response he got was "Who I am and the details of my physical life are not important." This was not just modesty or humility, traits that are invariable in spirit guides who return to teach, but also a reserve essential because of the human tendency to get caught up in detail, to romanticise, embroider and glorify the teacher at the expense of what is taught. Similarly, although raised as a Brahmin, his spiritual message was always universal, based on love and service, and never doctrinal. Whilst acknowledging the great spiritual teachers of the past, he never focused on their individualities or the religions created in their name, but only on the perennial truths they preached. No one, other than my mother, spent more time with Dr Letari than I; yet, during our discourses, he always manifested the same reticence regarding himself. Hence, what he chose to reveal to me was all the more precious.

He spoke of his death near Peshawar in 1914, and this only to explain how natural passing into the next life is. As previously mentioned, he was shot while assisting a man who had been wounded during a riot against the British. Colleagues struggled to save his life, but infection set in and he languished between life and death for a week before leaving the earth plane. When he first regained consciousness, he found himself reclining on a grassy embankment and seeing people familiar to him approaching. He recognised them as those dear to him, some from the life he had just left, who had predeceased him, others from whom he had parted at incarnation. The reunions were filled with joy, and love. For a time he rested while he became re-orientated to the spirit realm, but it was not long before he was approached by spirit elders, led by the Ramesôye, and asked if he would accept an important mission on the earth plane, one for which his experience and standing were suited. He was told that he would act as teacher and guide to a young boy who had incarnated in England a few months before his passing and that their united purpose would be to demonstrate the power of spiritual healing and to spread knowledge of homeopathy as *the* healing therapy for body, mind and soul. As always, the wishes and free will of the soul are respected. The choice always lies with the individual.

He told me that in accepting this task, which accorded so perfectly with his own aspirations, he experienced a moment of wry humour at the thought of himself, a young man fresh from life in north-east India, imprinted with the anti-British fervour of the area and so recently dispatched by a British bullet, now committed to entering intimately into the British life of his mediator. He found the dispensation apt, ideal for throwing off residual prejudice, which can cling tenaciously to the lower self. The years of preparation devoted by the spirit team to the rapid development of the young medium's psychic ability were also a time of preparation for Lejan Tari Singh. On the foundation of the knowledge and skill gained in spirit and during many lifetimes, he was groomed for the vital work that lay ahead. Spiritual healing, spiritual surgery, the science of spiritual medicine and homeopathy were thoroughly revisited as was the task of acquiring the greater fluency in English that he would require.

Just as we are never alone in our life experience, being always tended and supported by our unseen helpers, Dr Letari was not alone in the mission that centred round William. Although he was the pivotal figure, he was assisted by a number of gifted colleagues as well as by White Hawk, my father's 'gatekeeper'.

Festivals of spirit

At certain times of the year, coinciding with the commemoration of Christmas and Easter on the earth plane, spirits dedicated to various missions in the lower spheres withdraw for a time to their own realm and there attend festivals of their own. They meet with those they love, their teachers, imbibing anew their wisdom and partaking of their power. They hold counsel together, review what has been achieved and what remains to be done. Advice and further tasks are given and they commune with great spirits from the loftiest reaches of the higher heavens, who bring inspiration and vision of what is being planned by the Highest in the incessant contest between the forces of good and evil.

This time away from the material world is also replenishing. In harmonious conditions the returning soul enjoys the congenial companionship of those with similar tastes and pursuits. The circumstances for souls working on the earth plane can be compared with humans working at great depths in the ocean. The environment is foreign, taxing and exhausting. Periods of rest are essential. Dr Letari spoke of the invigoration and revitalisation he experienced when he returned to his own sphere and how essential it was, even though for only a short time, to throw off the heavy shroud necessary to function in the grosser dimensions close to earth and to experience and absorb the raptures and beauty of life in the spirit. In descending through the lower regions consciousness becomes attenuated, just as the diver's suit compresses the environment and shrinks the vision. In the case of the soul, the suit that must be donned is known as the astral body. The return to the higher levels necessitates leaving this vestment on the astral plane, a dimension just beyond the physical. Here it is sustained by the consciousness of the absent soul, otherwise it would disintegrate. On the soul's return it once again provides the means to descend to the lowest dimension of existence. During the short sojourn away from the heavy oppression of the earth's vibratory field, the soul's consciousness expands, but far more time would be required to fully register its immense capacity. A few days cannot restore what took years to attain. Contemplating such a diminution of consciousness, and the psychic claustrophobia it must entail gives us some conception of the immense sacrifice made by souls working in the dense milieu of earth.

I asked if these festivals of spirit, which in timing correspond so accurately with the major Christian festivals, were in any way related to the life and death of Jesus. Dr Letari told me that they had no connection to any scriptures, but hearkened back to the harvest festivals of ancient agricultural societies, which were held in thanksgiving for the blessings and bounty of the Great White Spirit and to invoke protection against the evils of famine and drought. These ancient sacraments also appealed for divine intercession against negative powers and celebrated the triumph of good over evil. Their timing was in rhythm with the vast cycles of nature, seasonal, planetary and cosmic. All the great souls active in caring for the planet derive from older earth races whose religions, stemming from hoary antiquity, were in harmony with nature's cadence. It was natural for them to adopt the traditional festival pattern of their past to celebrate communion with the creative power of the universe. Whereas the festivals held in the world of matter celebrated the emergence of new life and its harvesting, the festivals held in spirit provide opportunity to briefly withdraw from the lower spheres to assimilate new power from the infinite with which to bring spiritual illumination to the world. In this they are akin to the Eleusinian Mysteries, the most secret and sacred initiation rites of ancient Greece based upon the cult of Demeter (Mother Nature) and her daughter Persephone (Queen of the Underworld), who at the onset of Winter leaves her mother and descends, depleted, into the Underworld, and then, before the burgeoning of Spring, ascends replenished, bringing new life and vitality to the world – a resurrection! The spirit festival coinciding with the Jewish *Pesach* (Passover) and the Christian Easter is of particular significance in this respect. It is a celebration of the resurrection of spirit – a benediction upon all those striving for the resurrection of the world from sorrow, sadness and suffering – a time for revealing higher wisdom, when the learned can sit at the feet of the wisest of the wise. At the close, recharged with the joy of service, our guides return to us bringing the power of spirit into our midst.

At these special times, Dr Letari would take leave of us, but always with the assurance that if there were problems he would return to be with us. This very rarely happened.

The mediator

When I sat with Dr Letari on those special Thursday nights, my father was of course absent, out-of-his-body in the astral plane, a dimension of finer and higher frequency than that of the world of matter. After he returned at the end of a sitting and we shared a pot of tea together in the kitchen, he would invariably ask what Dr Letari and I had discussed. He had no memory of happenings on earth during his projection. Though unconscious to the world he had left, he was not in a passive state of sleep, but active and aware of his surroundings and everything that transpired. On a number of occasions he spoke to me about these experiences. His descriptions were well documented in *The Gift of Healing*.

> When I am going into a trance, I breathe in the yoga method taught to me by Dr Letari. Immediately I get a sensation as though I am falling, or being pulled backwards. As this sensation comes to a climax, I seem to be travelling through space at a terrific speed.
>
> I have opened my eyes many times at this point, but the only vision I have is of passing through a dense fog. Then quite suddenly, the fog clears and I am at a stile. I climb over this stile and immediately there is a voice speaking to me over my shoulder. The voice is always with me, explaining everything I see and everyone I meet. The stile seems to be on the edge of a very large field, which rises gradually to the form of a hill. I walk up the hill, and beyond it I visit many places.[1]

He related how he had often visited the 'children's land' where souls that had passed on early in life and remained caught-up in the child mode of expression dwelt. Here he had spoken to school-mates, many of whom he did not know had died before he met them there. He had also visited the famed Halls of Learning, which resembled the Acropolis at Athens. "It is always the same stile, the same hill, the same voice and beyond a large country with many different towns to visit."

On one occasion before going into trance for a group of sitters, my father engaged in a discussion about the nature of consciousness and how it gave reality to the type of spirit world the soul would experience. He was then asked to describe the nature of the dimension he entered when he was astrally projected; in particular, whether it was, or appeared to be, solid. He replied that if he could he would find out.

On his return from trance he gave them the following description:

> I arrived at my stile, the voice came to me, and it evidently knew my desire, because it said, "Feel the earth!" I did. It was solid. "Feel the grass beneath your feet!" I did. That was solid too, and even had dew on it. "Smell these flowers!" they were perfectly natural and had the usual perfume. In fact, everything about me was natural. Then I was told, "Feel your body." I did so. It was as solid as I am materially.
>
> Then the voice said, "Close your eyes; make your consciousness passive, or as you would do before preparing yourself for a trance state." I did. "Now feel the earth beneath your feet!" There was nothing. "Open your eyes." It wasn't dark, it wasn't light. "Feel your body!" It wasn't there. "Such is spirit" said the voice. "Just consciousness holding within it all experiences of your lifetime, all the joys and sorrows, your desires, achievements and failures, whence comes spiritual evolution. In your world of the material, you are able to examine matter, everything is matter. Therefore when thinking in spirit, you naturally build in your consciousness another material world."[2]

* * * * *

My psychic life

The expectation of many was that I would follow in my father's footsteps and become a trance medium with the same psychic gifts as my father, but as far back as I can remember I knew it was not the path I would walk. Dr Letari's full attention was given to tutoring me in the science of spirit and the science of homeopathy. As in the training of his mediator, he wished me to pass on this knowledge and experience to others. He told me that he and those close to me would give me all the assistance I would need in my practice and in my teaching. I recall him telling me, in my youth, that if I filled the drawers of my mind with knowledge, he would always be there to open them when I needed the information they contained, whether I was with a patient, analysing a case, lecturing or addressing a congress. To this day he has always been true to his word.

Astral projection

Although I have never developed clairaudience, clairvoyance or psychometric ability, I have been blessed not only with my singular upbringing, the example of my father and the tutelage of Dr Letari, but also with specific psychic experiences or archetypal dreams which have provided me at critical points in my life with essential knowledge, insights and cues to assist me in understanding and participating positively in my unfolding experience. Like my two illnesses, these stand out like milestones and signposts along my journey. The first of great significance to me occurred when I was thirteen or fourteen years of age. One morning, in the very early hours, my cat leaping onto my bed wakened me. I soon drowsed off again, but then became aware of slipping out of my body and rising above it. It was a pleasant sensation which I would have liked to persist, but no sooner had I focused on holding onto this sense of liberation, when I felt myself being drawn back, and this was associated with an alarming sensation. I felt as if I was passing through a very powerful force field, which created a shuddering vibration about me and within me. I felt buffeted and shaken, not physically, but on some deeper level, yet still external to the innermost me. While this was happening, I was conscious of being surrounded by shimmering light-waves, fluctuating rapidly in brightness and intensity, in rhythm with the quivering sheath of luminous turbulence that enclosed me. I felt overwhelmed by a vast energy, as if it would consume and immolate me. In a trice, I was back in my body, jolted awake with a shock, heart racing, chest heaving and adrenaline coursing through my body.

I landed running! I shot out of bed, hastened to my parent's room and despite the earliness of the hour and the likelihood of scaring them out of their wits, seized the shoulders of my father's sleeping form and shook him urgently. His return into the body was as abrupt as my own had been. In the South Africa of today, he would certainly have thought himself in the grip of an assailant, but in 1953–4 times were seemingly tranquil and he soon realised that it was his son's figure silhouetted above him. While my mother continued sleeping, he took me back to my room and we sat on the bed together. After I had described, as best I could, my psychedelic experience, he explained that what I had felt was my soul-self leaving my body, a nightly transition, which is usually unconscious. Because I had become conscious of the separation, my mind had stalled the process and for a moment I had been caught in the energy field between dimensions, hence the feeling as if an electric current was passing through and over me. He told me I could expect this phenomenon to happen again, and when it did, I should relax and just let the flow take me without trying to influence it.

He was proved right, it did happen again, in fact many times over the following years. I was a slow pupil, because time and again I would feel myself leaving my body, try to school myself into total passivity and compliance, with varying degrees of success, only to find the wonderful sensation receding and finally escaping me as I plunged back into the frenetic force field. Finally, one night, I was rewarded by finding myself completely free from my body and able to gaze upon it lying asleep on the bed. For quite a time that was all I managed, but the effect of repeated experiences upon a young mind was accumulative, instilling in me the irrefutable conviction of my non-physical nature. Simple as these exercises were, they provided me with more proof of the duality of life and the indestructibility of the soul than any evidence derived from the rich source that always surrounded me.

Characteristic of these tentative ventures onto the astral plane was their clarity, their defined realism, their unerring similitude, and my retention of full critical consciousness and volition, setting them apart from dreams and musings of the unconscious mind. From this initial projection, confined to the immediate proximity of my body, I graduated to floating out of the house without use of either window or door and viewing from above the surrounding neighbourhood that was so familiar to me. These more venturesome journeys out of the body were extremely infrequent, but none the less occurred with some regularity over the years. Eventually I was taken on longer, more distant excursions, flying with effortless speed over vast landscapes dotted with impressive buildings of remarkable architecture and smaller structures that I imagined to be habitations. I was conscious of not being alone and that those with me, sensed rather than seen, were escorting me.

A celestial concert

On a number of occasions there were specific destinations. One that stands out in my memory was joining a concourse of people wending their way towards an immense amphitheatre. On arrival, my unseen companions and I took our seats high up on terraces that extended downwards in serried ranks to a spacious stage below on which musicians were gathering.

Although we had no difficulty finding vacant seats, within moments the entire auditorium, which was open to the heavens, was filled to capacity. I was not conscious of the usual excited hum of voices common to such audiences on the earth plane, yet there was a tangible, anticipatory energy which surged and swelled about us. Hardly had I sensed this when the orchestra commenced playing, at first a simple refrain which slowly mounted in amplitude commanding more and more of my attention until quite suddenly there was only the music; music such as I have never heard before. Waves of exquisite sound ascended from the depths and swept over me and simultaneously, as if I too were an instrument, caused my entire being to resonate to every nuance of tonal expression. I was sitting in a symphonic ocean that coursed through me. I was one with the music. It was multi-textured and complex, a consonant concord of multiple harmonies caressing, entwining and interweaving, an intricate tapestry of celestial music that ravished my heart and enraptured my soul. Not only could I hear and feel the music, I could also see it. Every note was rendered visible by its corresponding colour. The orchestra created a beautiful musical colour-field, made up of multiple waves of excited and agitated colour, patterned perfectly to the composition, darting then flowing, blending then separating, expanding then contracting, forming sharp peaks and soft hollows, now light, now dark, now playful, now sombre; an ever-changing, dancing, shimmering, spectrum of sound that streamed out of the arena, flashed up to the heavens and swept over the countryside beyond. A sense of ineffable bliss pervaded me. I was spellbound, ecstatic and intoxicated; I could have immersed myself in its magnificence for eternity. Finally the music receded from me, ebbing away into a silence, which left me bereft, and very much awake, tears streaming down my cheeks.

This psychic event remains a treasured memory. It moved me so deeply that the visual and auditory images remain deeply etched. Unlike a dream they did not become nebulous with time, because they were received in full consciousness as a true and tangible happening of great import.

The music was pivotal to the significance of the experience. I have always loved what is loosely termed classical music, especially the Baroque, and particularly Bach and Handel, but my personal musical skills are elementary and limited to the role of an appreciative audience. All the promise I showed on the piano in Beaconsfield was lost when we emigrated. Even if we possess some psychic repository in which all we have ever heard is indelibly stored and accessible, the music I heard on that blessed occasion resembled no work I am familiar with nor reflected the style of any composer I have listened to. As I lay in bed, still charged with the powerful energy and intense emotions that had stirred me to the quick, I knew that I had been granted something infinitely precious. I had been permitted to look through a window into the great beyond, perceive my own immortality, and through compelling music, which could not have emanated from any source within myself, savour the rhapsody of the spirit realm.

Archetypal dreams

Throughout the years, and even to the present, I have been favoured with similar occurrences and occasionally important visitations, always experienced in the sleep state and always when for one or other reason they would prove beneficial or guiding. Latterly, the experiences of astral projection have diminished markedly and been replaced by archetypal dreams that require interpretation. These too have always occurred at critical points of dilemma or decision in my life. They present in parable form wisdom and instruction which when unravelled far surpass in scope and insight what any words or thoughts could convey. I waken from such a dream with a sense of wonderment and the question: "Now what was that all about?" Even while dreaming the archetypal dream, I am fully aware that what is unfolding before my inner eye holds great consequence for me. I am transformed from dreamer into alert observer. When they first commenced in my early thirties, I was fortunate to have a Swiss Jungian dream analyst, Mario Schiess, as a patient, who through his adept interpretation of these dreams introduced me to the fabulous world of the collective unconscious, enabling me to unite this concept with my interest in mythology and the earlier input of Ralph Twentyman.

Visitations

One of the visitations that touched me deeply occurred while I was boarding in Muswell Hill. My father had a much loved Boxer dog, Hector, named of course after the mythical Trojan hero of Homer's Iliad. When I left for my studies in England, he was already quite elderly, slow of movement and showing white about the muzzle, though still capable of bristling and stiffening his legs at the approach of other dogs. One night, I was aware of having passed into the astral dimension when I saw a young, magnificent Hector, as he was in his prime, with an intensely black muzzle, pure white chest and gleaming golden-brown fur, bounding towards me in delight, his eyes and face full of joy and excitement. In comparison with a common dream, everything was highly defined and crystal clear. The next moment, as large as he was, he was in my arms and licking my face. I could feel the wet warmth of his tongue and feel the heat, weight and muscular power of his body as he twisted and turned in expressing his love for me. When I awoke, I knew without doubt that Hector had passed into the spirit world, although my mother's last letter to me had not mentioned any deterioration in his health. This was soon confirmed; he had died unexpectedly on the very night of my dream.

Each psychic experience brought me in touch with a different aspect of the spiritual nature of life and its unbroken continuity. Through the music, I had touched indescribable sensory and emotional bliss, through Hector, I gained personal experience of what Dr Letari had told me regarding the more intense reality existing on the spirit dimension; that spirit to spirit was more real than physical to physical; and that the spirit world is not an indefinite, nebulous state populated by discarnate wraiths. I had also witnessed that after passing the threshold, we regain all our youth, beauty and vigour.

Another visitation, far more unexpected than the one I have just related, was the unheralded appearance of Arthur Richards. Although he was my godfather, he and I had never bonded emotionally and my last memory of him was as an eight-year-old sailing on his boat on the river Thames. Some four or five years after my father's death in 1972, he came to me. I was then in my mid-thirties and had just married Paddy, my second wife. I had not given the least thought to Uncle Arthur for years. He had passed to spirit in 1958, ten years after our departure for South Africa. Suddenly, without preamble, there he was, standing close to me looking just as I had last seen him, wearing a pin-stripe suit and tie. His demeanour was serious and sad as he told me that he regretted his behaviour towards my father at the end of their relationship and that he wished to apologise both to my mother and myself for being responsible for the rupture and the difficulties it had caused. Before leaving me, he once more stressed his wish that I should convey his thoughts and deep regret to Nancy. With that he disappeared and I have never seen him again.

Confirmation

When, at 67, I made my decision to discontinue full medical homeopathic practice in Pretoria and move to Cape Town in order to write, lecture and practise in a small way. Being still strong and vigorous and in full command of my clinical knowledge and skills, and therefore, well able to continue the work I was doing for many years to come, I suffered a sense of guilt; guilt at leaving all the remarkable patients in my practice; and guilt at shedding the responsibility. After forty-one years of intense practice there was a certain loss of identity and something akin to mourning. I had difficulty making the transition even though what I contemplated was creative and hardly retirement. As in the past, the Cosmos gave me encouragement and confirmation, and did so on two separate occasions, even before I had laid down my tools.

The Kingfisher

An archetypal dream

The first was a dream – an archetypal dream. As is the way with such dreams, I was asleep yet wide-awake, aware of my out-of-the-body state and acutely aware of the visual message that was being portrayed to me. Before me there appeared a hovering kingfisher, multi-coloured with flashing iridescent plumage. A second, then a third, then twenty or thirty soon joined it, and finally my entire vision was filled with these glorious birds, all suspended in the air, flapping their wings; a highly charged image replete with colour, avian beauty and incessant motion. The moment the vision ceased, I awoke with a sense of peace and upliftment and the knowledge that, in Dr Letari's words: "All is well!"

The collective unconscious in our depths is an ocean of images, concepts, patterns, metaphors and archetypes derived from humanity's accumulated impressions and interpretations of the phenomena of life down the ages; it is a repository of ancient lore and wisdom. The kingfisher is a universal archetype, embodying mystical and mythical meaning, qualities and attributes pooled in our unconscious through the intuitive insights of our ancestors.

To fathom the significance of my dream, I needed to subject it to careful analysis, as I do my patients' dreams. An acquaintance with mythical thinking is of great value in unveiling the hidden meaning of dream symbolism. I am a keen birdwatcher and knew that the kingfishers are classified in the bird family *Halcyonidae* (a number of southern African kingfisher species belong to the genus *Halcyon*, e.g. the Woodland and Grey-hooded kingfishers) and I also knew that this scientific name derived from an ancient Greek myth. So I first turned to the myth for insight into my dream.

The *Halcyon* was a legendary seabird, which later became identified with the kingfisher. According to myth, Alcyone, the daughter of Aeolus, lost her beloved husband Ceyx when he drowned in a shipwreck during a violent storm at sea. She found his body washed up on the shore and her grief was inconsolably. Her intense suffering and her devotion to his memory awakened the pity of the gods, who transformed the lovers into halcyons. These birds nested by the sea, or some say even on the sea. The waters were frequently so turbulent that many of the eggs and hatchlings were lost. From Olympus, Zeus, the God of Gods, saw the offspring of Alcyone and Ceyx being washed away by the waves each year, and was saddened. Out of sympathy, he restrained the winds and brought a calm, smooth sea, which lasted for seven days before and seven days after the winter solstice, the legendary time when the halcyon, or kingfisher, lays its eggs. This annual period of calm became known as '*halcyon days*' an expression, which has become idiomatic for calm, peaceful and tranquil times or a happy and carefree period in life. Also, because of the survival of the bird's progeny, the term denotes an ordained period of productivity and prosperity.

This kingfisher dream informed me that I had reached tranquil waters and that a period of happy creativity lay before me during which my affairs would prosper. The great number of kingfishers indicated abundance and success; it also emphasised the amount and diversity of the work that lay ahead, but in pleasant and congenial circumstances.

Archetypal dreams often feature animals, which hold archetypal or totemic significance for the dreamer. The shamans of old understood the esoteric and metaphorical import of these symbols and were, therefore, able to interpret the dreams that featured them. Such readings would provide not only wise instruction regarding unfolding events in the dreamer's life, but also insights into the dreamer's nature, prompting self-awareness. The practice of '*depth homeopathy*' necessitates the ability of the physician to think mythologically and to have the capacity to unravel and interpret dreams like the shamans of old. The 'like remedy' possesses the frequency required to touch the collective unconscious and evoke a healing response which sooner or later will produce dreams, which when correctly understood provide information about the dreamer's nature and perspective (delusions), and details invaluable to further remedy selection and assessment of progress. An archetypal dream can open up a complex case and prove conclusive to success.

If we scrutinise this very distinctive and attractive bird anthropomorphically with the intuitive eye of a shaman, we discover a wealth of insights of which we would otherwise remain ignorant.

The Kingfisher – an Archetype

The kingfisher displays, in its natural behaviour and physical attributes, traits, which are symbolic of the opportunities and challenges that are relevant to those affiliated to the archetype. It boldly dives headlong into water to catch small fish indicating a confidence to plunge into the unknown, enter unchartered territory and tackle new concepts without fear. This intrepid behaviour pertains particularly to water, which symbolises the emotions and the deep unconscious, denoting the desire and determination of the archetype to pursue self-knowledge, acquire occult wisdom and achieve spiritual illumination. They are often highly intuitive and psychically sensitive. The entire form of the bird is fashioned like a dart to penetrate the watery realm with maximum speed and minimum resistance. For this purpose it is endowed with a large dagger-like bill, which in many species is bright-red signifying passion of intent, and its poniard shape, a probing, curious, focused mind, able to penetrate obscure concepts and give attention to the finest detail. Compared with the rest of the bird, the head is large, a warning to the archetype to curb an ego capable of inflation. Its often strikingly colourful plumage, reputedly attained when the originally dull-grey bird, transported by inordinate pride, presumptuously flew too close to the sun, is similarly indicative of egotism and a love of self-display. The tight, compact body signals the need for this archetype to take regular physical exercise to offset inherited weaknesses. Their flight is rapid and arrow-like and those whose totem it is do not procrastinate and have the energy to accomplish various tasks efficiently without tiring. They are solitary birds that mostly nest in holes or tunnels dug in earth banks along rivers, lakes or man-made ditches. Some species nest in holes in trees. This indicates a need for privacy and solitude and time for contemplation and meditation. A few special friendships, or simply the relationship with their mate, suffice. They are often happier and healthier when living close to water. Kingfishers make distinct rattling or melodic piping calls, which carry over considerable distances. The archetype is often a gifted teacher able to convey knowledge and understanding in a clear, interesting and eloquent manner, and their message is likely to reach many ears. In its highest form, the kingfisher archetype becomes a 'fisher of men,' capturing aspirants in its persuasive, teaching net and inspiring them to emotional and spiritual growth.

The kingfisher has not been subjected to a homeopathic proving, but having the shape, speed and flight of an arrow; this avian archetype must be compared to an archer, an archetype with clear vision, accuracy of observation, unswerving focus, concentration and defined goals. The analogy evokes comparison with the Greek archer divinities, Apollo and his twin sister Artemis, and in turn with the noble metals associated with each: Aurum (gold) and Argentum (silver) respectively. So it is that from a dream the analyst is able to make important connections, gain insight into the nature of the dreamer and find indications for the selection of a remedy.

Archetypal analysis of this kind is identical to the Doctrine of Signatures (see Chapter 1) of which I will have more to say in the second volume of this series of titles. Identification with an archetype indicates both the potentiality and the vulnerability inherent to the image.

Once we are keened to the interested participation of the loving Cosmos in our affairs, we become alert to cues and clues with which this nurturing intelligence prompts us towards expressing our true selves. Receptiveness ensures that these prompts will be forthcoming, giving direction, encouragement and confirmation. Shortly after the kingfisher dream, I was invited to give a seminar to a group of homeopathic veterinary surgeons in Cork, southern Ireland. My wife, Paddy, accompanied me and during our stay we enjoyed and appreciated the wonderful hospitality of my Irish veterinary colleagues. Imagine the warm glow I experienced when we drew up before our hotel outside Cork and read above the main entrance: The Kingfisher Hotel. A few days later, we were invited to supper at the home of Tom Farrington our host and convenor of the seminar.

During the course of the evening, he had reason to open his laptop and the background display he had chosen for his computer was a beautiful photograph of the Common Kingfisher, *Alcedo atthis*.

Many years previous to these events, a young man of eighteen or nineteen, a patient of mine who was studying art, asked me if he could do a painting for me as an expression of his gratitude for the help I had given him and his mother. I thanked him, and, true to his promise, at his next appointment he presented me with an example of his work. It was a very respectable watercolour of the eye-catching South African Malachite Kingfisher, *Alcedo cristata*. Nothing happens without reason and oft times what we regard as trivial and insignificant may hold an important message. If we are alert, we will become conscious of a guiding influence in our lives and from this conclude that the role we play is significant, and, furthermore, that we are all of considerable consequence in the affairs of the Universe.

A psychic gardener

The second communication regarding my decision to retire from practice occurred on the 1st of December 2007, just two weeks before I passed my practice on to my son, Dorian. Our plans to move to Cape Town after my retirement necessitated the sale of the family home in Waterkloof, Pretoria, which we had occupied ever since our arrival in South Africa, some fifty-eight years before. The garden was filled with precious memories. Many of the trees that towered above the lawns and flowerbeds had been no taller than myself when first planted. There was a magnificent, bountiful avocado tree that had been grown from a pip and planted by my daughter Brigitte when she was seven years old. The matriarch of the garden was a lofty Australian Flame Tree, which in spring, having lost most of its leaves, became a spectacular display of bright, scarlet flowers. My father had a special relationship with this tree, and when, after a number of years, it had failed to blossom, he had a heart to heart talk with it, with the result that the following year it emerged in all its splendour. Whether his words stirred the spirit of the tree or not is immaterial. For us as youngsters, his reverence for the tree and his dialogue with it brought fantasy into reality and deepened our perspective of nature.

My parents always took great pride in the garden, which had been an acre of virgin veld when they first took occupation of the property in 1949. Father was a man of many abilities and among these was a practical turn of hand to which his years at the copper works had added great power of arm and shoulder. Every weekend, these attributes were put to good use in creating and maintaining, under my mother's watchful and more aesthetic eye, a garden of great beauty.

Although over time, there had been many changes in the general layout of the garden, there were certain features, which dated back to the earliest years. In the middle of the property, a grove of indigenous trees had stood. Father removed the trees in the centre and within the remaining circle laid down lawn. This area became aptly known as 'the circle' and was a favourite gathering point, variously used, depending on the season and time of day, for sunbathing, reading, writing, relaxing or having tea. However, it was also used at times for family sittings, particularly while Margaret and I were still young. Whatever changes were brought about in the rest of the garden, 'the circle' remained sacrosanct. Beneath the circle of trees were flowerbeds always home to columbines, fuchsias, azaleas and cannas, my mother's favourites. This tradition continued after her death.

When the garden was first laid out, mother created a number of fine rockeries, all built by my father. For the purpose, he imported lorry loads of attractive volcanic rock, which he arranged to form terraced flowerbeds. My little sister was far more involved in these activities than I, and father set great store by the time shared with his 'little princess,' placing the stones and laying paving. Later, when the garden took on a less formal appearance, these rockeries were cleared and the stones dispersed, but a large number were retained under the trees of 'the circle,' placed there for ornamental purposes.

Anyone who has faced the sale of a house upon which so much else depends will know how difficult it is to dovetail the event to coincide with a move or the purchase of a new abode. Yet, with the date for retirement set at mid-December, Paddy achieved the seemingly impossible when through her efforts, and a good deal of prayer, the sale of 350 Milner Street was finalised on the 2nd of November. Once the sale was sure and the realisation dawned that the home that housed so many special memories was no longer ours, a flood of nostalgic sentiment, particularly centred upon the garden, overcame us all. On the 17th of November, coinciding with the 80th birthday of Paddy's mother, Babs Weaving, we held a last family party at the house. Present were all William and Nancy's eight grandchildren and five great grandchildren.

My son Jason and my daughter Brigitte cut a heart on the bole of the flame tree within which, like lovers, they inscribed their initials. Margaret and I walked down to the circle and reminisced about our childhood and the times Dr Letari had spoken to us while we sat in the lotus posture on the lawn before him. We stood over the spot where he used to sit, a few metres away from the old, twisted tree against which a Greek-styled birdbath stood. Beneath the pedestal of kneeling nymphs was the spot where I had buried my father's ashes in December 1972, 35 years before. Margaret's eye alighted on a few of the old rockery stones which protruded from the soil here and there, some almost completely covered, others showing grey vestiges of the cement which she had helped my father apply when she was a child. Memories flooded back, and, with tears in her eyes, she exclaimed with great intensity that she must have the stones for her own garden; they could not possibly belong to anyone else. On searching amongst the plants and groundcover that obscured them, we found a considerable number, far more than we anticipated. In fact, collecting, removing and transporting them would prove quite a labour. Undeterred and enthused with her mission, Margaret arranged for a garden service to do the job.

On Saturday morning, 1st of December, a lady and her team of workers descended on the garden and began the arduous task of digging out and removing these very important stones. The previous evening, Paddy and I had returned from a very memorable trip to Japan where I had the privilege of lecturing to students of the Japan Royal Academy of Homeopathy (RAH). The experience had proved moving on many levels. It was our first visit to Japan, and, being during the last two weeks of November, coincided with the breath-taking autumn colours of the Japanese maple and *Ginkgo biloba* trees. This alone would have been sufficient to leave us with cherished memories, but to this was added a courtesy, generosity and hospitality that touched our hearts, and the joy of addressing highly appreciative audiences. I had been told that the Japanese were so polite and inscrutable that lecturers never knew whether they were approved of or not. My experience was quite the opposite. I lectured through a translator for three days to over 400 students. Apart from those in my Tokyo audience, the lecture was also simultaneously transmitted to students sitting in four other colleges. These were visible to me on TV monitors. My hostess Toraku Yui, Principal and founder of the RAH, a powerful personality filled with passion and love for homeopathy, set the stage for the seminar with fervent introductions and summings-up after each session. The content I had chosen was the fabrication of the basic archetypes of the homeopathic materia medica during the process of stellar evolution (which we will consider in Volume 2). Throughout the three days, I touched frequently upon our spiritual nature, and often emotions ran high. At one point, I had to pause due to my translator having to choke back her tears. There were very few men in my audience, but towards the close of the last day, during a break for refreshments, a Japanese gentleman sitting a few rows from the front, suddenly came up onto the platform, embraced me, looked into my eyes and said quietly: "I love you." With that he turned away and returned to his seat. This image lives with me and is relevant to what transpired in the garden that December Saturday in Pretoria.

The workers toiled all morning, while I attended to a backlog of correspondence in my study. At midday, having completed my work, I went down the garden to see how much progress had been made. As I approached the scene of activity, I saw that the lady in charge, who was totally unfamiliar to me, was sat on a chair in the middle of the circle, earnestly addressing my sister, who was standing nearby, raptly attentive to her every word. The seriousness of the scene brought me to a halt beside Paddy, where she stood next to the Grecian birdbath, in the shade of the old gnarled tree. I did not wish to intrude or interrupt, but my arrival drew the lady's attention. She looked at me, but seemed unfocussed, as if she was distracted by something she could either see or hear. She put her hand to her brow as though perplexed and exclaimed, "He is talking so much; he has so much that he wants to say; oh! He is talking so much!" Paddy turned to me and explained that the lady was a psychic and that while sitting in the circle she had become aware of my father's presence. He had made himself known to her and had already given a message to both Margaret and herself. The medium was sitting on the very spot where Dr Letari had sat so many times in the past, a spot hallowed by precious memories. Small wonder there were such powerful energies bearing down upon her. I said as much. The sound of my voice seemed to bring her into focus for she fixed her eyes upon me and began to channel my father's thoughts. The manner in which she spoke conveyed some of the urgency of my father's desire to communicate with us.

He told me that my decision to retire was wise and that I would now be embarking on a new career, through which I would be able to reach the ears of far more people and have a wider influence. He said that the Universe thanked me for the work that had been done and that he was proud of me. The medium then described a great number of lights she saw spreading outwards from me in all directions and my father explained to her that they represented the many souls that I would touch in one way or another. His final words to her were: "My son will never stop."

Paddy later related the message she had received. Father had thanked her for supporting and assisting me every step of the way. He told her how invaluable her help was and how those in spirit valued the vital role she played. It was a grateful message of thanks, very similar to that which Silver Birch had given to my mother so many years before. Those who know Paddy well and are aware of the vast amount of time and effort she has put into both my practice and my lecturing, will recognise it was well earned. He then said that she and those close to her were well protected.

Apart from the fact that the medium was unknown to me and that the channelling had been spontaneous and unsolicited, the use of the expression, "the Universe thanks you," was a significant phrase to me; it was in perfect keeping with Dr Letari and my father's cosmic perspective. The timing of the communication was also perfect. It allayed the doubts that had assailed me since deciding to leave practice and focused my vision on a broader future aligned with the purpose of my coming into the physical life. The vision the psychic had of the disseminating lights is an example of dream language in which an image can convey a far clearer and more potent message than any words. My father's urgency is understandable. Imagine the narrow window that synchronicity had provided for him to reach out to his loved ones to give them reassurance and encouragement at a critical time. That the opportunity should arise in 'the circle' sacred to the family was most fitting. The psychic who was involved came into my life unheralded and departed similarly, but I have subsequently heard that she is known for the accuracy of her mediumship.

Although the experiences of psychic phenomena I have described are personal, they are not unique, nor are they uncommon. Importantly, they evidence for all, the intimate immediacy of a world within a world, and the constant dual nature of our existence: physical, intellectual and emotional, yet essentially spiritual. The materialistic world impacts on us remorselessly and seductively, distracting our attention from the esoteric centre of our existence, which is the only reality. The more satisfied we become with the external world, possibly even to the degree of the arrogant complacency experienced by the scientific atheist, the less open we are to the love and promptings of the Cosmos which created us, treasures us and enfolds us. The emissaries of the Infinite are those special beings who walk our path, ever protecting, prompting and inspiring, and, when necessary, chiding us through the voice of our conscience. Our free will is inviolable. Spiritual energy and those who command it surround us, but it is we who must activate the switch, knock that the door may be opened and ask that help may be given!

References

1   Desmond AK. *The Gift of Healing*. London: Psychic Press; 1943. p55.
2   *Ibid.*, p56.

21

PASSING

A spiritual physician

My regular discourses with Dr Letari were of inestimable value and did much to shape my philosophy, my values, my homeopathy and my approach to patients. They extended from my return from England, at the end of 1966, until my father's death in December 1972, a period of six years. These meetings were built on the foundation, which Dr Letari had been putting in place ever since our first meeting in the material world when I was five years of age. The teachings I received were affirmed and consolidated by the example set by my parents.

My father possessed all the qualities a son would expect to find in a man committed to love and service through healing. He was a family man, a loving husband and father. One of his most striking attributes was the sense of confidence, calm, strength and safety one felt in his presence. We experienced this as a family. We felt that he was indestructible and that nothing could possible occur that he could not handle and overcome. We basked in his protective power. This sense of omnipotence extended to his patients. I have spoken to many of them, even after the passing of so many years there are still a number in the practice, and they all stress the faith and confidence he instilled, merely from having spoken to them. His, sometimes wicked, sense of humour was endearing. He was respected and held in high regard by all who knew him professionally. Those who knew him more closely loved him deeply.

He was a spiritual man, not a religious one. Even Spiritualism, which he respected, and to which he owed his original success and fame, was ultimately a means to an end: teaching the truth of survival after death and spreading knowledge of homeopathic medicine. He was particularly interested in the works of Swami Yogananda, e.g. *The Autobiography of a Yogi* and Swami Vivekananda, *The Yogas and Other Works*. Their teachings of Vedanta accorded fully with his own philosophy and the teachings of Dr Letari.

The eclectic

As a young man, he made an intensive study of the homeopathic materia medica and applied himself to maintaining this knowledge throughout his life. He enjoyed reading the great masters of the profession: Hahnemann, Hering, Allen, Bönninghausen, Nash, Kent, Farrington, Dunham and JH Clarke. He was eclectic in his therapeutic approach and studied the work of Johannes Gottfried Rademacher (1772–1849) and James Compton Burnett (1840–1901) and like them practised 'organ prescribing' – the selection of remedies based upon organ affinity – also referred to as 'organ drainage' therapy. He possessed all the editions of *Heal Thyself* edited by the lay-homeopath J Ellis Barker and all the volumes of *Homœopathy* edited by Margaret Tyler. All bear evidence of his close attention. Like Ellis Barker, he made good use of low potency prescribing, adding this method to his use of high and very high potencies. The wide sweep of his therapeutic techniques encompassed the use of homeopathic injectables, administered either subcutaneously or intra-dermally to indicated acupuncture points, or in the case of affected joints over the point of maximum tenderness. He made great use of the Wala range of injectable complexes for spinal and joint conditions.

Nosode therapy always featured high in his treatment strategy: the miasmatic nosodes, the bowel nosodes, nosodes of responsible organisms and auto-nosodes prepared from the patient's blood, serum or discharge. In certain cases, particularly those with autoimmune disease, he would take the patient's serum and run it up to the 200th potency and give this nosode to the patient once or twice per week as an adjunct to constitutional prescribing. In similar cases, he might increase the efficacy of a remedy by giving it simultaneously with the patient's own blood. He would draw up 1ml of the indicated remedy into a syringe, e.g. Rhus-tox 200, and then using the same syringe draw 4 ml of the patient's blood from the right arm. He would shake the syringe a few times to ensure a good mix of blood and remedy and then immediately inject the 5 ml mixture into the muscle of the opposite buttock.

Another adjunct he used when he deemed necessary was low potency complexes. These proved valuable for patients suffering from repeated specific infections often previously treated with many courses of antibiotics, e.g. chronic or recurrent cystitis. Along with the indicated constitutional remedy and possibly a miasmatic nosode, bowel nosode or infection-specific nosode, e.g. Tuberculinum, Sycotic-Co or E. coli 200, he would give a combination of remedies selected for the typical symptoms of the acute aggravation.

R$_x$ Aconitum (monkshood)   6X
       Berberis (barberry)   6X
       Cantharis (Spanish fly)   6X
       Equisetum (horsetail)   6X
       Eupatorium-purp (gravel root) 6X
       Uva ursi (bearberry)   6X

This low potency complex for cystitis would be given two or three times per day to improve resistance, while the prime constitutional remedy was given at selected intervals in higher potency. In the event of a flare up, the same remedy could be used more frequently, e.g. half-hourly. When such a complex worked well, he would review the formula and according to the patient's symptoms select the remedy in the complex he considered most likely to have brought relief and then use it exclusively for future attacks. Often in menopausal women, the cause of the vulnerability to repeated bladder infections is the consequence of low female hormones. In such cases, he would often add a remedy such as Folliculinum 12X to improve the hormone profile.

Likewise, in cases of asthma maintained on steroidal sprays (containing cortisone), bronchodilators, and anti-allergy remedies, he would often employ low potency complexes to assist the patient during the process of withdrawing drugs and establishing curative constitutional therapy. At the same time, he would counter the detrimental effects of the steroids with Cortisone 200 given daily or every other day. In some cases he would add a low potency mix of common asthmatic remedies to be used in a nebuliser or humidifier.

In addition to homeopathy, chiropractic was always an invaluable adjunct to his treatment of patients in both acute and chronic situations. The manipulative techniques he used were taught to him through Dr Letari. These differed in some ways from classic chiropractic, but not radically so. Most unique was his frequent use of the rapid muscular and spinal percussion therapy previously referred to. Realignment of joints was preceded by extensive soft-tissue work, which included both massage and percussion. This afforded him the opportunity, not only to prepare the patient for manipulation, but also, at the same time, to administer spiritual healing through laying-on-of hands. Apart from the obvious purpose of reducing spinal subluxations (minor dislocations), spinal articulation and manipulation was employed to directly affect the major chakra energy centres, which are particularly susceptible to spinal adjustment. The analysis of chakra function always constituted an important part of his diagnosis of a patient's condition. As we shall see later, this appraisal provided him with insight into the miasmatic predominance of a case and the organs or systems most affected. Equally, from the opposite perspective, miasmatic diagnosis and the identification of a specific organ problem would point to a related chakra imbalance.

He was innovative and, like Hahnemann in his Paris years, constantly experimenting with different healing methods. Central always to his treatment strategy, however, was the single remedy that covered the emotional and physical condition of the patient most similarly.

The development of the 'super-succussion' potentiser was an example of this experimental drive. Like Hahnemann, he believed that to be sure of the content and quality of the homeopathic medicines he prescribed, he should prepare and dispense his own remedies. To this end, he built on the well-stocked dispensary he had brought with him from England and eventually the Homœopathic Biochemic Laboratory came into being, supplying other practitioners with homeopathic remedies. He was convinced that trituration in the lower potencies was superior to succussion. He therefore procured ball mills with which to prepare triturates. He started with the biochemic tissues salts, but intended to extend the process to plant remedies. Even during the last year of his life, when his energy was ebbing away, his mind was filled with plans for the expansion and development of his manufacturing ambitions.

His results in practice were remarkable. He was intrepid, undaunted by the worst diagnoses, taking on cases where explanation for improvement by placebo effect, spontaneous remission or mistaken diagnosis would be laughable. His expertise extended to the treatment of acute conditions. He was as competent in dealing with otitis, tonsillitis and bronchitis as he was with rheumatoid arthritis. He was also a responsible physician. Because of his reputation for curing the incurables, many came to him with unrealistic expectations. He was aware of his and homeopathy's parameters, but he also knew that every case, even those that were terminal, could be assisted in some degree, if only to limit emotional and physical suffering.

The power behind the throne

My mother complemented him fully. In an introspective moment, Father once said to me, "My son, your mother is a far, far, better woman than I am a man!" This tribute speaks volumes. Their marriage was forged on a deep and abiding love and respect for one another. The trials my father endured strengthened the bonds between them and my mother, who was a confident woman with a good head for business, increasingly assumed an administrative role in all his affairs as the years passed. They were a very successful team and devoted to one another. Their compatibility extended from their common background and service to homeopathy to a passion for gardening and a shared taste in food, music and the arts. They were avid filmgoers and for years both Monday and Friday nights were devoted to the cinema. In their fifties, they took up ballroom dancing and this became a great joy for them; a pleasure they indulged regularly until father's health made it no longer possible. If there was a weakness in their union it lay in its strength. It was difficult to envisage the one without the other. How would either survive such a loss? This was to prove a valid concern.

Deteriorating health

> It is very necessary that you be careful. The power of the spirit flows, not in one continuous stream, but in well regulated measure, and you must close the tap again and again.

This warning of Silver Birch had not been without reason. Father was not careful. The tap was rarely closed. His drive to help others and promote homeopathy could not be halted or diminished. Probably, even before these cautionary words from the guide were uttered, damage had been done. The heavy schedule of repeated and often prolonged trance states, ectoplasmic surgery and healing extending over years exacted their penalty. Intense psychic work of this kind, especially when associated with healing, has a powerful effect upon the energy field of the body, impacting particularly upon the third or solar plexus chakra, which, true to its name, radiates power both psychically and physically. This chakra is also the seat of ego-power and is linked to our vitality, our drive, our ambition, our confidence and our will. The sequence of ordeals William had braved and overcome had further taxed this vital centre, which is intimately associated with the functions of the pancreas and the adrenal glands. The extreme demands accelerated inherited and constitutional tendencies and brought about a rapid and uncontrollable breakdown in his state of health.

Raised blood pressure, which first assailed him at 50, was the first sign of trouble. Apart from an occasional solitary cigarette that he nursed and cherished every now and again, he stopped smoking. Two years later, his blood sugar started to rise; diabetes was setting in. There was no family history of the disease. I had just returned from my studies in England, flush with medical and homeopathic knowledge and I was powerless. Once the collapse of pancreatic function had begun, it continued to deteriorate precipitously despite diet and combined homeopathic and orthodox oral medication. Within a short time, he was dependent on insulin injections to survive. No sooner was a successful regimen adopted than he swung out of control again and had to be re-evaluated. The specialist physician who attended him said his condition gave meaning to the old term, fragile diabetes. No answer was found, his sugar levels continued to swing unpredictably as did his blood pressure and the male family tendency to develop arteriosclerosis increased apace. Soon he developed the first signs of congestive cardiac failure. These were staved off for a time with a homeopathic complex of mother tinctures containing Crataegus (hawthorn), Cactus (night-blooming cereus) and Strophanthus (kombe seed), but there was no halting the inexorable collapse of his body.

In defiance of his illness, he pressed on with his practice as long as he could. His resolve to serve his patients was remarkable, but could not last. Finally his last reserves were exhausted and he had to capitulate. When he could no longer drive to his rooms, we knew his time for departure had come.

Passing

On the evening of 17 December 1972, William passed into spirit joining his beloved mentor Dr Letari and the team of spirit doctors that had worked with him for over forty years. Although only fifty-eight, he had lived a life packed with event, challenge and achievement and could look back on a life well spent in service to homeopathy and humanity

I recorded the séances my mother and I had with Dr Letari during the last months of my father's life; these remain treasured items in the family archive. The good Doctor had many words of advice for me about the future and many words of love and reassurance for my mother, who had suffered with my father every step of his decline, just as she had shared every step of his ascent to success. He told us that his mediator's arduous healing mission had contributed to his deteriorating health, but that given the impelling purpose, the public need and my father's drive there could have been no other outcome. Mother understood this fully as she did the fact that there is no such thing as death. Before retiring to bed on the night of father's passing, she noted in her diary, simply, "Bill died 11 p.m." She then scored through the word 'died' and wrote above it, "was reborn." Despite this conviction, her grief was to prove deep and inconsolable.

Father's funeral was held at the Pretoria crematorium on Friday, 22 December. Although for our mother's sake, Margaret and I wished to restrict the invitations to family and close friends, this proved impossible. He was a very public figure, had a huge practice and was loved and respected by so many colleagues, friends and patients. Everyone who knew him desired to pay their last respects. As at all his public lectures, the chapel was filled to overflowing. The ceremony, which honoured the passing of a very special person, was deeply moving. My mother's diary entry for that day reads, "Laid to rest so beautifully".

After the ceremony there was no chance of a quick escape; those wishing to express their sympathy and condolences surrounded us. In retrospect, the remembered images are gratifying. We were the recipients of so much empathy and love; but at the time the experience was harrowing, every tear in the eye of a sympathiser touched a resonating chord within. When it was over, the immediate family gathered at my home and we sat in the peace of the garden, seeking to fill a gaping void with togetherness.

We were prepared for my father's passing; it was not a shock; indeed, after such a painfully protracted though rapid deterioration in his health and strength, it came as release and relief; nonetheless, we were left stunned. It was as if our sun had set, never to rise again. I have much respect for the power of grief; it can be likened to the sea, for it is oceanic. It possesses unseen depths; it has its waves, it has its tides, and it has its calms, when all seems still and tranquil; but beneath, in its dark, unfathomable reaches monsters dwell. No emotion, other than continuous, prolonged fear, can prove as devastating to physical health. As a family, we had been richly blessed with personal evidence of the continuity of existence and survival after death, yet we were bereft. As my father so often said, at such times, the human state prevails, because even the deepest conviction of life everlasting does not fill one's arms or occupy the chair at the head of the table. As much as there is joy in reunion, there will be grief at parting. Our bereavement was doubled because in a moment my mother lost two husbands, and Margaret and I lost two fathers.

Emotions

My grief

His departure left a huge hiatus in my life both personally and professionally. His entire practice was now added to mine, so I was able to turn aside from grief and compensate for my loss through intense involvement in homeopathy and the sport I loved: long-distance road cycling. I became detached from the reality of my emotions, which I characteristically ignored and homeopathically neglected, and from the needs of my wife and family. The latter contributed to an estrangement between Annette and myself, which eventually resulted in our divorce, and Dorian and Troye, our sons, suffered from having an absent father. On the surface, I seemed to have taken my father's death in my stride, but in my depths all was not well.

My particular physical weakness after cerebral meningitis was a tendency to develop tonsillitis too easily from typical winter colds. This was amenable to acute homeopathic prescribing, so much so that I neglected considering its constitutional underpinning. True to form, during the winter following father's death I picked up a cold, which soon developed into a severe follicular tonsillitis, more severe than I had ever previously experienced. I had always managed to push my way through such infections without missing a day at practice, but this time, due to the severity of the attack, replete with a viciously sore throat, intermittent fever and utter prostration, I was forced to capitulate and take to my bed. My body was slow to react to the usually successful treatment. My throat gradually settled, but I began to develop alarming joint pains, most severe in my wrists, finger joints, knees and neck. A throat swab and blood tests revealed that I had developed rheumatic fever, a condition that can cause damage to the valves of the heart. The pathologist friend who did the tests was concerned that I should commence antibiotic therapy immediately. I had never resorted to antibiotics in the past, and I was sure that I would be able to cure myself homeopathically. It is said that the doctor who attempts to treat himself has a fool for physician. This may be true, but my doctor proved competent enough. I took the nosode Streptococcus in the 200th potency twice daily and Rhamnus californica (from the California coffee tree) 200 every two hours. Rhamnus is known for its ability to cure acute inflammatory rheumatism and to protect the heart against valvular damage. Once I commenced this regime, my condition rapidly improved.

I was soon back at work, free of pains, but somewhat lacking my usual vitality. Impatient to regain my fitness and typically unheeding of this residual tiredness, I started cycling again. For a few days I managed fairly well then I started to lose both strength and stamina and was forced to discontinue. I satisfied myself that I had no signs of heart involvement. I rested, treated myself and after a week, feeling better, risked another ride. This time, I managed no more than 12 miles (20 km) before I felt an unfamiliar tiredness overwhelming me. I turned about and rode home at a careful pace. I then backed off entirely from exercise, finding that I had only sufficient energy to see me through each day at my busy practice. Six weeks passed by in this way, and I began to increasingly look forward to the holiday Annette and I had planned for October in Umhalanga Rocks, near Durban in Natal. We had included my mother in these arrangements in the hope that a change of environment and time spent with her two grandsons would lift her spirits. The holiday came just in time because a few days before I closed practice, I started another infection, which knocked me off my feet. Although this time the infection seemed trivial, the exhaustion that attended the slightly sore throat and irritating cough I developed was profound. I was utterly prostrated and the drive to the holiday resort left me feeling like an invalid.

My joy

While the family, enjoyed time on the beach and other holiday activities, I remained confined to the environs of the hotel, unable to muster the strength to join them. I spent my time reading and relaxing, but instead of improving, I seemed to become wearier as the days passed. I had brought only the minimum of remedies with me, but this made little difference for by this stage the doctor and patient had truly merged into the fool. One evening, I felt even the short walk to the dining room would prove too far for me. Annette and the rest of the family decided to eat out for supper so I ordered a snack in our room, and then settled down on the bed intending to read. I had hardly managed a few pages when the tiredness I had felt all day overwhelmed me. After I had read the same paragraph a number of times without grasping its meaning, I gave in, turned off the lights and within seconds sleep overcame me.

Suddenly, I was aware of being on the astral plane, free of my body and standing beside the bed. Before me a figure materialised and I recognised my father standing some distance from me at the far end of the room. He was wearing the old-fashioned doctor's white coat, buttoned to the throat and reaching to the ankle, that he had worn in Leeds so long ago.

My memory of him was the attenuated, gaunt, ailing man whom I had so desperately wished to keep with us against my better judgement. I had a photograph, taken less than a year before his passing, which I cherished and kept on me. He and I are standing in front of his greenhouse. I have my arm about his shoulders and he is smiling and proudly holding up for the camera, one in each hand, two young tomato plants. He was not yet fifty-eight, but looked older than I do now at seventy-two. In the ten months since his death, I had often dreamed of him. The theme of the dreams was repetitive. He was desperately ill, ravaged by sickness and I was frantically trying to save him. My efforts were always fruitless. The emotions I experienced in those dreams were infinitely more intense than any I experienced during his years of illness, even when I stood beside my mother looking at his lifeless body in the hospital bed and my mother took his gold watch from his wrist and placed it on mine. I would waken from those dreams racked with sobs, feeling as if my heart had been torn out of my chest.

This haggard, broken person was not the figure I saw standing before me now. He was again in the full bloom of adult youth; surely no older than his late twenties or early thirties, yet vested with all the maturity, dignity and presence of a far older being. He was magnificent. Radiance streamed from him, lighting up the room. While time stood still, he looked at me silently and intently. I became aware that there was a vast power emanating from him and that I was standing in an ocean of love, which surrounded me, held me and permeated my entire being. He came towards me, took me in his arms and embraced me with infinite love and tenderness. I felt suspended in time and space, the deepest part of me caught in a beatific moment of ecstatic bliss. Still holding me in his arms, he expressed his love for me and told me the remedy he wished me to take: Aurum metallicum (gold). With that his presence, his power and his radiance slowly ebbed away, try as I might to hold him back. A moment later, I was awake, filled to overflowing with gratitude for the blessed visitation and weeping tears of joy.

That was the end of my grief. It was also the beginning of my recovery. I never looked back. I took the remedy he had advised. Within days of the psychic experience my strength and energy were restored. The photograph I had kept close to me for ten months now had only sentimental value and I packed it away with others from the past. In its place, I resurrected old studio portraits, taken in 1939 and the early 1940s at the time Richards was promoting the Hunslet Sanctuary. Father was not quite thirty years-of-age. These provide the closest resemblance to how he appeared to me in spirit. The one dearest to me, which was used most frequently by the *Psychic News* during his British heyday, stands on a small easel beside me as I type. In some measure it captures the combination of youth, strength and wisdom that his vision portrayed.

My mother's sorrow

My mother's sadness weighed heavily on the family. I hoped that she would derive as much benefit from my father's spirit appearance as I had. When the family returned to the hotel, I gave her a graphic and emotional account of what I had witnessed. She was deeply moved and uplifted, but the joy it brought her did not last. Her entire life had been devoted to William and his work, and her closeness to Dr Letari had been a constant inspiration to her, guiding and sustaining her through the long and arduous journey she had shared with my father. With their absence part of her died and even her grandchildren could not compensate for her loss. She went through the motions of life, administering the affairs of the Homeopathic Biochemic Laboratory, maintaining her friendships, taking up bowls and as always finding comfort in her immaculately groomed garden, but deep within, her grief was pervasive and persistent. Its erosive effect had dire consequences. Six years after father's death, she quite suddenly developed problems with her speech. It started with word hunting; difficulty in finding the correct words with which to express herself and the names of people well known to her. The glass of wine she so enjoyed each evening for the relaxation it afforded began to make her feel as if she had consumed an entire bottle. Suspecting a minor stroke, I referred her to a physician friend who specialised in neurology and he advised a brain scan, but she declined, telling him that "what would be would be" and that she was not concerned about any outcome her symptoms might indicate. A week later these had increased and I managed to persuade her to consent to the investigation if only for the family's sake. I was sat beside her when the result of the scan was made known: a brain tumour, suspected of being malignant and aggressive.

Transcending disease

I will never forget my mother's response. She turned to me with a radiant expression and there was laughter in her eyes, which had been absent for years, as she exclaimed, "Oh! David, I will soon be with your father!" She then gave me a very pointed look as she sternly said, while wagging her finger at me, "Don't you dare give me anything to hold me back." Surgery and radiation therapy were advised. These she proudly refused. It was remarkable to see how someone who had been given such a dread diagnosis could experience sustained elation when contemplating the inevitable consequence. She had no fear of death; she welcomed it with open arms.

I approached one of my teachers at medical school, an ex-professor of medicine, who had left academic medicine to return to private practice, and asked him if he would care for my mother when it became necessary to have her admitted to hospital. He kindly consented to do so and mother found in him a good friend, an older man whom she could talk to openly about her longing to be with "Bill" and her acceptance of her illness. She told him that it was her ticket for a wondrous journey that she looked forward to with excitement and anticipation. He was quite taken with her buoyancy and her unswerving conviction of survival after death. He told her that having seen the scans he agreed with her decision not to accept either surgery or oncology. He promised to make her passing as comfortable as possible.

Paddy was in the final weeks of her second pregnancy when my mother began to show her warning symptoms. Brigitte, our daughter was born on the 22 November. Mother was still at home and therefore had the opportunity of holding her new granddaughter in her arms. Using Silver Birch's words, one Lilley lady arrived just as another was about to depart. Within days of Brigitte's birth it became necessary to have mother admitted to hospital. She steadily deteriorated and finally became comatose, partly drug induced and partly due to her advancing condition. This continued for some days and we thought that she was already lost to us, but as often happens towards the end, when death is imminent, she unexpectedly rallied and broke through the coma with complete clarity of mind and speech. Paddy and I, together with Margaret and her husband Peter, were with her when this happened. She emerged as if from a deep sleep and when her thoughts had cleared, she looked at me most accusingly and demanded to know why she was still alive. I reassured her that it would not be long before she would be with my father. She remained completely lucid for a number of hours, during which she held court with a sense of humour and joyfulness, which had been absent for so long. While we should have been there to comfort her and lift her spirits, it was she who gave us encouragement and strength to face our sorrow. This short period provided us with our last image of her, smiling, teasing and light-hearted. She had returned to say goodbye and to dispel our grief with the knowledge that she was content and ready to leave the earth plane. During the night, she lapsed back into a coma from which she did not return.

She lived long enough for her brother, Wilfred Overton, who had witnessed the Helen Duncan materialisation séance, and his wife Nellie, to see her before she passed. Their holiday in South Africa from Leeds had been arranged almost a year before. Not knowing how much time there remained, we took them to the hospital from the airport. She was unaware of their presence, but it was of great importance to my uncle that he was able to kiss her farewell. In the early hours of the next morning, the 5th of December, five weeks after her diagnosis was made, she slipped away into the realm of spirit to be reunited with her beloved Bill and Dr Letari.

When, some days later, Paddy went to the hospital to collect Nancy's possessions, the matron in charge approached her. She felt she had to tell Paddy what a remarkable patient Mrs Lilley had been and how she had proved such an inspiration for all the staff that had nursed her. They had never before experienced a terminal patient possessing such complete conviction of life after death, welcoming the process of dying with serenity and displaying such a grateful, participatory attitude towards all that had to be done for her. She had been an example to everyone.

Eternal youth

It was six months before she came to me. As with my father's visitation, I found myself on the astral plane and there she was standing before me glorious and most beautiful, a golden girl-woman, her blue eyes dancing, her blonde hair loose and hanging in profusion to her waist, as I had never seen her before. I was surrounded by the power of her love and her rapture, which caressed and energised me. For a precious moment we embraced, then she withdrew, melting away into the ether; her exquisite face, bestowing upon me a tender glance of love, still lingers in my memory. No words were necessary. Her communication to me was at soul level, far removed from verbal expression. I woke glowing with warmth and my eyes overflowing with tears of joy. Although I have seen my father on a number of occasions, mother has never appeared to me again.

Messenger of Trust

My father touched the lives of many, bringing them a message of trust; trust in self, in life and in the creation. He brought healing to those who were deemed incurable and uplifted those who were spiritually bereft. His life was an example of complete commitment and dedication to the cause of spirit and to the cause of homeopathy, which he regarded as inseparable. His life was touched with mystery, a mystery that transported him from a Yorkshire village onto the main stage of life where he acquitted himself with accomplishment and honour. He left deep footprints that will endure for an age to come.

22

THE EGO-SELF:
THE DISEASE OF THE SOUL

Healing the soul

Through the histories of Samuel Hahnemann and William Lilley, I have been able to bring together two vital threads essential to the art of healing: the science of homeopathy and the science of spirit. We have considered the fundamental laws upon which homeopathy is based and contemplated the spiritual nature of the human being. From these deliberations, we understand that constitutional disease is a state of the soul, witnessed in the signs and symptoms of the mind and body, but most singularly in the unique profile of the patient's ego-self (ego-personality). The disease of the soul is expressed at its deepest level in the inherent and characteristic traits, emotions, feelings, values and behaviour of this psychological structure. *The ego-self is, therefore, that part of the soul that requires healing.* The healing of the soul is synonymous with the dismantling of the ego-self and resolving its intense attachments, and synonymous with the path of spiritual attainment, enlightenment or self-realisation, termed by Carl Gustav Jung – the process of individuation.

Life: an initiation

The life of the individual is a sacred initiation, a rite of passage, perfectly designed in every aspect to provide the soul in transit with the experiences and challenges essential for its spiritual unfolding. The elements that provide the rite of passage are the body, mind and constitution of the soul's physical vehicle, the situations, events and circumstances that arise in the course of the soul's physical life, the ego-self that cloaks the spiritual qualities of the soul and the constellation of beings with whom the soul interacts. All these elements are part of the soul's destiny and are therefore not random or subject to chance; they are ordained and synchronised to the responses of the soul, determined by its free-will and freedom of choice. They are tailored to the weaknesses and strengths of the developing soul, always with the objective of awakening it from its spiritual slumber. They may, therefore, be considered a divine prescription for the disease of the soul. Sometimes, the hardened nature of the ego-self is such that distressing and even tragic happenings may be required to bring realisation to the soul that this being with whom it identifies is actually its implacable adversary, bent, through means both devious and destructive, on maintaining its existence, usurping the sovereignty of the soul and impeding its growth: an enemy that must be overthrown.

Mythology and archetypes

The stage and setting for this conflict is created even to the meanest detail by the loving and healing power of the cosmic intelligence; the events choreographed to perfection to coax, urge and goad the soul into the role of hero for which it was created. In this scenario of predestined events and immortal actors playing out their divinely appointed roles, we enter the world of mythology and archetypes; a world portrayed in great works of art, sculpture, literature, poetry and music and dramatised in ballet, opera, plays and on film. It is the fertile world of our dreams, our imagination and our fantasy, rich with metaphor, allegory and analogy, seemingly a fiction, but pregnant with wisdom and meaning. It is also the world of the collective or universal unconscious in which the eternal archetypal themes and personages are to be found and into which our deep unconscious taps when energised by the advent of significant events or in response to homeopathic potencies with which the unconscious resonates. Fathoming the unconscious depths in either way causes images to surface wrapped in dreams, imaginings (delusions) and fears; images which relate deeply to the struggle between the true-self and the false- or ego-self. They are responses to influences, circumstantial and homeopathic, that can heal the soul and empower it in the protracted encounter with its perennial foe.

The mortal engagement is archetypal, the adversaries are archetypal and the combat has a rich mythological tradition. An example is the legend of St George and the Dragon; a heroic and iconic portrayal of the classic struggle between the forces of good and evil. Though familiar, and common in one form or another to the folklore of many cultures, the story is based on a far more profound and primal myth in which the god *Apollo* slays the monstrous serpent *Python* in the sacred precinct of the oracle at Delphi; a myth echoed in the slaying of *Medusa* by the hero *Perseus*. Often, a magnificent steed, sometimes winged, gifted with human speech and psychic powers accompanies the hero; a chthonic creature, able to guide and transport its rider (the soul) through the dark realms of the underworld (the unconscious) to confront and overcome the dragon (the ego-self) in its lair and achieve the priceless treasure it guards (the Self). The heroic horse (or other *familiar* or totem creature) is a metaphor for the forces aligned with the soul in its quest for spiritual perfection: grace, spirit inspirers (guardian angels), human seers and companions, and not least of all – *constitutionally selected homeopathic remedies*. The ancient Greek term *psychopomp*, 'guide of souls', perfectly describes the archetypal role played by the helpful beings, creatures and remedies that assist and mediate for the hero soul in its essential passage through the realms of the unconscious.

Such legends of valour and gallantry, cowardice and villainy, represent ancient analyses of the ambivalent human state depicted in archetypal form: allegories more graphic and visceral than the pragmatic appraisal of modern psychoanalysis. They depict the many and varied ways in which the archetypal struggle between the higher and the lower self is enacted within each of us. This battleground of the soul is the terrain on which the ego-based disease of the soul originates. Born of the clash of archetypal energies, disease is also archetypal; its effects manifested in the emotional and intellectual life and the physical constitution of the individual, first functionally and eventually structurally. To initiate a healing process, remedies must be able to act at the soul level of causation; to act at the deepest level they must be chosen for their archetypal relationship to the patient's ego-self and destined role. The major homeopathic remedies drawn from the mineral, plant and animal kingdoms are iconic and powerfully archetypal, e.g. Aurum (gold), Quercus (from the oak tree) and Lac leoninum (from the lion). When selected for their archetypal and remedial similarity to the circumstances, ego-profile and the symptoms and signs of the patient, they have the power to heal. They induce a curative cascade, initiated at the soul/ego interface, a cascade that permeates the entire constitution from the mental and emotional sphere to cellular level.

The battleground of the soul

Although the struggle for supremacy between the soul and the ego-self is expressed in terms of warfare between opposing forces, the imagery is allegorical. Within the text of the Hindu epic, *Mahabarata*, nestles a profound spiritual scripture: the *Bhagavad Gita – The Song of God*, comprising 700 verses of dialogue between the hero-prince Arjuna and his spirit guide Lord Krishna. The setting for the transmission of the divine message, which emerges from their dialogue and transcends religion, is fittingly the centre of a battlefield. This stage allegorically represents the terrain of the prolonged campaign that must be waged by the soul in its efforts to resolve the internal war between good and evil and overcome the tyranny of the ego-self, the cause of all its suffering and sorrow.

For the ego-self, and for the soul strongly identified with this tyrannical child conceived from its own fears, the battlefield is a reality. The ego-self gains recognition, identity and strength from the spotlight that opposition and conflict provides and in the face of its inflated image, the soul so often capitulates and lapses into acquiescence or slumber. The strategy the soul needs to employ in disempowering the ego-self, rather than resistance and struggle (so akin to the conventional medical model of treating disease, which only suppresses and drives disease deeper), must be after the fashion of the martial arts exponent: using the energy generated by the opponent to unseat him (so akin to the homeopathic model: using an energy most similar to cure disease). The self-serving, acquisitive energy of the ego-self needs to be redirected, channelled and sublimated through trust, love and service, thus enabling the soul to transcend the ego's selfish demands.

Ego intrigue

As we all experience, the ego-self does not easily yield its dominance. It fights tooth and nail for survival, using all the considerable means at its disposal – fear, attachment, diversion and seduction – to numb the soul to the siren call of the Self and to maintain the soul's identification with the ego. It feeds on the soul's lack of basic trust and swings the soul's focus, to varying degree, in either of two directions, a religious or scientific perspective, the extremes of which become fundamentalism. The central position between the religious or scientific inclination or bias is a neutral, apathetic, indifferent, 'live life as it comes' attitude: an indolence of the soul.

On the religious side, the ego-self lulls the soul into a state of unthinking, ingenuous dependency on texts, doctrines, rituals and traditions; the mediation of masters, saints and gurus; and redemption through the vicarious suffering of saviours. The ego-self eludes the attentions of the soul through enlisting the right anterior cerebral neo-cortex to its cause, with all its propensity for ungrounded, irrational conclusions based on romantic fantasy, wishful thinking and unrestrained imagination. While this female energy holds sway, the soul is mesmerised by the ego into believing myth to be fact. If the masculine left anterior neo-cortex should accept this delusion, another dimension of distorted ego thinking and perceiving is added, which at its worst may submerge the soul in the rampant passion of militant, religious fanaticism. In this pathological development, which is a manifestation of the ego-disease that afflicts the soul, we see the sweep of archetypal energy moving cerebrally from right to left. When this inner disease is vented externally, the somatic (physical) symptoms will be seen to move in the opposite direction: from left to right. These are signs of vital importance to the homeopathic physician, aiding in the choice of remedy, which through similarity weakens and eventually nullifies the insidious influence of the ego-self. This left to right movement of physical symptoms is a dominant characteristic of the serpent archetype, exemplified to its fullest extent in the remedy picture of the Brazilian bushmaster pit viper, *Lachesis muta*.

In this day and age, when left-cerebral dominance is strongly encouraged from our earliest school years and the importance of the arts is played-down, the ego-self easily recruits the intellect – the rational, masculine mind – into its service, duping the soul into disbelief with persuasive arguments against the existence of a loving, caring Supreme Intelligence. For the soul viewing life through the filters created by the materialistic, earth-bound ego-self there is no divine playwright, choreographer or composer creating, orchestrating and conducting the play of world events; life remorselessly unfolds driven by merciless, insentient, universal forces acting arbitrarily without purposeful design. Whereas the problems stemming from religion's repression of the soul are often mitigated by morality and faith, the arid doctrine of reductionism extolled by scientific atheists leaves the soul almost entirely under the command of an arrogant, blinkered ego-self that struts its materialistic philosophy, viewing with contempt any belief in a spiritual dimension. The ego stills the small voice of the soul by convincing the soul that it does not exist. The masculine intellect overrides the sensibilities of feminine intuition; the logic of the left anterior neo-cortex inhibits the imaginative creativity of the right anterior neo-cortex. Here the archetypal energy sweeps cerebrally from left to right resulting in somatic symptoms that commence on the right and move to the left, a symptom characteristic of the key remedy picture of Lycopodium (club moss or wolf's foot).

Lachesis and Lycopodium are central remedies of the homeopathic materia medica and therefore pivotal to the treatment of disease at the level of the ego-self. They are frequently called for, they are compatible and complement one another well, and, as seen in the movement of their healing energy, together embrace a wide spectrum of human emotion, especially centred about the critical interplay between the masculine (right) and the feminine (left) principles; conflict, turbulence and imbalance in the fundamental relationship of these principles lies at the root of so much human distress and suffering. Two major remedies, Carcinosin (a nosode prepared from breast cancer) and Lac caninum (a sarcode prepared from dog's milk), stand shoulder-to-shoulder with Lachesis and Lycopodium in this regard; both are noted for their affinity for constitutions showing a shift of symptoms back and forth, from one side to another; both are more inclined to produce, and therefore cure, symptoms commencing on the left side, migrating to the right and then swinging back to the left, showing their kinship with the injured feminine: a theme that is central to human disease. These four cardinal archetypal remedies stand at the very core of the homeopathic arsenal and will be studied comprehensively as we delve deeper into the healing of the soul.

The scientific atheists are unwittingly in league with the ego-self when they assert that matter is the only reality. They would respond with incredulity if informed that their campaign to erase religious faith and replace it with the cold doctrine of a soulless existence in a soulless universe empowers the ego-self at the expense of the soul and must contribute to ego-based disease. Similarly the dependency, bigotry, exclusiveness and superstition fostered by religious teachings represses the development of the soul, sows the seeds of difference and division, invites partisanship and conflict and plays into the propensities of the ego-self: the disease from which the soul suffers.

When, in the narrative of the *Bhagavad Gita*, Prince Arjuna stands in his chariot on the sacred battlefield of Kurukshetra between opposing forces of kinsmen, he is dismayed at the prospect of a bloody, fratricidal war and turns to his divine charioteer Krishna for counsel. This is the scenario facing the homeopathic physician wishing to practise *depth homeopathy*. No matter the nature of the disease that presents, the opposing forces arrayed behind the symptoms and signs are those of the clash between the soul and the ego-self, the hero and the usurper, blood brothers locked in combat. This knowledge is of inestimable value to the physician in giving counsel and selecting the indicated remedy; and also to the patient, because the overcoming of disease necessitates gaining ascendency over the whims, needs and intrigues of the ego-self. Treatment at this level is directly related to the spiritual unfoldment of the patient and has to be a project in which physician and patient collaborate with a common goal. Ideally, both should be conversant with the spiritual nature and purpose of life and perceive the healing power of disease. Homeopathic remedies align with this power and take the patient forward physically and spiritually.

Although this life is seemingly so tangible and real, in contrast to the greater Reality that supports and projects it, it is an illusion. Life's reality lies in its potential to challenge our complacency and provide opportunities for us to gain experience, exercise morality, give service and regain sovereignty over the ego. In this sense it is real and deeply meaningful, but, paradoxically, it is also grand theatre, unfolding dramas not only in the life of individuals, but often on a massive scale, as in the two World Wars. In a moment, a tsunami, a volcanic eruption or an earthquake can kill thousands and leave destruction, poverty, homelessness and famine in their wake. Despite appearances, the calamity, including all the bereavement, suffering and hardship it brings, does not possess the reality we weight it with. The happening is an illusion, an essential fiction, providing a stage for the immortal actors on the platform of life to fulfil their roles. The response to the happening is the personal reality of the actor; the opportunity for spiritual growth provided by the happening is the reality within the fiction. No one can die, all the participants are immortal; life on the earth plane is always transient and as precious as it may seem cannot be compared with our natural life in the spirit world. The experience of all those directly or indirectly involved in any disaster or tragedy, is as it needs to be, perfectly designed to catalyse change, to stir the soul and awaken it from its ego induced slumber, to provide it with circumstances that will induce it to rise above the interests, demands and preferences of the ego-self and concern itself with loving and serving others.

The ego is characteristically self-indulgent, self-centred and complacent, attached to pleasure and power, steeped in the senses, fixed in its habits and resistant to any change that discomforts or displeases it. When life ruffles its feathers, it becomes petulant, impatient, intolerant and resentful. Like a spoilt child, the ego-self has a sense of expectation and entitlement; it is a fair weather friend of fortune. At first, the shocks of life may harden and embitter the ego-self, arousing hatred against God and humanity, often driving it to perpetrate despicable acts and atrocities: impingements and transgressions which paradoxically transpire according to spiritual laws; laws which are impenetrable to us, since we lack the vantage point to survey and analyse the inexorable co-ordinates of destiny, which with immaculate precision bring people together at a fateful moment. Life never tires in its ceaseless efforts to dethrone the ego-self and prompt the soul to come out of hibernation. It may take lifetimes, many shocks and much coercion, but eventually the trials which the ego-self and soul are subjected to will weaken even the most recalcitrant ego-self and move the tardy soul to realise and express its nobility.

Maya – the illusion of life

In Sanskrit, the language of the ancient Hindu scriptures, the illusion of life is called *maya*. A simple parable related by the great spiritual teacher Vivekananda illustrates the illusory nature of life encompassed by this word. When attempting to grasp the ineffable workings of the cosmic intelligence, we have to resort to myth rather than logic to explain the inexplicable. In this sphere of understanding, myth transcends logic. I shall quote the seer's story of *maya* as he related it.

> **The Story of *Maya***
>
> A legend tells how once Nārada said to Krishna, 'Lord, show me māyā.' A few days passed, and Krishna asked Nārada to make a trip with Him towards a forest. After walking several miles, Krishna said, 'Nārada, I am thirsty; can you fetch some water for Me? 'I will go at once, Sir, and get you water.' So Nārada went.
>
> At a little distance there was a village. He entered the village in search of water and knocked at a door, which was opened by a most beautiful young girl. At the sight of her, he immediately forgot that his Master was waiting for water, perhaps dying for want of it. He forgot everything and began to talk with the girl. Gradually the talk ripened into love. He asked the father for the daughter, and they were married and lived there and had children.
>
> Thus twelve years passed. His father-in-law died; he inherited his property. He lived, as he seemed to think, a very happy life with his wife and children, his fields and his cattle, and so forth. Then came a flood. One night the river rose until it overflowed its banks and flooded the whole village. Houses fell, men and animals were swept away and drowned, and everything was floating in the rush of the stream. Nārada had to escape. With one hand he held his wife, and with the other two of his children; another child was on his shoulders, and he was trying to ford this tremendous flood. After a few steps, he found the current was too strong, and the child on his shoulders fell and was borne away. A cry of despair came from Nārada. In trying to save that child, he lost his grasp upon the others, and they also were lost. At last his wife, whom he clasped with all his might, was torn away by the current, and he was thrown on the bank, weeping and wailing in bitter lamentation.
>
> Behind him there came a gentle voice: 'My child, where is the water? You went to fetch a pitcher of water, and I am waiting for you. You have been gone quite half an hour.' 'Half an hour!' Nārada exclaimed. Twelve whole years had passed through his mind, and all these scenes had happened in half an hour!
>
> And this is māyā. In one form or another we are all in it. It is a most difficult and intricate state of things to understand. It has been preached in every country, taught everywhere, but only believed in by a few, because until we get the experience ourselves we cannot believe in it.[1]

The Song Celestial

In the *Bhagavad Gita*, Lord Krishna, the spirit guide of Arjuna, reveals to the prince – when he is reflecting with despair on the possible death of beloved family members and close friends – the deathless, eternal, indestructible nature of the soul and its spirit (the *Atman*: the divine essence of the soul).

> Your words are wise, Arjuna, but your sorrow is for nothing. The truly wise mourn neither for the living nor the dead.
>
> There was never a time when I did not exist, nor you, nor any of these kings. Nor is there any future in which we shall cease to be.
>
> Just as the dweller in this body passes through childhood, youth and old age, so at death he merely passes into another kind of body; the wise are not deceived by that.
>
> Feelings of heat and cold, pleasure and pain, are caused by the contact of the senses with their objects. They come and go, never lasting long. You must accept them.
>
> A serene spirit accepts pleasure and pain with an even mind, and is unmoved by either.
>
> That which is non-existent can never come into being, and that which is can never cease to be. Those who have known the inmost Reality know also the nature of *is* and *is not* (the difference between what is Reality and what is illusion).
>
> That Reality which pervades the universe is indestructible. No one has the power to change the Changeless.
>
> Bodies are said to die, but That which possesses the body is eternal. It cannot be limited, or destroyed. Therefore you must fight (overcome the limitations and lies of the ego-self).[2]

> Know this Atman (Spirit; Self)
> Unborn, undying,
> Never ceasing,
> Never beginning,
> Deathless, birthless,
> Unchanging for ever.
> How can it die
> The death of the body
>
> Worn-out garments
> Are shed by the body:
> Worn-out bodies
> Are shed by the dweller
> Within the body.
> New bodies are donned
> By the dweller, like garments.

> Not wounded by weapons,
> Not burned by fire,
> Not dried by the wind,
> Not wetted by water:
> Such is the Atman ...[2]

Arjuna then asks Krishna how one might identify a soul that has freed itself from bondage to the ego-self; how might one recognise such a person? Krishna emphasises the dispassionate, unattached nature of such a soul; qualities at total variance with the inclinations of the ego-self.

> Not shaken by adversity,
> Not hankering after happiness:
> Free from fear, free from anger,
> Free from the things of desire.
> I call him a seer and illumined.
> The bonds of his flesh are broken (the bonds of the ego-self,
>   the senses and the body).
> He is lucky and he does not rejoice:
> He is unlucky, and he does not weep.
> I call him illumined.
>
> The abstinent run away from what they desire
> But carry their desires with them:
> When a man enters Reality,
> He leaves his desires behind him.

Krishna warns of the seductive power of the ego-self, which should never be underestimated.

> Even a mind that knows the path
> Can be dragged from the path:
> The senses are so unruly.
>
> Thinking about sense-objects
> Will attach you to sense-objects:
> Grow attached, and you become addicted;
> Thwart your addiction, it turns to anger;
> Be angry, and you confuse your mind;
> Confuse your mind, you forget the lesson of experience;
> Forget experience, you lose discrimination;
> Lose discrimination, and you miss life's only purpose.
>
> When he has no lust, no hatred,
> A man walks safely among things of lust and hatred.
> To obey the Atman (hearken to the inner voice of the Self)
> Is his peaceful joy:
> Sorrow melts
> Into that clear peace ...

> The wind turns a ship
> From its course on the waters:
> The wandering wind of the senses
> Cast man's mind adrift
> And turn his better judgement from its course.
> When a man can still the senses
> I call him illumined.
> The recollected mind is awake
> In the knowledge of the Atman
> Which is dark night to the ignorant:
> The ignorant are awake in their sense-life
> Which they think is daylight:
> To the seer it is darkness.
>
> Water flows continually into the ocean
> But the ocean is never disturbed:
> Desire flows into the mind of the seer
> But he is never disturbed.
> The seer knows peace:
> The man who stirs up his own lusts
> Can never know peace.
> He knows peace who has forgotten desire.
> He lives without craving:
> Free from ego, free from pride.[3]

This ancient text, dating back to between 500 and 200 BCE, provides a very clear exposition of the task of the soul on the path of self-realisation. The advice is not in the form of religious dogma or creed, it is couched in simple terms giving spiritual advice on how the soul should escape and rise above the sly seductions of the ego-self and achieve the Atman (Self). Central to this endeavour is mastering the emotions, motives and addictions of the ego-self and moving away from a life embroiled with the senses and enslaved by the body. This reaching out to the Self is a process of sublimation, not conflict. Conflict represses, accentuates and perpetuates; sublimation transcends, resolves and heals. This healing of the soul, and the associated healing of the mind and the body, necessitates the dissipation of the ego-self: a continuous transformation extending through lifetimes. Once the soul sincerely resolves to escape the thrall of the ego-self, homeopathic treatment can most powerfully address the deepest issues upon which the ego-self is based and sustained. Homeopathy, soul medicine, stands beside us like Krishna, the divine charioteer, ministering to us in times of dilemma and distress, lightening the burden of our inherited, imprinted, conditioned, constitutional and miasmatic traits, removing the ego-filters that distort our vision, and, as psychopomp, transporting us through the dimensions of the unconscious, even to the depths of our personal abyss, that we may confront and triumph over the baleful ego-dragon that mantles the sublime purity of our divinity: the treasure of all treasures.

References

1   Vivekenanda. *The Yogas and Other Works*. Revised Edition. New York NY: Ramakrishna-Vivekenanda Center; 1953. pp238–239.
2   Prabhavananda S. *Bhagavad-Gita – The Song Of God*. Prabhavananda S. Isherwood C (trans). London: The New English Library Limited; 1972. pp36–37.
3   Prabhavananda S. *Bhagavad-Gita – The Song Of God*. Isherwood C (trans). London: The New English Library Limited; 1972. pp44–42.

> The second volume of *Healing the Soul – The Archetype and the Psyche* – will introduce the reader to the collective unconscious, the realm of the universal archetypes – the fundamental role models, innate tendencies or quintessential paragons of human nature that through resonance mould and transform the personal unconscious and pattern the focus, values, behaviour and destiny of the individual – and conduct the reader into the mysterious, intangible domain of the psyche to become conversant with its structure and its dynamics, the better to understand and challenge the adversary that every soul must confront and overcome on the path to health and Self-realisation: the delinquent ego-self – the innate cause of all disease.

INDEX

absent healing 309, 311, 314–315, 326–327, 331, 334, 335, 336, 337, 344–345, 357, 413, 419–420, 428, 481–482
acupuncture 536
Adelaide, Queen 237
Aitken, Sir Maxwell (Lord Beaverbrook) 371–372
alchemy 34, 55, 57, 94–95
Alkali Pneum 76–77
Allen's Encyclopaedia 322, 536
allergies 39, 123, 201, 202, 225, 265, 267, 275, 441, 537
Allied Health Professions Council of South Africa (AHPCSA) 497–498
allopathy *see* orthodox medicine
Altrincham City Council ban on spiritualist meetings 416–418
American Indians 376–377, 386
  see also Silver Birch; White Hawk
American Institute of Homeopathy 205
American Medical Association 37, 205
analgesics (painkillers) 41
analytical psychology *see* Jung, Carl Gustav
Anhalt-Köthen, Duke and Duchess of 110, 112–113, 148, 150–151
anima and animus 3, 4
anthroposophy 232–233, 509, 510
antibiotics 132, 246, 463–464
apartheid politics 514
apothecaries, restrictions on homeopathic practice 108–109
archetypal dreams 520, 523–524, 525–526, 550

archetypes 1, 88, 397, 467, 478, 504, 505, 560
  anima and animus 4
  cuttlefish 4, 510–511
  dog 21, 433
  of the four humours 25, 45–46, 50
  kingfisher 525–528
  and mythology 550–551
  serpent 200, 553
  see also ego/soul interface; individuation
Aristotle 44, 50
Arkwright, Dr Thomas 432
arsenic poisoning 39, 40, 65
arthritis 258, 280, 354–355, 421, 435, 466–467, 493
artistic genius 246, 383, 394–395, 397, 426, 450
asthma 201, 202–203, 225, 267, 275, 537
astral projection 298–299, 330, 384, 394–395, 459, 517, 518, 519, 520–524, 543–544, 547
atheism 6–7, 229–231, 233–235, 253, 365, 377, 400, 491, 532, 552, 553, 554
atopy (allergies) 39, 123, 201, 202, 225, 265, 267, 275, 441, 537
auras 341–342, 385, 424, 428, 446, 449
autoimmune diseases 35, 241, 280–281, 354–355, 421, 435, 466–467, 493, 536, 539–540
Avicenna 50
Avogadro Constant 99–100, 220, 260, 273
Axham, Dr FW 358, 359

Bach flower remedies 324
Barbanell, Maurice 26, 365–367, 376–377, 378–379, 439
    The Psychic News 328, 372–373, 403, 412, 414, 431–432, 439
    see also Silver Birch
Barbanell, Sylvia 366–367, 376, 403
Barker, J Ellis 536
Barker, Sir Herbert 358–359
basic trust 10, 28, 29, 552
Baum, Prof Michael 236–239, 243, 247, 254, 260, 266
Baumgärtner 194, 195
Beaverbrook, Lord (Maxwell Aitken) 371–372
bereavement and grief 134, 349–350, 354, 355, 363, 395, 408, 541–543
Bhagavad Gita – The Song of God 551–552, 554, 557–559
Bibliotheca Classica 2
Blackie, Dr Margery 216, 507–508
Blake, Helen 26
blood poisoning (septicaemia) 504–505
bloodletting 44, 46, 66, 68–69, 107, 155, 178
boereraad 459
Boericke, William 219, 224
Boger, Dr CM 143
Bonaparte, Louis, King of Holland 140
Bonaparte, Napoleon see Napoleonic Wars
Bönninghausen, Dr Clemens Maria Franz von 139–147, *140*, 153–154, 189, 211, 213, 214, 221, 322
Bönninghausen, Karl 147, 189–190
Borgia family 39
Borland, Dr Douglas 508
Boyer, Dr Ronald 14, 15, 16, 20
Bradford, Dr Thomas Lindsley 67, 145, 147, 189, 218
Bradley, Dennis 368–369, 370, 371
British Association of Homeopathic Veterinary Surgeons (BAHVS) 19
British Faculty of Homeopathy 13, 17–18, 19, 20, 21, 500
British Homeopathic Journal 3, 209, 510

Brown, Mr W 308
bruising 43, 274
Brukenthal, Samuel von 62–63
Brunnow, Ernst George von 111, 129
Burnett, Dr James Compton 536

caffeine 41, 131, 135–136, 221, 237, 284
cancer 229, 235, 237–238, 238–239, 244, 258, 308–309, 312–313, 340
    see also Carcinosis Miasm; nosodes
Carcinosis Miasm 130, 134, 435
cause and effect 381–382, 396–398, 427
centesimal scale of dilution 97–101
chakras 300, 341–342, 343, 421, 465, 499, 537–538, 539
Charles, Prince of Wales 237–238, 239
Cheltenham 334–345, 356, 455
chicken pox 122, 462
children's land 518–519
chiropractic 320, 340, 498, 537
cholera 150–153, 250
choleric humour 25, 45, 46, 50
Christian fundamentalists 239–240
Christianity 48, 392, 393, 399, 401, 499–500
chromotherapy see colour therapy
chronic disease causation theory 117–136, 204, 414, 434, 435, 441
    Carcinosis Miasm 130, 134
    Psoric Miasm 120–123, 125–126, 127–128, 129, 130–132, 133–134, 135–136
    Sycotic Miasm 120–121, 123, 125, 126–128, 132, 133, 135, 462–463, 465, 466, 467, 508
    Syphilitic Miasm 120–121, 124, 125, 126, 127–128, 130, 132–133, 135
    Tuberculosis Miasm 130, 134
Churchill, Winston 21, 352, 371–372, 433
cinchona experiment 67–68
City Centre practice (South Africa) 470, 472, 512, 514
    see also Sanctuary

clairaudiency 291, 298, 309, 326, 330, 348
clairsentience 385, 399
clairvoyancy 291, 298, 309, 341–342, 350
  see also individual clairvoyants
Clarke, HC 197, 321–322, 332
Clarke, John Henry 508, 536
Clarus, Professor Dr 88–89, 107–108, 195–196
clinical trials see provings; randomised controlled trials (RCT)
Close, Stuart M 322
coal miners, treatment with sulphur 504–505
codeine 41
coffee 41, 131, 135–136, 221, 237, 284
collective unconsciousness 3, 523, 525, 526, 527, 550–551
colour therapy 341–343, 377, 449
common cold 39
consciousness 3, 232–233, 268, 272–273, 384, 386, 427, 428, 431, 517, 519
constipation 41, 72, 312
continuum of disease 51, 118–121, 133–135, 204, 269, 435, 465
  see also Psoric Miasm
contraceptive pill 243–245
Cook, Grace 377
Cook, Trevor 64
cosmos 9–10, 34, 232, 394, 528, 532
Coulter, Catherine 200
cow pox 73
  see also vaccinosis
Cowperthwaite, AC 322
Croserio, Dr 182, 185
Cullen, William 67
curative effect, definition of 257–262
  see also Law of Direction of Cure; quantum science and homeopathy; remedies, methods of employment
cycles in nature and the soul 27, 391, 393–395, 517

cystitis 276, 536–537

Darwin, Charles 228, 230
  see also natural selection
David, Pierre Jean 175
Dawkins, Prof Richard 229–231, 233, 234, 238, 240, 243, 247, 254
death see life after death
depth homeopathy 526, 554
Desmond, Keith Arthur 315, 340, 343, 345, 347, 348, 407–408, 408–409, 410, 432, 515
  The Gift of Healing 431–432, 438, 440–441, 518
diabetes 202, 203, 241, 466, 539–540
Diamond, John 240
diarrhoea and vomiting 39–40, 40–41, 152, 249
Dickens, Charles 363
Digby, Berkeley 12–13, 14
dilutions see potentisation
Dionysos 391
direct-voice mediumship 368–372, 376
discord and disunity in homeopathic community 114, 118, 129–130, 148, 153–160, 218–219
disease, as a natural process 257–259
disease causation theory see chronic disease causation theory
disease continuum 51, 118–121, 133–135, 204, 269, 435, 465
  see also Psoric Miasm
divine beneficence 34, 390–400
Doctor in the House 5–6
Doctrine of Signatures 43–44, 527
Down syndrome 508
Doyle, Sir Arthur Conan 362–363, 368, 370, 371
DPT immunisation (diphtheria, pertussis, tetanus) 466
dreams see archetypal dreams
Dudgeon, Dr Richard 93, 214
Duncan, Helen 350–355, 415, 417
Dunham, Dr Carroll 147, 322, 536
dynamisation see potentisation
dysentery 39

ectoplasm 348–350, 351, 353–354, 384, 414–416
ectoplasmic surgery 479–480, 483–488
ectoplasmic voice box 368–372
eczema 123, 201, 202, 225, 265, 275, 441, 492
Edwards, Harry 415–416
ego/soul interface 4–5, 7, 10, 21, 28–29, 36, 200, 261–262, 294, 319, 323, 549–560
   see also evil, relativity of
Einstein, Albert 94
elements see humours
Eleusinian Mysteries 517–518
emotional trauma 134
emotions see ego/soul interface
emotions and colour 342–343
Empedocles 44
endocrine glands 427
epilepsy 49, 253, 466, 490–491, 493–494
Ernst, Dr Edzard 236, 237, 254, 260
euthanasia 420
Everett, Dudley 215, 467, 501, 511
evil, relativity of 398–400
evolution see natural selection
eye, iris 342

Farrington, H 322, 536
Farrington, Tom 528
Fates 199–200, 398
Feda 371
feminine and masculine 4, 376, 464, 552–553, 554
festivals of spirit 516–518
fever 253
Fickel, Dr 159
Findlay, Arthur 328, 365
Flint, Leslie 369
fluxion machines 219–220, *220*
foetus 428
Foubister, Dr Donald 508–509
Fraudulent Mediums Act 418
   see also Witchcraft Act (1735)
Frazer, Peter 8

free will 25, 381, 390, 397, 398, 399, 496, 516, 532, 550
Freemasons 62, 110, 310, 331–332, 471
French Academy of Medicine 173
Freud, Sigmund 509
Friederich Augustus I, King of Saxony 107

Gaia 199
Galen 25, 43, 44, 45–46, *45*, 49, 50, 65
Galileo Galilei 37, 239
Gallic Homeopathic Society 174
gastroenteritis 39
Gerdsdorff, Heinrich August von 175
Gerson diet 238
Ghost Club 363
Goethe, Johann Wolfgang von 106
Gohier, Louis 163–164, 186
gonorrhoea 100, 120–121, 123, 124, 126–127, 132, 435, 462, 463, 465
   see also Sycotic Miasm
Gould, Stephen Jay 228–229, 231–232
Graves, Robert 2
Great Spirit 376, 377, 380, 381, 383, 389, 390, 401, 406, 407, 437, 517
The Greater World 308–309, 317
Greek and Roman myths see mythology
Greek medical schools 44
grief and bereavement 134, 349–350, 354, 355, 363, 395, 408, 541–543
Griesselich, Dr Philip Wilhelm Ludwig 166
Gross, Dr Gustav Wilhelm 129, 147, 205, 208, 209, 210
Guizot, Minister 173, 184
Gutman, William 510

Haehl, Richard
   on Hahnemann 72, 87, 100, 110, 118, 129–130, 143–144, 157, 181, 224
   on Mélanie d'Hervilley 161, 167–168, 187, 189, 190
Hahnemann, Dr Christian Friedrich Samuel

childhood and education 59, 61–63
marriage to Henriette Kuchler 64, 148–150
family 60, 64, 65, 70, 75, 77, 85, 110, 112, 149, 150, 158, 168, 169, 172, 183, 186, 187
early practice and writing 63–73, 75–90
later practice and writing 105–115, 139
marriage to Mélanie d'Hervilley and practice in Paris 161, 165–191
death and will 169–171, 185–189
portraits and personal effects 33, 63, 111, 180
Alkali Pneum 76–77
and Bönninghausen 142–144
cholera treatment 150–153, 250
Chronic Diseases: Their Peculiar Nature and Their Homeopathic Cure 117–136, 204
cinchona experiment 67–68
and Clarus 88–89, 107–108, 195–196
and Hering 195–196
insanity treatment 69
jubilees 148, 154, 183–184
Law of Similars 37–43, 44, 72–73, 101–102, 248–254, 259, 269, 425, 444
and Leipzig Hospital 154–160
Materia Medica Pura 82–83, 110, 127, 142
olfaction 284
Organon 42, 73, 78–81, 94, 110, 117, 118, 129, 142, 143, 152, 165, 180–181, 190, 212–213, 221, 222, 224, 322, 443, 448
and the origins of homeopathy 33–34, 36, 53
on orthodox medicine 64–65, 66–67, 68–69, 72, 79–80
and potentisation 93–102, 179, 181, 211, 217–218, 221–225, 276
and Prince Karl of Schwarzenburg 105–109

provings (pathogenetic trials) 80–83
scarlet fever treatment 75–76
typhus treatment 86
Halcyon 525–526
Hale, Edwin 423
Halls of Learning 519
Halstead, Arnold *327*, 328
Handley, Rima 168, 172, 189, 190
Harmsworth, Alfred Charles William, 1st Viscount Northcliffe 367–368, 371, 372
Harris, Sam 234
Hartmann, Dr Franz 87–88, 88–89, 89–90, 111, 158
hay fever (rhinitis) 39, 201, 225, 275
Haynel, Dr August 112
'healing controversy' 440–450
heart conditions 54–55, 276, 342, 542
Hector (William Lilley's dog) 523–524
Heisenberg's Uncertainty Principle 268
Hephaistos (Vulcan) 504
Hering, Dr Constantine 147, 181–182, 189, 193–205, *193*, 322
and Jenichen 205, 209, 210, 213–214
Law of Direction of Cure 201–204, 423, 441, 444
Surinam and Lachesis 196–201
hero's quest 390, 395–396, 550–552, 554
herpes 462
Hervilley, Marie Mélanie d' 147, 161–191
early life 161–165
marriage to Hahnemann 165–189
life after Hahnemann 182, 189–191, 193
Hesiod 199
high potencies *see* potentisation
Hindu mythology 341, 511, 551–552, 555, 556–560
Hippocrates 25, 42, 44, 45, 46, 248, 252
Hitchens, Christopher 234
Hitler, Adolf 21, 332, 433
hives (urticaria) 275
Holocaust (Nazi) 389, 397–398

Homeopathic Biochemic Laboratory 538
Homeopathic College of Pennsylvania (HCP) 181, 201
homeopathic injectables 536
homeopathic remedies
  correct usage 284
  location of 43
  sources and categorisation of 277–282
  stability, storage and sensitivity 282–284
  Aconitum (monkshood) 537
  Adonis vernalis (pheasant's eye) 276
  Allium cepa (red onion) 39, 282
  Antimonium tartaricum (tartar emetic) 249
  Apis (honey bee) 454
  Argentum nitricum 11
  Argentum (silver) 3, 43
  Arnica montana (leopard's bane or bruise-wort) 43, 274, 275, 476, 480
  Arsenicum album (white arsenic) 39–40, 40–41, 249, 461
  Aurum (gold) 3, 98, 125, 544, 551
  Belladonna (deadly nightshade) 75, 76, 102, 109, 454
  Bellis perennis (common daisy) 509
  Berberis aquifolium (mountain grape) 423, 537
  Bryonia alba (white bryony) 152, 252, 321
  Cactus (night-blooming cereus) 540
  Calc-carb (calcium carbonate) 9–10
  Calc-phos (calcium phosphate) 482
  Calc-sulph (calcium sulphate) 94, 480
  Calendula officinalis (marigold) 274, 482
  Camphora (camphor tree) 151–152, 249, 277
  Cantharis (Spanish fly) 537
  Capsicum (Cayenne pepper) 454
  Carb-sulph (carbon sulphate) 504–505
  Carbo vegetabilis (vegetable carbon) 152, 277
  Carcinosin (cancerous breast tissue) 280, 508–509, 554
  Causticum 94, 422
  Ceanothus americanus (red root) 274
  Chelidonium majus (greater calendine) 43
  Cinchona (Peruvian bark) 67–68, 194–195, 425
  Coffea cruda (unroasted coffee) 41
  Cortisone 200 537
  Crataegus (hawthorn) 342, 540
  Cuprum metallicum (copper) 3, 152, 249, 478
  Digitalis purpurea (foxglove) 54–55
  E. coli 536
  Echinacea angustifolia (purple coneflower) 482
  Equisetum (horsetail) 537
  Eupatorium-purp (gravel root) 537
  Ferrum (iron) 3, 478
  Folliculinum 509, 537
  Fucus vesiculosis (sea kelp) 243
  Gelsemium 11
  Guaiacum 125
  Hepar sulph 94
  Hydrastis canadensis (golden seal) 43
  Hypericum perforatum (St John's wort) 274
  Ipecacuanha 41, 68
  Lac caninum (dog's milk) 21, 509, 554
  Lac leoninum (lion's milk) 551
  Lachesis (Brazilian pit viper) 102, 196–201, 281, 454, 553–554
  Lactuca virosa (wild lettuce) 164
  Latrodectus mactans (black widow spider) 342
  Lycopodium (club moss) 9–10, 102, 553–554
  Mahonia aquifolium (oregon grape) 422–423
  Malandrinum (grease of horses) 422, 461, 462
  Mercury 65, 102, 126, 133, 241
  Mezereum 125
  Nitric acid 125, 127, 132, 511

Nux vomica (strychnine tree) 474
Opium (poppy) 41
Phosphoric acid 152
Phosphorus 482
Pulsatilla pratensis (meadow anemone) 252
Pyrogen 480
Quercus (oak tree) 551
Rhamnus californica (California coffee tree) 542
Rhus toxicodendron (poison oak) 152, 321, 536
Selenium 204
Sepia (cuttlefish) 43, 281, 509, 510–511
Silicea (quartz) 98, 102, 482
Solanaceae (nightshade) 3, 454
Stannum (tin) 478
Stramonium (thornapple) 42
Streptococcus 542
Strophanthus hispidus (kombe seed) 276, 540
Sulphur 3, 9–10, 125–126, 132, 204, 265, 483, 504–505
Sycotic co 422, 536
Symphytum officinale (comfrey or knitbone) 482
Tellurium 204
Thuja occidentalis (Northern white cedar) 100, 126–127, 132, 422, 461–462, 463, 465, 511
Tuberculinum 280, 482, 536
Twelve Tissue Salt Remedies 276, 324, 340
Uva ursi (bearberry) 537
Venus mercenaria (edible clam) 510
Veratrum album (white hellabore) 40–41, 84–85, 152, 249
homeopharmaceutics 302, 498
Homer 1, 523
Homer, Mrs E 442
homesickness 454
hostility to homeopathy
 in Hahnemann's day 37, 86–89, 102, 105, 107–109, 145–146, 151, 159–160
 modern day 227–231, 235–240, 244, 260, 265, 432, 489–497
hostility to spiritual healing 343–345, 352, 405, 416–418
House of Divinity *see* Sanctuary
House of Ramesôye *see* Sanctuary
HRT (Hormone Replacement Therapy) 242–245
Hubbard, Dr Elizabeth Wright 511
hubris, medical 5–6, 51, 377
Hufeland, Chistoph Wilhelm Friedrich von 66, 72, 78, 151
Hughes, Dr Richard 322
humours 25, 44–46, 49, 50, 65, 93, 241
hyperaesthesia 424–425
hyperthyroidism 281
hypothyroidism 241–242, 243, 276, 281

immortality 28, 34, 95, 198, 269, 337, 383–384, 390–391, 412, 463
 see also ego/soul interface; life after death
immunisation 35, 281
 DPT and MMR 466
 Smallpox 73
 vaccinosis 461–467
individualisation 54, 78, 79, 250–252, 267
individuation 95, 198, 269, 549
infinitesimal doses *see* Law of the Infinitesimal Dose
inherited disease *see* chronic disease causation theory
insanity 42, 49, 69, 258
insomnia 41
iris of the eye 342
isopathy 278
Itch Miasm *see* Psoric Miasm

Jackson, Desmond 481–489, 494
Jahr, Dr Georg Heinrich Gottlieb 184, 186
jaundice 43
Jenichen, Caspar Julius 205–214, 215

Jenkins, Dr Michael 18–19, 20
Jenner, Dr Edward 73
Jesus 401, 450, 517
Jewish community 251, 365, 366, 470, 518
Jung, Carl Gustav 3, 95, 198, 314, 509, 549
   see also Schiess, Mario

Kabbalah 392
karma *see* cause and effect
Kayne, Dr Lee 22, 23
Kayne, Dr Steven 21–23, 25–26
Kent, Dr James Tyler 143, 199, 219, 225, 322, 508, 536
Kleinert, Georg Otto 114
Koch, Robert 121
Koenig, Karl 510
Korsakoff, General von 207, 217–219, 220
Krishna 552, 554, 556, 557, 558, 559
Krishnamurti, Jiddu 232

Lachesis (Brazilian pit viper) 196–210
Law of Direction of Cure 34, 80, 201–204, 423, 441, 444
Law of Similars 37–41, 72–73, 101–102, 194, 248–254, 259, 269, 425, 444
   see also Doctrine of Signatures
Law of the Infinitesimal Dose 93–102, 117, 146, 152–153, 259–261, 263–265
laying-on-of-hands 301, 304, 314, 320, 348, 387, 418–419, 421, 426, 428, 431, 434, 435, 445, 483, 537
Lead Kindly Light 294
Leah, Frank 407–411, 440
Leckridge, Dr Bob 17, 18, 19, 20
left and right sides of the body 39, 464–465, 553–554
Leipzig
   battle of 85–86
   Hospital 154–160
   Medical Faculty 62, 87–90, 195–196

Leonard, Gladys Osborne 363, 371
Leopold II of Austria 69
Lepato, David 457, 485
leprosy 125, 127–128
Letari, Dr
   absent healing 331, 335, 336, 337, 419–420, 481–482
   colour therapy 341–342
   ectoplasmic surgery 479–480, 483–488, *484*
   festivals of spirit 517
   Frank Leah's portrait 409–411, *411*, 440
   guidance of Dr David Lilley 11, 391, 412–413, 476–477, 498–499, 512–514, 518–520, 535, 540
   guidance of William Lilley 299–302, 320–321, 323, 345, 347–349, 404, 470–471, 499, 514–515
   'healing controversy' 431, 440–450
   laying-on-of-hands 314, *318*, 320. 348, 418–419. 426, 428, 431, 434, 435
   lecturing and teaching 414, 425–428, 434–436, 457–458
   life story 515–516
   and Margaret Lilley's baptism 439
   and Nancy Lilley 305–306, 404
   and Oliver Lodge's telepathic experiment 364–365
   role of responsible healers 418–420
   treatment of David Lilley's meningitis 452–455
   treatment of William Lilley's dog bite 475–476
   and William Lilley's military tribunal 332, 333, 334, 335–337
   see also Sanctuary
Letari House *see* City Centre practice (South Africa)
Letari Nursing Home (Bulstrode St, London) 355–362, *356*, *360*, 403–404, 420–425, 460, 467–468, *468*, 472
Lethière, Guillion 163, 186
Levin, Dr S 477–478

Li Chu 290, 291, 292, 293
life after death 379–380, 382–384, 390–391, 503–505, 543–544, 547
  see also reincarnation
like cures like *see* Law of Similars
Lilley, Dr David
  childhood and education 339, 361–362, 433, 451–452, 455, 460–461, 468, 498, 499–500
  introduction to and training in homeopathy 1–7, 500, 507–511
  early practice 7, 512
  lecturing and teaching 7–23, 530
  European holiday 500–501
  family life 469, 542–543, 546
  grief on father's death 541–544
  retirement from practice 524–526, 528–533
  and Dr Letari 11, 412–413, 476–477, 498–499, 512–515, 518–520, 535, 540
  inspiration for *Homeopathy Healing the Soul* 23–29, 477–479
  meningitis 452–455
  psychic experiences 520–533
  vaccinosis 461–467
Lilley, Jesse 297, 361, 502–505
Lilley, Margaret Tara 439, 500, 501, 511, 529, 530, 531, 546
Lilley, Nancy 304–307, *305*, 339, 404, 438, 538–539, 540, 544–545, 545–547
Lilley, Paddy 17, 524, 529–530, 531, 532, 546
Lilley, Sarah Ellen (Sally) 290–294, 295–297, *330*, 361, 469, 470, 502
Lilley, Thomas 328, *330*
Lilley, William Henry
  childhood and introduction to spiritualism 289–292, 293–297
  marriage to Nancy Overton 304–307, 538–539
  homeopathic training 301–302, 321–323, 339–340, 341, 347–348, 502
  early practice 302–304, 307–309

South Africa practice 457, 459–461, 467–472
  deterioration of health and death 501–502, 513, 528–533, 539–541
  description and photographs of *289*, 318, 327, 330, 344, 468, *484*, *497*
  court cases 489–497
  dog attack injuries 473–477
  eclectic methods of healing 536–538
  exemption from military service 332–337
  'healing controversy' 440–450
  and Helen Duncan séance 353
  Law of Direction of Cure 202–203
  and Oliver Lodge's telepathic experiment 364–365
  other spirit guides 331
  and potentisation 214–216, 423, 498, 536–537, 538
  and Ramesôye 296–299, 318–319
  and Silver Birch 405–407, 436–438, 539
  as a spiritual physician 471, 535, 547
  and White Hawk 294–296, 298, 319, 377
  see also Letari, Dr; Richards, Arthur Charles; Sanctuary
Lilley, William Henry (senior) 324–325, *327*, *330*, 332, *360*, 361, 469–470
Lindlahr, William Henry 471
Linnaeus, Carl 199
Lippe, Dr Adolph 147
liver disease 43, 312–313, 422
LM potency scale 179, 181, 212–213, 221–225
Lodge, Oliver 363–365, 368, 371
London Evening Standard (on the Letari Nursing Home) 357
Louise Auguste, Princess of Prussia 172–173
Lutheranism 48, 59, 94

magnetic healing 447, 449
Mahabarata see Bhagavad Gita – The Song of God

Malan, Dr HV 179–180, 212
malaria 67, 68
mania 42, 49
martial arts 552
masculine and feminine 4, 376, 464, 552–553, 554
materialisation 349–355, 415
materialism 227, 374, 376, 386, 532, 553
   see also hostility to homeopathy; hostility to spiritual healing
maya 556
measles 122, 250–252, 267, 466
Mees, LFC 510
melancholic humour 25, 45–46, 50
Mendel, Gregor 121, 133
meningitis 314–315, 452–455, 462–463
menopause 242–245, 537
menstruation 41, 43
mental symptoms 203–204
metals 3, 48, 94–95, 509–510
miasms *see* chronic disease causation theory
Michelangelo 426
MMR immunisation (measles, mumps, rubella) 466
Moiloa, Robert 20
Moirai 199–200, 398
Moore, Frances 438
Mossdorf, Dr Theodore 112
Mowatt, Anna Cora 176–177
Mozart, Wolfgang Amadeus 450
Müller, Dr Moritz 153, 154, 155, 156–157, 157–158, 159
Müller, Johann 61
multiple sclerosis (MS) 280, 358, 466
musculo-skeletal conditions 321
mythology
   and archetypes 550–551
   Greek and Roman 1, 2, 3, 95, 199–200, 299, 390, 391, 396, 398, 455, 504, 509–510, 517–518, 525–526
   hero's quest 395–396
   Hindu 341, 511, 551–552, 555, 556–560

mythos and logos 231–232, 233, 259
Norse 455

Napoleon III, Emperor of France 147, 189
Napoleonic Wars 83–84, 85–86, 105
Nash, Dr EB 322
National Health Service (NHS) 237, 239
Native American Indians 376–377, 386
   see also Silver Birch; White Hawk
natural disasters 555
natural selection 34, 231, 234, 254
natural theology 230
nature and healing 25, 44, 54–56, 258–259, 435
Nelson & Co homeopathic pharmacy
   see Everett, Dudley
Neo-Platonism 48
nervous system 424–425
Newtonianism 34, 227, 236, 239, 260, 263, 266, 270
non-overlapping magisteria (NOMA) 228–229
norovirus 40
Northcliffe, Lord 367–368, 371, 372
nosodes 267, 279–281, 461, 482, 508–509, 536, 542, 554
numinosity 269

olfaction 284
opium 41, 72, 164
organ prescribing 536
Orphism 391
orthodox medicine 4–5, 6–7, 34–35, 40, 50–51, 152, 261, 312–313, 387
   antibiotics 463–464
   immunisation 281, 465–466
   methods of remedy employment 241–248
   randomised controlled trials (RCT) 54, 238, 239, 247–248, 265–270, 272
   use of psychic diagnosis 404–405
   see also hostility to homeopathy

orthodox religions 377, 379, 380,
    391–392, 393, 400–402, 425, 472,
    554
osteopathy 340, 358–359, 502
out of body experiences *see* astral
    projection
Overton, Cyril 306–307
Overton, Nancy *see* Lilley, Nancy
Overton, Wilfred 328, 353, 355, 546

paediatric homeopathy 271, 508
painkillers (analgesics) 41
palaeontology 228
Paley, William 230
Palfreyman, Joseph 291, 292
palliative effect *see* orthodox medicine
Paracelsus 24–25, 43, 46–57, *47*, 68, 70,
    95, 205, 245, 273, 423
Parish, WT 445–447
Pasteur, Louis 121
pathogenic trials *see* provings
patient-physician relationship 268–269
Pelikan, Wilhelm 510
percussion therapy 321, 537
personality types *see* archetypes
Peters, Alfred 363
Peters, Dr Sidney John 440–450
phlegmatic humour 25, 45, 50
phyletic gradualism 228
placebo effect 7, 82, 108, 146, 238, 266,
    269, 270–273
planetary evolution *see* cosmos
Plato 391
poisons 39, 40, 41, 44, 51, 65, 164, 342,
    424–425, 504–505
    see also Lachesis (Brazilian Pit-Viper)
potentisation 93–102, *97*, 260–261,
    273–275, 423
    Avogadro Constant 99–100
    fluxion machines 219–220, *220*
    Hahnemann's LM potencies 179,
        181, 212–213, 221–225
    indications for higher potencies
        276–277
    indications for lower potencies
        275–276, 536–537

Jenichen's high potencies 205–214,
    215
Korsakoff's single bottle 207,
    217–219, 220
and telecommunications analogy
    263–264
William Lilley's super-succussion
    214–216, *216*, 220, 222–223, 498,
    538
Powell, Evan 371
Pretoria News (on W Lilley's cases)
    490
provings 102, 249, 322, 510
    Cinchona 195
    on the healthy 80–83, 89–90, 95–96,
        241
    Lachesis 197
    and RCTs 269–270, 272
    Thuja 126–127
Psoric Miasm 120–123, 125–126,
    127–128, 129, 130–132, 133–134,
    135–136
psychic art 407–411
Psychic News 328, 365, 372–373, 379,
    544
    and David Lilley 412
    and Dr Sidney John Peters 440–441
    and Dr Letari 410, 415, 416, 418,
        419–420, 431
    and William Lilley 337, 347, 359,
        362, 403, 405–406, 413, 414,
        420–425, 436–437, 439, 455
psychic rod *see* ectoplasm
Psychic Truth (on the 'healing
    controversy') 441, 442
psychokinesis 370
psychometry *see* absent healing
Puhlmann, Dr Gustav 161–162
punctuated equilibrium 228
pyrexia 253
Pythagoras 44

quantum science and homeopathy
    262–285
Quarin, Dr 62
quinine poisoning 424–425

quinquagesimillesimal see LM potency scale

rabies 122
Rademacher, Johannes Gottfried 536
radiatory healing 447, 449
Raeside, Dr John 508, 510–511
Ramesôye 296–299, 318–319, 323, 341, 499, 515
randomised controlled trials (RCT) 54, 238, 239, 247–248, 265–270, 272
Reality *see* ego/soul interface
Red Cloud 376
reincarnation 27, 391–396, 427
religion and science 53, 228–235
religion, orthodox 377, 379, 380, 391–402, 425, 472, 554
religious fundamentalism 232–233, 239–240, 552
remedies, methods of employment 241–254
   application of Law of Similars 248–254
   no matching to disease 241
   opposing force (*contraria contrariis curentur*) 245–248
   supplementation, substitution or replacement 241–242
Renaissance 39, 394, 397
repertory systems 12, 142–143
rheumatic fever 542
rheumatoid arthritis 280, 354–355, 421, 435, 466–467, 493
rhinitis (hay fever) 39, 201, 225, 275
Richards, Arthur Charles
   first meetings with William Lilley 310–315
   and David Lilley, psychic visitation 526
   and Helen Duncan séance 353
   as mentor for William Lilley 331–332, 434, 458
   and Silver Birch 405, 436–437
   visitation 524
   and William Lilley's military tribunal 333–334, 335

   and William Lilley's move to South Africa 457, 460, 468, 469, 470, 471
   see also Sanctuary
Richet, Charles 350
right and left sides of the body 39, 464–465, 553–554
Roberts, Estelle 369, 376–377
Roberts, HA 322
Rose, Dr Barry 13, 17, 18
Rosicrucianism 392
Ross, Mrs 469
Royal Family (British) 90, 237–238, 239, 432, 433, 508
Royal London Homeopathic Hospital (RLHH) xiv, 3, 7, 239, 507–511

Sanctuary
   Hull 337–339, 460
   Hunslet (Leeds) 315, 317–321, *318*, 323–337, *327*, *329*, *330*, 413, 460, 471–472
   Letari Nursing Home (Bulstrode St, London) 355–362, *356*, *360*, 403–404, 420–425, 460, 467–468, *468*, 472
   Putney 460, 469, 470
   Tudor Lodge (Cheltenham) 339–345
   see also City Centre practice (South Africa)
Sanders, Henry 365, 366
sanguine humour 25, 45, 46, 50
Sanskrit literature 341, 511, 551–552, 555, 556–560
sarcodes 281–282, 509, 554
scabies 129, 131, 134, 280
scarlet fever 75–76, 109, 122
Schiess, Mario 523
Schüssler, Dr Wilhelm 276, 324, 340
Schwarzenburg, Prince Karl of 105–108
Schweikert, Dr Georg August Benjamin 155, 158, 159
scientific atheism 6–7, 229–231, 233–235, 377, 491, 532
Scotland Yard 405
Second World War 332–339, 352, 361–362, 432–433, 435, 450

Index   573

self *see* ego/soul interface
self-realisation *see* individuation
senses, physical 386
septicaemia 504–505
serial dilution 97, 98, 99, 100, 101, 206, 208, 215, 216, 219, 220, 260, 263, 264, 280
serial killers, homeopathic psychological profiling 19
Sevar, Dr Raymond 20
shadows 3, 198, 401
Shakespeare, William 254, 295, 391, 395, 424
shamans 43, 526
Shaw, George Bernard 358–359
Silver Birch 366–367, 372, 373, 375–379, 439
  guidance of William Lilley 405–407, 436–438, 445–446, 539
  message and teachings 379–402, 472
Singh, Lejan Tari *see* Letari, Dr
Skinner Potentiser *220*
sleep *see* archetypal dreams; astral projection
small pox 73, 122, 421
  see also vaccinosis
Smit, HP (Lassie) 459–460, 469, 474, 475, 476, 485–486, 488, 513
Smith, E 442
snakes *see Lachesis* (Brazilian pit viper)
Society of Homeopathic Physicians 19, 148, 478
Solomon, Elizabeth 20
soul 26–28, 34, 35, 53–54, 56–57, 298–299, 419–420, 424, 425, 427, 435, 448–449, 451, 463–464
  see also ego/soul interface; Silver Birch
South African Complementary Medical Association (SACMA) 14
South African Faculty of Homeopathy 13, 20–21
South African naturopathic and homeopathic college 470–471
speech 385
spirit *see* soul
spirit festivals 516–517

spleen 274, 422
spontaneous remission 108, 123, 238, 271
St George and the Dragon 550
stage fright 11
Stahl, Dr Georg 42, 43
Staines air disaster 511
Stapf, Dr Johann Ernst 90, 129, 147, 148, 205, 208, 209, 210, 214, 217, 237
Steiner, Rudolph 232–233
steroids 355, 421, 441, 537
Stewart, Albert 351
Stoerck, Dr Anton von 42
stress 253
subjective plane of existence 4, 261–262
succussion
  fluxion machines 219–220
  and Hahnemann 96–98, 100, 101, 212–213, 222–223
  and Jenichen 206, 207–208, 209, 210
  and Korsakoff 217, 219
  Lilley's super-succussion 214–216, 221, 538
suffering and spiritual growth 387–398
superbugs 35, 40, 235, 246
suppositories 284
Suss-Hahnemann, Dr Leopold 183, 186, 189
Swaffer, Hannen 328, 367–374, 375–376, 379, 401, 405, 417–418, 436–438, 445, 472
Swayne, Dr Jeremy 18, 26
Sycotic Miasm 120–121, 123, 125, 126–128, 132, 133, 135, 462–463, 465, 466, 467, 508
symbolism *see* archetypal dreams; archetypes
symptoms as expression of healing power 249–254
synchronicity 2, 12, 17, 22, 23, 56–57, 167, 273, 314, 532
syphilis 65, 120–121, 123, 126, 128, 129, 132–133, 241
Syphilitic Miasm 120–121, 124, 125, 126, 127–128, 130, 132–133, 135

Tafel, Prof. LH 145
tar remedies 441
tautopathy 279
tea 131, 135–136, 221
telekinesis 370
telepathy 363–365
tetanus 466, 474–476, 477
Theosophical movement 232
thyroid conditions 241–242, 243, 276, 281
token-object reading *see* absent healing
Tolkien, JRR 396
tonsillitis 257, 542
trituration 98–99, 100, 197, 212, 221–222, 538
trust, basic 10, 28, 29, 552
tubercular meningitis 314–315
tubercular osteomyelitis 481–489
tuberculosis 125, 141, 312
Tuberculosis Miasm 130, 134
Tübingen, Dr Riecke 108–109
Tudor Lodge (Cheltenham) *see* Sanctuary
Twelve Tissue Salt Remedies 276, 324, 340
Twentyman, Dr Ralph 3, 509–510, 523
Two Worlds 365, 486–488
  see also 'healing controversy'
Tyler, Dr Margaret 508, 536
typhus 86

unconsciousness 1, 3–4, 231, 299, 384, 459, 520, 523, 525, 526, 527, 550–551, 559
urinary tract diseases 276, 422–423, 536–537
urticaria (hives) 275
uterine conditions 43

vaccinosis 461–467
Valiantine, George 368

Van Rhijn, Dr Anton 20
Vedas 341, 375, 535
Veith, JM 152
venereal diseases *see* gonorrhoea; syphilis
Vesalius, Andreas 46
veterinary homeopathy 146, 271
Vettriano, Jack 329
Victoria, Queen 90
visitations *see* life after death
Vivekananda, Swami 535, 556
vomiting and diarrhoea 39–40, 40–41, 152, 249

Wala homeopathic injectables 536
war and disease 435, 450
Ward, Mrs H 308, 309
Watson, Tom 471
Wauters, Ambika 343
Weir, John 432
Westmoreland, Mrs 297, 302–303, 309, 333
Wheeler, John A 268
White Eagle 377
White Hawk 294–296, 298, 319, 377, 516
Whitmont, Edward 3, 510
Williams, Dr David 13, 26
winter vomiting 40
Wismar homeopathic dispensary 214
Witchcraft Act (1735) 352, 416–418
World War II 332–339, 352, 361–362, 432–433, 435, 450

Yogananda, Swami 535
Yorkshire Copper Works Brass Band 307
Yorkshire Evening News (on The Sanctuary) 325–328, 333–334

Zukav, G 268